Psychosocial Aspects of Disability

Insider Perspectives and Counseling Strategies

Irmo Marini, PhD, CRC, CLCP, is Professor and PhD Coordinator of the Rehabilitation Counseling Program, Department of Rehabilitation, at the University of Texas-Pan American in Edinburg, Texas. Dr. Marini obtained his PhD in Rehabilitation from Auburn University in Auburn, AL, and a master's degree in Clinical Psychology from Lakehead University in Thunder Bay, Ontario, Canada. He is the 2010 recipient of the American Rehabilitation Counseling Association's James F. Garrett distinguished career in research award, and recipient of the National Council on Rehabilitation Education's 2009 distinguished career award in education. Dr. Marini is coeditor of *The Professional Counselor's Desk Reference*, has authored and/or coauthored over 65 refereed journal publications, and contributed 13 book chapters on rehabilitation counseling psychology and forensic rehabilitation topics. He is former President of the American Rehabilitation Counseling Association and former Chair of the Commission on Rehabilitation Counselor Certification.

Noreen M. Glover-Graf, PhD, is a Professor in the Department of Rehabilitation at the University of Texas-Pan American. She holds a doctorate degree in Rehabilitation Counseling from the Rehabilitation Institute at Southern Illinois University. She has over 30 publications primarily in the areas of spirituality, sexual abuse, and trauma-related disability.

Michael Jay Millington, PhD, is the Director of the National Clearinghouse of Rehabilitation Training Materials, editor of the *VEWAA Journal*, and research assistant faculty at Utah State University. Since 1985 he has worked and grown in the rehabilitation counseling profession as a practitioner, manager, academic, and advocate. He has published 38 articles and book chapters in areas of interest and expertise primarily on topics of employment and disability. Current academic pursuits include evolving social network models and their potential application in knowledge translation, counseling, and case management. He cofounded the Louisiana Business Leadership Network and was proudly among those in Louisiana who helped to restore the community in the aftermath of hurricane Katrina. He believes in the power of community, the basic goodness of humanity, and the moral superiority of dogs.

Psychosocial Aspects of Disability

Insider Perspectives and Counseling Strategies

Irmo Marini, PhD, CRC, CLCP
Noreen M. Glover-Graf, PhD
Michael Jay Millington, PhD

SPRINGER PUBLISHING COMPANY

NEW YORK

Springer Publishing Company, LLC
11 West 42nd Street
New York, NY 10036
www.springerpub.com

Acquisitions Editor: Sheri W. Sussman
Composition: Techset

ISBN: 978-0-8261-0602-5
E-book ISBN: 978-0-8261-0603-2

13 14 15/ 5 4 3

The author and the publisher of this Work have made every effort to use sources believed to be reliable to provide information that is accurate and compatible with the standards generally accepted at the time of publication. The author and publisher shall not be liable for any special, consequential, or exemplary damages resulting, in whole or in part, from the readers' use of, or reliance on, the information contained in this book. The publisher has no responsibility for the persistence or accuracy of URLs for external or third-party Internet Web sites referred to in this publication and does not guarantee that any content on such Web sites is, or will remain, accurate or appropriate.

Library of Congress Cataloging-in-Publication Data

Marini, Irmo.
    Psychosocial aspects of disability : insider perspectives and counseling strategies / Irmo Marini, Noreen M. Glover-Graf, Michael Jay Millington. -- 1st ed.
      p. cm.
    Includes bibliographical references and index.
    ISBN 978-0-8261-0602-5 (pbk.) -- ISBN 978-0-8261-0603-2 (e-book)
  1.   People with disabilities--Psychology. 2.   People with disabilities--Rehabilitation--Social aspects.
3.   People with disabilities--Counseling of. I. Glover-Graf, Noreen M. II. Millington, Michael Jay. III. Title.
    BF727.P57M37 2011
    362.4–dc23

                                                                                          2011024003

Special discounts on bulk quantities of our books are available to corporations, professional associations, pharmaceutical companies, health care organizations, and other qualifying groups.

If you are interested in a custom book, including chapters from more than one of our titles, we can provide that service as well.

For details, please contact:
Special Sales Department, Springer Publishing Company, LLC
11 West 42nd Street, 15th Floor, New York, NY 10036-8002
Phone: 877-687-7476 or 212-431-4370; Fax: 212-941-7842
Email: sales@springerpub.com

Printed in the United States of America by Maple-Vail Manufacturing Group

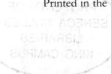

We would like to extend our appreciation initially to Phil Laughlin, former senior editor at Springer, for returning to Irmo after his first book and asking if he had any other projects in the works that Springer may be interested in. After Phil left, Executive Editor Sheri Sussman took over the project, and like Phil, made the task as stress-free as possible. We are honored to have had Sheri's mentoring, advice, and continuing support with this project. Sheri's resume of being the editor on countless rehabilitation counseling textbooks is a testament to her intrinsic interest and dedication to improving the lives of persons with disabilities.

Irmo, Noreen, and Michael

I would like to thank my family who continue to think I can fly long after I stopped being able to walk. Your confidence and support of me and Darlene are matched only by my love for each of you. To my students, past, present, and future, who give me so many good reasons to get out of bed every morning and who continue to teach me just as much as I do them. To all my colleagues and friends who have nourished my mind over the years, thank you for your support. And to my friends with disabilities and newfound friends through this project, thank you for the opportunity and wisdom you have shared with me. Finally, to my wife Darlene, who inspires and supports me, you epitomize all that a partner should be.

Irmo

To my mother, Margie Graf, who has taught me through example the meaning of hard work, perseverance, and dedication. And, to my three girls Jayme, Rory, and Amy, who give me the gifts of their love and joy. Also, special thanks to my friends Nina, Moose, and Jason, who pulled me away from my computer for walks, conversation, and coffee. Finally, I wish to acknowledge the students who searched databases and compiled a mountain of organized literature.

Noreen

To Emma and the Bean.

Michael

Contents

Foreword

What a marvelous and amazing textbook. Drs. Marini, Glover-Graf, and Millington have done a remarkable job in the design of this highly unique book, which comprehensively and very thoughtfully addresses the psychosocial aspects of the disability experience. These highly respected scholars have produced a major work that will be a central text in rehabilitation education for years to come and be particularly helpful and instructive for students learning about the impact of disability on individuals and families.

This book has many innovative features that I believe are noteworthy. Probably the most unique aspect of the book is that every chapter is followed by a personal story and perspective of an individual with a disability that relates to the chapter content. These pointed and well-written personal stories, from an "insider perspective," will greatly assist students in hearing and understanding the material at a different level and applying it to real people, rather than simply reading text content. The book is also distinguished from others through the sociological perspective taken in the historical account of how people with disabilities have been treated and perceived over time. Typically this content is found in other foundational texts and it is very helpful to have this type of review in this book, as it sets the stage and establishes the context for the content that follows.

In relation to the substantive content of the book, the authors have done a very thorough job of exploring societal attitudes, cultural perspectives, and sexuality, and in reviewing the seven most commonly discussed theories of adjustment, adaptation, and coping with disability and applying these conceptual frameworks to both congenital and adventitious disability experiences.

The book also provides information on how other professional disciplines perceive and are trained to view disability, in order to provide students with a better understanding of the total rehabilitation process and interdisciplinary approaches. The authors also uniquely discuss the medical and psychosocial aspects of caregiving in this country and highlight some of the most difficult decisions individuals and families may have to make in this process. A review of positive psychology is also included, where questions about why some people with disabilities thrive and adapt after injury or chronic illness, while others do not, are explored in some depth. In another unique and innovative aspect of this book, the authors provide a discussion of counseling strategies and interventions directed at assisting individuals with disabilities and their families to cope and adapt, including a discussion of the ethical issues and responsibilities for counselors in this critical process.

I believe this text has clearly addressed some of the limitations found in other books that cover similar content. I wholeheartedly endorse this exceptional work by these scholars and hope that students preparing for helping roles in the area of disability and rehabilitation, including rehabilitation counselors and other related disciplines, have the opportunity to use this book in their advanced studies.

Michael J. Leahy, PhD, LPC, CRC
Professor and Director
Office of Rehabilitation and Disability Studies
Department of Counseling, Educational Psychology and Special Education
College of Education
Michigan State University

Preface

Like many people without disabilities, I went through the first 23 years of my life with somewhat ambivalent feelings about those with disabilities. Basically, I did not have an opinion of them as a whole because I had never really been exposed to anyone with a disability and was too self-absorbed. What little knowledge (or lack of it) that I did possess, I realize now was stereotypical, prejudicial, and fraught with misconceptions. When I did see someone with a disability, I often felt compelled to offer help or money. As an able-bodied person, I felt good about periodically doing things like giving money to Jerry's Kids in the Labor Day Muscular Dystrophy Telethon, opening doors for people in wheelchairs, and pretending not to be anxious in "their" presence. Yes, I thought I was pitching in and doing my part for this group of disenfranchised persons, all the while unknowingly disempowering them. Then one day, without warning, I became "one of those people."

At age 23, during the second period of a Lakehead University varsity hockey game that I was playing in Thunder Bay, Ontario, Canada, I was tripped up into the end boards, slamming headfirst with no real time to react. In an instant, I catapulted away from the boards and lay on my back with my helmet cutting into my nose. My neck was immediately broken and I lay there paralyzed from the chest down, somehow knowing it right at that moment, yet somehow fully believing that I would be alright in a few weeks. The other team's physician was heard to have later said he thought I would not make it through the night. With the excruciating pain I felt running through my neck and the immense fear that was beginning to overwhelm me, I was not really sure I wanted to live.

My subsequent 11 months of hospitalization and rehabilitation that followed was initially riddled with setbacks. Three weeks after the accident, I was transferred to Toronto for surgery and rehabilitation. My girlfriend Darlene (now my wife) quit her job to be with me. My sister also came for three weeks but had to return home with no news of improvement. After a neck fusion to replace my shattered vertebrae, my lung collapsed a few days following surgery putting me into respiratory arrest. After being revived, I was placed on a respirator for a month. During that time, I lay in bed with a halo vest (circular plate screwed into your forehead and attached with bars to a hard plastic vest which wears like hockey shoulder pads), most times too fatigued to try to breathe on my own. Two friends bused the thousand miles to see me and one remained to coach and pester me off the respirator. One of the first lessons I learned as someone with a disability was that the love and support of friends, family, and significant others are immeasurable.

Nevertheless, I continued with complications of pneumonia and bladder infections. I was in intensive care for over two months, and once moved to a regular room, finally had the opportunity to sit up in a wheelchair for the first time. Having looked at nothing but the ceiling for so long and wearing a halo vest not allowing me to gaze downward, I wanted to see my image in the mirror. As I was wheeled in front of it, I gazed in disbelief and then began sobbing uncontrollably. I was devastated at how much weight I had lost. Having been a bodybuilder since age 12 and an athlete playing all sports practically since I left my mother's womb, I could not believe that I had lost 45 lbs of muscle mass on my arms, chest, and legs. Over a decade of hard work was gone in a couple of short months. I grieved the loss of who I once was, feared the thought of what was to be, and wanted to die. At the same time, there was still some part of me that denied the severity of my injury and still believed I would walk again.

Darlene's stability, dedication, and faith in me kept me going, as did the daily calls and periodic visits from family and friends 1,000 miles away. When I finally was released to Lyndhurst rehabilitation hospital in Toronto after four months of bedrest, I began to re-learn daily living activities we typically master by age 4, such as eating, brushing, and dressing. Daily muscle strengthening exercises as well as occupational therapy helped to alleviate some of my dysthymia; however, things were not happening quickly enough. The local and national media took great interest, sensationalizing mine and Darlene's dedicated love story about a hockey player who would have committed suicide had it not been for the love of his former-model girlfriend. But none of the notoriety mattered. I was still in a wheelchair.

After almost 11 months of institutionalization, I had gained back about as much mobility as I ever physically would. I had an incomplete C5–C6 tetraplegia, essentially paralyzed from my chest down, having shoulder, bicep, and wrist extension functioning still remaining. In my last media interview, which I gave shortly before returning to Thunder Bay with Darlene in December, the last question I was asked was if there was anything else I wanted to say about my ordeal that no one else had yet queried me about. I thought about it for a long second, then slowly responded by saying that despite all the hard work and recovery I had made over the past 11 months, I would not be "walking" out of the hospital. I otherwise felt healthy but I was paralyzed for life. In my mind it seemed like I had failed. I knew that things would never be the same. In the rehabilitation hospital I was with many people my age who were also now in wheelchairs. It was a sanctuary from the outside world because we were all in the same situation; nobody stared at you, nobody judged you, and nobody discriminated against you. I also realized that I was afraid to go home. I was afraid of what people would think, and how they would react to me in a wheelchair. Although I was still the same person I was before, I realized that many people would not see it that way. I was plagued with other worries as well. Would I be able to have sex and father a child? Would I be able to work or was I to collect disability for the rest of my life and be accountable to quarterly social worker visits? How would others relate to me? How often would I be sick and re-hospitalized? Would I have to live in a nursing home? Who would take care of me? How could I replace my interest and love of playing sports? What was I going to do now that I was no longer physically able to do anything? I was terrified at what lay ahead and pictured that life as I knew it was over. There was not going to be a happy ending to my story.

What I have learned in the past 30 years as a former athlete turned wheelchair-user and now scholar in the field of rehabilitation counseling psychology for the past 21 years is comprised in this book. Many of my earlier concerns have been, and continue to be answered. Now, however, as a researcher and professor, I have other questions about the psychosocial aspects of disability. What are the dynamic differences between those persons with disabilities who appear to do well or succeed versus those who never really adjust following a trauma? What are the differences between those persons born with a disability versus those who acquire them later in life? Why are some persons with disabilities plagued by secondary complications, whereas others with similar disabilities are not? What are the cultural differences regarding disability, and how do families respond to a loved one with a disability? These and other related topics are explored in this book.

What sets this psychosocial text about disability apart from the numerous others we have read is that this is the first to truly allow counselors and other related health professionals to "*walk a mile in our shoes*" and to learn from the writings of 16 people with disabilities across North America. As such, parts of the book are devoted to the compiled short stories of people with various disabilities regarding their experiences as to what life is like living with each of their conditions. These enriched stories from persons who are deaf, blind, have albinism, mental illness, tetraplegia, paraplegia, poliomyelitis, head injury, spinal muscular dystrophy, multiple sclerosis, and others are shared along with counseling guidelines for working with persons with similar disabilities. What readers will quickly realize is that these are people first and foremost who have lives, and whose disability happens to be but one of many traits or qualities possessed by them and not the salient feature defining them. The remainder of this book deals with a number of issues and strategies for counseling persons with disabilities. Having taught, researched, and read extensively on this topic for over two decades, I think this text covers what my colleagues Noreen Glover-Graf and Michael Millington and I believe are the pertinent and current topics in the field. Part One explores disability from a sociological perspective or those factors external to the person. Topics here include: Chapter 1, the history of how persons with disabilities have been viewed and treated in society throughout the centuries to the current day and into the foreseeable future; Chapter 2, attitude formation, societal attitudes, and myths about disabilities and improving our social consciousness; Chapter 3, culturally different issues and attitudes toward disability; and Chapter 4, attitudes toward disability by specific special interest and occupational groups.

Part Two focuses on the psychology of disability surrounding the individual and his or her family. Specific chapters address: Chapter 5, theories of adjustment to disability by the individual; Chapter 6, family adaptation across cultures toward a loved one who is disabled; Chapter 7, sexuality issues and disability; and Chapter 8, the psychosocial world of the injured worker.

Part Three addresses a mixture of pertinent topics concerning psychosocial issues of disability. These include: Chapter 9, quality of life across the life span for persons with disabilities; Chapter 10, implications of social support and caregiving on loved ones with a disability; and Chapter 11, thriving versus succumbing to disability: Psychosocial factors and positive psychology.

Part Four focuses on counseling strategies and insights when working with persons with disabilities and their families. Chapters include: Chapter 12, which counseling theories and techniques work best with different disability populations and why; Chapter 13, counseling with families; Chapter 14, ethical responsibilities in working with persons with disabilities and duty to educate; Chapter 15, basic do's and don'ts in counseling persons with disabilities; and Chapter 16, what we counsel, teach, and research regarding the needs of persons with disabilities: What have we been missing?

And as noted earlier, interwoven at the end of each chapter are "Insider Perspective" short stories from persons with various types of disabilities across North America. Contributors were solicited through advertisements and word of mouth, requesting that they focus their experiences to address the following six areas: (a) basic demographic information about themselves and their disability, how/when it happened, education, age, marital and living arrangement status, employment or history of; (b) how they perceive they have been treated by society (in public places, hospitals, social occasions, etc.) overall as well as specific instances that may occur every now and then; (c) what ways they have used to adapt or respond to their disability, which could include aspects of one's personality, family support, and finances; (d) if and when they felt as though their situation (which may/may not have had anything to do with their disability) became difficult to deal with at times, and if so, what generally triggered these feelings; (e) what they believed to be the greatest assets and the greatest barriers in their lives; and (f) what key message/advice would they want to convey to soon-to-be counselors or health professionals regarding working with people with disabilities.

Viewing the world from their eyes and in their own words is perhaps the most profound aspect of this or any other psychosocial textbook to date. Readers will be struck by the fact that these are ordinary people generally leading otherwise "normal" lives with bumps in the road along the way. Some stories are longer than others, as each accounts for different life experiences and focuses on different dynamics occurring in their lives. Although we have only included 16 of the more intimate of these personal accounts, there were over 40 submissions in the original call for stories. This book is dedicated to getting their word out to anyone interested in this topic.

Finally, disability is discussed as a social construct throughout this text, which addresses disability from a minority model perspective. The perceived shortcomings of persons with disabilities to adequately function in society are viewed more as a failure of our society to fully accept and integrate persons with disabilities. Historically, persons with disabilities have been marginalized and dehumanized, and thus not considered worthy of equal status afforded its nondisabled majority members. As with other minority groups, these sentiments take time to change people's perceptions. Where ignorance or misinformation has guided people's thinking, education and contact with persons with disabilities have generally produced a positive attitude change. However, where blatant discrimination, prejudice, and ethnocentricity exist, attitude change then becomes questionable. This book is dedicated to those students, practitioners, academics, and interested others who may be uneducated or misinformed.

Irmo Marini, PhD, CRC, CLCP

Acknowledgments

Projects of this magnitude are never done without a great deal of assistance. As such, we would like to thank doctoral student Amber Feist, who spent countless hours finding us easily over 800 journal articles, books, and book chapters on these topics, and provided feedback on several chapters. A special thank you also to Darlene Marini, who inputted about half of the references with great diligence and patience. The project would have taken an additional several months if not for her assistance. And to Sheri W. Sussman, whose time and careful editing eye strengthened the book immeasurably.

We would also like to acknowledge the 16 individuals who were kind enough to share their stories with readers and truly give meaning to the research that surrounded their experiences. Patricia Moniot, Linda Napolitano, Elvia Prieto Armendariz, Miriam Kimmelman, Michael Hoenig, Francia Malone, Jennifer Addis, Gino Sonego, Dave Shannon, Richard Daggett, Verne Sanford, Kristine Stebler, Michael Hineberg, Kathleen Prime, Patricia Konczynski, and Shannon Nettles: Thank you for making our book come to life.

PART ONE

Disability From a Sociological Perspective

ONE

The History of Treatment Toward Persons With Disabilities

Irmo Marini

OVERVIEW

For persons born in the last half of the 20th century, it might appear as though persons with disabilities have always seemingly been treated with kindness and a helping hand. Historically, this indeed sometimes was the case in certain parts of various countries by certain entities such as the church and other non-profit organizations. Some cultures even revered persons with disabilities and held them in high esteem. Gallagher (1995), for example, stated that among the Dahomeans of West Africa, infants born with disabilities were believed to be the result of supernatural forces and said to be good luck in some instances. Indeed, adults with deformities were often selected as state constables. Also, among the Chagga of East Africa, children with disabilities were believed to satisfy evil spirits, which in turn safeguarded others from misfortune (Obermann, 1965).

Unfortunately, these views were but isolated incidences. Generally, the history of treatment and attitudes toward persons with disabilities has often been marked by societal fears, intolerance, ambivalence, prejudice, and ignorance regarding disability. Taken in total, throughout the ages, persons with disabilities have been subjected to infanticide, starved, burned, shunned and isolated, strangled, submerged in hot water, beaten, chained and caged, tortured, gassed, shot, sterilized, warehoused and sedated, hanged, and used as amusement (Chubon, 1994; Gallagher, 1995; Sand, 1952). Surprisingly, many of these practices continued up until the end of World War II, and although this inhumane treatment was drastically curtailed in the last half of the 20th century, atrocities toward persons with disabilities still continue in various parts of the world today. Gostin (2008) indicates that despite the 1991 United Nations adoption of Principles for the Protection of Persons with Mental Illness (World Health Organization, 2005) as well as the 2006 United Nations Convention on the Rights of Persons with Disabilities, persons with mental illness throughout the world are still treated inhumanely and are living under deplorable conditions, including in prisons, on the streets, and in asylum-type settings.

Exactly why persons with disabilities have been historically treated so inhumanely is a complex question with many answers: however, most notably, they are devalued and perceived as less than human (Gostin, 2008). Depending on the era, infants with disabilities were put to death for economic or spiritual reasons (Chubon, 1994). Among the Jukun of the Sudanese Kingdom, children with deformities were abandoned in caves or bushes because they were believed to be possessed by evil spirits. Plato and Aristotle sanctioned infanticide for eugenic and economic reasons, believing that infants with disabilities would burden the system's resources (Gallagher, 1995).

EARLY CIVILIZATION (BC–AD 500)

There exists some evidence that persons with severe disabilities sometimes survived a number of years during early civilizations (Lowenfeld, 1975). Archeological and anthropological skeletal finds suggest that persons with spina bifida lived dating back to the Neolithic period (Sigerist, 1951). Venzmer (1968) reported evidence of disability during the Old Stone Age, again with the remains of persons with spina bifida being found as well as osteomyelitis, congenital hip dislocation, and spinal tuberculosis. With physically disabling conditions such as these, it is obvious that even back then, it would seem likely that loved ones must have taken care of their disabled members. Since no evidence of adaptive aids such as wheelchairs or walkers exists, it is believed that nondisabled family members may have carried their disabled loved ones from place to place.

Although it appears that some persons with disabilities survived during these earlier times, due to the lack of medical understanding and technology, persons with congenital disabilities either died of complications such as infections shortly after birth or were killed for economic, eugenic, or religious reasons (Deutsch, 1949). The Greeks believed the body and soul were one entity and that a blemish to the body (disability) also signified a blemish to the soul (Dickinson, 1961). Infanticide of infants with physical disabilities was practiced for eugenic reasons as advocated by Plato, and economic reasons as sanctioned by Aristotle (Deutsch, 1949). The body and soul connection by the Greeks also led to religion-based fears, as many believed that a disability signified punishment from God for having sinned (Turner, 1987). This belief was especially true for persons with mental illness who were believed to be suffering from demonic possession. The Greek physician, Hippocrates, however, rejected this premise and instead believed that the cause of mental illness was due to environmental reasons and brain impairment (Coleman, 1964). As a result, Hippocrates established the first sanitarium for what turned out to be well-off families who had a member with mental illness. Other persons with mental illness did not fare as well and were often starved, chained, whipped, caged, or put to death (Sand, 1952). For both the Greeks and Romans, infants with disabilities were routinely killed or abandoned. Greeks who became disabled later in life, however, were permitted to live and often became beggars, whereas some persons with mental retardation were owned by wealthy Romans for amusement as court jesters (Kanner, 1964).

Sigerist (1951) identified four differing attitudes toward disability during this early period. The ancient Hebrews viewed disability as punishment from God for having sinned. The Greeks considered disability a matter of economics and social status, and thus persons with disabilities (who often were beggars) were viewed as socially inferior; however, the Christians viewed disability as a curse or as being possessed, thereby needing prayer and charity. Today, despite the fact that many view disability primarily in a clinical sense as an organic chronic illness or disease, there are still others who believe disability to be caused from having sinned.

MIDDLE AGES (AD 600–AD 1500)

The Middle Ages were dominated primarily by the principles of Christianity. The Scripture in the Old Testament linked sin against God with chronic illness and disability (Gallagher, 1995). A reference to persons with disabilities found in Leviticus 21:18 that states, "he is unclean, and thus may not be a priest, or even approach the altar" conveys an unfavorable attitude about disability. In Samuel 5:8 it is written that "The blind and the lame shall not come into the home." Byrd (1990) enlisted the assistance of pastors in Alabama to cite the number and type of listings relating to disability in the Bible. The top five terms and their frequency of use were "blind" mentioned 93 times, "sick" cited 88 times, "afflicted" cited 88 times, "leprosy" noted 67 times, and "drunken" cited 50 times. Ultimately linked from the Bible to the present day is the notion that a person's disability can be healed if he or she has faith in God and repents of his or her sins. Gallagher (1995) cites the biblical passage where Jesus states to a blind man, "I have healed you, go and sin no more," implying, or at least interpreted as, sinning had caused the blindness.

Medicine and the medical profession were poorly regarded, because physicians were not well trained and often ineffective in treating persons with various diseases. The public opposed human dissection, and thus medical knowledge and understanding slowed considerably during this period (Rubin & Roessler, 1995). Chubon (1994) noted that medicine became a moral issue because disability continued to be largely viewed as punishment from God. Physicians were replaced by monks and priests, whose initial practices were humane. Persons with disabilities were treated in monasteries and hospitals where methods such as exorcism, prayer, incantations, magical herbs, and laying on of the hands were used (Obermann, 1965). Despite best efforts, the monasteries-hospitals were too few to meet the needs of the poor, the homeless, and those with disabilities.

With these noble efforts to treat persons with disabilities, Christianity's reach only went so far. Lowenfeld (1975) reported that the German and Slavic people of Central Europe continued to abandon and kill persons with disabilities who could not care for themselves. Since the plight of persons with disabilities was viewed as God's punishment, no attempt was made to find out the underlying cause of the disability. Coleman (1964) noted that humane treatment of persons with disabilities gave way to more inhumane treatments once again as the Middle Ages progressed. Persons with disabilities were feared and tortured, whipped, immersed in hot water, and starved in an effort to rid the person's body of the devil (Safilios-Rothschild, 1970). It was indeed contradictory for the Catholic Church to be compassionate and benevolent to persons with disabilities on the one hand, and yet at times be inhumane and cruel on the other. These human behaviors likely reflect individual interpretations and personal attitude differences among people rather than the will of the Catholic Church itself.

THE RENAISSANCE PERIOD (AD 1500–AD 1700)

During the period between 1500 and 1700, attitudes began to change regarding disability and treatment modalities. Coleman (1964) noted how the view of persons with mental illness as possessed slowly changed to them being viewed as sick or ill. Chubon (1994) stated that knowledge regarding the cause and symptoms of disability and illness began to be studied again, and physicians were allowed to dissect and study human cadavers. Persons with mental illness and mental retardation began being sent to the ever-growing number of asylums rather than monasteries. The asylums unfortunately offered no treatment or therapy, and instead functioned as prisons, some of which literally chained and caged noncompliant or acting-out patients (Coleman, 1964). During the great witch hunts between 1480 and 1680 reported in the *Malleus Maleficarum* book known as *The Hammer of Witches* (Kramer & Sprenger, 1971), it is estimated that between eight and 20 million people, mostly women, were tortured and put to death as witches in Europe. A good portion of this population often had a mental illness or visible disability or disfigurement. The book identified how to spot witches by their impairment or by giving birth to children with impairments.

Despite some of the inhumane treatment that continued for persons with mental illness and mental retardation, there were some positive steps toward rehabilitating persons with disabilities during this period as well. Obermann (1965) cites how persons who were deaf were taught how to write during the 15th century and later were taught how to speak and read as well. Sand (1952) additionally notes how persons who were deaf and blind were taught how to communicate by forming letters on their arms.

EARLY AMERICA (1776)

For the settlers in the 13 colonies, disability was perceived as God's punishment. Persons with mental illness or related acting-out behavior were often persecuted and burned or hanged like witches. For the most part, however, disability was viewed as a moral problem, often bringing disgrace to families who had a disabled loved one (Chubon, 1994). Physicians continued to be trained poorly or were self-trained and often treated illnesses such as influenza, yellow fever, and typhoid fever by having patients drink different concoctions (Miller, 1966). This was also a period where "bleedings" (boring a hole in the head to release poisons from fever) occurred (Weisberger, 1975). Persons with mental illness from wealthy families were typically kept at home if they were nonviolent; however, if they were violent, they were locked up and essentially treated as criminals (Deutsch, 1949).

In 1752, Benjamin Franklin aided the Quakers in establishing the first colonial hospital in Philadelphia (Miller, 1966). Although this hospital was designed to treat all disorders, including mental illness, the quality of care was lacking (Grob, 1973).

A second hospital was built in 1791 in New York. A few years later in 1798, the first Marine Hospital service was opened to treat merchant seamen with disabilities, and this eventually evolved into the U.S. Public Health Service (Singer, 1928). Also during the 1760s–1780s, the first three medical schools in the United States were opened. Dr. Benjamin Rush trained some 3,000 doctors during this period and believed that disease could be driven from the body. Rush also believed in and practiced bleeding as a form of treatment for fever.

THE INDUSTRIAL REVOLUTION (1700–1900)

The Industrial Revolution between the 1700s and 1900 brought some interesting developments concerning persons with disabilities. First was the changing infrastructure of the United States as urbanization began to flourish, leading to the building of more hospitals. This also led to greater advancements in treating persons with various illnesses. Second, there was mechanization and the development of factories, primarily in these urban areas. Factory working conditions were often likened to those of present-day sweat shops, whereby workers were given few breaks, had to meet stringent quotas, and were generally supervised in a coercive, authoritarian manner (Cheit, 1961; Chubon, 1994). Indeed, industrial capitalism was geared to having healthy able-bodied persons able to work long hours in mass production lines, thereby excluding persons with mental and physical limitations from these types of work environments (Turner, 2006).

With industrialization came a new type of prevalent disability: injured workers. Workers who were injured on the job were often customarily fired if they could no longer produce, leaving them no recourse but to sue their employers since workers' compensation legislation did not yet exist. Historically, the first workers' compensation legislation was passed in Germany in 1884, Hungary in 1887, Great Britain in 1897, and in the state of Maryland in the United States in 1902 (Worrall & Appel, 1985). Workers' compensation is best defined as an agreement between employer and employee, in that an employer will automatically cover medical and wage replacement benefits for employees injured on the job, regardless of who is at fault. In turn, injured workers agree not to sue their employer. Prior to this legislation, however, employers virtually won all lawsuits brought against them by injured employees due mainly to three existing tort laws: the doctrines of "contributory negligence" (a worker contributed to his or her injury), "assumption of risk" (a worker knew the risks of the job and voluntarily did it anyway), and "fellow servant" (an injury occurred as the result of a coworker's negligence). These laws most often heavily favored the employer, and the burden of proof was with the employee (Berkowitz, 1960; Cheit, 1961).

In other arenas, services for persons with disabilities continued to improve. Thomas Gallaudet, a theologian by education, became interested in working with the deaf population and studied educational methods in teaching persons who were deaf in Europe (Holbrook, 1957). Later, with the help of Congress, Gallaudet raised money to open the first U.S. school for educating persons who were deaf in Hartford, Connecticut in 1817. Similarly, for persons who were blind, the first attempts to educate and vocationally prepare this population occurred in Paris in 1784 by Valentin Hauy. Between 1791 and 1827, six other institutions for persons who were blind were opened in the United Kingdom (Nelson, 1971). The first institution for the blind was eventually opened in the United States in 1832 by Dr. Samuel Howe. By 1887, Howe's success and his public relations efforts led to the opening of similar schools in over 30 states (Holbrook, 1957). In France, there were about 60 schools for deaf children by 1870, primarily run by Catholic congregations, starting with the two oldest and state-protected schools in Paris and Bordeaux founded in 1760. This proliferation of deaf schools stemmed from the fact that there were believed to be twice as many deaf children as there were blind (Buton, 2006). Interestingly, the majority of Parisian teachers were deaf themselves. Although the majority of the deaf population favored teaching French Sign Language (FSL), French education administrators pushed for teaching deaf students oral methods, which was ultimately passed by the Milan Congress in 1880 and immediately introduced that year. As a result, the majority of deaf-mute teaching candidates were banned until FSL was finally reimplemented in France in the 1990s.

Persons with mental illness during this time did not fare as well. Mental illness was not only misunderstood and feared by many persons, it was also seen as incurable (Rubin & Roessler, 1995). In the United States, Dr. Benjamin Rush advocated for the humane treatment of persons with mental illness by surrounding them with pleasant conditions and conversation with others. Rush's plea, however, went largely unacknowledged as persons with mental illness continued until recently (1960s) to be institutionalized with little or no psychological treatment and often under brutal living conditions. It was only after researcher Dorothea Dix investigated over 100 of these psychiatric hospitals and made her findings public that more humane treatment and living conditions came into effect (Holbrook, 1957). By 1860, Dix's impact led many state legislatures to provide funds to build more hospitals that provided humane treatment to persons with mental illness. Unfortunately, deinstitutionalization has resulted in thousands of persons with severe mental illness being confined in prisons or homeless in the streets without any assistance of any kind and no access to medication or counseling (Gostin, 2008).

Prior to the latter half of the 19th century, most persons with physical disabilities such as muscular dystrophy and spinal cord dysfunction died due to various complications such as pneumonia and infections. This was generally the case until the development of antiseptic surgery by Joseph Lister in 1865, which greatly increased survival rates (LaRue, 1972). Obermann (1965) noted that the first three hospitals for persons with physical disabilities were opened between 1863 and 1884 in Philadelphia and New York. In 1893, the Industrial School for Crippled and Deformed Children was established in Boston, representing a first in the United States to vocationally train this population for jobs. Similar schools flourished after the polio epidemic of the 1940s (Chubon, 1994).

As developments for persons with disabilities continued to slowly improve in most industrialized countries, there was concomitantly a growing philosophical and far-reaching issue that began to emerge. Persons with various disabilities had experienced differential types of treatment, depending on what their disabilities were up until this point. How people viewed persons who were perceived as weak or different became clear in the years shortly following Darwin's infamous 1859 book, *Origin of*

Species. Darwin's work set the stage for a barbaric movement that unfortunately continues in some parts of the world today.

THE SCIENCE OF EUGENICS

Smart (2009) noted that Sir Francis Galton, Karl Pearson, and Sir Ronald Fisher were all eugenicists and statisticians in academe. Galton originally coined the term "eugenics," which is defined as "the study of hereditary improvements of the human race by controlled selective breeding" (Smart, 2009, p. 4). Galton essentially believed that society could be ruined if less intelligent people out-reproduced those of greater intelligence, and espoused that government should encourage the rich to reproduce and prevent the less intelligent poor from doing so. Galton and his colleagues were statisticians who developed statistics still used today concerning the normal distribution curve and what is considered to be the "norm." Their books, Galton's *Hereditary Genius* (1887) and *Inquiries into Human Faculty and its Development* (1883), as well as Fisher's *Genetical Theory of Natural Selection,* all delved into the concept of natural selection and selective breeding. Darwin's 1859 *Origin of Species* specifically dealt with natural selection but addressed the concept only as it pertained to plants and animals. Gallagher states, "Darwin held that the members of a species will have various and sundry variations, and that these variations will, in one way or another, influence the ability of the individual member to survive" (Gallagher, 1995, p. 44).

Twelve years later in 1871, Darwin's focus expanded from plants and animals to humans, with his second book titled *The Descent of Man* in which he stated:

> We civilized men, on the other hand, do our utmost to check the process of elimination; we build asylums for the imbecile, the maimed, and the sick; we institute poor-laws; and our medical men exert their utmost skill to save the life of everyone to the last moment ... Thus the weak members of civilized societies propagate their kind. No one who has attended to the breeding of domestic animals will doubt that this must be highly injurious to the race of man.

One of Darwin's followers, Herbert Spencer, actually coined the term "survival of the fittest" and applied Darwin's principles specifically to humans. In Spencer's 1884 book titled *Social Statics: Or the Conditions Essential to Human Happiness,* he stated that "under the natural order of things society is constantly excreting its unhealthy, imbecile, slow, vacillating, faithless members" (Spencer, 1884, p. 355). Both Spencer and Darwin's principles, along with Mendelian laws of heredity and genetics, became extremely popular with the public, politicians, academics, and physicians regarding the ideal order of the biological world (Gallagher, 1995). Fine (1956, as cited in Rubin & Roessler, 1995) noted that Spencer believed "it was better for society to allow the poor and weak to perish than to sustain their existence and encourage their multiplication through government-supported public relief and health programs" (Rubin & Roessler, 1995, p. 17).

Spencer's Social Darwinism philosophy increased in popularity. It was an ethnocentric view advocated almost exclusively by White Anglo-Saxons of North European descent (Alemdaroglu, 2006). They believed that the wealthy and powerful were genetically superior to the poor and that poor people did not have the genetics or ability to ever be successful; hence, failure breeds failure. They believed welfare programs propagated failure and was dangerous to the health of the human race (Gallagher, 1995). As this movement grew, social scientists and others aiming to validate Social Darwinism held conferences and published numerous books and periodicals on the topic.

Richard Dugdale's 1874 study typified such works when he pieced together the family tree of the Jukeses and Kallikaks. Dugdale traced six generations of the Jukes family (but failed to take into account those members who succeeded or did well) and found that of the 709 Jukes or those married to them, 76 were convicted of crimes, over 200 collected charity or relief benefits, 128 were prostitutes, and 18 owned houses of prostitution (Gallagher, 1995). The Kallikak family situation was somewhat different but also supposedly strengthened Spencer's philosophy. During the Revolutionary War, Martin Kallikak had an illegitimate son by an apparently "fee-bleminded" girl. The son, who came to be known as "Old Horror," spawned 480 descendants over several generations, 143 of which were classified as feebleminded, 82 died in infancy, 33 were prostitutes, 24 were alcoholics, 3 had epilepsy, and 3 were criminals (Gallagher, 1995, p. 49). Kallikak later married a Quaker girl from a reportedly good family and many of their descendants became doctors and lawyers. Although many of the Social Darwinism advocates were in agreement as to who the weaker of the species were (i.e., criminals, prostitutes, and persons who were blind, paralyzed, developmentally disabled, mentally ill, or had epilepsy), there remained some controversy as to who else was considered hereditarily unfit.

In 1900, Duncan McKim came forward with a book titled *Heredity in Human Progress*, and essentially claimed that heredity was responsible for "insanity, idiocy, imbecility, eccentricity, hysteria, epilepsy, the alcohol habit, the morphine habit, neuralgias, nervousness, Saint Vitus dance, infantile convulsions, stammering, squinting, gout, articular rheumatism, diabetes, tuberculosis, cancer, deafness, blindness, deaf-mutism and color blindness" (cited in Gallagher, 1995, p. 50). McKim's views began to show the confusion in thinking as to who the weaker of the species actually were.

Several years prior to this, two new medical procedures, salpingectomy (tying a woman's fallopian tubes) and vasectomy (tying the *vas deferens* of the male), were found to be an effective and humane way of sterilizing individuals. Around the same time in 1896, Connecticut became the first state to forbid persons considered to be "feeble-minded, imbeciles or having epilepsy" to marry or have sexual relations. Anyone breaking this law could find themselves facing a 3-year prison sentence. Other states followed suit with similar legislation and indeed expanded the list of disabilities to include persons believed to be "insane, syphilitic, alcoholic and certain types of criminals" (Haller, 1963, p. 47). Kansas passed similar laws in 1903, New Jersey and Ohio in 1904, and Michigan and Indiana in 1905. Public support continued to grow for the program, which soon expanded into sterilization.

On another front during the last 30 years of the 19th century, a different kind of social discourse was occurring in the United States involving ethnicity, gender, and disability. Coco (2010) described San Francisco as having passed what came to be known as the "ugly act" in 1867 to remove unsightly beggars, most of whom had disabilities, off the streets. The law passed in a number of Western and mid-western states over the next 40 years, with Chicago's Municipal Code Ordinance of 1911 stating:

> No person who is diseased, maimed, mutilated or in any way deformed so as to be an unsightly or disgusting object or improper person be allowed in or on the public ways or other public places in this city, or shall therein or thereon expose himself to public view, under a penalty of not less than one dollar nor more than fifty dollars for each offense. (Chicago Municipal Code sec. 36034)

Coco (2010) further noted that when persons with disabilities were picked up off the street, they were sent to the Cook County poorhouse in Chicago, which had deplorable living conditions. Records from 1884 showed that 30,130 disabled persons resided in these poorhouses compared with 22,896 able-bodied persons. Among those with disabilities, 4885 were described as lame or crippled, 7780 as simply "sick," 2600 with epilepsy, and 1648 as paralytic. Astonishingly, the last ugly law arrest occurred in 1974, before it was finally repealed in Chicago later that year (Kraut, 2010).

The first federal Immigration Act of 1882 prohibited U.S. entry to any "lunatic, idiot or any person unable to take care of himself or herself without becoming a public charge" (Baynton, 2001, p. 45). The "public charge" terminology allowed immigration officials wide latitude for discriminating against undesirable immigrants, even when a visible disability could not be determined. The Act to limit persons with disabilities was further strengthened in 1891, when the words "likely unable" replaced the term "unable." The 1907 law was even more exclusive in denying entry into the United States for anyone judged "mentally or physically defective, such mental or physical defect being of a nature which *may affect* the ability of such alien to earn a living" (Baynton, 2001, p. 45). The whole intent of the immigration legislation was to exclude not only the disabled but also other perceived undesirable groups as well. The 1924 Immigration Act saw the institution of ethnic quotas wildly and subjectively tied to disability. Almost half of southern and eastern Europeans were described by "experts" as feebleminded. Jewish immigrants were viewed as neurotic, Slavik immigrants described as slow-witted, and the Portuguese, Greeks, and Syrians viewed as undersized, of poor physique, and physical degenerates.

African American slaves had already experienced Anglo-Saxon prejudice some 70 years earlier as some writers alleged that African Americans were intellectually inferior and therefore should not be set free because they could not care for themselves. A number of physicians such as John Van Evrie, Samuel Cartwright, Samuel Forrey, and John Nott during the 1840s and 1850s all wrote in prominent medical journals linking disability to African Americans. Van Evrie warned about race-mixing leading to abnormal and deformed offspring, supposedly resulting in the deterioration of moral and intellectual endowments. Cartwright differentiated and attributed two types of mental illness toward African Americans: one that was accompanied by body lesions that decreased one's desire to work and engage in mischief, and another that caused slaves to run away from their masters (Baynton, 2001, p. 177). Forrey, writing in the *New York Journal of Medicine* in 1844, noted higher rates of insanity, deafness, blindness, and idiocy among free slaves that was not captured in the census. Nott, a year earlier, had compared Caucasian women with Black women in the *American Journal of Medical Sciences*, indicating that White women possessed lily skin, silky hair, and a Venus form, whereas Black women were wenches with odorous skin, a woolly head, and animal features (Baynton, 2001). Forrey also saw many peculiar similarities among the American Indians.

Unfortunately, American women were not spared from being deemed disabled and inferior as well. Cynthia Russett wrote that "women and savages, together with idiots, criminals, and pathological monstrosities were a constant source of anxiety to male intellectuals in the late 19th century" (as cited in Baynton, 2001, p. 41). A common belief (among White males) during the time was that women possessed physical, intellectual, and psychological flaws and were often irrational with a high rate of hysteria. Neurophysiologist Dr. Charles Dana noted that if women were enfranchised to vote, this would lead to an approximate 25% increase in insanity due to their delicate nervous stability.

Back in the early 20th century, countries such as Denmark, Canada, and Switzerland passed sterilization laws for persons with disabilities and undesirables such as criminals. Similar to the United States and Germany, these movements were largely the agenda of well-educated, elitist middle- and upper-class Anglo-Saxons who generally held positions of power (e.g., attorneys, physicians, politicians, academics). Although the eugenics movement was very popular with some elitists in Europe, France, and Turkey in the ensuing years, the move for sterilization and blocking marriages of certain groups were largely defeated by opposition from the church, the working class, and public health institutions in those countries (Alemdaroglu, 2006). In Turkey, forced sterilization and abortion are against Muslim values and beliefs, whereas most French eugenicists believed individuals' environments played a key role in their upbringing, and therefore future offspring could have a better life if living conditions were improved.

Regardless of other international laws and religious beliefs, it was the state of Indiana that finally passed the first U.S. sterilization laws of criminals, imbeciles, and rapists in 1907. By 1926, sterilization laws had passed in 23 other states and were affirmed by the U.S. Supreme Court in 1927 (Kanner, 1964 as cited in Rubin & Roessler, 1995). Gallagher (1995) noted that there was some confusion and variation as to who qualified for sterilization from state to state, but that most state laws had expanded to sterilize persons with mental retardation, mental illness, and epilepsy. Several states also sterilized persons considered alcoholic, homosexual, drug abusers, and repeat criminals. The state of Missouri, for example, even sterilized chicken thieves. Even though the sterilization laws in the United States peaked in the 1920s, the practice continued into the 1950s and remained on the law books of 17 states until the 1980s. It is estimated that over 60,000 disabled and so-called unworthy able-bodied Americans had been forcibly sterilized by 1958 (Gallagher, 1995). The infamous 1927 Supreme Court decision re: *Buck v. Bell* permitted the sterilization of Carrie Buck who was believed to be incompetent and genetically inferior. Justice Oliver Wendell Holmes in his decision wrote, "Three generations of imbeciles are enough" in reference to Buck's mother having been institutionalized and Buck described as promiscuous (Buchanan, 2007; Carlson, 2009; Smith, 1999).

Despite popular public and legislative support of the sterilization program, a group of ministers representing the Social Gospel Movement opposed Social Darwinism, arguing that the survival of the fittest mentality was against biblical teachings and that the Social Darwinism sentiment would promote selfish behavior and disregard for fellow human beings. But not all Social Gospelers were in agreement, as many held firm to the notion that disability and illness were related to sin and defects within the individual (Hofstadter, Miller, & Aaron, 1959 as cited in Rubin & Roessler, 1995). In the end, despite the fact that the laws forbidding certain people to marry were never actually enforced and thus had little effect, psychologically the damage had been done regarding how society perceived and dehumanized persons with various disabilities. As a result, Gallagher (1995) notes that many persons with disabilities and their families during this period became ashamed or embarrassed of their conditions, and many became shut-ins and feared public ridicule.

EUGENICS TO AN EXTREME: EXTERMINATION

As the United States sterilization laws peaked during the 1920s, Germany passed its first sterilization law in 1933 (Gallagher, 1995). Leading up to Germany's sterilization laws were the popular opinions of several people who influenced the debate on Social Darwinism. The Germans, much like the Americans, were anxious to preserve their racial heritage. However, Germany's anti-Semitic views misconstrued the primary philosophy of Social Darwinism. Whereas Darwin and Spencer focused on heredity and the weaker of the species, some German thinkers extended these principles to justify genocide of the Jews.

One of the earlier influential thinkers in Germany was the famous biologist and social scientist Ernst Haeckel, who in 1899 wrote *The Riddle of the Universe*. This text went through 10 editions and sold extremely well. In it, Haeckel wrote:

> Such ravaging evils as consumption, scrofula, syphilis, and also many forms of mental disorders are transmitted by inheritance to a great extent and transferred by sickly parents to some of their children, or even to all of their descendants ... hundreds and thousands of incurables-lunatics, lepers, people with cancer, etc., are artificially kept alive ... without the slightest profit to themselves or the general body ... Now, the longer the diseased parents, with medical assistance, can drag on their sickly existence, the more numerous the descendants who will inherit incurable evils, and the greater will be the number of individuals again, and over the succeeding generations, thanks to that artificial medical selection, who will be infected by their parents lingering, hereditary disease. (as cited in Gallagher, 1995, p. 56)

Clearly, Haeckel believed that certain disabilities were incurable and passed on through hereditary means. He believed this population to be a drain on the economy, and a commission was established to determine which persons with deformities, mental illness, and other diseases should be allowed to live or die for what he referred to as "redemption from evil." Haeckel also advocated for humanitarian reasons that certain persons with disabilities should be killed at birth (Gallagher, 1995). This sentiment was essentially mirrored by another German scholar who followed Haeckel, Professor Heinrich Ziegler. Ziegler focused more on persons with mental retardation, epilepsy, and alcoholism, stating that these persons were primarily responsible for moral decay, murders, and other crimes. Ziegler believed that since crime was hereditary, it was pointless to try to rehabilitate or retrain criminals since they were incurable. He believed that all wrongdoers (e.g., drunks, vagrants, the poor, people with mental retardation or paralysis, and criminals) should be locked away for life and out of sight from the public (Gallagher, 1995).

In 1920, German psychiatrist Alfred Hocke and lawyer Karl Binding wrote what is believed to be a very influential book of its time for Germany: *The Permission to Destroy Life Unworthy of Life*. Both were professors who also believed in Social Darwinism; however, their views regarding natural selection and preservation of the race elevated to a new level. They argued that the medical profession should be allowed to administer a painless death to certain people for racially "hygienic" reasons (Gallagher, 1995). Hocke and Binding's book became influential primarily because a young Adolf Hitler was intrigued by their ideas and in fact endorsed the book.

Through films dealing with topics on euthanasia of persons with disabilities, documentaries depicting persons with severe mental retardation living in dismal conditions, and other types of propaganda, German society was ready in the late 1920s to embrace a sterilization law. Gallagher (1995) notes that even Nazi schoolroom textbooks illustrated the perceived low value of disabled lives. A mathematics text titled *Mathematics in the Service of National Political Education* cites the following problem: "If the building of a lunatic asylum costs 6 million marks, and it costs 15,000 marks to build each dwelling on a housing estate, how many of the latter could be built for the price of one asylum?" Another problem read, "How many marriage-allowance loans could be given to young couples for the amount of money it cost the state to care for the crippled, criminal, and insane?" (cited in Gallagher, 1995, p. 61).

It was only after the Nazis had assumed full authority in the legislative block that the sterilization program in Germany became law in 1933. During the fall of the same year, the Ministry of Justice under the Nazi-controlled German penal code proposed a law to authorize euthanasia. The news spread and in the United States, the *New York Times* cited details of the proposal . . . "It shall be made possible for physicians to end the tortures of incurable patients, upon request, in the interests of true humanity." The proposed law, however, was never passed due to outcries from the Catholic and Lutheran authorities (Gallagher, 1995). Despite the failure of the euthanasia proposal, the concept continued to be supported and discussed among politicians, physicians, and scholars. All the while, between July 14, 1933, and September 1, 1939, the Nazis reportedly sterilized 375,000 persons classified as congenitally feebleminded (203,000), schizophrenic (73,000), epileptic (57,000), and acute alcoholic (28,000), and those diagnosed with manic-depression, hereditary deafness, hereditary physical deformity, and hereditary blindness. During the same period, Hitler was secretly meeting with Nazi doctors, politicians, attorneys, and scholars to discuss and establish the systematic extermination of German citizens with disabilities.

Finally, on September 1, 1939, Adolf Hitler signed a secret order (unbeknownst to the public) to deliver what was termed "final medical assistance" to German citizens with disabilities. Specially selected physicians were made aware of the T4 killing program and how it was to be carried out. Persons with disabilities were described as "useless eaters" and "unprocessed inferiors" who drained the economy and burdened society without contributing anything in return. Gallagher (1995), in having reviewed Washington archives as well as the 1946 Nuremberg trial proceedings, notes how efficient the killing program was run. Essentially, unknowing physicians across Germany were asked to provide lists of their patients with various disabilities. These patients were subsequently rounded up and exterminated, first by gas or injection, and eventually toward the latter part of the program, also by starvation, experimentation, and shooting. Those persons with disabilities already in institutions were exterminated in much the same way. In the majority of cases, families were sent an urn of ashes with a letter regretfully indicating that their loved one had died of a contagious disease, and therefore had to be cremated for health and safety reasons.

Despite the remarkable organization of, and initial efficiency in carrying out Hitler's secret order, it soon became fraught with problems. First, there was confusion as to who should be placed on "the list." Although Hitler initially excluded German war veterans with disabilities from being exterminated, toward the end of the program in 1941, this was no longer the case. Second, although the program initially began as one in which German citizens with disabilities were exterminated in a non-painful manner, toward the end of the program they were being starved and shot to death. Third, some citizens who were placed on "the list" were arguably not disabled, especially when considering, for example, those with a single episode of reactive depression over the loss of a loved one but otherwise productive individuals. As Gallagher states, "When the German doctors decided to kill their insane patients, they destroyed the lives of many productive, valuable citizens." (Gallagher, 1995, p. 41). Hence, the age-old debate regarding who was considered to be the weaker of the species resurfaced and was just as riddled with contradictions as it was in earlier times. By the time the German public became aware of, as well as outraged by, the final medical assistance program, 2 years had gone by and an estimated 300,000 German citizens and war veterans had been exterminated. Under extreme pressure from both the public and the church, Hitler put an end to the killing of German citizens with disabilities in August 1941.

KEY LEGISLATION AND ATTITUDES IN THE UNITED STATES DURING THE 20TH CENTURY

Despite the fate of German citizens with disabilities abroad and the popularity of Social Darwinism, more humane treatment and services for persons with disabilities were slowly occurring in the United States. As World War I was ending, the implementation of the 1917 Smith–Hughs Act designed to provide funds for vocational training for dislocated industrial workers became law. There was also some recognition that persons with certain disabilities had potential for vocational training (MacDonald, 1944). This was followed up with the 1918 Soldier's Rehabilitation Act, which was established to vocationally rehabilitate veterans with disabilities (Obermann, 1965). Arguments regarding the need for a similar civilian program failed to be mandated until 2 years later, when the 1920 Smith–Fess Act was passed. The Federal Board of Vocational Education administered the program at the federal level and offered a 50–50 matching state fund split to entice states to participate (Rubin & Roessler, 1995). Watson (1930, as cited in Chubon, 1994) noted how the war positively influenced attitudes toward persons with disabilities as well as increased advances in orthopedic surgery.

Obermann (1965) cited the attitudes of the vocational rehabilitation field during the 1920s as paternalistic toward people with disabilities, and social service employees held stereotypical views of persons with disabilities. It was generally believed that such persons were incapable of making vocational decisions; therefore, vocational rehabilitation workers were viewed as all-knowing, not-to-be-questioned specialists who would make decisions for clients with disabilities. These attitudes have become more popularly known as stemming from the medical model paradigm and unfortunately are still held by some helping professionals today (Trieschmann, 1988).

Politically, little else happened in securing greater funding for persons with disabilities until President Franklin Delano Roosevelt (FDR) took office in 1932. Roosevelt had taken office in the midst of the Great Depression and was intent on providing economic relief for the disadvantaged, poor, and homeless. He did this by signing into law the historic Social Security Act of 1935, which also made the federal vocational rehabilitation program permanent. Roosevelt himself had contracted polio at age 39 in 1921 and was keenly aware of not only the lack of services but also the attitudes toward people with disabilities (Rubin & Roessler, 1995). In his book *FDR's Splendid Deception* (1994), Gallagher describes how FDR had an understanding with the news media that he was to never be photographed or filmed sitting in his wheelchair. Although Roosevelt ambulated by wheelchair and leg braces, he was always photographed or filmed standing at the podium or in his car meeting the public without any assistive device. Roosevelt believed that the public would perceive him as a weak leader should it ever be known that he was disabled. With his condition, FDR also experienced a great deal of pain and spent much of his time in the therapeutic warm spring pools in Warm Springs, Georgia, which he later purchased and ran in 1927. Roosevelt spent so much time here, it became known by insiders as the "Little White House." Despite his disability experience, Roosevelt did not specifically have a disability agenda. His interest was more with the poor and disadvantaged, and he even proposed a 25% reduction in funding the vocational rehabilitation program: an effort that did not pass Congress. It is ironic to note that FDR's disability secret and fears of being discovered and perceived as weak is not how the public remembers him today. Having brought America through the Depression, passed the historic Social Security Act, and brought the United States through

World War II, FDR is believed by many to be one of the greatest presidents this country has ever had.

World War II had a significant impact on the services, treatment of, and attitudes toward persons with disabilities. A major development was the fact that over 12 million Americans went into the military, which freed up jobs in the civilian economy (Levitan, Mangum, & Marshall, 1976). Yelin (1991) cited that in all of the 20th century, persons with disabilities had the highest employment rate during World War II. Yelin noted how the simple principles of supply and demand dictated what employers needed to do during the period. Persons with disabilities were hired in many of the factories that made products for the war. Unfortunately, once the war was over, many of the able-bodied males and females who returned home ultimately displaced employees with disabilities, once again increasing the high unemployment rate of this population, which continues to hover around 70% to the current day.

Following World War II, there continued to be medical advances that improved the life expectancy of certain disabilities, especially those with physical impairments such as spinal cord injury. Legislatively, the 1943 Bardon–LaFollete Act extended rehabilitation services to persons with mental retardation and mental illness. In addition, the first federal-state rehabilitation program for the blind was approved, and continues today as its own separate program. Services for persons with mental retardation and mental illness were further expanded in the 1954 Vocational Rehabilitation Act Amendments (Parker & Szymanski, 1998). This Act also saw first-time funding for three universities to prepare training rehabilitation professionals to provide primarily vocational counseling for persons with disabilities.

Although other disability-related legislation ensued over the next two decades, the next key disability legislation came about with the 1973 Rehabilitation Act. Prior to this, the United States experienced the long overdue growing pains of the civil rights movement, culminating in the Civil Rights Act of 1964. This Act mandated equal treatment and opportunities for African Americans and other minorities. The women's rights movement also occurred during this period, again demonstrating the effectiveness of peaceful, social activism as a powerful way to facilitate social change through federal government intervention (Rubin & Roessler, 1995). Also during the 1960s, consumerism and the consumer rights movement led by Ralph Nader demonstrated that consumers needed to be actively involved in the type and quality of services they received. These movements had a significant impact for persons with disabilities who also continued to be disenfranchised from participating in employment, housing alternatives, and voting, as well as socially.

The Rehabilitation Act of 1973 was historic for several reasons. The first was the fact that then President Richard Nixon was not a fan of vocational rehabilitation and wanted to cut funding. He also previously twice vetoed bills to establish independent living centers, but finally agreed to fund a comprehensive needs assessment and six independent living center demonstration projects in 1973 (Rubin & Roessler, 1995).

Second was the establishment of Client Assistance Programs (CAPs), designed to advise clients of various services, and for counselors to act as ombudsman or mediator in situations where clients experienced problems in obtaining services for which they might be entitled. The Rehabilitation Act of 1978 gave further strength to CAPs by including assistance for legal remedies to ensure the rights of clients with disabilities. The third key aspect of this 1973 legislation was the implementation of the Title V Sections 501–504. Section 501 of the Act limited discrimination in any federal hiring, placement, and advancement of "qualified" persons with disabilities in employment. In addition, affirmative action plans had to be developed for each government agency. Relatedly, Section 503 of the Act limited discrimination by private employers who received federal funds of $2,500 or more. Although these actions were initially good first steps, private businesses that did not use federal funds were still allowed to discriminate against hiring qualified persons with disabilities. The fourth key aspect of the 1973 legislation involved Section 502, where the Architectural and Transportation Barriers Compliance Board was established to ensure compliance with the Architectural Barriers Act 1968. This Section also involved investigating transportation and housing barriers/needs as well as promoting the use of the international accessibility symbol in all public buildings (Jenkins, Patterson, & Szymanski, 1998). Section 504 addressed equal opportunity and discrimination against persons with disabilities in education programs, health care, housing, and employment. Regarding the employment provision, an individual could not be found unqualified if a reasonable accommodation could otherwise make the individual qualified to perform a particular job unless it caused the employer undue hardship (Rubin & Roessler, 1995). Again, although these were encouraging changes toward ensuring the civil rights of persons with disabilities, they were limited to only those entities receiving federal funds.

The Independent Living Movement

The independent living movement essentially evolved as persons with disabilities learned from the social activist movements concerning minority civil rights, consumerism, and women's rights. Leading up to the independent living movement, many persons with disabilities were becoming frustrated with how society both viewed and treated them. Persons with all types of disabilities found themselves trying to negotiate an able-bodied world in which public phones were inaccessible to those who were deaf, buildings and transportation were inaccessible to those with physical disabilities and blindness, and segregation in schooling existed for those with mental and physical disabilities, especially those of ethnic minority status (Sue & Sue, 1999). Many persons with disabilities were also angered by societal attitudes of them being incapable, sick, and helpless (DeJong, 1979a). Those with disabilities began to realize that in many instances, they knew what was best for themselves and that rehabilitation and medical professionals were not empowering them to live independently. Echoing this notion, DeJong (1979b) cited three propositions that essentially described the philosophy of independent living: (a) consumer sovereignty—people with disabilities know best what their needs are; (b) self-reliance—people with disabilities must rely on themselves for their own self-interests; and (c) political and economic rights—people with disabilities have the right to participate in economic and political life (Nosek, 1998).

DeJong (1979b) conceptualized the independent living movement as a paradigm in direct opposition to the medical model or traditional rehabilitation paradigm. In comparing the two, the independent living paradigm views environmental barriers and societal attitudes as the definition of what the problem is, whereas the medical model paradigm views the individual's disability and functional limitations as being the problem. The person with a disability is viewed as the "patient," with its implications of passively and unquestionably accepting what the professional advises in the medical model paradigm; however, in the independent living paradigm, the individual is viewed as a "consumer" of services, thereby needing to be informed of alternatives in order to select what he or she believes is the best alternative. Also within the medical model paradigm, the physician or rehabilitation counselor is supposedly all-knowing and in control of making decisions he or she believes are in the best interest of the patient; however, in the independent living paradigm, the consumer is in control of ultimate decisions concerning his or her welfare. In solving the problem, the medical model paradigm views the rehabilitation team (physicians, therapists, rehabilitation counselor, etc.) as having the ability to minimize the physical or mental impairments. Under the independent living paradigm, the solution revolves around self-help, advocacy, peer counseling (from others with disabilities who have negotiated the system in the community), and the removal of environmental obstacles and societal attitudes. Today, these extreme viewpoints have moved closer to the center in that consumers are more often being included and consulted in decisions about their welfare by the rehabilitation team.

The earliest origins of independent living came in 1962, when four students with physical disabilities at the University of Illinois at Champaign-Urbana advocated to be moved into a home with attendant care rather than remain in a nursing home. After President Nixon funded the first six Centers for Independent Living (CIL) demonstration projects in 1973, the one located in Berkeley, CA assisted several students with physical disabilities to also relocate from the University health center wing to apartment housing with attendant care services (Nosek, 1998). Today, there are approximately 400 CILs in the United States offering by mandate for federal funding at least four core services: peer counseling, information and referral, independent living skills training (essentially activities of daily living), and community advocacy. Many CILs across the country offer other services, such as housing assistance, transportation services, equipment maintenance, attendant care or referral, financial and legal advice, community awareness in education, interpreter services, and other types of assistance (Nosek, 1998). In addition, many of the staff at the Centers should ideally be persons with disabilities, including its Executive Director; however, this is not always the case. Further, the Board of Directors for the Centers must consist of at least 51% of persons with disabilities in order to continue to receive federal funding (Marini, 1994).

Psychosocially, the independent living movement and employees of CILs have done much to empower persons with disabilities to live independently and accept control over decisions in their lives. Groups such as the Americans with Disabilities for Attendant Programs Today (APAPT) have forged ahead with effective demonstrations to create accessible transportation in various cities, and more recently have campaigned against forcing persons with disabilities of all ages who need assistance with activities of daily living to go into nursing homes. ADAPT and others have advocated for the reallotment of some of the money earmarked for nursing homes to go toward a federally funded community-based attendant care program in which persons with disabilities can choose where they want to live. Several demonstration projects have shown this to be a cost-effective and preferable option for persons with disabilities.

Other Key Disability-Related Legislation

Other key legislation occurring in the 1970s was the 1975 Education for All Handicapped Children Act (subsequently called the Individuals with Disabilities Education Act of 1991). This Act provides equal rights and equal opportunities in education for students with disabilities in the "least restrictive environment" (e.g., mainstreamed or integrated into a regular classroom as much as possible). The Act also calls for an Individualized Education Plan (IEP) designed to follow, assess, and treat students with disabilities throughout their public schooling, whether the service is therapy, career counseling, or specialized teaching/tutoring. In addition, a student is monitored and prepared for transition from school to work with a vocational rehabilitation counselor as part of the transition team. Research had previously shown that over 80% of all special education graduates were neither employed nor in school 1-year postgraduation, with long waiting lists for entry into sheltered workshops.

The 1978 Rehabilitation, Comprehensive Services, and Developmental Disabilities Amendments Act expanded reader services for persons who are blind and interpreter services for those who are deaf, and established independent living services as part of the state-federal rehabilitation program. The National Institute of Handicapped Research (now retitled as the National Institute on Disability and Rehabilitation Research) was established, as was the National Council on the Handicapped (renamed the National Council on Disability). The Rehabilitation Act Amendments of 1986 established supported employment services, primarily for those with psychiatric disabilities, mental retardation, and head injuries. Also in 1986, the Air Carrier Access Act made Section 504 clear to all federally funded airlines that they could not discriminate against persons with disabilities. Similarly, the 1988 Fair Housing Act Amendments was the first federal law that extended nondiscrimination mandates to the private sector, regardless of whether they received federal funding (West, 1991). This mandate was intended to ensure accessibility standards for all new multifamily dwellings.

The 1990 Americans with Disabilities Act (ADA) is considered to be the most significant civil rights legislation for persons with disabilities to date (West, 1991). Leading up to its passage, there was overwhelming evidence collected by Congress confirming that persons with disabilities had historically been segregated and discriminated against in employment and social participation. Rubin and Roessler (1995) noted that there were 11 public hearings where testimony was gathered as well as 63 public forums covering all 50 states. Some of Congress's concluding results at the time indicated the following: (a) there were over 43 million Americans with disabilities and this number was growing due to an aging population; (b) persons with disabilities had historically been segregated and discriminated against in areas of employment, education, housing, transportation, communication, recreation, public accommodations, institutionalization, voting, health services, and access to public services; (c) census data and national polls indicated that persons with disabilities were disenfranchised socially, vocationally, economically, and educationally; (d) persons with disabilities were treated as a minority group without equal rights or opportunities, ultimately costing the United States billions of dollars to keep this population dependent and nonproductive.

Despite business and other lobbying groups advocating against the ADA due to fears of its costs and that small businesses would suffer financial hardship making accessibility accommodations, President George Bush signed the bill into law on July 1st, 1990. The ADA contains five Titles. Title I concerns employment and both strengthened and expanded the 1973 Rehabilitation Act against discrimination of "qualified" (must be able to perform the essential functions of the job) persons with disabilities in hiring, training, discharge, and promotion policies (Adams, 1991). The Act was expanded to businesses with 25 or more employees in 1992, and again in 1994 for businesses with 15 or more employees (West, 1991). Employers had to make reasonable accommodations for employees with disabilities unless such changes would cause the employer undue hardship (financial hardship or an accommodation that would negatively affect the business). Employers were also prohibited from asking questions about one's disability in a job interview or having them submit to a medical exam without making all job applicants do the same.

Title II of the ADA contains two Subtitles. Subtitle A extends Section 504 of the 1973 Rehabilitation Act prohibiting discrimination against persons with disabilities in state and local government public entities receiving federal funds that provide programs, activities, or services (West, 1991). Subtitle B requires public transportation systems and facilities receiving federal funds to become accessible. This includes new railway cars as well as local and national route buses. Despite Subtitle B's intended mandate, many smaller cities and rural areas continue to have inaccessible public transportation due to the presumed undue hardship it would cause the municipalities.

Title III deals with prohibiting discrimination against persons with disabilities concerning public accommodations, covering all entities where the general public has full access to services and enjoyment. This is inclusive of all theaters, sports facilities, hotels, restaurants, museums, auditoriums, parks, day-care centers, gymnasiums, and so on (West, 1991). Architectural barriers must be removed unless business owners can show undue hardship in making the required changes. Excluded from the Title III mandate are religious entities such as churches and private clubs. Unfortunately, as late as 2008, many persons with physical disabilities still report that the top causes of frustration and anger for them are environmental barriers and negative business attitudes toward making the necessary accommodations mandated now some 20 years later (Marini, Bhakta, & Graf, 2009).

Title IV of the Act pertains to increased access to telecommunications for persons who are deaf. This involves the availability of dual-party relay service systems where those persons using a telecommunication device for the deaf (TDD) could communicate through the phone via an operator trained with the system (Hearne, 1990). Accompanying this legislation was the Television Decoder Circuitry Act of 1990 requiring all new televisions larger than 13 inches to come equipped with close captioning.

Title V covers miscellaneous provisions that include personal behaviors not covered by the ADA. These include individuals who are currently engaging in illegal drug use, homosexuality, bisexuality, transvestism, transsexualism, pedophilia, exhibitionism, voyeurism, gender identity disorders, compulsive gambling, kleptomania or pyromania, and other substance abuse disorders resulting from illegal drug use (Jones, 1991). Title V also requires the Architectural and Transportation Barriers Compliance Board to set out guidelines on how historic buildings will be made accessible. Section 507 requires a study be conducted by the National Council on Disability regarding access by wheelchair users in wilderness areas. A confusing point about provisions in Title V is that no effective-date section was included; however, others argue that the enactment date was effective after the ADA was signed into law.

During the past two decades, Americans with disabilities have forged ahead in testing the ADA and "tweaking" it to fight for their civil rights. They have fared better in some arenas than in others. Blackwell, Marini, and Chacon (2001) researched the number and types of ADA lawsuits since the Act's inception and found that persons with disabilities were experiencing poor success with Title I filed complaints. Herman (2000) cited a 2000 issue of *Mental and Physical Disability Law Reporter*, which indicated that employees won their discrimination lawsuits only 5% of the time during the past decade. Individuals who instead had the Equal Employment Opportunity Commission (EEOC) handle their case fared a little better as 15% of these cases were in favor of the employee. The primary reason cited for the poor success rate was attributed to employees' ignorance regarding court procedures and technical legal requirements of the ADA for those claiming workplace discrimination. Another interesting finding was that the majority of Title I complaints were from existing employees with less severe disabilities attempting to keep their jobs as opposed to new applicants suing for discrimination.

Other areas of the ADA that have been consistently challenged pertain to Title III on public accommodations. Marini (2000a, 2000b, 2002c; Marini et al., 2009) cite numerous cases and consumer frustration regarding businesses electing to fight the finer details of the ADA by challenging it in court. Airlines have been sued for not allowing wheelchair users to store their chairs in the closet. In addition, flight crews have forgotten disabled passengers onboard for extended periods after the plane has landed. In other areas, the first movie theater chains that began building stadium-style seating initially only designated the very front row of the theater (arguably the worst seats in the house) for wheelchair users. The courts have upheld wheelchair user complaints, concluding that persons with disabilities must be afforded "similar lines of sight" (equal access to the best seats, which have been determined to be 1/3 to 1/2 the way from the front row) as nondisabled patrons (Gilmer, 2000). Other Title III legal battles include international cruise ships not having to abide to the Americans with Disabilities Act regulations despite the fact that they dock and pick up U.S. passengers constantly, or major retail stores crowding their aisles with merchandise racks, thereby restricting wheelchair access. Hotels have also been sued for not securing prior reservations of accessible rooms. Wheelchair users complained of being stranded upon arriving at hotels where they had previously reserved an accessible room, only to find the room had been rented out. Similarly, various hotel chains have been sued for inaccessibility, or for too few rooms designated as accessible (Marini, 2000a). Finally, in sports, the U.S. Supreme Court ruling on *PGA (Professional Golf Association) Tour, Inc. v. Martin* permitted professional golfer Casey Martin to ride in a golf cart between shots at Tour events. Association officials had argued that allowing Martin to ride a cart while other golfers could not gave Martin an unfair advantage (Blackwell et al., 2001). The Court ruled, however, that under the ADA, this was a reasonable accommodation for Martin to be able to play the game. Martin's disability makes it painful for him to walk long distances and places him at risk of injury.

Today, most cases are mediated without going to court, as businesses make required changes that they have ignored for the past 20 years. However, some continue to not only flagrantly violate the law but also fight making the required changes until mandated by the courts. Blackwell et al. stated, "Although the government can legislate laws, it cannot legislate peoples' stereotypical or sometimes prejudicial attitudes. These attitudes result from misunderstanding and discrimination, and result in low expectations about things people with disabilities can achieve" (Blackwell et al., 2001, p. 405).

IMPLICATIONS AND THE FUTURE OF DISABILITY: REVISITING DARWIN AND EUGENICS

Have we learned from our past? As we begin to enter a new era of being able to determine that a mother's unborn fetus carries the gene for a congenital disability such as mental retardation or muscular dystrophy, parents and their physician can decide early on whether to abort and start over. The gene(s) responsible for later-in-life neuromuscular diseases, such as Alzheimer's or Huntington's disease, will soon be able to be eradicated as well. Similarly, extracting stem cells from aborted fetuses or growing them in a Petri dish may help millions of people with neuromuscular diseases such as Parkinson's as well as spinal cord injury and other disabilities. Couples today can also choose to have a designer baby by being impregnated with eggs for sale by a supermodel if they desire (Wilson, 1999). Smart (2009) cited an October 1999 Associated Press story about a *Playboy* photographer who started a website selling supermodel eggs. In just the first morning of bidding, 5 million people visited the site with the highest bid for an ovarian egg from the supermodel listed at $42,000. In another process called preimplantation genetic diagnosis, parents can choose to have their unborn fetus genetically altered for eye or hair color. Cloning also appears to be inevitable. Some scientists indicate that various diseases and disabilities may be eradicated by harvesting and extracting healthy cloned body parts and implanting them in their disabled host. Finally, a number of surveyed physicians have anonymously indicated that they have assisted terminally ill patients to end their lives as well as having not provided life-sustaining assistance for newborns with severe congenital disabilities (Singer,

1995). Are these changes viewed as a step forward or backward in human development? This is not easily answered. Olkin (1999) states that by preventing babies with disabilities from being born, and due to advertising or charity drives portraying the "suffering" of persons with disabilities, society negates the very existence of those with congenital disabilities and conveys the message of the disabled being better off not existing at all than to exist with a disability. As Olkin who was born with polio indicates however, most people with disabilities would not have chosen to be aborted and do not consider themselves to be suffering.

In the first few pages of her book *Disability, Society, and the Individual* (2009), Julie Smart contemplates, "What is normal?" She indicates that normal is often defined as the absence of deviance or disability. *Webster's Dictionary* defines the word *normal* as "conforming with or constituting an accepted standard, model or pattern; esp., corresponding to the median or average of a large group in type, appearance, achievement, function, development, etc." (*Webster's Dictionary*, 1980, p. 970). Smart (2009) argues that typically the majority culture or those in power are the ones who define what is normal. This was also the mindset a century ago among primarily White Anglo-Saxon male academics, politicians, and physicians in power who contemplated who the weaker of the species were who should be prevented from procreating. Similar logic also epitomized Nazi Germany's extermination program in pursuit of the superior race in the 1930s and 1940s.

We continue to revisit this issue today as eugenicists proclaim the decline of civilization. Van Court (1998) notes that civilization depends on innate intelligence and that ancient civilizations fell when intelligence declined. Of course there is no empirical way to prove this assertion. Herrnstein and Murray, in their controversial 1996 book *The Bell Curve*, conclude that with the sample they studied, a majority of social problems occurred when the average IQ in their sample dropped three points from 100 to 97. Princeton University professor, Peter Singer continues to draw criticism from disability advocates for his views that fetuses with genetically detected disabilities should be aborted and that parents should have the right to terminate the life of their severely disabled infant within 30 days of its birth (Marini, 2002b).

Recently, the science of eugenics has focused more on IQ arguments and the science of "dysgenics." Dysgenics refers to the study of fewer intellectually superior scoring people having children, while more those with lower IQs have children (Lynn & Van Court, 2004; Lynn & Vanhanen, 2002; Van Court, 1998). Specifically, in Lynn and Vanhanen's (2002) book *IQ and the Wealth of Nations*, the authors argue that the decline of IQ has correlated with an increase in crime, high unemployment, greater poverty, and dependence on welfare by many single mothers. Conversely, of the 81 countries assessed, those with higher IQs had higher levels of education, had greater economic success, and made more contributions to their social infrastructure.

Ironically, due to medical advances, the life expectancy and quality of life for persons living with disabilities in industrialized nations will continue to improve from a medical perspective for those who can afford health care. To this end, the United States will continue to arguably have a "survival of the economically fittest" mentality if universal health care is not soon realized. For the estimated 76 million baby boomers presently transitioning to retirement, the golden years may not be something to look forward to in view of increasing health care costs. In 2010, President Obama became the first president since FDR to pass a major health reform bill, but with health insurance companies arguably still largely in control and Congress currently controlled by Republicans looking to repeal health care, the resulting impact remains to be seen.

Finally, as far as our current medical capabilities to genetically screen out and abort fetuses with a potential disability gene, it is difficult to think of a world without the likes of Franklin D. Roosevelt, Steven Hawking, Beethoven, Albert Einstein, Stevie Wonder, Wilma Rudolf, and the thousands of other gifted persons born with congenital disabilities who have undoubtedly positively influenced the human condition. Nevertheless, the Darwin debate continues today in the eugenics guise of genetic screening and humankind's ongoing quest for the perfect being.

REFERENCES

Adams, J. E. (1991). Judicial and regulatory interpretation of the employment rights of persons with disabilities. *Journal of Applied Rehabilitation Counseling, 22*(3), 28–46.

Alemdaroglu, A. (2006). Eugenics, modernity and nationalism. In D. M. Turner & K. Stagg (Eds.), *Social histories of disability in deformity* (pp. 126–141). New York, NY: Routledge.

Baynton, D. C. (2001). Disability and the justification of inequality in American history. In P. K. Longmore & L. Umansky (Eds.), *The new disability history: American perspectives* (pp. 33–57). New York, NY: New York University Press.

Berkowitz, M. (1960). *Workmen's compensation: The New Jersey experience.* New Brunswick, NJ: Rutgers University Press.

Blackwell, T. M., Marini, I., & Chacon, M. (2001). The impact of the Americans with Disabilities Act on independent living. *Rehabilitation Education, 15*(4), 395–408.

Buchanan, A. (2007). Institutions, beliefs, and ethics: Eugenics as a case study. *Journal of Political Philosophy, 15*(1), 22–45.

Buton, F. (2006). Making deaf children talk: Changes in educational policy towards the deaf and the French Third Republic. In D. M. Turner & K. Stagg (Eds.), *Social histories of disability in deformity* (pp. 117–125). New York, NY: Routledge.

Byrd, E. K. (1990). A study of biblical depiction of disability. *Journal of Applied Rehabilitation Counseling, 21*(4), 52–53.

Carlson, E. A. (2009). Three generations, no imbeciles: Eugenics, the Supreme Court, and *Buck v. Bell. Quarterly Review of Biology, 84*(2), 178–180.

Cheit, E. F. (1961). *Injury and recovery in the course of employment.* New York, NY: Wiley.

Chubon, R. A. (1994). *Social and psychological foundations of rehabilitation.* Springfield, MA: Charles C. Thomas.

Coco, A. P. (2010). Diseased, maimed, mutilated: Categorizations of disability and an ugly law in the late nineteenth-century Chicago. *Journal of Social History, 44*(1), 23–27.

Coleman, J. C. (3rd ed.) (1964). *Abnormal psychology and modern life.* Chicago, IL: Scott, Foresman.

DeJong, G. (1979a). Independent living: From social movement to analytic paradigm. *Archives of Physical Medicine and Rehabilitation, 60*, 435–446.

DeJong, G. (1979b). *The movement for independent living: Origins, ideology, and implications for disability research.* East Lansing, MI: University for International Rehabilitation, Michigan State University.

Deutsch, A. (2nd ed.) (1949). *The mentally ill in America.* New York, NY: Columbia University Press.

Dickinson, G. L. (1961). *Greek view of life.* New York, NY: Collier Books.

Gallagher, H. G. (1995). *By trust betrayed: Patients, physicians, and the license to kill in The Third Reich* (rev. ed.). Arlington, TX: Vandamere.

Gilmer, G. (2000). A stadium seating update. *New Mobility, 11*(87), 18–21.

Gostin, L. O. (2008). "Old" and "new" institutions for persons with mental illness: Treatment, punishment or preventive confinement? *Journal of the Royal Institute of Public Health, 122*, 906–913.

Grob, G. N. (1973). *Mental institutions in America: Social policy to 1875.* New York, NY: Free Press.

Haller, M. H. (1963). *Eugenics: Hereditarian attitudes in America thought.* New Brunswick, NJ: Rutgers University Press.

Hearne, P. G. (1990). The Americans with disabilities act: A new era. In L. G. Perlman & C. E. Hansen (Eds.), *Employment and disability trends and issues for the1900s* (Switzer Monograph No. 14). Alexandra, VA: National Rehabilitation Association.

Herman, R. N. (2000). The American's with Disability Act: Ten years later. *Paraplegia News, 54*(7), 12–14.

Hofstadter, R., Miller, W., & Aaron, D. (1959). *The American republic since 1865* (Vol. 2). Englewood Cliffs, NJ: Prentice-Hall.

Holbrook, S. H. (1957). *Dreamers of the American dream.* Garden City, NY: Doubleday.

Jenkins, W. M., Patterson, J. B., & Szymanski, E. M. (1998). Philosophical, historical, and legislative aspects of the rehabilitation counseling profession. In R. M. Parker & E. M. Szymanski (Eds.), *Rehabilitation counseling: Basics and beyond* (pp. 1–40). Austin, TX: Pro Ed.

Jones, N. L. (1991). Essential requirements of the Act: A short history and overview. In J. West (Ed.), *The Americans with Disabilities Act: From policy to practice* (pp. 25–54). New York, NY: Milbank Memorial Fund.

Kanner, L. (1964). *A history of the care and study of the mentally retarded.* Springfield, MA: Charles C. Thomas.

Kramer, H., & Sprenger, J. (1971). *The Malleus Maleficarum of Heinrich Kramer and James Sprenger.* Dover, DE: Dover Publications.

Kraut, A. M. (2010). The ugly laws: Disability in public. *Journal of American History, 97*(1), 214–215.

LaRue, C. (1972). *The development of vocational rehabilitation programs, 1880–1940: A case study in the evolution of the public services in the United States (Working Paper No. 188/R5014).* Berkley, CA: Institute of Urban and Regional Development, University of California.

Levitan, S. A., Mangum, G. L., & Marshall, R. (1976). *Human resources and labor markets.* New York, NY: Harper & Row.

Lowenfeld, B. (1975). *The changing status of the blind.* Springfield, MA: Charles C. Thomas.

Lynn, R., & Van Court, M. (2004). New evidence of dysgenic fertility for intelligence in the United States. *Intelligence, 32*, 193–201.

Lynn, R., & Vanhanen, T. (2002). *IQ and the wealth of nations.* Westport, CT: Praeger Publishers.

MacDonald, M. E. (1944). *Federal grants for vocational rehabilitation.* Chicago, IL: University of Chicago Press.

Marini, I. (1994). Identified service and training needs of centers for independent living in southeastern United States. *Journal of Rehabilitation, 60*(1), 47–51.

Marini, I. (2000a). ADA continues to be tested and "tweaked". *SCI Psychosocial Process, 13*(2), 69–70.

Marini, I. (2000b). ADA report card 10 years later. *SCI Psychosocial Process, 13*(4), 83–84.

Marini, I. (2002b). Ashcroft challenges Oregon's death with dignity act. *SCI Psychosocial Process, 15*(2), 94.

Marini, I. (2002c). Argus study may impact wheelchair seating. *SCI Psychosocial Process, 15*(1), 39–40.

Marini, I., Bhakta, M. V., & Graf, N. (2009). A content analysis of common concerns of persons with physical disabilities. *Journal of Applied Rehabilitation Counseling, 40*(1), 44–49.

Miller, J. C. (1966). *The first frontier: Life in colonial America.* New York, NY: Dell. (Original printing 1952.)

Nelson, N. (1971). *Workshops for the handicapped in the United States.* Springfield, MA: Charles C. Thomas.

New World dictionary of the American language (2nd ed.). (1980). New York: World Publishing Co.

Nosek, M. A. (1998). Independent living. In R. M. Parker & E. M. Szymanski (Eds.), *Rehabilitation counseling: Basics and beyond* (3rd ed., pp. 107–141). Austin, TX: Pro-ed.

Obermann, C. E. (1965). *A history of vocational rehabilitation in America.* Minneapolis, MN: T.S. Denison.

Olkin, R. (1999). *What psychotherapists should know about disability.* New York, NY: The Guilford Press.

Parker, R. M., & Szymanski, E. M. (1998). *Rehabilitation counseling: Basics and beyond* (3rd ed.). Austin, TX: Pro-ed.

Rubin, S. E., & Roessler, R. T. (1995). *Foundations of the vocational rehabilitation process* (4th ed.). Austin, TX: Pro-ed.

Safilios-Rothschild, C. (1970). *The sociology and social psychology of disability and rehabilitation.* New York, NY: Random House.

Sand, R. (1952). *The advance of social medicine.* London, UK: Staples Press.

Sigerist, H. E. (1951). *A history of medicine.* New York, NY: Oxford University Press.

Singer, C. (1928). *A short history of medicine.* Oxford, UK: Clarendon Press.

Singer, P. (1995). *Rethinking life and death.* New York, NY: Oxford University Press.

Smart, J. (2009). *Disability, society, and the individual.* Austin, TX: Pro-Ed.

Smith, J. D. (1999). Thoughts on the changing meaning of disability: New eugenics or wholeness? *Remedial and Special Education, 20*(3), 131–133.

Sue, D. W., & Sue, D. (3rd ed.) (1999). *Counseling the culturally different: Theory and practice.* New York, NY: John Wiley & Sons, Inc.

Trieschmann, R. B. (1988). *Spinal cord injury: Psychological, social, and vocational rehabilitation.* New York, NY: Demos Publications.

Turner, B. S. (1987). *Medical power and social knowledge.* Beverly Hills, CA: Sage.

Turner, D. M. (2006). Introduction: Approaching anomalous bodies. In D. M. Turner & K. Stagg (Eds.), *Social histories of disability in deformity* (pp. 1–16). New York, NY: Routledge.

Van Court, M. (1998). *Future Generations Mission Statement.* Retrieved from http:\\eugencis.net\\papers\ mission.html.

Venzmer, G. (1968). *Five thousand years of medicine.* New York, NY: Taplinger.

Watson, F. (1930). *Civilization and the cripple.* London: John Bale and Danielson, Ltd.

Weisberger, B. A. (1975, December). The paradoxical Doctor Benjamin Rush. *American Heritage Magazine, 27*(1), 98–99.

West, J. (1991). *The Americans with Disabilities Act: From policy to practice.* New York, NY: Milbank Memorial Fund.

Wilson, J. (1999, October 20). Egg salesman defends web venture. *The Herald Journal,* pp. 1–10.

World Health Organization. (2005). *WHO manual on mental health legislation.* Geneva, Switzerland: Department of Mental Health and Substance Dependence, WHO.

Worrall, J. D., & Appel, D. (1985). *Workers' compensation benefits: Adequacy, equity, and efficiency.* Ithaca, NY: ILR Press.

Yelin, E. H. (1991). The recent history and immediate future of employment among persons with disabilities. In J. West (Ed.), *The Americans with Disabilities Act: From policy to practice* (pp. 129–149). New York, NY: Milbank Memorial Fund.

INSIDER PERSPECTIVE
The Story of Patricia E. Moniot

I am writing to let people know that life can be lived despite a mental disability, and they are not alone. There are others who have survived rock-bottom conditions of life and built a productive lifestyle with the help of professionals, other mental health consumers, and supportive family and friends.

My particular brand of disability is bipolar affective disorder, manic-depressive illness. The disease first manifested itself in 1968, after my graduation from college. I had earned my BA in mathematics and was preparing to attend the University of Detroit, where I had a fellowship for my PhD. However, I had a serious bout of manic-depressive illness, and my parents drove me back to Jamestown and soon put me into Gowanda Psychiatric Center for 2 months in 1968 because they had no health insurance.

I knew something was wrong when my parents and I stepped off the elevator. A young man lounging against the wall was grinning ghoulishly at me. His eyes flashed a greeting: Welcome to Gowanda's Little Shop of Horrors. I felt like a new, uninitiated inmate of an insane asylum for the first time. My impulse was to turn and run, but the elevator had gone down, and the doors were locked. I clung to my belief that I was only physically ill, in danger of dying, and in a true hospital where I would receive the best and quickest care.

In the doctor's office, I told Dr. Battersby that I felt like I was going to die. By reading upside down, I was able to see the doctor write "hypochondria" on my admission form. I would later wonder why a hypochondriac would be given 900 mg of Thorazine and 900 mg of Stelazine on the first day, before any tests had been given.

My parents, full of misgivings, left for home. Two nurses took me in to a large, white room to be admitted. I was feeling faint and nervous. They couldn't get a blood pressure reading on me with either of two blood pressure machines. Next, they told me to take off all my clothes, including my glasses and watch. I had never been naked in front of anyone, and I could not see without my glasses. In terror, I refused to strip unless they got me a robe. The nurses were angry, but they did give me a robe. When they unfolded a sheet on the floor and tied up all my belongings in it, I didn't know that they needed to mark everything; I thought they were trying to cause me grief and pain.

After I was weighed and my temperature was taken rectally, they deposited me in a single room. I felt for a moment that I was going to be okay: I had a room and nurses to take care of me. That's what I thought! In fewer than five minutes, a barefoot old hag of a patient shuffled into my room and made off with my shoes and glasses. I was forced to run after her and grab them back. Then the nurses told me to go into the day room and get acquainted with the other patients. I was shocked by what I saw.

The kleptomaniac who had taken my glasses and shoes was shuffling around, gathering up all the ash trays and dumping them into the window sills. There were bars on the windows, which let in very little air. The room was blue with smoke from patients' and nurses' cigarettes. There was a stench of urine. Several women in nightgowns were sitting around with their heads hanging down. I felt like I had died and gone to hell, rather than being treated in a hospital, as I had expected.

I was unable to walk down the halls, because I was light-headed, dizzy, and restless. In order to cross the day room floor, I had to run. To go to the dining room, I had to crawl on my hands and knees, unless I could hold onto the arm of a patient. I was so utterly humiliated by this crawling that I would always end up crying and losing my appetite.

The bathroom was a long white room with a row of 20 toilets along one side. There were no lids, seats, doors, or partitions in the toilets. Therefore, there was no privacy. Toilet paper was locked up in the nurses' station.

We patients were herded around for medication, meals, and allocation to our cots in the wards. During a blizzard, we found that the wind was blowing drifts of snow into our bedrooms, and there were only a few blankets available.

One of the patients was very obese and had to be helped off the toilet and off her chair. The nurses were always yelling at her. One day the lady had a heart attack and collapsed on the day room floor. For three hours the nurses walking by would kick her in the side and say, "Get up, Michaeline! Get up you lazy pig!" Finally, a nurse checked her vital signs and started to yell, because the lady was not alive, and the nurses were in trouble. After that, we did not feel secure that we would get well and leave the hospital alive. I did't think that the nurses liked us; all they wanted to do was smoke cigarettes in the nurses' station.

After being in Gowanda for 2 months, I worked hard on my own to learn to walk. I started to say things to please the doctor, who appeared twice weekly to ask me how I was doing. I do not remember any therapy that helped me. Aggressive patients dominated the group meetings. To help my coordination and concentration, I learned to crochet and do other crafts each day; and I made myself slippers and doll clothes. I think that the knowledge that my family, who visited me every weekend, would be waiting for me, and that the other patients were kind to me, kept me going and were the most important factors in my recovery.

From 1968 to 1973, I tried to establish my residence in Buffalo and get a job. However, I returned again and again to Buffalo's institutions and lived briefly in various group homes.

After 5 years in institutions and group homes, my parents brought me home and put me to bed. I remained in depression for 3 solid years, never leaving my room, except for meals and personal needs.

In 1976, I was invited to play the organ at our church. At last there was a light at the end of the tunnel. I was inspired to try moving into the sunlight, and my depression lifted through the healing influence of music.

Soon I moved into a tiny attic apartment in Jamestown. I started out with three old saucepans and a floor lamp donated by my mother. At the time, I was thrilled with these awesome gifts. Looking back, I think a "coming out shower" would have been better. I lacked many living skills that I was not taught in hospitals, such as lighting pilot lights, assembling appliances, and setting digital clocks. The Friendship Peer Support Line and the Southwestern Independent Living Center were helpful in managing questions like these.

In my tiny attic apartment, I felt isolated. I coped by calling the Crisis Line, taking walks, and visiting the library. I became restless. I asked about a volunteer clerical job at Jamestown General Hospital. A wonderful lady named Helen took me under her wing and taught me outpatient billing. One year later, I went from volunteer to paid employee by passing a Civil Service test and by demanding to be hired when an opening occurred. I worked there for 12 years, learning to use a computer and how to deal with the public, especially the elderly or disabled.

My counselor advised me to seek job training through the PIC (Private Industry Council) programs. The first step was to take an aptitude test; I found high scores in clerical and music interests. The counselor, John Theismann, was polite and elevated my self-esteem by his attitude of respect. He placed me in a keyboarding class, where I was uplifted by a quick increase in typing and computer skills and had a good time.

In a few weeks PIC placed me in a supported position at the United Way Project DIAL office. My supervisor there, Judith Brentley, trained me gently to perform referrals to agencies by means of using a computer. Eventually, I was able to produce a volunteer training manual for office use.

The entire PIC program was positive and made me feel competent. The job was a steppingstone. Years later, when I had won other positions, PIC declared me a success and put my name in their Hall of Fame.

Another program in which I was rehabilitated was VESID, the State Education Department of Vocational and Educational Services for Individuals with Disabilities. The VESID program trained me in clerical skills at the Niagara Frontier Vocational Rehabilitation Center in Buffalo, NY. My clerical supervisor regarded me as intelligent and worthy of obtaining a secretarial position. The VESID personnel were kind and patient, even though my behavior was altered by medication problems. My self-esteem rose when I could type 65 words per minute, and I produced a regular newsletter, *The Rehab-Ability News*, written by disabled clients. I felt comforted by the feeling that the personnel cared and believed in me. I used my clerical skills in all the jobs I have had since then. In my present position, I send invoices to both PIC and VESID to cover the transportation costs of other clients participating in these programs.

In 1985, I was correctly diagnosed with bipolar affective disorder and I have been well ever since on lithium, learning to drive a car and living independently. My goal is to remain employed and to continue my volunteer work.

My favorite ways of thanking God for bringing me through these obstacles are playing the piano in nursing homes, working in agencies that provide services for the elderly and disabled, advocating for handicapped people through writing on their behalf, surprising the lonely and poverty stricken with special cards and gifts, and being supportive by phone to housebound friends. These activities are my way of adding joy and meaning to my life.

Writing has become one major outlet for my energy, a way to capture on paper memories of long ago, and a way to share an account of my ongoing recovery from mental illness. Like the large, light snowflakes on the first day of winter, my ideas drift down and land upon my notebook with almost no effort at all.

I have a message to mental health professionals about the needs of their clients and patients. It may well be misunderstood by anyone who has not experienced mental illness himself, although the disabled have shown that they understand. Here is a list of our needs in counseling sessions:

1. Give the patient a large appointment card that is not likely to be lost; or use a calendar page with appointments and family events marked on it.
2. Praise the patient when he/she makes it on time to your office.
3. Offer the patient a free cup of coffee or other drink, for it may be difficult for him to talk at length. Having coffee is a symbol of friendliness.
4. Be on time yourself; this will set a good example for promptness. The patient has a schedule, too, and his time is valuable.
5. Do not label the patient "discourteous" or "lazy" if his illness contributes to his inability to show up. Believe that he really is sick and cannot always get to a phone. Do not expect the patient to think correctly at all times.
6. Be careful not to complain about how much money is lost when a patient fails to show up. This promotes resentment and guilt.

7. Explain about the waiting list; the patient will realize that his peers may be denied treatment because he did not call to cancel his appointment.
8. Contact friends or relatives who can be relied on to remind the patient of his/her appointment.

I will close with a list of 10 most urgent needs of consumers who were deinstitutionalized and are now living independently in the community:

1. Preventing a problem from becoming a full-blown crisis.
2. Coping with small-scale manic or depression moods.
3. Discussing living skills.
4. Regaining a sense of safety or security.
5. Obtaining comfort in the middle of the night.
6. Choosing services through referral information.
7. Confiding feelings about relationships.
8. Confessing fears and deciding if there is a real crisis.
9. Relaxing with "shrink" jokes and using humor to minimize anxiety about treatment.
10. Unburdening memories of the old institutions.

We just want a vehicle where we can express our thoughts and feelings in a friendly, nonjudgmental atmosphere. We want others to deal with us on the strength of our character, not by our labels as mental health consumers.

DISCUSSION QUESTIONS

1. How many of you believe we should put a limit on the number of children for those who do not contribute to society (e.g., collect disability, on welfare) can have?
2. What is your opinion regarding physician assisted suicide? Under what conditions would it be okay, and are we on a slippery slope?
3. Should we allow embryonic stem cell surgery to help treat neuromuscular diseases and other disabilities?
4. Is genetic testing a good idea and what would you do if you were told your child was going to have Down's syndrome?
5. If you could select your unborn baby's characteristics, what would you choose (e.g., eye color, gender, height, IQ, hair color, skin color)?

EXERCISE

A. The class represents politicians, academics, physicians, and attorneys from 1895 debating who comprises the weaker of the species who should start being sterilized. Four examples are brought up: (a) a welfare single mother of four children; (b) a physician who has epilepsy; (c) a professor who is paralyzed from an accident and requires an attendant; and (d) a physically healthy homeless male.

TWO

Societal Attitudes and Myths About Disability: Improving the Social Consciousness

Irmo Marini

OVERVIEW

Where do people get their information from when it comes to disability? Since the majority of Americans are not college graduates and there are no designated courses in public schools dealing with disability, our information most often comes from a variety of questionable sources. In this chapter, we explore the concept of attitudes, the sociological aspects of how attitudes toward persons with disabilities are formed, and what many of the myths and misconceptions are about disability. Finally, we will discuss ways to enhance attitudes and the social consciousness toward disability.

ATTITUDES DEFINED: COMPONENTS AND CONCEPTS

It is first important to understand that some researchers argue that the concept of "attitude" is too abstract to accurately measure. It is further compounded by the fact that unless respondents' answers to attitude surveys are anonymous, many people respond in a way they believe to be *socially desirable* (Antonak & Livneh, 1988). In other words, people will claim they have positive attitudes toward persons with disabilities (even if they do not), because to state otherwise is not socially acceptable and considered to be prejudice. Attitude survey studies have further been criticized due to poorly validated measures being used, violations of internal validity, poor theoretical referents (not supported by theory), and making causal relationships from correlational studies (Antonak & Livneh, 1988, 2000; Chubon, 1994; Yuker, 1988). Regardless of such complaints, there have been hundreds of empirical studies devoted to studying attitudes toward disability (see Yuker, 1988).

Although there is no single definition pertaining to the concept of attitudes, there are certain commonalities that exist among these definitions (Ostrom, Skowronski, & Nowak, 1994). Plotnik defines attitude as "any belief or opinion that includes a positive or negative evaluation of some target (object, person, or event) and that predisposes us to act in a certain way toward the target" (Plotnik, 1996, p. 540). Ostrom et al. (1994) state that any definition of attitude shares three features: an *evaluative* feature that involves whether we like or dislike an object, person, or event; a *target* at which the attitude is aimed; and a *predisposition* to behaving or acting a certain way toward the target. For example, if an individual likes or admires (evaluation feature) persons with spinal cord injuries (target feature), he or she is more apt to approach and talk to such an individual as opposed to avoiding her (predisposed feature).

Eagly, Mladinic, and Otto (1994) also differentiate the fact that attitudes have three components to their makeup. As with other aspects of human behavior, attitudes involve a cognitive, affective, and behavioral component. The *cognitive* component includes our beliefs and thoughts. The *affective* component pertains to the feelings or emotions that are conjured up when we think about a target (object, person, or event). The *behavioral* component again predisposes us to act in a certain way. So, in the case of persons with antisocial personality disorder, some people "believe" that those with antisocial personality disorders are rude and uncaring toward others. This may cause some people to "feel" anger toward persons with personality disorders and, in turn, also "behave" rudely or totally avoid contact with this population.

Ostrom et al. (1994) further distinguish between three ways in which attitudes influence or function for us in our daily lives. A previously formed attitude *predisposes* us to behaving a certain way when encountering or anticipating an encounter with a target. We *interpret* new events or situations we encounter, which assists us in categorizing the target and deciding how to behave next time (i.e., "I don't like scary movies, therefore, I will avoid going to them). We then *evaluate* or assess the new encounter, which, in turn, helps us form our opinions or beliefs about the target.

As such, attitudes function to minimize our discomfort in negotiating our environment from day-to-day because we continuously interpret and evaluate it, generally acting in ways that minimize our discomfort unless we have little choice, such as in a job interview or taking an exam. For example, some people feel uncomfortable or anxious about passing homeless persons without giving them money. This may lead them to avoid making eye contact or ignoring a homeless person as they walk by. Still others may believe that homeless persons are lazy (predisposition/interpretation/cognition), causing them to defiantly walk past a homeless person and give them a dirty look (behavior).

Finally, it is important to note that people are not always consistent in the three components that form attitudes. An individual's beliefs and affect toward another person or group of people may be very different from how he or she outwardly behaves. In situations where people perceive they have little control, they may behave in a way that is socially desirable and appear to like the person. For instance, an employee who despises his boss may nevertheless be outwardly very friendly to her for some perceived ulterior reason (e.g., being promoted or avoiding being fired). Having laid the foundation for how attitudes are defined and developed, we now turn our attention to attitude formation regarding persons with disabilities.

ATTITUDES TOWARD DISABILITY: POSITIVE, NEGATIVE, OR AMBIVALENT?

Inherent Problems in Attitude Measurement

There has been a great deal of debate among researchers as to not only whether we can accurately measure attitudes toward disability but also whether peoples' attitudes are positive, negative, or ambivalent (Antonak & Livneh, 2000; Makas, 1988). The answer to this question is too complex to ever be able to make generalizations about society as a whole. Chubon (1982), in a critical review of the literature on attitude measurement during the 1970s, found numerous problems with the findings researchers were making. First, only 60 of the 102 articles he reviewed were empirical studies; the remaining were editorials or conceptual papers having no empirical basis. Second, in the empirical studies, there appeared to be differing attitudes based on the type of disability being studied. For example, Sowa and Cutter (1974) found that persons with alcohol or substance abuse problems were viewed more negatively by some professionals. Tringo (1970) also found that respondents ranked physical disability more positively than sensory impairments or brain injury. As such, attitude surveys, many of which often essentially cluster all disabilities into one homogeneous group, contained little meaningful value. Chubon (1982) also noted that many attitude instruments were poorly validated and had poor internal validity, a sentiment also echoed by Antonak and Livneh (1988). Finally, a number of studies used college students as participants, which again had limited generalizability to the attitudes of the general public (Comer & Piliavin, 1975; Fichten & Bourdon, 1986; Makas, 1988).

Beatrice Wright (1988) further argued that scientists have a predisposed "fundamental negative bias (p. 3)" when conducting attitude studies about disability. She indicated that some measurement instruments themselves are laden with negatively biased labels (e.g., former mental patient, amputee). Researchers also tend to make the disability the most salient aspect of the survey without accounting for other factors that help form our attitudes toward others, such as age, education, physical appearance, socioeconomic status, and so on (Antonak & Livneh, 2000). Many of the attitude survey instruments focus solely on the disability. Wright (1988) further noted how people tend to rate relationships with a stranger more negatively than with someone they know. In other words, it is inaccurate to conclude that participants necessarily have a negative attitude toward persons with disabilities solely based on administering a survey where the disability is the most salient feature and where the person with the disability is a stranger.

We must take into account the effect of the stranger relationship. Indeed, this argument was confirmed in the 1991 Lou Harris poll, which showed that able-bodied persons had more favorable attitudes toward persons with disabilities when they knew someone with a disability (Harris, 1991). A third criticism Wright (1988) asserted pertains to negatively loaded statements about disability in surveys that connotes something negative about disability (e.g., persons with disabilities should pay more for auto insurance). This example alludes to the myth that persons with disabilities are unsafe drivers, and Wright argues that such negatively laden statements perpetuate stereotypes. A fourth fundamental negative bias committed by researchers deals with ignoring findings that do not meet statistical significance. Researchers become so motivated to obtain statistically significant findings (which show differences and increase chances of publication) that they ignore the meaningfulness of obtaining no differences. Findings showing how persons with disabilities are similar to able-bodied persons have typically been ignored. As Goffman (1963) observed, persons with disabilities are stigmatized as being "different" and therefore reduced or discounted as a people. This was further confirmed in the 1992 Harris survey where a majority of respondents reported that persons with disabilities were viewed as fundamentally different from those without disabilities.

Harold Yuker, in his 1988 book *Attitudes Toward Persons with Disabilities*, supported Wright's (1988) argument that researchers have a knowing or unknowing negative bias in developing and interpreting attitude survey findings by making the disability the most salient aspect of the survey, while ignoring other factors that social psychologists have long since shown affect people's attitudes. Yuker and others describe what some of these other important factors are.

Physical attractiveness

Research suggests that people rated as more physically attractive create more favorable impressions than those rated less attractive (Longo & Ashmore, 1995). Physically attractive people are also generally perceived to be more kind, intelligent, interesting, responsive, likable, competent, sociable, outgoing, and poised and more likely to be promoted in their jobs (Eagly, Ashmore, Makhijani, & Longo, 1991; Longo & Ashmore, 1995; Yuker, 1988).

Competence

Persons viewed as being competent are perceived as being more attractive and credible (Yuker, 1988). Like physical attractiveness, there is no empirical evidence to support the assumption that attractive persons are indeed any more competent or intelligent than persons perceived to be unattractive. Nonetheless, many in society continue to perceive persons with disabilities as incompetent. Wright (1983) described the concept of "spread" pertaining to how some persons without disabilities assume that someone with a physical disability may also be mentally retarded. This belief often plays out, for example, when a nondisabled person goes to a restaurant with someone who uses a wheelchair, and the waiter asks the nondisabled partner what the wheelchair user would like to order, thus erroneously perceiving the wheelchair user as mentally unable to order for himself or herself.

Social skills

Social poise, including nonverbal behavior and the ability to interact with others, is also perceived as more attractive and likable (Gresham, 1982). Good social skills have been demonstrated to be important in mainstreaming children as well as in employment and promotion (Collmann & Newlyn, 1957; Oberle, 1975). Conversely, poor social skills have been shown to lead to rejection or negative attitudes toward persons with mental retardation (MacMillan & Morrison, 1980).

Other important factors that influence attitudes that are not considered in attitude measurements are the relationship of age, education, socioeconomic status, and personality variables (Antonak & Livneh, 2000; Yuker, 1988). We tend to like and feel more comfortable with others who are similar to us. Therefore, being of the same ethnic background, age, education, and socioeconomic status, all have an influence on our attitudes (Gosse & Sheppard, 1979; McGuire, 1969; Rabkin, 1972; Sue & Sue, 1999).

ATTITUDES TOWARD DISABILITY

There exists a plethora of empirical and anecdotal studies and books documenting that, for the most part, attitudes toward people with disabilities most often tend to be negative in nature (Chan, Livneh, Pruett, Wang, & Zheng, 2009; Chubon, 1994; Donaldson, 1980; Livneh, 1988; Olkin, 1999; Wright, 1988). The next section addresses 15 commonly perceived origins or causes of negative attitudes, also identifying studies related to positive attitudes and those that indicate attitudes toward disability in general as neither positive nor negative, but rather ambivalent.

Mackelprang and Salsgiver (2009), for example, discuss common stereotypical attitudes toward persons with disabilities covering a variety of themes. First, is the notion that persons with disabilities are perpetual children, citing the March of Dimes telethon and "Jerry's kids," referring to how Jerry Lewis portrays people with muscular dystrophy, regardless of their age. This sentiment is also evident in the medical model paradigm, in which some physicians treat their disabled patients as children. Second, is the stereotype that people with disabilities are objects of pity, as evidenced again in telethons, but also in news and media coverage where common descriptors such as "tragedy" and "victim" are overused. Third, is the notion that people with disabilities are a menace or threat to society. This is portrayed in numerous movies and television characters, including psychotic serial killers in television police dramas (Byrd, Byrd, & Allen, 1977). Group homes for those with developmental and intellectual disabilities are often vehemently protested against by concerned parents who fear for their children's lives because they believe these populations will sexually assault or attack their children. Fourth, is the perception that disabled persons are sick and incompetent, and therefore need to be cared for. They are also relieved of any responsibility to contribute to society because they are incapable of doing so. A fifth stereotype centers around disability as a psychological and economic burden to society, consuming resources without providing anything in return. This sentiment is very similar to the ones held by the Nazis and eugenicists, which ultimately led to confinement, sterilization, and extermination.

Origins of Negative Attitudes

Livneh (1991) and others have postulated a number of reasons regarding the origins of negative attitudes toward persons with disabilities. These are discussed or combined with other plausible reasons as to why persons with and without disabilities may possess less favorable attitudes toward those with disabilities. In all, 15 different hypotheses are proposed.

1. *Attributional origins*: Plotnik defines attributions as "the things we point to as the causes of events, other people's behaviors, and our own behaviors" (Plotnik, 1996, p. 537). Studies have shown that European Americans tend to attribute blame to internal reasons (i.e., Jack did not get the job because he lacked the qualifications), whereas persons of minority tend to attribute blame to external or environmental factors (i.e., Jack did not get the job because the employer discriminated against him) (Sue & Sue, 1999). Similarly, individuals who are perceived as having caused their own disability receive more negative appraisals than those perceived as not having contributed to their situation (Bordieri, 1993; Marantz, 1990; Murphy, 1998; Obermann, 1965; Zola, 1983). In general, military veterans are viewed more positively, whereas persons with alcohol and substance abuse disorders, HIV/AIDS, and mental illness are viewed more negatively because of a common belief that their disability was self-inflicted or results from a weak personality (Bickenbach, 1993; Hayes, Barlow, & Nelson-Gray, 1999; Safilios-Rothschild, 1982).

2. *Blaming the victim*: Wright (1983) defines the concept of blaming the victim, which, although sounding similar to attributional origins in definition, is distinctively different. Blaming the victim for his or her circumstances is not just limited to disabilities considered to be self-imposed (i.e., substance abuse). It is a psychological safety mechanism designed to minimize our fears and anxiety as to why something bad cannot happen to us. If I can justify to myself that I am a better driver than my reckless neighbor who was recently in an accident and fractured his neck, it serves to minimize my fears that such events can randomly occur anytime and happen to anyone.

3. *Disability as a punishment for sin*: Despite its early origins in beliefs, some people continue to believe that disability is a punishment from God for having sinned (Byrd, 1990). This may be especially true for those who follow the teachings of the Bible closely. As noted in Chapter 1, there are passages in the Bible that allude to persons being healed of their disability by repenting their sins (Gallagher, 1995). Meng (1938, as cited by Livneh, 1991) cited three unconscious mechanisms of punishment for sin attributions. These relate to the belief that either the individual has sinned, he or she is disabled unjustly and therefore is now motivated to sin, or, projecting one's own sinful impulses onto the person with a disability, he or she is evil.

4. *Anxiety-provoking situations*: Several research studies have explored the reported anxiety persons with and without disabilities express in unstructured (or even structured) interactions (Albrecht, Walker, & Levy, 1982; Kleck, 1968; Marinelli, 1974; Marini, 1992). Anxiety or discomfort is typically experienced when people are in ambiguous social situations where they do not know what to say or how to behave (Albrecht et al., 1982). Nondisabled persons often have an irrational fear of unintentionally offending someone with a disability that might upset them (i.e., telling a person who is blind that you went to "see" a movie last night). In Leary's (1990) literature review regarding social anxiety, he indicated that people initially assess a social situation in terms of its costs and rewards. If the perceived costs of an anticipated interaction outweigh the rewards, individuals will most likely avoid

the interaction altogether. As such, if persons with or without disabilities perceive that an interaction with the other has little value or reward attached to it, and the anticipated interaction provokes discomfort or anxiety, social avoidance will likely occur (Piliavin & Piliavin, 1972). Kleck (1968) demonstrated how persons without disabilities held less eye contact and ended interactions sooner with persons with disabilities than they did with those without disabilities.

5. *Childhood influences*: Livneh (1991) and others also believe that young children are influenced as they grow up in forming attitudes toward others (Vash & Crewe, 2004). Sometimes when children hurt themselves for doing something they should not be doing, parents scold them by saying "God punishes you when you are bad," which can later be misconstrued when encountering someone with a disability. The authors state how young children are sometimes scurried away from interacting with someone with a disability in public; however, this action thwarts the child's natural curiosity and leaves him or her with a sense that "these people" (with disabilities) are somehow different and need to be avoided. Thus, if children grow up having had little opportunity to interact and learn about people with disabilities, they tend to fear what they do not understand and tend to derive their attitudes from prevailing myths or misconceptions (Begab, 1970).

6. *Sociocultural conditioning*: Livneh (1991) discussed several societal and cultural norms that have had a negative impact on attitudes toward disability. Western society is almost obsessed with physical appearance and the "body beautiful" concept (Buss, 1999). Seligman (1993) described how Americans spend billions of dollars each year on self-improvement programs and products, such as dieting, exercise devices, workout videos, cosmetic facial creams or surgery, hair coloring, liposuction, gastric bypass surgery, plastic surgery, and so on. Television commercials and magazine ads depict young, athletic, healthy, medically inadvisably thin, physically attractive people promoting consumer products; however, none of the actors are persons with disabilities (Smart, 2009). As noted in Chapter 1, some people will pay thousands of dollars for a supermodel's ovarian egg. Western society also admires persons who are successful and wealthy. Many celebrities, athletes, and musicians are highly admired and publicized in our culture (Safilios-Rothschild, 1968). Few people with disabilities seemingly fall into this esteemed category, and instead are perceived as objects of charity, many of whom are poor, helpless, sick, and incapable of making decisions (Biklen, 1986; Olkin & Howson, 1994).

7. *Psychodynamic factors*: Pertain to views held by nondisabled persons toward those with disabilities in relation to unconscious psychological processes developed during childhood. Wright (1960, 1983) first described *requirement of mourning*, where an individual with a disability is expected to grieve the loss of body function and preinjury way of life. Nondisabled persons may inherently expect persons with disabilities to experience ongoing sadness, and, if they do not, they are accused of being in denial and may draw criticism from others (Dembo, Leviton, & Wright, 1956). Another psychodynamic variable relates to living in a *just world*: the perception that people generally get what they deserve (Walster,

1966; Yamamoto, 1971). We rationalize or justify why someone becomes disabled as either punishment for some misdeed (much like childhood influences) or because he or she was inept (attributional blame), which safely justifies why such an injury will not happen to us. This serves to reduce existential anxiety over the randomness of events and the fear that bad things can indeed happen to good people. This is similar to Wright's *blaming the victim* concept. The concept of *spread* is another unconscious origin of negative attitudes, whereby it is assumed that a disability envelops or spreads to define all aspects of the individual (Wright, 1960, 1983). Someone with a physical disability is believed to be mentally impaired as well; thus, the disability becomes the single most salient defining feature of the individual.

8. *Existential angst*: Smart (2009) describes the fear nondisabled persons experience in becoming disabled themselves. Being in the presence of someone with a disability reminds us of our vulnerability to also acquire a disability. Schilder (1935) viewed this unconscious fear as a threat to one's body image. This is similar to why many people do not like going to hospitals, nursing homes, or funerals or making their will. In all instances, we may experience discomfort in contemplating our own deterioration and eventual death. For some nondisabled persons, disability brings these unpleasant thoughts into consciousness, and such thoughts can be disturbing. Therefore, as a defense mechanism, some persons without disabilities may prefer to avoid those with disabilities to repress these fears (out-of-sight, out-of-mind) (Siller, Chipman, Ferguson, & Vann, 1967). Siller et al. (1967) further discuss the concept *fear of contamination*, whereby nondisabled persons fear that by interacting with someone with a disability, they too might become disabled, or by marrying someone with a disability, their offspring will be disabled. There is also a perceived related stigma that there must be something wrong with a nondisabled person if he or she has to associate with someone with a disability.

9. *Aesthetic aversion*: Livneh (1991) describes aesthetic-sexual aversion in relation to what society finds visually pleasing or repulsing to the eye. Certain disabilities, such as amputation, facial disfigurement, and deformity, are perceived as repulsive to look at, despite the fact that we have a morbid curiosity to stare. The conflicting cognition of wanting to stare and concomitantly look away generates discomfort. Aesthetics relates to the concept of beauty as in the eye of the beholder, and as discussed earlier, Western society dictates that beautiful people are those who are deemed physically attractive, thin, wealthy, and successful.

10. *Minority status*: Despite an estimated 54 million persons reporting a disability (2000 U.S. Census) in the United States, persons with disabilities are marginalized and disenfranchised more than any other group in North America. As a member of a minority group, societal perceptions of people with disabilities are that they are poor, helpless, sick, and incapable (Biklen, 1986; Mackelprang & Salsgiver, 2009). Being an ethnic minority, having a disability, and being female triples misperceived stereotypes and is statistically evidenced by disparities in

employment rates, education levels, and poverty levels (Szymanski, Ryan, Merz, Trevino, & Johnston-Rodriguez, 1996; Wright, 1988).

11. *Prejudice-inviting behavior*: Wright (1960) described how some persons with disabilities behave in a way that strengthens negative stereotypes toward them. This includes acting fearful, helpless, passive, and dependent, not standing up for oneself, and seeking secondary gains, such as acting helpless to receive attention (Livneh, 1991). Such behaviors confirm society's views that persons with disabilities need to be cared for and are inferior.

12. *Disability-related factors*: Livneh (1991) and others described several disability-specific factors that suggest some disabilities or dynamics are viewed more negatively than others (Safilios-Rothschild, 1970). There are inconclusive results as to whether nondisabled persons have more negative attitudes toward certain disabilities as opposed to others (Goodyear, 1983; Schmelkin, 1984; Stovall & Sedlacek, 1983). Schmelkin (1984) concluded that preferences toward disability could not be hierarchically ranked due to the multidimensionality factors related to it (e.g., severity, cause, gender, age, type of disability). Smart (2009) asserts, however, that a hierarchy of stigma does exist toward disability, backed by several studies indicating that of four disability categories, persons with physical disabilities are least stigmatized, followed by those with cognitive disabilities, those with intellectual disabilities, and those with mental illness (Antonak, 1980; Charlton, 1998; Tringo, 1970). It further appears that individuals believed to have caused or contributed to their own misfortune are rated more negatively. Weiner, Perry, and Magnusson (1988) found that persons with physical disabilities were not viewed as having caused their disabilities, but those with emotional and behavioral disabilities were to blame due to perceptions of being weak-willed. Yamamoto (1971) found that curable and predictable disabilities were viewed less negatively than those that were chronic or unpredictable. There is also some support that the more severe, visible, and aesthetically aversive a disability is, the less favorable the attitudes may be (Shontz, 1964; Siller, 1963). Olkin (1999) noted that in initial contacts with someone with a disability, appearance and severity of the disability do influence attitudes. However, initial negative attitudes can be diminished once the individual with a disability becomes better known and is able to demonstrate the disability is but one trait. If the person with a disability is perceived as being attractive and competent, and possesses good social poise, these factors create more positive attitudes.

13. *Media portrayals of disability*: Perhaps the most influential factor in facilitating and perpetuating negative attitudes toward disability is the effect of the media (Anderson, 1988; Black & Pretes, 2007; Byrd et al., 1977; Hadley & Brodwin, 1988; Marini, 1992). Television, newspapers, and magazines often reinforce negative stereotypes about disability. Byrd et al. (1977) found that of 64 shows depicting disability, 51 were police dramas, movies, and comedies that made scant effort to educate viewers, and in a majority of the police dramas, the character with the disability often was a psychopathic killer. In a later study, Byrd (1989) found that 49 of 67 characters portrayed in 302 films had abnormal personalities.

Other characteristics of portrayals indicated that in over 50% of the films, the person with a disability was portrayed as being a victim, over 50% of the characters with disabilities were not given an occupation, and the fate of the character with a disability was given a negative or neutral ending in 67% of the films. The absence of persons with disabilities in media also conveys a different message. Persons with disabilities are rarely seen in television commercials or magazine advertisements (Smart, 2009). The absence of persons with disabilities enjoying themselves, purchasing and consuming goods, and socializing in restaurants or other public venues indirectly conveys the message that people with disabilities do not get out much and are sick and helpless. Similarly, the typical language reporter's use in newspapers and magazines pertaining to persons with disabilities also facilitates negative attitudes, while sensationalized news headlines often perpetuate society's fears about persons with mental illness. Whenever someone with schizophrenia injures or murders someone, and despite the fact that persons with mental illness are statistically less violent than the general population (Gostin, 2008), the lay public generalizes and fears all persons with schizophrenia. In addition, journalists and reporters often cover disability stories by making the disability the salient focus of the story, to titillate the reader's emotions with the use of common descriptive words such as "victim," "tragedy," or "courage," depending on the story angle (Margolis, Shapiro, & Anderson, 1990). In addition, since telethons receive more donations when viewers are made to feel for the recipients (e.g., muscular dystrophy telethon), it comes as no surprise when nondisabled Americans indicate the most common sentiments they feel toward persons with disabilities are pity and/or admiration (Lou Harris & Associates, 1991).

14. *Demographic variables related to nondisabled persons*: A number of researchers have explored factors related to nondisabled persons and their attitudes toward disability. Findings reveal the following: (a) Females tend to have more positive attitudes toward persons with disabilities than do males (Antonak & Livneh, 2000; Chesler, 1965; English, 1971a). (b) Young children (age 6) show a preference for playing with nondisabled children (Weinberg, 1978), whereas persons in late childhood and adulthood appear to have more positive attitudes than older persons (Ryan, 1981). (c) Persons with higher levels of education generally have more positive attitudes (Tunick, Bowen, & Gillings, 1979). (d) Overlapping with education is socioeconomic status, where several studies have shown that those with higher incomes typically manifest more favorable attitudes (English, 1971b; Whiteman & Lukoff, 1965), although Olkin (1999) notes that this is not always the case. Livneh (1991) further noted that certain personality traits may predispose some persons to possess negative attitudes; however, Yuker (1994) warned against conducting such studies due to the futility in being able to change one's personality. Nevertheless, several studies have suggested that persons who were ethnocentric possessed poorer attitudes (Wright, 1960), as do persons with higher levels of anxiety in ambiguous or uncertain situations (Cloerkes, 1981; Fichten & Bourdon, 1986; Marinelli & Kelz, 1973). Further, nondisabled persons with a higher self-concept appear to possess more positive attitudes than those with a

lower self-concept (Jabin, 1966; Yuker, 1962). Finally, persons with a more positive body image and scoring high on ego strength also possessed more positive attitudes toward disability than those with low ego strength and poor body image (LeClair & Rockwell, 1980; Noonan, Barry, & Davis 1970; Siller, 1964).

15. *Perceptions of burden*: Without any prior knowledge or experience, many nondisabled persons automatically assume that disability connotes a "burden." Olkin (1999) noted how many researchers studying disability in families are biased from the onset regarding their findings, and look for the burdening and stressing aspects of caring for someone with a disability. She cited numerous studies with the word "burden" in the title and suggested that the simple repetition of these ideas permeates consciousness. Olkin further noted that many parent–child studies where the child is born with a disability are conducted sometime shortly after the birth of the child when parents are most distressed. Such findings, she argues, are negatively skewed as the parents attempt to come to terms with the situation. In opposing research discussed in Chapter 10, many caregivers do not perceive their loved one as a burden, are less depressed or stressed than was previously hypothesized, feel a sense of purpose in caring for their loved one, and overwhelmingly would choose to care for their disabled loved one at home rather than placing the person in a nursing home (Bogdan & Taylor, 1989; Lawrence, Tennstedt, & Assmann, 1998; Smart, 2009).

Positive Attitudes or Traits Ascribed To People With Disabilities

Although studies of positive attitudes toward persons with disabilities are much fewer in number than those dealing with negative attitudes, the findings nevertheless are consistent with other studies in that people without disabilities often make assumptions about groups they have little knowledge about. As such, these perceived positive characteristics about people with disabilities are no more accurate than are the negative traits ascribed to them.

Persons with disabilities are sometimes ascribed angelical traits, despite the apparent paradox of attitudes that disability is a punishment for having sinned. Mitchell (1976) had respondents rate counselor effectiveness by viewing videotaped interviews of counselors who were wheelchair users versus counselors who had no disability. The counselors who used wheelchairs were rated more effective and positively by both male and female respondents; however, female respondents rated the counselors in wheelchairs significantly more effective in areas of empathic understanding, level of regard, and congruence.

Comer and Piliavin (1975) compared the attitudes of a group of persons without a disability versus persons who were disabled for some time, versus those who had acquired a disability within the past year. Participants were asked to rate photographs of a White male using a wheelchair, one with an amputation, and a third picture of a nondisabled Black male. The nondisabled participants rated the two persons with disabilities as more intelligent, sensible, and admirable. Conversely, respondents who were disabled for a long time rated the nondisabled person more positively than respondents who became recently disabled. The authors suggested that those who were injured for a long time realized that there were no saintly qualities to being disabled as are sometimes bestowed upon persons with disabilities for assumedly being courageous in dealing with adversity.

As noted earlier, pity and admiration are common emotions expressed toward those with disabilities. One might initially think that inspirational stories in which persons with disabilities have accomplished some goal would enhance development of positive attitudes toward disability. Zola (1991), however, described the double message meaning after watching media reports on Franklin Delano Roosevelt and Wilma Rudolph. He explained how the message that is directly conveyed to the general public is that people with disabilities can accomplish great things (e.g., become President or an Olympic runner). Unfortunately, the indirect double message conveyed is that if others with disabilities are not successful, it is their own failure, weakness, or lack of motivation. This concept of blame relates back to how the majority culture tends to blame the individual, whereas persons in minority cultures often tend to attribute blame to external causes (Sue & Sue, 1999). Smart (2009) refers to disabled heroes as "super crips," a term used primarily by persons with disabilities to describe those who have overcome insurmountable odds to succeed.

It has become apparent that more contemporary writers addressing the psychosocial issues of persons with disabilities have philosophically approached the topic from a *Social Constructivist* viewpoint (Chubon, 1994; Chan et al., 2009; Mackelprang & Salsgiver, 2009; Smart, 2009). Social psychologists and sociologists have been addressing disability from this viewpoint for some time. The social construct model of disability (a.k.a. the minority or environmental model) posits blame for the handicapping elements of a disability with faults in the environmental and attitudinal barriers imposed by society (Blackwell, Marini, & Chacon, 2001; Graf, Marini, & Blankenship, 2009). Situations such as employment discrimination or opposing the building of a halfway house for persons with mental illness are examples of attitudinal barriers, whereas being unable to enter a restaurant with stairs if you use a wheelchair exemplifies an environmental barrier to social participation. The World Health Organization (WHO, 1980) defines "disability" as the consequences of impairment in terms of functional performance, while "impairment" refers to abnormalities of body structure and appearance with organ or system function resulting from any cause. This, in turn, may or may not lead to a "handicap," defined as disadvantages experienced by the individual as a result of impairments and disabilities. Handicap thus reflects an interaction with, and adaptation to, an individual's surroundings or environment. In other words, an individual may have a disability (spinal cord injury) caused by an impairment (paralysis), but is not otherwise handicapped in crossing a street if there are curb cuts. He does, however, become handicapped from crossing the street if there are no curb cuts.

Are People Really Ambivalent Toward Disability?

Several researchers argue that the general public's attitudes toward disability are mainly ambivalence because they essentially have not formed an opinion one way or another (Makas, 1988). Persons who have little or no contact with persons with disabilities likely do not give the issue much thought (out-of-sight, out-of-mind) until a situation presents itself. Makas (1988) argued that many nondisabled persons misunderstand what even constitutes a positive attitude. She developed a 37-item multidimensional attitude survey, the *Issues in Disability Scale* (IDS, formerly titled Modified Issues in Disability Scale), where the questions are worded in such a neutral way that the survey taker is unable to answer in a socially desirable manner. In one study, comparing the responses of persons with disabilities versus those without disabilities, nondisabled respondents scored significantly differently in their response to the question, "If a person with epilepsy becomes angry with people over little things, it should be overlooked because of his/her disability." Respondents with disabilities expressed essentially not feeling sorry for someone with epilepsy, whereas those without a disability perceived the anger and frustration someone having epilepsy might feel (making the disability salient), thereby believing that such behaviors are acceptable considering the circumstances. Another example is the question, "For a severely disabled person, the kindness of others is more important than any educational program." Once again, respondents with disabilities viewed education as a means to earn equal status and likely interpreted the kindness of others as paternalistic, whereas those without disabilities viewed being kind as a sign of compassion. On a more subconscious level, in viewing the importance of kindness over education, persons without disabilities may be expressing the negative belief that persons with disabilities are unlikely to complete an educational program, and therefore, kindness and charitable donations are indeed more important.

Katz, Hass, and Bailey (1988) opined that attitudes toward disability are ambivalent due to conflicting cognitions of wanting to help and wanting to avoid an encounter. Although there exist a number of studies indicating the anxiety many nondisabled persons have in interacting with someone with a disability (wanting to avoid), some studies indicate that where there is a clearly defined need to provide assistance, the likelihood of an interaction increases (Stephens, Cooper, & Kinney, 1985). Stephens et al. (1985) found that nondisabled persons spent more time and gave more assistance in helping a wheelchair-using female look for a lost earring, when compared with a female without a disability. Stephens concluded that the social obligation toward helping someone who is perceived as not being able to help himself or herself overrides interaction anxiety or the desire to avoid the situation. It may be that we are so conditioned to offer some sort of assistance toward those with disabilities (e.g., open the door, give to charity, volunteer time) that when an opportunity to simply interact with someone with a disability occurs, many nondisabled persons basically do not know what to say or do. Another potential barrier to interacting for individuals regardless of having a disability or not is simply the perception of not having anything in common with the other person and basically little to talk about (Leary, 1990).

Overall, it is likely that attitudes toward persons with disabilities depend on many of the factors discussed earlier. Measuring attitudes is too complex to generalize the results of any one study or combination of studies and relate them to the general population (Antonak & Livneh, 1988, 2000). Indeed, some people with and without a disability do possess negative attitudes to varying degrees, ranging from blatant prejudice to simple ignorance and misinformation. Similarly, some persons with and without disabilities possess positive attitudes toward those with disabilities. Research indicates that in many instances, such persons have had previous contact with or exposure to someone with a disability that was a positive experience (Chan et al., 2009; Yuker, 1988). Finally, people without disabilities who have had limited or no exposure to those with disabilities may not harbor any preconceived positive or negative attitudes because they have not given the topic much thought. These individuals are simply ambivalent or apathetic to the subject and may be influenced by education and exposure to persons with disabilities. The next section focuses on improving the social consciousness toward disability.

Improving the Social Consciousness Regarding Attitudes Toward Disability

Havranek (1991) has indicated that although we can mandate legislative changes to improve access and equal rights for persons with disabilities, we unfortunately cannot mandate people's attitudes. Bowe (1978) further claimed that the greatest barrier facing persons with disabilities today is societal attitudes. Despite the numerous civil and human rights laws, discrimination and indifference still exist. As such, and having reviewed the common reasons how and why people possess negative attitudes toward disability, it becomes important to explore what factors and conditions are necessary to potentially enhance people's attitudes. Research findings essentially delineate such studies into three general categories: (a) increased contact and familiarity with persons with a disability; (b) providing accurate education and information that minimize misconceptions about disability; and (c) mixing contact with education, or essentially having the educator be a person with a disability.

Contact

Within the realm of exploring attitudes toward disability lie a number of studies pertaining to the influence of contact with or exposure to someone with a disability. Yuker (1988) found that of 274 studies relating to contact between someone with and without a disability, 51% of the studies suggested that participants' attitudes became more positive, 39% of the studies were inconclusive, and 10% of the studies reported that participants had a more negative attitude after contact. Yuker believed that certain factors must be present for a positive change in attitude to occur. He surmised from his analysis that persons with disabilities must be perceived as possessing good communication and social skills, be perceived as competent, and be willing to self-disclose some information about their disabilities in an unemotional manner. Yuker further concluded that the interaction must be reciprocal and not a one-sided conversation, where each participant gains some reward from the interaction.

The concept of each participant gaining something from the interaction was discussed earlier concerning Leary's (1990) research on social anxiety. Leary believed that we regularly cognitively assess whether we have something to gain from an anticipated social interaction, regardless of whether someone has a disability. If the individual perceives nothing can be gained from the interaction, he or she will tend to avoid the situation. When a disability is then entered into the equation, we know from other studies that many nondisabled persons feel anxious in not knowing what to say or how to behave, and therefore are likely to avoid the interaction altogether (Albrecht et al., 1982; Kleck, 1968; Marinelli & Kelz, 1973; Piliavin & Piliavin, 1972). Wright (1988) described the stranger phenomenon (we may avoid first-time interactions with nondisabled persons for the same reasons), and that researchers must be careful in analyzing such findings so as to not make the disability salient.

Albrecht et al.'s (1982) finding that some people feel anxious in not knowing what to say or how to behave has also been linked to an irrational fear that many nondisabled persons have: namely, the myth that a person with a disability may become emotional about his or her situation. Evans (1976) concluded from his review of previous attitude studies that nondisabled persons likely have conflicting thoughts of not wanting to offend, wanting to approach due to curiosity while concomitantly wanting to avoid due to discomfort, and trying not to stare or say the wrong thing. He recommended that it is largely up to the person with a disability to put others at ease about the disability. This is accomplished by explaining a little bit about the disability and how it was acquired. In addition, if the person with the disability can talk about the disability in an unemotional manner, this conveys that the person is "okay" with his or her situation. This strategy serves to minimize the curiosity many nondisabled persons may have about the story behind the disability as well as indicating that the person with the disability can talk about it without becoming emotional. Sagatun (1985) found, however, that although nondisabled persons liked it better when the person with the disability initiated contact first and acknowledged his or her disability, persons with disabilities preferred the nondisabled person to initiate contact and ask about the disability rather than having to volunteer that information. Persons without disabilities seem to prefer those with disabilities to acknowledge their situation, to more or less get it out of the way, whereas many persons with disabilities do not like volunteering such information if it does not "fit" into the flow or context of the conversation. These findings are further supported in studies by Belgrave (1984), Belgrave and Mills (1981), and Evans (1976).

Finally, as noted by Yuker (1988), Donaldson (1980) concluded that in order for positive attitudes to ensue from social contact, the individual with the disability must be perceived as having "equal status" in relation to age, education, competence, and occupation. It should be noted that these same qualities, as well as the factors Yuker (1988) cites regarding possessing good social skills, are basically the same factors necessary for anyone to decide whether he or she is interested in becoming acquainted with someone, regardless of disability status.

Environmental factors may also be related to changing attitudes. Stewart (1988) placed two students with physical disabilities in a weight training class and pre-post tested the class after 10 weeks regarding their attitudes toward disability, compared with a control group class without any students with disabilities. Findings were significant in that attitudes became more positive for the class with the two students with physical disabilities. Conclusions drawn from this study indicate that regular contact in an equal status environment where similar interests are perceived and engaged in is likely to enhance attitudes toward disability.

Education

Newspaper, television, and movie coverage regarding disability has traditionally conveyed more misinformation and stereotypes than accurate information (Black & Pretes, 2007; Marini, 1992). News stories about disability are typically human interest stories that depict persons with disabilities as victims of some tragedy or conversely stories of courage in which the individual with the disability has accomplished something "in spite of" the disability.

Aside from pure media entertainment or human interest stories that have done little to educate the public about disability, rehabilitation researchers have used attitude surveys after having participants view films to determine whether educational films regarding disability can enhance participants' attitudes. Researchers have found that when participants viewed an educational or humorous film regarding disability designed to change attitudes, participants' attitudes statistically were more positive following the film when compared with a control group (Elliott & Byrd, 1984; Matkin, Hafer, Wright, & Lutzker, 1983). Sadlick and Penta (1975) found similar significant results after rehabilitation nursing students were shown a film of 10 former patients with tetraplegia who were employed and doing well compared with a no-film control group. The film group scored a more positive attitude on Osgood's Semantic Differential Scale (Osgood, Suci, & Tannenbaum, 1957) both immediately after the film and again 10 weeks later. Antonak (1982) also conducted a similar study with similar results using lay persons who viewed a slide presentation of persons with disabilities performing various activities of daily living independently in their homes. Researchers of these studies recommended avoiding pretesting attitudes as it can invalidate findings by tipping participants off and having them answer in a socially desirable fashion at posttesting (Antonak, 1982; Matkin et al., 1983).

There are unfortunately still other researchers or therapists at universities, colleges, and rehabilitation centers who continue to use experiential sensitivity exercises, such as the disability-for-a-day or class period activities in which students/employees must ambulate in a wheelchair, wear earplugs, or use a blindfold. Although seemingly a good exercise for students to experience and better empathize with persons with disabilities, some researchers arguably have found that this exercise creates more negative attitudes than positive for several reasons. Wright (1978) was the first to criticize these activities by arguing that such exercises make the disability salient and demonstrate the initial frustration anyone in a new situation would experience. Participants are often not informed about how someone with a disability generally grows accustomed and adapts to their situation, and eventually learns to problem solve everyday barriers without a second thought. The exercises by themselves, however, focus on the daily frustrations and "contribute to disabling myths about disabilities" (Wright, 1980, p. 174). Wilson and Alcorn (1969) had students simulate being blind, deaf, or paralyzed via wheelchair and found no significant change in attitude toward persons with disabilities.

Grayson and Marini (1996) conducted a wheelchair-using exercise for an experimental group of rehabilitation counseling graduate students in which they were required to wheel a quarter-mile to the cafeteria, order and drink a beverage, then wheel back to the main building. A control group did not participate. Both groups completed a qualitative survey about disability. A significant *t*-test finding showed that the experimental wheelchair-using group perceived greater differences between persons with and without disabilities, indicating that persons with disabilities must have a harder time in society. Another significant difference between groups was that the sensitivity group further indicated that "persons with disabilities must get frustrated often . . . must feel different from being stared at so much . . . and, must be preoccupied with how accessible certain places must be." Without correcting such beliefs, counselors are likely to have preconceived notions regarding such clients, and spend unnecessary time probing these otherwise irrelevant issues. If such exercises are to be utilized in training, debriefing is highly recommended. Instructors need to acknowledge how participant feelings of frustration are most common during the first several months following a trauma as the individual learns to adapt to his or her situation, but that most persons with disabilities learn to cope with and minimize daily hassles over time (Grayson & Marini, 1996; Silver, 1982; Wright, 1980). Similar findings have been most recently confirmed using meta-analysis, where more than half of the studies analyzed showed disability simulation exercises as having either a negligible effect or a negative effect in changing attitudes (Flower, Burns, & Bottsford-Miller, 2007).

Education and Contact

Perhaps the strongest method of enhancing attitudes toward disability is to have the messenger or educator be a person with a disability. Aside from being perceived as a more credible source of information, the exposure or contact with someone perceived as having "equal status" facilitates attitude change (Yuker, 1988, p. 27). Scheiderer, Marini, and Hall-Gray (1995) pre-post tested two separate classes using the Modified Issues in Disability Scale (Makas, 1988) at the beginning and end of the semester. One class was taught by a professor who used a wheelchair, and the other was taught by a nondisabled instructor. Although there were no differences between groups at pretest, results were significant at posttest, indicating more positive attitudes in the class that had the instructor with the disability. Chesler and Chesney (1988) further discuss the benefits of self-help groups regarding persons with disabilities educating and assisting persons with disabilities. Overall, these authors cite the benefits of networking, sharing emotional experiences, gaining access to information, learning new coping skills and resources, contributing to the welfare of others, and mobilizing to advocate for change. Finally, Chan et al. (2009) delineate several other methods of attitude change, including persuasion, disability simulation, affirmative action, and impression management. Persuasion becomes most effective when the message contains strong and cogent arguments that are similar to the attitudes held by the individual. Disability simulation exercises discussed earlier must have a built-in debriefing component after the simulation to be effective, otherwise participants' perceptions may become more negative due to first-time frustrations attempting to negotiate the physical environment (Flower et al., 2007; Grayson & Marini, 1996). Such debriefings must include an acknowledgment that the majority of persons with disabilities generally adapt to their environment and circumstances over time. Regarding affirmative action, although mandated by laws such as the Americans with Disabilities Act, laws themselves in all likelihood have mixed results regarding positive or negative attitude change. Positive changes can occur because more persons with disabilities have access to the social environment, therefore increasing contact with others, which often leads to more positive attitudes. Conversely, for individuals who are not in favor of federal mandates regarding disability rights, this may facilitate even greater negative attitudes (McMahon, Hurley, Chan, Rumrill, & Roessler, 2008). Finally, protests have been shown to be somewhat effective in changing behaviors (e.g., government legislation, damaging media portrayals); however, research is lacking regarding whether positive attitude change necessarily follows (Corrigan et al., 2001).

Conclusions Regarding Attitudes

With the 1990 ADA allowing for greater social and employment interaction between persons with and without disabilities, nondisabled persons continue to be exposed to persons with disabilities in a variety of situations every day. As researchers have found in at least 50% of instances, this daily exposure or contact is likely to enhance attitudes and minimize interaction strain (Corrigan et al., 2001; Yuker, 1988). Depending on the circumstances of the interaction, however, a nondisabled person's attitudes could become more negative or not change demonstrably. Researchers have found that when the interaction is more structured, such as someone with a disability asking for assistance, there is a greater likelihood that an interaction will take place, especially since the behavior of helping persons with disabilities is engrained in our culture. If, however, there is no clear reason or cause for someone without a disability to approach and initiate a conversation with someone who is disabled, then the likelihood of such an interaction becomes less likely. This is due not only to the stranger phenomenon (Wright, 1988) but also to anxiety over not knowing what to say, how to behave, and irrational fears that the person with the disability may become emotional, causing further awkwardness (Albrecht et al., 1982; Evans, 1976; Leary, 1990; Marini, 1992). In a potential interaction situation, we cognitively weigh the rewards and costs of the interaction consciously and/or subconsciously. If we perceive there is nothing to gain from an anticipated interaction and experience anticipatory anxiety thinking about the encounter, we will likely avoid the situation.

When initial contacts between persons with and without disabilities do occur, it often is up to the person with the disability to place the nondisabled person at ease during the interaction (Evans, 1976; Marini, 1992). This may be accomplished by voluntarily self-disclosing a little information about how one came to be disabled, and doing so in a matter-of-fact, nonemotional way. This not only satisfies the nondisabled person's curiosity, but also suggests that the person with the disability is comfortable with his or her situation. Unfortunately, many persons with disabilities would rather not self-disclose particulars about their disability unless specifically asked about it or if it seems relevant to the conversation. Allport (1954) noted a number of conditions that generally facilitate positive attitudes when contact occurs. These factors include the following: (a) perceived equal status (e.g., education, occupation); (b) the contact is necessary to achieve a desired goal; (c) the contact is promoted by some authority or social climate; (d) the contact is intimate; (e) the contact is pleasurable; (f) the contact is by choice; (g) the contact is selected over other rewards; and (h) the contact is to complete some functional goal or activity.

Despite the numerous suspected origins regarding negative attitudes toward persons with disabilities, nondisabled persons who are not blatantly prejudiced and unwilling to change their attitudes may only require greater exposure and accurate information regarding disability. With the 1990 ADA representing the greatest civil rights legislation for persons with disabilities in U.S. history, persons with disabilities now enjoy greater access to employment, education, and social participation than ever before. This increasing exposure and contact with persons with disabilities in equal status or similar interest situations over time has seemingly continued to enhance positive attitudes toward those with disabilities, but still is perceived by many with disabilities to have a long way to go.

REFERENCES

Albrecht, G. L., Walker, V. G., & Levy, J. A. (1982). Social distance from the stigmatized: A test of two theories. *Social Science Medical, 16*, 1319–1327.

Allport, G. W. (1954). *The nature of prejudice.* Cambridge, MA: Addison-Wesley.

Anderson, P. M. (1988). American humor, handicapism, and censorship. *Reading, Writing, and Learning Disabilities, 4*, 79–84.

Antonak, R. F. (1980). A hierarchy of attitudes exceptionality. *Journal of Special Education, 14*, 231–241.

Antonak, R. F. (1982). Development and psychometric analysis of the scale of attitudes toward disabled persons. *Journal of Applied Rehabilitation Counseling, 13*(2), 22–29.

Antonak, R. F., & Livneh, H. (1988). *The measurement of attitudes toward people with disabilities.* Chicago, IL: Charles C. Thomas.

Antonak, R. F., & Livneh, H. (2000). Measurement of attitudes towards people with disabilities. *Disability and Rehabilitation, 22*(5), 211–224.

Begab, M. J. (1970). Impact of education in social work students' knowledge and attitudes about mental retardation. *American Journal of Mental Deficiency, 74*, 801–808.

Belgrave, F. Z. (1984). The effectiveness of strategies for increasing social interaction with a physically disabled person. *Journal of Applied Social Psychology, 14*(2), 147–161.

Belgrave, F. Z., & Mills, J. (1981). Effects upon desire for social interaction with a physically disabled person of mentioning the disability in different contexts. *Journal of Applied Social Psychology, 11*, 44–57.

Bickenbach, J. E. (1993). *Physical disability and social policy.* Toronto, ON: University of Toronto.

Biklen, D. (1986). Framed: Journalism's treatment of disability. *Social Policy, 16*, 45–51.

Black, R. S., & Pretes, L. (2007). Victims and victories: Representation of physical disability on the silver screen. *Research & Practice for Persons with Severe Disabilities, 32*(1), 66–83.

Blackwell, T. M., Marini, I., & Chacon, M. (2001). The impact of the Americans with Disabilities Act on independent living. *Rehabilitation Education, 15*(4), 395–408.

Bogdan, R., & Taylor, S. (1989). Relationships with severely disabled people: The social construction of humanness. *Social Problems, 36*, 135–148.

Bordieri, J. E. (1993). Self blame attributions for disability and perceived client's involvement in the vocational rehabilitation process. *Journal of Applied Rehabilitation Counseling, 24*(2), 3–7.

Bowe, F. (1978). *Handicapped America: Barriers to disabled persons.* New York: Harper & Row.

Buss, D. M. (1999). *Evolutionary psychology: The new science of the mind.* Boston, MZ: Allyn & Bacon.

Byrd, K. (1989). A study of depiction of specific characteristics of characters with disability in film. *Journal of Applied Rehabilitation Counseling, 20*(2), 43–45.

Byrd, E. K. (1990). A study of biblical depiction of disability. *Journal of Applied Rehabilitation Counseling,* *21*(4), 52–53.

Byrd, E. K., Byrd, D., & Allen, C. M. (1977). Television programming and disability. *Journal of Applied Rehabilitation Counseling, 8*(1), 28–32.

Chan, F., Livneh, H., Pruett, S., Wang, C. C., & Zheng, L. X. (2009). In F. Chan, E. De Silva Cardoso, & J. A. Chronister (Eds.), *Understanding psychosocial adjustment to chronic illness and disability: A handbook for evidence-based practitioners in rehabilitation* (pp. 333–367). New York, NY: Springer.

Charlton, J. I. (1998). *Nothing about us without us: Disability oppression and empowerment.* Berkeley, CA: University of California.

Chesler, M. A. (1965). Ethnocentricism and attitudes toward the physically disabled. *Personality & Social Pyschology, 2*(6), 877–882.

Chesler, M. A., & Chesney, B. K. (1988). Self-help groups: Empowerment attitudes and behaviors of disabled or chronically ill persons. In H. E. Yuker (Ed.), *Attitudes toward persons with disability* (pp. 230–245). New York, NY: Springer.

Chubon, R. A. (1982). An analysis of research dealing with the attitudes of professionals toward disability. *Journal of Rehabilitation, 48,* 25–30.

Chubon, R. A. (1994). *Social and psychological foundations of rehabilitation.* Springfield, IL: Charles C. Thomas.

Cloerkes, G. (1981). Are prejudices against disabled persons determined by personality characteristics? *International Journal of Rehabilitation Research, 4*(1), 35–46.

Collmann, R. D., & Newlyn, D. (1956). Employment success of mentally dull and intellectually normal ex-pupils in England. *American Journal of Mental Deficiency, 61,* 484–490.

Comer, R. C., & Piliavin, J. A. (1975). As others see us: Attitudes of physically handicapped and normals toward own other groups. *Rehabilitation Literature, 36,* 206–221.

Corrigan, P. W., River, L., Lundin, R. K., Penn, D. L., Uphoff-Wasowski, K., Campion, J. et al. (2001). Three strategies for changing attributions about severe mental illness. *Schizophrenia Bulletin, 27,* 187–195.

Dembo, T., Leviton, G. L., & Wright, B. A. (1956). Adjustment to misfortune: A problem of social psychology rehabilitation. *Artificial Limbs, 3,* 4–62.

Donaldson, J. (1980). Changing attitudes toward handicapped persons: A review and analysis of research. *Exceptional Children, April,* 504–514.

Eagly, A. H., Ashmore, R. D., Makhijani, M. G., & Longo, C. C. (1991). What is beautiful is good but . . . : A meta-analytic review of research on the physical attractiveness stereotype. *Psychological Bulletin, 110,* 109–128.

Eagly, A. H., Mladinic, A., & Otto, S. (1994). Cognitive and affective bases of attitudes toward social groups and social policies. *Journal of Experimental Social Psychology, 30,* 113–137.

Elliott, T. R., & Byrd, E. K. (1984). Attitude change toward disability through television: Portrayal with male college students. *International Journal Rehabilitation Research, 7,* 330–332.

English, R. W. (1971a). Correlates of stigma toward physically disabled persons. In R. P. Marinelli, & A. E. Dell Orto (Eds.), *The psychological & social impact of physical disability* (pp. 162–182). New York, NY: Springer.

English, R. W. (1971b). Correlates of stigma toward physically disabled persons. *Rehabilitation Research & Practice Review, 2,* 1–17.

Evans, J. H. (1976). Changing attitudes toward disabled persons: An experimental study. *Rehabilitation Counseling Bulletin, 19,* 572–579.

Fichten, C. S., & Bourdon, C. V. (1986). Social skill deficit or response inhibition: Interaction between disabled and nondisabled college students. *Journal of College Students Personnel, 27,* 326–333.

Flower, A., Burns, M. K., & Bottsford-Miller, N. A. (2007). Meta-analysis of disability simulation research. *Remedial and Special Education, 28*(2), 72–79.

Gallagher, H. G. (1995). *By trust betrayed: Patients, physicians, and the license to kill in The Third Reich* (rev. ed.). Arlington, TX: Vandamere.

Goffman, E. (1963). *Stigma: Notes on the management of spoiled identity.* Englewood Cliffs, NJ: Prentice-Hall.

Goodyear, R. K. (1983). Patterns of counselors' attitudes toward disability groups. *Rehabilitation Counseling Bulletin, 26*, 181–184.

Gosse, V. F., & Sheppard, G. (1979). Attitudes toward physically disabled persons: Do education and personal contact make a difference? *Canadian Counselor, 13*, 131–135.

Gostin, L. O. (2008). "Old" and "new" institutions for persons with mental illness: Treatment, punishment or preventive confinement? *Journal of the Royal Institute of Public Health, 122*, 906–913.

Graf, N. M., Marini, I., & Blankenship, C. (2009). 100 words about disability. *Journal of Rehabilitation, 75*(2), 25–34.

Grayson, E., & Marini, I. (1996). Simulated disability exercises and their impact on attitudes toward persons with disabilities. *International Journal of Rehabilitation Research, 19*, 123–131.

Gresham, F. M. (1982). Misguided mainstreaming: The case for social skills training with handicapped children. *Exceptional Children, 48*, 422–433.

Hadley, R. G., & Brodwin, M. G. (1988). Language about people with disabilities. *Journal of Counseling and Development, 67*, 147–149.

Harris, L. (1991). *Public attitudes toward persons with disabilities.* New York, NY: Louis Harris and Associates.

Harris, R. W. (1992). Musings from 20 years of hard-earned experiences. *Rehabilitation Education, 6*, 207–211.

Havranek, J. E. (1991). The social and individual costs of negative attitudes toward persons with physical disabilities. *Journal of Applied Rehabilitation Counseling, 22*(1), 15–21.

Hayes, S. C., Barlow, D. H., & Nelson-Gray, R. G. (1999). *The scientist–practitioner: Research and accountability in the age of managed care* (2nd ed.) Needham Heights, MA: Allyn & Bacon.

Jabin, N. (1966). Attitudes towards the physically disabled as related to selected personality variables. *Dissertation Abstracts, 27*(2-B), 599.

Katz, I., Hass, R. G., & Bailey, J. (1988). Attitudinal ambivalence and behavior toward people with disabilities. In H. E. Yuker (Ed.), *Attitudes toward persons with disabilities* (pp. 47–57). New York, NY: Springer.

Kleck, R. (1968). Physical stigma and nonverbal cues emitted in face-to-face interaction. *Human Relations, 21*, 19–28.

Lawrence, R. H., Tennstedt, S. L., & Assmann, S. F. (1998). Quality of the caregiver–care recipient relationship: Does it offset negative consequences of caregiving for family caregivers? *Psychology of Aging, 13*(1), 150–158.

Leary, M. R. (1990). Anxiety cognition and behavior: In search of a broader perspective. *Journal of Social Behavior and Personality, 5*(2), 39–44.

LeClair, S. W., & Rockwell, L. K. (1980). Counselor trainee body satisfaction and attitudes toward counseling the physically disabled. *Rehabilitation Counseling Bulletin, 23*(4), 258–265.

Livneh, H. (1988). A dimensional perspective on the origin of negative attitudes toward persons with disabilities. In H. E. Yuker (Ed.), *Attitudes toward persons with disabilities* (pp. 35–46). New York, NY: Springer.

Livneh, H. (1991). On the origins of negative attitudes toward people with disabilities. In R. P. Marinelli & A. E. Dell Orto (Eds.), *The psychological & social impact of disability* (pp. 111–138). New York, NY: Springer.

Longo, L. C., & Ashmore, R. D. (1995). The looks–personality relationship: Global self-orientations as shared precursors of subjective physical attractiveness and self-ascribed traits. *Journal of Applied Social Psychology, 25*, 371–398.

Mackelprang, R., & Salsgiver, R. (2009). *Disability: A diversity model approach in human service practice.* Pacific Grove, CA: Brooks/Cole.

MacMillan, D. L., & Morrison, G. M. (1980). Correlates of social status among mildly handicapped learners in self-contained special classes. *Journal of Educational Psychology, 72*, 437–444.

Makas, E. (1988). Positive attitudes toward disabled people: Disabled and nondisabled persons' perspectives. *Journal of Social Issues, 44*(1), 49–61.

Marantz, P. R. (1990). Blaming the victim: The negative consequences of preventive medicine. *American Journal of Public Health, 80*, 1185–1187.

Margolis, H., Shapiro, A., & Anderson, P. M. (1990). Reading, writing, and thinking about prejudice: Stereotyped images of disability images of disability in the popular press. *Social Education, January*, 28–30.

Marinelli, R. P. (1974). State anxiety in interactions with visibly disabled persons. *Rehabilitation Counseling Bulletin, 18*, 72–77.

Marinelli, R. P., & Kelz, J. W. (1973). Anxiety and attitudes toward visibly disabled persons. *Rehabilitation Counseling Bulletin, 16*(4), 198–205.

Marini, I. (1992). *The use of humor to modify attitudes, decrease interaction anxiety and increase desire to interact with persons of differing abilities.* Unpublished doctoral dissertation, Auburn, AL: Auburn University.

Matkin, R., Hafer, M., Wright, W., & Lutzker, J. (1983). Pretesting artifacts: A study of attitudes toward disability. *Rehabilitation Counseling Bulletin, 5*, 342–348.

McGuire, W. J. (1969). The nature of attitudes and attitude change. In G. Lindsey & E. Aronson (Eds.), *The handbook of social psychology* (Vol. 3, pp. 136–314). Reading, MA: Addison-Wesley.

McMahon, B. T., Hurley, J. E., Chan, F., Rumrill, P. D., & Roessler, R. (2008). Drivers of hiring discrimination for individuals with disabilities. *Journal of Occupational Therapy, 18*, 122–132.

Meng, H. (1938). Zur sozialpsychologie der Krperbeschadigten: Ein beitrag zum problrm der praktischen psychohygiene. *Schweizer Archives fr Neurologie und Psychiatrie, 40*, 328–344. (Reported in Barker, R. G., et al., 1953.)

Mitchell, J. C. (1976). Disabled counselors: Perception of their effectiveness in a therapeutic relationship. *Archives of Physical Medicine Rehabilitation, 57*, 348–352.

Murphy, M. A. (1998). Rejection, stigma, and hope. *Psychiatric Rehabilitation Journal, 22*, 185–189.

Noonan, J. R., Barry, J. R., & Davis, H. C. (1970) Personality determinants in attitudes toward visible disability. *Journal of Personality, 38*(1), 1–15.

Oberle, J. B. (1975). The effect of personalization and quality of contact on changing expressed attitudes and hiring preferences toward disabled persons (Doctoral dissertation). *Dissertation Abstracts International, 37*, 2144A.

Obermann, C. E. (1965). *A history of vocational rehabilitation in America.* Minneapolis, MN: T.S. Denison.

Olkin, R. (1999). *What psychotherapists should know about disability.* New York, NY: The Guilford Press.

Olkin, R., & Howson, L. (1994). Attitudes toward and images of physical disability. *Journal of Social Behavior and Personality, 9*, 81–96.

Osgood, C. E., Suci, G. J., & Tannenbaum, P. H. (1957). *The measurement of meaning.* Chicago, IL: University of Illinois.

Ostrom, T. M., Skowronski, J. J., & Nowak, A. (1994). The cognitive foundations of attitudes: It's a wonderful construct. In P. G. Devine, D. L. Hamilton, & T. M. Ostrom (Eds.), *Social cognition: Impact on social psychology.* New York, NY: Academic Press.

Piliavin, J. A., & Piliavin, I. M. (1972). Effect of blood on reaction to a victim. *Journal of Social Psychology, 23*, 353–361.

Plotnik, R. (1996). *Introduction to psychology* (4th ed.). Pacific Grove, CA: Brooks/Cole.

Rabkin, J. G. (1972). Opinions about mental illness: A review of the literature. *Psychological Bulletin, 77*, 153–171.

Ryan, K. M. (1981). Developmental differences in reactions to the physically disabled. *Human Development, 24*, 240–256.

Sadlick, M., & Penta, F. B. (1975). Changing nurse attitudes toward quadriplegics through use of television. *Rehabilitation Literature, 36*(9), 274–278.

Safilios-Rothschild, C. (1968). Prejudice against the disabled and some means to combat it. *International Rehabilitation Review, 14*, 8–10.

Safilios-Rothschild, C. (1970). *The sociology and social psychology of disability and rehabilitation.* New York, NY: Random House.

Safilios-Rothschild, C. (1982). Social and psychological parameters of friendship and intimacy for disabled people. In M. G. Eisenberg, C. Griggins, & R. J. Duval (Eds.), *Disabled people as second-class citizens* (pp. 40–51). New York, NY: Springer.

Sagatun, I. J. (1985). The effects of acknowledging a disability and initiating contact on interaction between disabled and non-disabled persons. *The Social Science Journal, 22*(4), 33–43.

Scheiderer, B., Marini, I., & Hall-Gray, E. J. (1995). The effect of contact on attitudes toward persons with disabilities. *SCI: Psychosocial Process, 8*(3), 102–105.

Schilder, P. (1935). *The image and appearance of the human body.* London, UK: Kegan Paul, Trench, Trubner.

Schmelkin, L. P. (1984). Hierarchy of preferences toward disabled groups: A reanalysis. *Perceptual and Motor Skills, 59*, 151–157.

Seligman, M. E. (1993). *What you can change & what you can't.* New York, NY: Knopf Inc.

Shontz, F. C. (1964). Body-part size judgement. *VRA Project No. 814, Final Report.* Lawrence, KS: University of Kansas. (Reported in McDaniel, J. W., 1969.)

Siller, J. (1963). Reactions to physical disability. *Rehabilitation Counseling Bulletin, 7*(1), 12–16.

Siller, J. (1964). Reactions to physically by the disabled and the non-disabled. *American Psychologist, Research Bulletin, 7*, 27–36.

Siller, J., Chipman, A., Ferguson, L. T., & Vann, D. H. (1967). *Studies in reaction to Disability: XI. Attitudes of the non-disabled toward the physically disabled.* New York, NY: New York University, School of Education.

Silver, R. L. (1982). *Coping with an undesirable life event: A study of early reactions to physical disability.* Unpublished doctoral dissertation. Evanston, IL: Northwestern University.

Smart, J. (2009). *Disability, Society, and the Individual.* Austin, TX: Pro-Ed.

Sowa, P. A., & Cutter, H. S. (1974). Attitudes of hospital staff toward alcoholics and drug addicts. *Quarterly Journal of Studies on Alcohol, 35*, 210–214.

Stephens, M. A., Cooper, N. S., & Kinney, J. M. (1985). The effects of effort on helping the physically disabled. *The Journal of Social Psychology, 125*(4), 495–503.

Stewart, C. C. (1988). Modification of student attitudes toward disabled peers. *Adapted Physical Activity Quarterly, 5*, 44–48.

Stovall, C., & Sedlacek, W. E. (1983). Attitudes of male and female university students toward students with different physical disabilities. *Journal of College Student Personnel, 24*, 325–330.

Sue, D. W., & Sue, D. (3rd ed.) (1999). *Counseling the culturally different: Theory and practice.* New York, NY: John Wiley & Sons, Inc.

Szymanski, C. R., Ryan, C., Merz, M. A., Trevino, B., & Johnston-Rodriguez, S. (1996). Psychosocial and economic aspects of work: Implications for people with disabilities. In E. M. Szymanski & R. M. Parker (Eds.), *Work and disability: Issues and strategies in career development and job placement* (pp. 9–38). Austin, TX: Pro-ed.

Tringo, J. L. (1970). The hierarchy of preference toward disability groups. *Journal of Special Education, 4*, 295–306.

Tunick, R. H., Bowen, J., & Gillings, J. L. (1979). Religiosity and authoritarianism as predictors of attitude toward the disabled: A regression analysis. *Rehabilitation Counseling Bulletin, 22*(5), 408–418.

Vash, C. L., & Crewe, N. M. (2004). *Psychology of disability* (pp. 288–299). New York, NY: Springer.

Walster, E. (1966). Assignment of responsibility for an accident. *Journal of Personality and Social Psychology, 3*, 73–79.

Weinberg, N. (1978). Preschool children's perceptions of orthopedic disability. *Rehabilitation Counseling Bulletin, 21*, 183–189.

Weiner, B., Perry, R. P., & Magnusson, J. (1988). An attributional analysis of reactions to stigmas. *Journal of Personality and Social Psychology, 55*, 738–748.

Whiteman, M., & Lukoff, I. F. (1965). Attitudes toward blindness and other physical handicaps. *Journal of Social Psychology, 66*, 135–145.

Wilson, E. E., & Alcorn, D. (1969). Disability simulation and development of attitudes toward the exceptional. *Journal of Special Education, 3*(3), 303–307.

World Health Organization. (1980). *International classification of impairments, disabilities, and handicaps: A manual of classification relating to the consequences of disease.* Geneva, Switzerland: World Health Organization.

Wright, B. (1960). *A physical disability: A psychological approach.* New York, NY: Harper & Row.

Wright, B. A. (1978). The coping framework and attitude change: A guide to constructive role playing. *Rehabilitation Psychology, 4*, 177–183.

Wright, B. A. (1980). Developing constructive views of life with a disability. *Rehabilitation Literature*, *41*, 274–279.

Wright, B. (1983). *Physical disability: A psychosocial approach* (2nd ed.). New York, NY: Harper & Row.

Wright, B. A. (1988). Attitudes and the fundamental negative bias: Conditions and corrections. In H. E. Yuker (Ed.), *Attitudes toward persons with disabilities* (pp. 3–21). New York, NY: Springer.

Yamamoto, K. (1971). To be different. *Rehabilitation Counseling Bulletin, 14*(3), 180–189.

Yuker, H. E. (1962). *Yearly psychosocial research summary.* Albertson, NY: Human Resources Center.

Yuker, H. E. (1988). *Attitudes toward persons with disabilities.* New York, NY: Springer.

Yuker, H. E. (1994). Variables that influence attitudes toward persons with disabilities: Conclusion from that data. *Psychosocial Perspectives on Disability. A Special Issue of the Journal of Social Behavior and Personality, 9*, 3–22.

Zola, I. K. (1983). Developing new self-images and interdependence. In N. M. Crewe & I. K. Zola (Eds.), *Independent living for physically disabled people* (pp. 49–50). San Francisco, CA: Jossey-Bass.

Zola, I. K. (1991). Communication barriers between "the able-bodied" and "the handicapped." In R. P. Marinelli & A. E. Dell Orto (Eds.), *The psychological and social impact of disability* (3rd ed., pp. 157–180). New York, NY: Springer.

INSIDER PERSPECTIVE
The Story of Linda Napolitano

I am a physically disabled woman, born in 1951. My disability is called spinal muscular atrophy (SMA). I've been in a wheelchair since I was approximately 11. SMA is a neuromuscular condition, which results in progressive weakness throughout the muscles in the body. There are different types of SMA. The type I have is slowly progressive and I have a "normal" life span. At my birth, my parents were told they had a healthy baby girl. When I began walking, I walked slowly, never ran, and fell down quite a bit, as I lost balance very easily. I remember becoming very fatigued when I was still able to walk. By 11 years, it had become impossible. At that time, doctors were unable to actually put a name to my condition. We were told it was neuromuscular, related to muscular dystrophy. It wasn't until I was in my late 20s that my condition was labeled.

I went to a regular high school and graduated in 1969. Although I never graduated college, I took classes on and off, throughout my late 30s and early 40s, in a homebound program. The classes were taken over the phone. There was a speaker in each class I took and we could hear each other and were able to correspond.

I worked for over 20 years with the Nassau County Department of Recreation and Parks on Long Island. I did office work, as I had been trained in secretarial skills in high school. I finally had to resign at the age of 41. I was tiring more easily and the weakness in my arms had progressed considerably.

I have never married or had children. I live in my own apartment in my parents' home. I have had a home health aide for the past 6 years. She is with me most of the day. In the evenings, my family helps me out. I have taught myself to use the computer and I do my writing on it. I usually write essays having to do with disability or personal experiences.

I do feel a difference in the way I'm treated by society now as opposed to 20 or 30 years ago. I remember times in the past being discriminated against because of my being in a wheelchair. One time, I was turned away from a movie theater because I was told that my chair would block the aisle and that I was a fire hazard. Another time I wasn't permitted to use a dressing room in a department store because "carriages" weren't allowed in dressing rooms. I think that people staring at me was more prevalent then. I believe that, in general, people have become more accustomed to seeing the disabled out in public, mainstreaming into society. I still do find that there are attitudes that need changing concerning the physically disabled. I have found that much of society does not look at me as an adult and I feel I am being talked down to as if I were a child. I am very rarely referred to as a woman. I believe that has to do with the fact that I, like many physically disabled people, am dependent in many ways. Many of us, especially those who have been disabled since childhood, have not married or moved out of our parents' homes, and so we have not "grown" up and moved away from Mom and Dad. We may need their help, physically and/or financially.

Because I am seen as child-like, I have always appeared younger than my age, and have never married or had children; I am also not seen as a sexual being. It's amazing how many people, after reading an article I wrote on sexuality and the disabled, have told me that they never thought of the disabled as having sexual feelings. They say that I've enlightened them. I will admit that not everyone denies or ignores the fact that the disabled have sexual feelings, but I have found it is still common, especially among the older generation.

Throughout my life, so many people have said to me, "How do you do it?" or "How do you cope?" My first reaction has always been, "What choice do I have?" I have learned that I can choose to be miserable all of my life by feeling sorry for myself or I can try to make the best of it with the gifts that I have been given. These gifts are being able to use my brain and experience feelings. I communicate well with my speaking and writing. I'm not saying that I don't get depressed. I'm saying that depression doesn't rule my life. I've always maintained a cheerful attitude. I have a great sense of humor, which has been extremely important in saving my sanity. I believe that without laughter, this would be a miserable existence.

I have been fortunate in having a family. My parents are both alive and in pretty good health. They have always taken good care of me. I have two siblings (a brother and a sister), a sister-in-law, a niece, and a nephew. I am close with my family. I also have some cousins and friends I am close with. It's important knowing that I have people who care about me and whom I can talk to.

Another way I have learned to deal with my situation is by praying. I am not what I consider to be a very religious person. I am more a spiritual person. I believe that Jesus gives me strength and I've come to realize we all have a purpose on earth.

Several years ago, I went into therapy. I felt I needed to talk with a professional who was not personally involved with me—someone who could be objective. I was holding lots of feelings inside that needed to be expressed. Therapy was very helpful in raising my self-esteem. I used to feel that because I physically wasn't able to do much for anyone, that no one needed me. My therapist helped me to see that there are other ways that friends and family need me, such as the love, support, and advice I give them.

Mentally and emotionally, I believe I'm very strong and have coped pretty well with my disability. There are times, though, when I feel as if my situation is getting too difficult to handle. I feel stressed from worrying about who's going to care for me. If my regular health aide is ill or on vacation, the health care agency sends substitutes. My biggest concern is whether or not the substitute aide will be able to lift me and otherwise be a responsible and reliable caregiver. I'm also concerned about my parents caring for me. They are naturally aging, and it is becoming more difficult for them.

Another stressful situation I face is my progressive weakness. I live with the insecurity of not knowing when or if I will become weaker and exactly what I will no longer be able to do. I'm usually reminded of this when I realize there is something new I'm having difficulty doing, such as lifting up a glass or the phone. My condition isn't one day I'm able to do something, the next day I can't. It's realizing that certain things I used to do are now becoming more difficult.

I believe that the hardest thing I've had to cope with in my life is loneliness. I have never been married and never had a long-term relationship. While it is true that all love relationships have problems and lots of time and energy are involved in maintaining them, there is no denying that people with disabilities have a much more difficult time in finding and keeping relationships. In my experience, I have found that most men run from an involvement with me. Unfortunately, when I was younger, I was shy and uncomfortable with my situation, so when there was a guy showing interest in me and in starting a relationship, I wouldn't focus too much on my disability and problems we may encounter. I wouldn't encourage him to be open and talk about his feelings and concerns about a possible involvement with me. As a result, guys would become uncomfortable and probably sense my uneasiness, and so no real relationships developed. Therapy and maturity has helped me realize that it is vital to be open and honest. I am more comfortable with myself now and recently had a very honest relationship with a man. We discussed my disability and the problems associated with it at great length. We also discussed both of our feelings and some possible problems we may face. Unfortunately, we are not together, mainly because of some problems we did face that became a great obstacle. This relationship, even though it was short-lived, was the best I ever had. I attribute that to the fact that we were so open, honest, and comfortable with each other.

Coping with my loneliness is so very difficult because there are no substitutes for a loving and intimate relationship. Keeping busy helps one not to think too much, but the loneliness is always present. Sometimes, I feel lonelier in a room filled with people, especially being around couples, even more so then when I'm alone.

No matter how depressed I become, I never let those feelings consume me for great periods of time. I become frustrated and anxious. I cry and feel sorry for myself, but it doesn't last. I'm strong. I hate feelings of self-pity. But I am also human, and even though there are moments I give in to self-pity, I refuse to live my life that way. It does me no good feeling miserable and unhappy, and it hinders me from moving on, growing, experiencing, and enjoying some simple pleasures in life. My biggest pleasure in life has been being an aunt. Having missed the opportunity of having children and desperately wanting motherhood, I have children in my life that I love and who are part of me.

I feel the greatest barrier in my life has been my fear of taking chances. Once I become comfortable in a way of life, I don't want changes. An example of this was going from using a manual wheelchair to a motorized one. The motorized chair would make life easier for me and for those caring for me, plus it would give me greater independence. I was deathly afraid of using this new chair and resisted for a long time. Even though I thought I wanted to be independent, I was afraid of trying something new. I'm not certain if my fear of risk-taking is environmental (my family are worriers, afraid of changes) or if it stems from my insecurity of not knowing what further progression will take place with my disability and who will take care of me. I believe it's all of those things.

In working with people with physical disabilities, it is extremely important that counselors treat us with respect and dignity. We are faced with indignities on a daily basis, especially having people taking care of our personal needs. Don't talk down to us as if we are children. We are adults with adult problems. We think and feel exactly like every other human being. We are just physically weaker and may not be able to perform the simple tasks that most people do. Don't patronize us. Don't just nod "yes" at everything we say or at feelings we express. If you are not disabled, you don't really know how we feel. Don't pretend that you do. There are times you may say, "No, I don't know exactly how you're feeling, but I can try to understand." I know I would appreciate someone listening and trying to understand rather than saying that he or she knows precisely what I'm feeling. Always focus on a person's abilities, strengths, and talents. Don't dismiss our need to discuss feelings concerning our weaknesses, though. They are very real and need expression. Encourage the physically disabled, as anyone else should be encouraged, to appreciate the gifts they have and to use them to the best of their abilities. I believe that all of us, disabled and able-bodied, have something to give and we all learn from one another.

DISCUSSION QUESTIONS

1. What types of social interactions make you nervous? Recall an individual you were with the last time this occurred, and describe how you felt, behaved, and what your thoughts were during the interaction?
2. Which type of disability do you believe you would feel *most and least* comfortable socially interacting with, and describe your reasons why?
3. Discuss common stereotypes of various disabilities and where or how such views originate.
4. Have students discuss who their circle of friends include and what their friends have in common with them?

EXERCISES

A. Have students select and watch three movies over the course of the semester, then write a two-page reaction paper for each about how the person with the disability was portrayed. They should address whether the disability was made salient, whether the person was a hero or victim, whether he or she was sexually active, and whether he or she was employed; how the person was treated by others; and if there was a happy ending for the individual.

MOVIE LIST: 1. *Children of a Lesser God*; 2. *Whose Life Is It Anyway?*; 3. *Coming Home*; 4. *The Waterdance*; 5. *One Flew Over the Cuckoos Nest*; 6. *Edward Scissorhands*; 7. *If You Could See What I Hear*; 8. *Born on the Fourth of July*; 9. *My Left Foot*; 10. *Brady Story*; 11. *Forrest Gump*; 12. *Rainman*; 13. *Scent of a Woman*; 14. *Nell*; 15. *Lorenzo's Oil*; 16. *Philadelphia*; 17. *What's Eating Gilbert Grape?*; 18. *At First Sight*; 19. *Mask (with Cher)*; 20. *The Other Sister*; 21. *Frida*; 22. *I Am Sam*; 23. *Something About Mary*; 24. *As Good As It Gets*; 25. *Door to Door*; 26. *Gattaca*; 27. *Hunchback of Notre Dame*; 28. *Powder*; 29. *A Beautiful Mind*; 30. *Girl Interrupted*; 31. *Pumpkin*; 32. *The Ringer*; 33. *Murderball*; 34. *The Doctor*; 35. *Reign Over Me*; 36. *Home of the Brave*; 37. *Million Dollar Baby*; 38. *Passion Fish*; 39. *Ray*; 40. *The Sea Inside*; 41. *Vanilla Sky*; 42. *Awakenings*; 43. *Sling Blade*; 44. *The Music Within*.

B. Have students participate in a disability sensitivity exercise (e.g., wear a blindfold, use earplugs, use a wheelchair) and perform some activity around campus; then have them discuss their experience as well as the strengths/weaknesses of such activities.

THREE

Culturally Different Issues and Attitudes Toward Disability

Michael Jay Millington

OVERVIEW

Counseling people with disabilities has evolved in its constructs from medical models that focus on pathology within the individual, to functional models that focus on economic viability of the individual, to socio-political models that focus on the handicapping dynamics of the external environment (Smart, 2009). We have evolved science and practice sufficiently to understand that disability is a social construction (Shakespeare & Watson, 1997). The meaning of disability emerges from the interaction between the person and the society (Michailakis, 2003); it varies across groups and changes over time. The sociopolitical lens highlights the issue of power, its use, and its abuse (Szymanski & Trueba, 1994); the minority experience under a dominant culture (Hahn, 1988); and the role of culture as a context (Hershenson, 2000) for empowerment, research, and the development of more effective practice. In this chapter we will consider the changeable nature of disability from this postmodern, multicultural perspective and explore its implications for serving diverse populations in diverse cultural settings.

We will use the idea of attitudes as an organizing concept. Attitudes are affectively charged cognitions, predisposing a class of stereotypical behaviors toward a referent in social situations (Triandis, 1971). Attitudes are a cultural artifact of social learning (Livneh, 1988). Attitudes toward disability vary as a function of the context, the nature of the disability, and the interaction of the two (Gordon, Minnes, & Holden, 1990). We are primarily concerned with attitudes toward people with disabilities because they are historically charged with negative biases (Wright, 1988) that can ultimately influence the efficacy of service and inclusion of people with disabilities (Marinelli & Dell Orto, 1999).

Attitudes are a psychological artifact of culture. Individual attitudes toward people with disabilities vary widely across the general population, but they are influenced by the values, beliefs, and experiences of the individual's community. What we think about people with disabilities, what we expect, and how we treat people with disabilities is taught to us in the home, the church, and the school

(Joe & Miller, 1987). Attitudes that direct individual response to disability become, in the aggregate, attitudinal themes that direct the community response, with powerful implications for rehabilitation counseling service delivery and outcomes. It follows that different cultural influences create different community attitudes. Counselors move in a world where the meaning of disability is contextually defined and in flux. In the evolving multicultural society, it is incumbent upon professionals to broaden their understanding of the phenomenon of disability across the cultural landscape and to consider how best to respond on behalf of the client and the profession in any given situation.

To this end, we will review disability themes from four representative ethnic groups: Hispanic Americans, African Americans, Asian Americans, and Native Americans. We will provide a brief overview of their history, worldview, and traditional perceptions of disability and the community response. Each group will be considered from multiple subgroup perspectives, to get a sense of the range of attitudes extant within. We will attempt to provide some commentary and synthesis along the way and in conclusion.

HISPANIC ROOTS

Hispanic American is a term that was created by the U.S. Census Bureau to categorize a spectrum of Spanish-speaking ethnic groups that populate the Americas. It is not universally embraced by the peoples labeled, some of who prefer Latin American, Latino, Latina, Chicano, or Chicana (Hays, 2008). For the purposes of this chapter, we will use the term Hispanic American to refer to persons with ethnic roots in Cuban, Mexican, Puerto Rican, and Dominican cultures, as well as all of the cultures represented in Central and South America.

Hispanic Americans come from many different countries of origin, each with their own history and particular cultural influence. They are unified by a common language, Spanish, and distinguished by their dialects, idioms, and vernacular. Within the U.S. experience, they are differentiated by class and level and quality of acculturation/enculturation. First-generation immigrants tend to speak Spanish only, bilingualism occurs among the second generation, and English-only speakers are common in the third generation. Often a hybrid "Spanglish" is spoken with shifting and local usage.

What can be said of Hispanics in general, by way of contrast with the dominant White U.S. culture, is that they tend to be collectivist in a very family-centered way. They value socialization and time spent building relationships as opposed to keeping to an agenda and timetable. Communication is less direct, more circumspect, (i.e., low context; Brice, 2002). Hispanic Americans tend to be emotionally expressive and oriented to the present rather than the future or past.

Becoming Hispanic American

One of the primary differences between Hispanic American groups is the history of their immigration. The first Mexican Americans were created by a shift in borders following the Mexican War (1846–1848). Large swaths of the Southwest were part of Mexico until the border was established at the Rio Grande. Economic and political turmoil within Mexico generated a wave of immigration in the early 1900s to 1930 and the onset of the Great Depression. The government deported many Mexican immigrants and their American-born children, or placed them in detention camps. Need for cheap labor in dangerous conditions to serve the war effort in World War II reversed this policy and led to the second wave of Mexican day laborers, migrant farm workers, and immigrants—legal and otherwise.

The first substantial wave of Cuban immigrants was political refugees seeking temporary asylum in the United States following the communist revolution (ca. 1959). These were high-level government and military officials, landowners, and the wealthy elite. They did not expect to stay long in the United States and formed a tight-knit community in Miami, where they waited and agitated for the overthrow of Fidel Castro. They became very influential in the politics of southern Florida, and the federal government, through covert military acts, espionage, and economic embargo, underwrote their cause. Liberal immigration policies encouraged the second wave (ca. 1970–1980) of skilled working-class immigrants. As the Soviet Union's support of the Cuban economy dwindled and stopped, a third wave of mostly unskilled immigrants came to escape growing poverty (Brice, 2002).

El Salvador is the smallest and most densely populated country in Central America with a history of rebellion and oppression. In early colonial history, the indigenous tribes of the region were annihilated through slaughter and disease and appropriated through interbreeding by the conquistadors. In the 20th century, a farmer's (campesino) uprising (ca. 1932) met brutal suppression, 30,000 deaths, and the destruction of much of the agrarian economy. Protracted civil war devastated El Salvador's agrarian economy (ca. 1973–1992). The war pitted wealthy ruling families, with the support of the U.S. military, against a united leftist coalition of the poor. A wave of El Salvadoran immigration followed as a response to poverty, war, and the organized crime that followed in its wake (Batres, 2001).

The Dominican Republic shares a common early history with Haiti as they inhabit the same island (Hispaniola). The genocide of the indigenous people, the early introduction of slaves from Africa, and the establishment of European colonies are the same. The split with Haiti in 1844 and the Spanish language set it on a different path. In the 20th century, 30 years of dictatorship ruined the infrastructure of the Dominican Republic and fueled the first wave of political dissidents (ca. 1930–1960) immigrating to the U.S. Growing poverty in the rural areas forced people to the cities, and massive unemployment and social degradation in the cities led to a second wave of immigrants seeking economic relief. Today, it is a poor country saddled with insurmountable national debt. Immigrants tend to be single family members tasked with raising income for the family back home, with the expectation of an eventual return (Lopez-De Fede & Haeussler-Fiore, 2002).

The United States was a magnet for Hispanic immigrants and recognized as a haven from political upheaval and a path to better economic circumstance for much of the 20th century. In a more limited and conflicted sense, it remains so today. The role of U.S. political and economic adventurism in creating the conditions that lead to immigration is less often reported. Also overlooked for much of this history has been the relationship of Hispanic migrant workers to the economy of the Southwest and, by agricultural extension, the rest of the country. Hispanic workers provided for their families by taking hard labor jobs on the farm (see

Breeding, Rogers, Harley, & Crystal, 2005) and in other industries; jobs that others would not do, at a wage that others would not take, under conditions that others would not bear (Shorris, 1992). This labor economy created affordable produce, profitable farms, and a shadow work force of illegal immigrants who could neither complain about exploitation nor organize against it.

Hispanic Americans have a long history as descendents of the original Americans and have been part of this nation's history since its inception. They are well represented in educational mastery, economic success, political power, and class. They are the largest U.S. "minority" at 12.5% according to the 2000 census.

The Family

Although Dr. Glover-Graf addresses family and culture more definitively in Chapter 6, I will address the topic more globally here. Family is the center of Hispanic American life. It is more important than either the individual or the larger community. Hispanic families are traditionally extended generationally with well-defined roles within. The elders (grandparents) hold a place of honor and respect. Often they are sought for advice. In Cuban families, family elders retain ownership of the family's most valuable possessions (e.g., the business, the boat, the tractor, the land). Elders contribute as stewards of familial wealth rather than through physical labor. The head of household is the adult male (father) who is the primary wage earner and around whom family supports revolve. The family's task is to maximize the earning potential of the head of household. The adult female (mother) is responsible for the home and the raising of the children. The oldest male child is recognized as the future head of household and groomed accordingly. The oldest female child is expected to share in the task of raising younger siblings. Children grow up in a highly protective and supervised home, remaining more deeply dependent upon the family hierarchy for a much longer period of time than their cohorts in the dominant culture. Dominican children do not leave the familial home until they are married, and if they do not marry, they are not likely to leave at all (Lopez-De Fede & Haeussler-Fiore, 2002).

Machismo is an unavoidable term in the discussion of family roles, but it is poorly defined and even more poorly understood. The term itself has a very recent 20th century etymology and no stable core. At the center is the concept of an idealized masculine worldview and deportment. To some it is the patriarchic duty of protecting the family, instilling and enforcing the right values in the home, and the education of the young. To others it is the rejection of all feminine values, and baser interpretations of what it means to be a man (aggression, sexual promiscuity, etc.). What they have in common is the strong expectation of a narrowly defined identity for the male (husband, father, colleague) and the potential for shame and conflict if the role is compromised (Lopez-De Fede & Haeussler-Fiore, 2002).

Women are similarly idealized in role and value. Women are the stewards of the family and home. In a Catholic world, the primacy of Saint Mary holds the mother of Christ in reverence and through the Virgin of Guadalupe a strong symbol of the ideal. The values projected upon this ideal of the feminine tend to be quiet, dutiful submission to the male and chaste piety. Failure to live up to the ideal can result in public and private (De Paula, Lagana, & Gonzalez-Ramirez, 1996) sanction and shame.

Religion and Worldview

The Hispanic world is overwhelmingly Catholic and Catholicism plays a central role in individual identity, the function of the household, and the relationship of the family to the community . . . all aspects of life (Falicov, 1998). The Catholic Church hierarchy plays an important role in the structure of the community. Priests and saints act as intermediaries to the divine through ritual acts, and the petitioning of the saints for favor, blessing, or miraculous intervention is commonplace. Often this petition takes the form of a negotiation, acts of devotion in return for healing, for example. Catholicism has been a refuge for the oppressed in Central and South America and sometimes an advocate for social justice up to and including a liberation theology, such as that which sustained the campesinos in El Salvador (Boff & Boff, 1987).

Threads of African and Indigenous religion and spiritualism run through Hispanic cultures (Kemp, 2005). Some have been subsumed within the local Catholic tradition. For example, the Mexican goddess Tonantzin is subsumed in the icon of our Lady of Guadalupe (Poole, 1996). The Day of the Dead is subsumed in the celebration of All Soul's Day (Brandes, 1997). Santeria is a Caribbean confluence of African Yoruba and Catholic religious systems that replaced the pantheon of Saints with more approachable and Earth-bound minor deities who will protect the individual and respond positively to acts of devotion. In Santeria, everyone has a contract with a spirit before birth. Fulfilling the contract brings rewards; to fail is to be punished (Brice, 2002).

Disability in the Family and Community

There is a general lack of research into Hispanic American attitudes and beliefs concerning disabilities. What has been done is largely dated, potentially biased (see Ruiz & Padilla, 1977), and does not take the heterogeneity of the population into consideration (Graf, Blankenship, Sanchez, & Carlson, 2007; Salas-Provance, Erickson, & Reed, 2002). Hispanic Americans understand and accept the premise of Western medicine, but understanding is couched in a religious worldview. Health, either good or bad, is a dispensation from God. And so disability is often construed as punishment, a test, or simply "God's will." The implication being that you somehow deserve your lot in life or that it was your destiny (Alvarez & Ruiz, 2001).

Psychological states (worry, anger, fear), environmental conditions (bad air, germs, bad food, imbalance of cold and hot, etc.), and supernatural agents (Lafitte, 1983) conspire to cause illness and disability. Mothers are often held responsible for the congenital disabilities of their offspring, as it is assumed that they violated a taboo (e.g., eating the wrong food, witnessed a horrific event, or encountered a disfigured person) while pregnant (Brice, 2002). Psychiatric disabilities are the most prone to supernatural explanation, usually attributable to evil spirits or witchcraft (Molina, Zambrana, & Aguirre-Molina, 1994).

Response

The family is responsible for caregiving. Each member of the family has a role to play (Trevino & Szymanski, 1996). They provide all of the support, if possible, including nurturance, home remedies, and spiritual petitions for relief. Seeking help outside of the family is a sign of weakness (Smart & Smart, 1991) and incompetence (Hanline & Daley, 1992). Families tend to draw inward, to protect the family member, especially children to the point of overprotection (Rivera, 1983). Sheltering and isolation is seen as a way to protect the family member (and the family) from a world that they believe will stigmatize them, shame them, and offer them nothing of value (Lopez-De Fede & Haeussler-Fiore, 2002).

Religious coping involves drawing strength directly from one's faith. The observation of ceremony and ritual add to the psychological wellbeing of the individual and family (Abraido-Lanza, Vasquez, & Echeverria, 2004). Religiosity increases the perception of control over something that it ultimately the Will of God. Because God intervenes directly in the lives of people, the family believes in the potential for miraculous cures and devotion as a means to the miracle (Weisman, 2000).

There are folk healers in the Mexican tradition (Glover & Blankenship, 2007) who holistically treat problems in body, mind, and spirit. They are considered to be divinely inspired to provide natural and supernatural remedies. Herbs and medicinal plants may be ingested or topically applied in combination with massage and ceremonial intervention in the spirit world. Folk healers are most commonly used when conventional medicine and prayer have failed to produce the desired result (Zavaleta, 2000).

Hispanic American women play the central role in caregiving, are most informed about service, and most likely to seek it. Help is sought from the family outward. Case in point, mental health is enmeshed in the inter-relationships of the family (Vera & Conner, 2007). Mental health is "taught" parent to child in terms of harmony and interdependence. Promoting mental health moves outward into the community. Mental health is provided through local community resources (e.g., day care, parks with programs). Mental health is operationally defined as having jobs nearby, knowing that you are providing for your family, and keeping them safe. Outside of the family, Hispanic Americans prefer to turn to trusted individuals, family friends, clergy, or peers in the community. Hispanic women will willingly try everything *but* mental health services (Vega, Kolody, & Aguilar-Gaxiola, 2001) as they are highly stigmatizing to the individual and the family. However, the more familiar she is with mental health services (through the experiences of friends) and the less attributable the mental illness is to supernatural causes and moral failing, the more likely mental health services will be engaged (Alvidrez, 1999).

AFRICAN AMERICAN ROOTS

The term African American is a categorical aggregate of people with diverse geographic African origins, ethnic influences (e.g., West Indian, Haitian, Spanish, and Native American), and community histories in the United States (Lee, Blando,

Mizelle, & Orozco, 2007). The overwhelming majority of African Americans are English-speaking citizens with a generational claim to the country that dates back to the first European colonies. Others are relative newcomers who speak French, Creole, Spanish, or Portuguese and immigrated to the United States via South American countries and the Caribbean. Still others come directly from the African continent with cultures and dialects too numerous to mention.

They have come for different reasons, at different times, and are established in all strata of society. An African American middle class is well established and the professional and affluent classes are growing (Edwards & Polite, 1992). Still, an out-sized proportion of the African American community struggles with poverty. The progress and continuing challenge of the African American community is the legacy of a struggle for civil rights and full community inclusion in a society that condoned slavery for hundreds of years, enforced oppression through law and acts of terrorism, and even now continues to wrestle with its prejudices and myriad micro-oppressions. African American subgroups may differ in their response to this legacy, but they follow the same arc. They tend toward strong family ties and respect for familial authority (Robinson & Howard-Hamilton, 1994). Religion is a central organizing force in extended families and networked communities. African Americans are generally wary of authority figures in the dominant White culture (Monteith & Spicer, 2000; Whaley, 2001) and often negotiate the dominant culture as a world distinct from their own (Diemer, 2007).

Becoming African American

The original African American immigration, if the term can be preserved here, was borne of the slave trade. The Spanish first shipped African slaves to Cuba and Hispaniola in the 1500s to replace the indigenous populations that were exterminated in the colonization of the New World. The slave trade was a commercial enterprise that enriched plantation owners for nearly 400 years. Slaves were cargo and treated as such with no regard for family or tribe in their placement. Indeed, any semblance of community expressed among slaves was seen as a threat to commerce and the safety of the slave owners. From emancipation, to Jim Crow, to the Civil Rights Movement and beyond, the history of African American life is a narrative of resistance and resilience.

Haiti (Jacobson, 2003) is the northwest third of the island of Hispaniola, which was one of the earliest and largest plantation colonies in the Caribbean. African slaves were brutally suppressed for fear of an uprising, which eventually came in 1791 with the wholesale slaughter and destruction of French colonial infrastructure in the north. This led to a full-scale revolution and the eventual independence of Haiti in 1804. This was a pyrrhic victory for the freed slaves who were left with a devastated agriculture, nonexistent commerce, an unskilled and uneducated populace, and a dictatorial regime. The history of Haiti hence has been a succession of oppressive governments, revolutions, and coups around a class struggle between the aristocracy of mulatto elites and the impoverished populace. Over time, the Haitian rainforest was burned for charcoal, leaving the infertile soil exposed and prone to mudslides in the hilly terrain.

Between hurricanes, a recent earthquake, and a cholera epidemic it is a devastated land, the poorest in the Americas, with the lowest in health (Arthur, 2002), earnings, and education, and little hope for rising out of its Third World status in the foreseeable future (Jacobson, 2003).

Haitians first immigrated to the United States in the 1800s, forming communities in Louisiana, Baltimore, and Philadelphia. The first modern immigration wave took place as upper class mulattos and rural landowners fled political upheaval and violence in the 1950s and 1960s. Less skilled workers began to immigrate in the 1960s to fill low-wage jobs left by Vietnam War draftees. Haitian "boat people," also fleeing state-sponsored terrorism and extreme poverty, arrived unwanted in the 1980s and were detained in camps in New York and Texas. Many of those who managed to stay did not return after political turmoil in Haiti subsided (Jacobson, 2003). The fact that Haitians were rejected and treated as illegal immigrants while Cuban refugees were welcomed and assimilated has been a long-standing sore point for Haitians.

Jamaica was colonized by Spain (ca. 1494), seized by Britain (ca. 1655), and granted independence in 1962. The culture of Jamaica developed against a backdrop of slavery, oppression, and the fight against both over the course of centuries. Escaped slaves formed independent communities in the island interior, surviving colonist attempts to destroy them. Slave revolts in 1831 set political action in motion that resulted in the abolition of slavery by the British Parliament in 1834, but did little to change the political, social, or economic conditions of the newly freed. Slowly, a middle class emerged, though much of the gains were lost again in the great depression (ca. 1930s). An unsuccessful workers revolt led to labor organization and greater political representation. While there have been Jamaican communities in New York and New Jersey since the late 1800s, immigration to the United States did not become significant until the 1970s and 1980s. Middle-class Jamaicans fleeing political unrest early on and the professional class fleeing the growing criminal threat of drug traffickers and organized crime were challenged in finding comparable employment abroad. Employed in the United States and yet unable to return to the lives they had left, they worked as they could to support their families in Jamaica and worked toward reuniting the family in the United States (Miller, 2002).

The Family

The extended family is the center of life with an emphasis on group survival. Family members are protective of their own and tend to define problems in terms of external threat rather than internal fault or conflict (Boyd-Franklin, 2003). The identity of the individual is negotiated in the context of interdependence and contribution to the family (Lee et al., 2007). Multigenerational households are common, with grandparents acting as head of household. Traditional gender roles are followed in that women are responsible for taking care of the family, but women are often the heads of household, by economic necessity or matriarchic tradition. Aunts and uncles living in close proximity will serve as surrogate parents, providing emotional and financial support, and receive the same level of respect as biological parents (Miller, 2002). Kinship bonds often extend informally to friends and neighbors (Jacobson, 2003).

Within this collectivist theme, class influences family structure. In Haiti, class is sharply delineated by language and economics. The French-speaking ruling class retained the lion's share of public resources within the urban centers and segregated their education system accordingly. The Creole-speaking people of Haiti are rural, and left with few resources and little opportunity for education and advancement. In Jamaica, the upper and middle classes are also concentrated in the urban centers and delineated by church affiliation. The Anglican Church provides an organizing center for the community of the wealthy; the Baptist Church serves the same function for the poor. Each holds the other in some level of contempt (Miller, 2002). The wealthy tend to cleave to a more European standard of traditional marriage, proscribed spousal partnership, and nuclear families. Cohabitation is more common among the poor. Children may continue to live in the family home well into adulthood, out of economic necessity (Jacobson, 2003).

Religion and Worldview

Religion is the central organizing structure of the community. Its function goes beyond the spiritual. The church is an important gathering place (Miller, 2002), where the community exercises charity for families in need (Boyd-Franklin, 2003) and advocacy in the struggle for parity (Miller, 2002). Advocacy has been strong in the African American church from the beginning. For instance, the African Methodist Church was founded in response to discrimination in the Methodist Church and as a protest against slavery in Pennsylvania in the early 1800s. African American churches are predominantly Christian and represented in many denominations.

In the Caribbean, a heritage of African cosmology influences Christian worship. In Haiti, for example, voodoo provided spiritual support for the slave uprisings and early political movements. Catholicism is now the majority religion (90%) in Haiti, but the pantheon of voodoo spirits still abide syncretically within the canon of the saints and in ceremonies that have incorporated them. While voodoo is not commonly practiced among Caribbean immigrants, its African origins still resonate through their spiritual worldview in a complex cosmology of supernatural spirits that can intervene in their lives and must be respected (Jacobson, 2003).

Disability in the Family and Community

As we investigate the attitudes of African Americans toward people with disabilities, it is important to look at the special circumstances that the history of an enslaved people in America created around this issue. The American version of slavery was particularly dehumanizing: "African Americans were thought to have good mental health if they were subservient (being controlled and docile), whereas protesters were categorized as deranged and mentally ill" (Wilson, 2005, p. 157). The psychology of the time pathologized the African American experience to justify the oppression of African Americans first through slavery and later through every social outlet, including education, health, and employment (Wilson, 2005).

Mental illness carries stigma exacerbated by that history. In a qualitative study (Matthews, Corrigan, Smith, & Aranda, 2006) African Americans identified good mental health as being stable, in touch, positive attitude, resilient, and in good spiritual health. Stress and trauma were reported as the primary reason for mental health problems in general, but religious leaders attribute mental illness, at least in part, to spiritual intercession (e.g., demons). Overall, mental illness was seen as unresponsive to treatment. Appraisals of life with mental illness were consistently negative. Positive appraisals, when they occurred, were usually attributable to spiritual intervention. The stigma of mental illness is socially contagious, capable of diminishing the standing of those who associate with people with mental illness. Compassion carries the risk of sharing in the consequences of stigma.

Jamaican perception of disability depends upon the cause of the disability and the worldview of the perceiver. Because God punishes the wicked and rewards the good, disability is often seen as the consequence of sin. Disability thus attributed becomes a public shame for both the person with a disability and the family. Disabilities acquired by observable means under circumstance beyond the control of the person generate the most compassion; disabilities acquired through negligence generate the least compassion. Illnesses that cannot be explained otherwise may be construed as the work of evil spirits or witchcraft (Leavitt, 1992). Mental illness is often thought to be a vengeful act of an enemy who attached a ghost to the person spirit.

Haiti perspectives on disability are similarly defined in terms of shame and further charged with the propensity for community rejection and abuse. What may be considered a disability in the United States is often attributed to personal failing in Haiti. Public response to personal failing is actively negative and exclusionary. Children with developmental disabilities are seen as especially devastating to the family's hopes for the future because of high expectations that education is the solution to current economic hardship. Disabilities, developmental or acquired, are mysterious and dangerous and not readily discussed. If a woman bears a child with a disability, the man may impregnate another woman to demonstrate that the disability is attributable to the mother and not to him. Often, the mother of the child with a disability is abandoned (Jacobson, 2003). A spirit curse, punishment of a Christian god, or a spell cast by an enemy, disability is often thought to be supernatural in origin. Many Haitians are afraid of people with disabilities, as if they are contagious, whether the disability is mental or physical (Jacobson, 2003).

Response

Turner and Alston (1994) identified four basic strengths that support the African American family's response to physical disability, namely, strong kinship bonds, role flexibility, religious orientation, and education/work ethic. Where extended families are intact, the family member with a disability is supported from within. Family roles are flexible and adaptable to need. New tasks are taken on easily within the role or shared as a community task. Grandparents, spouse, uncles, and aunts may all take on the duties as head of household should the need arise. Neighbors supervise the young in public settings. The extended family tends to be active in family affairs whether they are in close proximity or living at a distance. Active participation in church spirituality is pursued as a way of coping individually and collectively with the consequences of mental illness. The church provides a social gathering place and a resource for support such as pastoral counseling, community outreach, and charitable giving. It is the hub of the social support network where extended families connect and share. Education/work ethic links hard work and education instrumentally to attainment of the good life, and families come together to support achievement of its members (Turner & Alston, 1994):

> The African-American spirit to excel, despite seemingly insurmountable odds, will greatly benefit African Americans who are disabled in the career retraining aspect of rehabilitation. As a means of motivating African Americans with disabilities in their efforts to reenter the work world, health and human service professionals can nurture this instinctive tendency to excel in life. (Turner & Alston, 1994, pp. 919–920)

The strong family focus dictates that the problems associated with disability are resolved as close to home as possible. This support strategy facilitates inclusion for people with physical disabilities and challenges for people with mental illness.

The African American community expects self-reliance and stoic silence about mental health problems. Seeking help is embarrassing and stigmatizing (Matthews et al., 2006). Mental health services are only appropriate in cases of extreme need and seen as ineffective and unresponsive. Avoidance is fueled by expectations of loss and ill treatment within the system. Psychotropic medication is mistrusted and hospitalization is feared. Once labeled, the person is thought labeled for life. The label portends reduced opportunities and a bleak economic outlook. Medication and its side effects are thought to be a permanent burden that carries the risk of addiction (Cooper et al., 2003). It is clear why parents will fight the labeling process to the point of avoiding service. The resistance to outside intervention can be ameliorated somewhat with the inclusion of familiar and trusted figures, especially church officials and spiritual counselors (Snowden, 2001). Depending on racial identity and attitudes toward Whites, some clients are more comfortable with counselors with a similar ethnic background (Ferguson, Leach, Levy, Nicholson, & Johnson, 2008).

Jamaican families tend to resolve their family issues in-house before they seek help in their community, and they seek help in their community before they seek help in the form of government services (Miller, 2002). Family interventions may include reading bible passages and use of talismans and animistic ritual to ward off the evil ghosts. Children with congenital disabilities are closeted away from public view, to protect them from abuse and to avoid shaming the family. They may maintain a passive "sick role" all of their lives. Deep conflict arises where demand for chronic care exceeds the family's ability to provide. Institutionalization for any family member is a failure of the family obligation and a public humiliation, to the point that abandonment is a possible and preferable option. Little is expected from people with mental illness, care is meager, and abuse is historically common. When help is sought it is the woman's task to find it. They tend not to trust the experts, will challenge their conclusions, will demand to be heard, and will confront anything they feel is unjust (Miller, 2002).

Haitian families hold a similar hierarchy of responses. The family as a group makes decisions and, where possible, they use family support systems to provide for the family member. Children with disabilities are loved but considered worthless in the family's economic struggle, which takes precedence over other concerns. When outside help is needed, the family turns to religion and, in contrast to the Jamaican response, public institutions. However, Haitians turn to state-sponsored support looking for a cure rather than an extended rehabilitation process with limited outcomes (Jacobson, 2003).

ASIAN ROOTS

The term Asian American was coined and used originally by community activists to replace the Western vernacular "Oriental," which was thought to be racist and colonial. It has since become both a categorical identifier for the Census Bureau and a unifying label adopted by Asian Americans in pursuit of civil rights. The fatal beating of Vincent Chin in 1982, and the subsequent acquittal of his admitted murderers (Yip, 1997) galvanized the loose confederation of varied ethnic Asian American communities and charged this label with identity politics. It refers to American citizens with heritage in a wide range of nations and cultures spanning the Far East, Southeast Asia, and Indian subcontinent. The range of difference could hardly be larger. Asian American heritage includes Japan, China, India, Korea, Pakistan, Indonesia, Philippines, Bangladesh, Malaysia, and Vietnam. Religion includes Christianity, Buddhism, Hinduism, Sikhism, and Islam. Languages and dialects are numerous beyond mention.

Asian Americans, particularly of East Asian descent, tend to have strong collectivist groundings where work satisfaction emerges from contribution to the group, not the celebration of self (Henderson & Chan, 2005). Interpersonal relationships and protocol are exacting and require constant monitoring and maintenance (Xie & Leong, 2008). They value conformity, self-discipline, emotional restraint, and deference to age and authority (Kim, Atkinson, & Yang, 1999) in contrast to, and in conflict with, the individualistic, informal, and irreverent popular U.S. culture (Atkinson, 2004). Asians have been labeled the "model minority" based on stereotypical expectations of high academic skills and deferential demeanor. The stereotype is offensive and wrong (Wong & Halgin, 2006). Asian Americans fare no better in GPA than Whites and share the same employment struggle—along with the added struggle against the stereotype itself. The "model minority" is misunderstood and seeking to change that status.

Becoming Asian American

The first Asian immigrants to the United States were likely Chinese (Liu, 2001). Early immigrants were wealthy merchants and skilled tradespersons, who settled on the West Coast and were generally well respected for their demeanor and work ethic. In the 1800s, many unskilled Chinese laborers were hired to work in the gold mining towns and mines, and on the transcontinental railroad. The Chinese were willing to work hard and long in harsh conditions for little pay, taking jobs others would not, and taking these jobs in agriculture, mining, railroad, and service. They were subject to growing racial hatred and became the target of violence when the job market made it difficult for Whites to find work. As scapegoats for the economic ills of the times, the violence increased and began to threaten the employer who hired them. Laws were passed to ban further immigration of Chinese and the population dwindled (Chan, 1998). Changes in legislation in the 1930s allowed merchants' families to immigrate. Large families coalesced in "Chinatowns," while first wave laborers left the mines to start businesses. In 1943, further relaxation of immigration law allowed many older men to return to China to find wives, bringing mostly female immigrants. In 1965 flat annual quotas (20,000) allowed for entire families to immigrate, mostly working class early on; later more immigrants were from educated families who came over as students and stayed to work. In 1978, normalized relations with China and additional quotas for Taiwan and Hong Kong created an influx of students and scholars.

Over 5000 years of dynastic history in Korea ended when it was colonized by Japan in 1910. Korea was liberated from Japanese rule following World War II, only to become a pawn in a proxy war as Korea was split into the communist north and democratic south. Thus it has remained since the end of the Korean War in 1953. When we speak of Korean immigrants to the United States, we are speaking overwhelmingly about South Korea. The first wave of Korean immigrants came through Hawaii (ca. 1903–1920) to escape Japanese colonial oppression. They came as plantation laborers and "picture brides" for plantation laborers until anti-Asian polices were passed, stopping all immigration. Immigration was renewed during the Korean War for military family members and adopted orphans. In 1965, the loosening of immigration quotas brought a surge of middle class and educated Koreans to the United States. As South Korea has become more prosperous, immigration has slowed (Kim-Rupnow, 2001).

The U.S. colonization of the Philippines following the Spanish American War in the early 1900s created two paths by which Filipinos could immigrate. The sons and daughters of the ruling elite, and later the highly educated civil service workers, were brought to the United States to receive an education. Some stayed, others returned but maintained contacts in the United States. Less educated or less socially connected Filipinos became plantation/farm laborers in Hawaii and California. The early laborers suffered the brunt of the racism targeting Asian Americans in California due to their economic position and lack of representation (Melendy, 1972). During World War II, working class Filipinos were recruited from the communities close to military bases and, in turn, they tended to build distinct Filipino communities near military bases in the United States. In 1965, change in immigration policy favored the professional class from urban centers. All of these groups came to pursue better economic circumstances, but with varying expectations (De Torres, 2002).

Vietnam was conquered and colonized in 1885 by the French, invaded and occupied by the Japanese in 1945, embroiled in a 30-year long civil war, and suffered through a decade of strife before slowly becoming a stable country, hub of economic trade in Asia, and trading partner with the United States (Hunt, 2002). Immigration to the United States is closely tied to and shaped by the Vietnam War and its aftermath.

At the end of the war, thousands of South Vietnamese fled with the American forces. The fall of Saigon and the rise of the unified Socialist Republic of Vietnam abruptly halted this practice until another massive wave several years later, as villagers, rice farmers, and fishermen (Phan, Rivera, & Roberts-Wilbur, 2005) struggled to escape political persecution and extreme poverty. Political prisoners, Amerasians (offspring of soldiers), and those with relatives in the United States were allowed to immigrate. In total, nearly 1 million refugees immigrated to the United States (Hunt, 2002).

The Family

Family is the basic social unit, transcending the individual in many traditions (Liu, 2001). With the group's well being at the center, harmony and balance are the measures of wellness. Harmony in the home, leads to harmony in the community, leads to harmony in the nation. Harmony is sustained through well-established roles for husband, wife, daughter, son, grandparents, and so on, and these roles are defined by subordination to authority and interdependence (Kim-Rupnow, 2001). There is hierarchy in the roles, but the hierarchy tends to serve the family unit rather than the head of household. Parents sacrifice for their children, particularly in education. Children, in turn, are obligated to support their aging parents (Kim-Rupnow, 2001). Roles are gender and age based. Father takes the lead. Mother follows. Older siblings are responsible for helping in raising their younger siblings (De Torres, 2002) who, in turn, are taught to show respect and obedience. Assertiveness, particular among the young is rude. Frank expression of emotions or needs is discouraged, especially for men (Kim-Rupnow, 2001). Sacrifice and sublimation of one's own ego for the sake of the family is the rule. Improper behavior of the individual shames the person and the family (Hunt, 2002). Family is extended multigenerationally (Liu, 2001). There is a reverence for age. Family concept moves outward from the extended family to the community, and obligations and benefits go with it. Community is a tightly knit group that will help members find work, support, education, and housing. Being faithful to the family and the local community that supports you is a source of pride.

Compared with other Asian groups, the traditional Filipino family is perhaps less reserved and formal in their inter-relations and more democratic in their approach to dealing with family decisions. Filipino families engage in complex social relationships with extended family networks of both blood and affiliation (e.g., godparents) through which favors are traded and obligations are served. Social obligations and family grudges can be passed down generationally and revisited in family gatherings (De Torres, 2002). Pinoys (individual Filipinos) living alone is rare. Core families stay together until married off, even longer if economically necessary. Employed elder siblings support younger siblings, avoiding marriage until younger siblings are through with their education. The youngest daughter takes care of the parents (De Torres, 2002).

The collectivist Indian family may be contrasted against other Asian groups by the extent of the patriarchal emphasis. Family property is held in common, but the male head of household is the sole decision-maker on matters of property and family. Beyond the patriarch, males of all age are to be respected and obeyed. Women tend to join their husband's family and inherit subservient positions (Pinto & Sahu, 2001). The relationship of the family to the community at large is still influenced by an ancient caste system that sets the social and economic parameters of appropriate behavior and association. Castes are a formalized class system that reserve the best schools, homes, jobs, and ultimately wealth and influence for the upper castes and relegates the lower castes to powerlessness, poverty, and exclusion (Pinto & Sahu, 2001).

Religion and Worldview

Asian Americans are well represented in populations of every major religion in the world. Religious or spiritual foundations are manifold and finding commonality is a challenge. Confucianism has been an influential philosophy in its focus on the primacy of harmony and the role of social relationships, particularly family relationships. The acceptance of fate and one's role in society is an important aspect of Confucian philosophy. Taoism literally means, "The Way" or the path, and it refers to a metaphysical view of the natural order of the universe and the human's proper role in it. It is a holistic perception of reality in that nothing exists except in relation to everything else. It counsels that events will fall into harmony if we do not try to impose our order upon it. The yin and yang of the Tao represent a never-ending cycle of change, a dance between the two prime principles, male and female. The transcendent is always before you in the everyday. Balance is found by being present in the unfolding moment, by not attempting to force your will upon the world but responding spontaneously and authentically to the moment. In Buddhism, the emphasis is on the pursuit of enlightenment rather than its simple acceptance. Buddhists believe that the soul is reincarnated, born over and over again into a world of suffering, birth, life, and death. Suffering is caused by desire to have and control things. The end of suffering comes through a disciplined approach to living a moral life, to strengthen one's mind, and to seeking enlightenment. Hinduism recognizes a transcendent supreme deity and a pantheon of gods, goddesses, and avatars that are manifestations of the godhead. The cycle of life, death, and rebirth moves the soul forward through many lifetimes and karma follows the soul. The path is toward a higher state. Your position in life is perceived as a natural consequence of your karmic debt or reward. The path to enlightenment has Earthly pursuits of righteousness, material prosperity, and gratification of the sensual, but culminates in a renunciation of the material world for the spiritual life (Pinto & Sahu, 2001).

Disability in the Family and Community

Disability is seen as disharmony, which is a threat to the natural Confucian order of things. Stigma is often high in Chinese communities (Lam, Tsang, Chan, & Corrigan, 2006), indeed the common Chinese term for disability translates as "useless" or "sick" (Liu, 2001). Lay theories abound as to the cause of disability, from retribution for sins of a past life (Liu, 2001), to eating lamb while pregnant (Lam et al., 2006). While any disability of any kind is stigmatizing, the most severe response has historically been reserved for people with mental illness. Mental illness is attributed to weak moral character, and so their behavior brings shame to the family.

In India, disability is punishment for misdeeds in past lives (karma). Congenital disability is accepted as karmic fate, although little help is forthcoming. Indians see their children as an investment in the future, especially the male children. A child with developmental disability is not seen as a good investment of time, money, or effort. They are loved, but no effort is made to make them independent. Acquired disabilities are more sympathetic, particularly if there is hope that former productivity can be regained. Disability is a family affair and the women shoulder the burden. Empowerment is selfishness. Individuals are admonished to live for the family, especially the females (Pinto & Sahu, 2001).

In Korea (Kim-Rupnow, 2001) and Vietnam, disability is caused by supernatural agents, punishment from God, curses from evil forces, or punishment for the sins of your ancestors. Oftentimes it would be divined that mother did something wrong during pregnancy, failing to eat right or breaking a taboo. Educated Koreans are more likely to believe in genetic and biological causes. Koreans tend to see developmental disabilities as karmic retribution, bringing shame to the person and family. As a sign of retribution for sins, the family member with a disability is often isolated from the public. Acquired disabilities may been seen in a positive light if they are seen as sacrifice for the common good, and others seek to regain their role (Kim-Rupnow, 2001). In Vietnam, the congenitally blind are thought to have spiritual vision, special powers to see into the future and the past; they are often employed as psychics at the temple or in the marketplace. Vietnamese attitudes toward disabilities have been especially shaped by our war. Following the war and in the aftermath of landmines, people with all nature of physical disability were very common and without stigma. Agent Orange created both congenital and acquired disabilities and a new generation of "victims of the war." These are also held faultless and without shame.

Asian Americans are generally more accepting of acquired disabilities than congenital physical or mental illness (Wang, Chan, Thomas, Lin, & Larson, 1997). Mental illness is associated with weak character or blamed on evil spirits, or punishment of the gods. Mental illness is shameful and worse, reflects badly on the family and ancestors (Ho, 1984). It is not generally discussed in family.

Response

Those with a scientific background seek solutions. Those with a spiritual background seek healing. Many pursue both. Noting the coping strategies of Chinese families, Lam et al. observed:

> The prime source of coping relies on oneself, including facing the problem and devising a solution; enduring and persevering; striving; and having confidence. It is generally believe [sic] that if one has the willpower; one should be able to overcome the problem. The second major source of coping is help from one's family and social network. The third source is form shamanism and folk religions. The final coping strategy is doing nothing and letting nature take its course, an approach which is greatly influenced by Taoist philosophy. (Lam et al., 2006, p. 276)

Believing strongly in the mind-body connection (Hampton, Yeung, & Nguyen, 2007), they will often integrate medical care with spiritual healing. People with mental illness often prefer Chinese spiritual healers to physicians (Lam et al., 2006). Institutionalization is an agreeable and often preferred treatment of people with mental illness, and group homes for people with developmental disabilities are disliked by many Chinese Americans. Where services are available, they may be underutilized because, as a group, Asian Americans have a higher tolerance for psychological discomfort of stress and anxiety (Zhang, Snowden, & Sue, 1998).

Help seeking is mitigated or encouraged by community pressure (Christopher, Skillman, Kirkhart, & D'Souza, 2006) as well as support. Chinese Americans and Korean American seek medical treatment for mental illness. Koreans offer religious ritual along with Western medicines. Korean systems recognize disabilities stemming from the human body, mind, and environment. Filipinos dealing with developmental disabilities turn to the church for support with little expectation. Others go to folk healers looking for compassion when nothing else works (De Torres, 2002).

NATIVE AMERICAN ROOTS

The term "Native American" is an ethnic label coined by the United States Government to categorize the original inhabitants of the North American continent. It is not a term that is universally accepted by those to whom it is applied. Generally speaking, individuals identify more with their tribe than an appellation assigned to them by outsiders, but it is a serviceable and nonpejorative term that has fallen into common use.

The Native American rubric spans more than 500 distinct cultural entities (Hays, 2008), over 300 sovereign reservations and more than 250 different languages (Sanderson, 2001). Over 60% of self-identified Native Americans are of mixed heritage and vary in level of acculturation (Trimble, Fleming, Beauvais, & Jumper-Thurman, 1996). The origins of the indigenous tribes arc into prehistory and their inter-tribal relationships are exceedingly varied. They were geographically dispersed across the continent, and their cultures reflect the environments in which they lived, from nomadic hunter gathers to settled agrarians.

This expansive range of cultures challenges our ability to generalize, but there are some strong commonalities that transcend tribal affiliation. Native Americans value living in harmony within themselves, with others, and with nature. The individual identity is anchored in place, specifically the reservation or ancestral lands. They have a deep spiritual connection with the natural world. Strong tribal bonds and a collectivist mindset put the needs of the family and tribe above the personal (Sue & Sue, 1999). Native Americans live in a world of relationships and experience in the present. The world is not linear and ruled by time. Traditions are honored. Elders are revered leaders in the community. Native Americans are deferent in their communication and seemingly taciturn in conversation—often because of a desire to understand before they speak and to respond with great care (Clark & Kelley, 2001). Native American culture is propagated through matriarchal systems, oral history, traditional healing methods, and an abundance of ceremonies that bind people, mark occasions, teach lessons, circumscribe time, heal the spirit, and otherwise reaffirm the tribal identity. They are united across tribes by a shared history of oppression, racism, and a learned wariness of White dominant culture and society (Garrett, 1999; Garrett & Herring, 2001).

Becoming Native American

Native American history of the United States begins in genocide, a continuation and expansion of the extermination of tribes through the Western Hemisphere by Europeans since 1492 (Churchill, 1998). In an inexorable ethnic cleansing of civilization from east to west, in the name of manifest destiny, for the acquisition of real estate and natural resources, unaccounted millions were killed and driven off of their land. A catalog of broken treaties documents the duplicity of the government. Blood was on the hands of the common people as well; pioneers, ranchers, miners, all who swept westward for plunder. They killed with guns, with small pox, and with alcohol (Garrett & Carroll, 2000). By the 1900s there were roughly 250,000 Native Americans left. The country was conquered, the indigenous people expunged, and the prosperity of the Whites assured.

In 1924, Calvin Coolidge signed a bill that gave citizenship to the survivors of the Native American holocaust. Now they could be citizens of the United Sates of America . . . but they could not be Indians. Through the Bureau of Indian Affairs government efforts to eradicate the Native American way of life turn cultural. The bureau moved to kill their languages and religious ceremonies. The bureau outlawed traditional governance. They removed children from their homes and sent them to boarding schools, where they were brutalized physically, emotionally, and spiritually. Without resources, the people became dependent upon a government that was systematically shaming them into extinction. Poverty, unemployment, alcoholism, suicide, violence, and disease threatened to destroy the people from within. And yet, they persevered. Resistance evolved into a social/political movement that achieved civil rights for Native Americans in 1968 and self-determination in 1975. That movement continues today. Tribes continue to reclaim their heritage (Archambault, 2001), press for justice, and advocate for solutions to social problems borne of oppression (Lomay & Hinkebein, 2006).

The Family

The traditional definition of family among Native Americans differs qualitatively from Western models, and is even rather unique compared with other ethnic expressions of extended family systems (Light & Martin, 1996). Family includes biological (blood) kinship, both nuclear and extended, and social kinship (nonblood) in the home, clan, tribe, and beyond (Lomay & Hinkebein, 2006). Kinship bonds create massive social networks that provide economic, social, and logistical support to family members (Rowley & Rehfeldt, 2002).

Bonds between the individual and family, family and tribe are forged in an often-complex web of ceremonial relationships. Family systems are matriarchal in some tribes (Thomason, 2000) and more patriarchal in others, but the overarching values are interdependence (Red Horse, 1983) and egalitarian, with all roles taking a place of honor in the tribe. Native American women's traditional role is based in the care and nurturance of others (Gilligan, 1993) and the stewardship of culture and tradition (Allen, 1986). They are in charge of childrearing, domestic tasks, and the overall concerns of the family (John, 1988). They wield great power in the home and through the network of family relationships. The role for Native American men is primarily outside of the home as provider for the family and in leadership roles in the clan or tribe, such as medicine man or representative in tribal council. Elders hold a special place of honor in the family and the community. With age come wisdom and the collection of oral history, language, songs, dances, ceremonies, and the personal virtues of patience and generosity. Elders often hold healing positions and other positions of authority earned through their years of experience. Children are the focus of the family and their care and education is largely a communal activity. Aunts and uncles (blood and nonblood) discipline the children. Elders will provide cultural knowledge. Grandfathers teach the young men. Grandmothers teach the young women. Roles are taught by observation, modeling, and practice. History is taught through stories. Children are allowed freedom and discipline tends to be light, so as not to break their spirit. Everything is learned against the backdrop of community and spirituality. While traditional roles are clearly defined, role shift has been common and not stigmatizing.

Religion and Worldview

Native American spirituality is practiced as a way of life, integrated into every aspect and moment of community (Atwood, 1991). There is a supreme creator who has provided the natural world and the life within it. All living things have a spirit and move in a spirit world. Because it is the handiwork of the creator, the world and it spirits are sacred and to be honored accordingly (Lomay & Hinkebein, 2006).

The human condition is threefold: body, mind, and spirit. Together with the natural world, these constitute the anchors of the circle of life, what the Cherokee call the four winds (Dufrene, 1990). The circle metaphor echoes outward through a series of concentric circles represented by the individual spirit, the family/clan, the natural world and the network of relations beyond the clan, and finally the spirit world. As persons move through the circle of life, they seek harmony with their place on the path and their relationship with the world at every level (Garrett & Carroll, 2000). Harmony of individual and tribe is pursued through the observation of complex systems of ceremony, ritual, and instruction and walking, as the Navajo say, in the beauty way. The most important pursuit in life is not the acquisition of things, but the cultivation of relationships. In the Native American worldview, we are all one; connected, interdependent, and responsible for maintaining our own harmony and balance . . . for our own wellbeing, and the wellbeing of the tribe (Locust, 1985). Traditional spirituality and beliefs persist independently for some and in concert with adopted Western, mostly Christian, religion (Lomay & Hinkebein, 2006) for others.

Disability in the Family and Community

The Western concept of disability does not translate well into the Native American worldview. There is often no word equivalent. Its closest interpretation would describe a person who has a limited social network and dysfunctional interpersonal relationships in the community (Locust, 1994; Pichette, Garrett, Kosciulek, & Rosenthal, 1999), or a person who exhibits moral weakness (Rowley & Rehfeldt, 2002). Many conditions that Western thought perceives as disabling are simply functional descriptors. For example, a person diagnosed with Down's syndrome simply "thinks slowly." The tribe is more concerned that the person be supported according to his or her needs and give to the community according to his or her abilities. Where the concept of disability in Western thought immediately focuses on the difference implied by the characteristics of impairment, Native American thought does not. As Locust (1994) points out, ". . . [tribal] life was like a flowing stream, and the disabilities of tribal members merely stones which the water encountered. The water flowed around and over the stones, perhaps rippling a bit here and there, but incorporating the stones within itself and continuing on as before. A stone—or many stones—did not make the running water less a stream" (Locust, 1994, p. 3).

Wellness is harmony in body, spirit, mind, and community. Unwellness is disharmony in the same. Natural unwellness results from the breaking of taboos. Unnatural unwellness is the consequence of malicious manipulation of supernatural forces, that is, sorcery (Locust, 1985). Unwellness can be brought on by bad dreams, gambling, sexual activity, ignoring ceremonies, contact with the dead, or the transgression of ancestors (Rowley & Rehfeldt, 2002). Talking about an illness or disability may cause it or make it worse (Rowley & Rehfeldt, 2002). Mental illness can be caused by the desecration of holy objects. Epilepsy is caused by incest. Mental wellness, posits Gone (2008), is tied to the land, often the reservation, and the constellation of relationships that move upon it. The reservation is part of the person in body and spirit. Leaving the reservation is a struggle with identity (Anderson & Ellis, 1995). Living in two worlds is an existential challenge (Rayle, Chee, & Sand, 2006) that can lead to spiritual unwellness.

Breaking taboos is not necessarily an intentional act; one may be totally unaware of having done so, particularly in the case of congenital disabilities. Pregnant women are admonished to respect a great many taboos, such as stepping over a snake (Hopi), contact with bear scat (Apache), sitting under a tree that has been hit by lightening, witnessing an eclipse, and so on, all of which are thought to cause birth defects (Joe & Miller, 1987). For the child born with a congenital disability, the body is compromised, not the spirit. There is a lack of stigma associated with congenital disabilities. The person born with such a disability is due respect, inasmuch as the spirit had its reasons for choosing to enter the world in this form.

Response

Native American healing is concerned with the "why" of an illness or impairment rather than the "what" (Joe & Miller, 1987). The visionary healer seeks the cause, that is the broken taboo and the offended spirit behind the illness (Locust, 1994). The purpose is to restore balance in body, mind, and spirit. The instrument of healing is the canon of intricate rituals and ceremonies acquired over a lifetime of study (Lomay & Hinkebein, 2006). Native American medicine's priority is not to cure, but to heal. The Western cure assumes a fix that will return one to a previous state. Native American medicine seeks to reestablish balance and harmony under the current circumstances. This results in a different interpretation of the relationship between person and disability. It is possible that behavior judged symptomatic of mental illness in Western medicine may be construed as signs of a vocational (shamanic) calling in Native American medicine (Schacht, 2001). Many who would be labeled with a disability by Western services are absorbed by the Native American culture and never seen. The tribal community takes care of its own in the name of harmony. People with obvious, visible, and severe disabilities are often fully engaged and included in all aspects of community life (Schacht, 2001). For members with severe disabilities, the family finds meaningful work within the community that is within the person's ability. Whatever work is found is enough to provide dignity and a place of honor in the tribe (Joe & Miller, 1987). Invisible disabilities, such as learning disabilities, are greeted with skepticism and distrust. Family often sees the diagnosis of a learning disability as a problem in the school, not in the person . . . or the family (Joe & Miller, 1987). Trepidation in dealing with government service is based in history. State sponsored services can become taboo in and of themselves.

The interface between Western and Native American medicine requires special attention. While it is easy for them to fall into conflict, it has been shown that they can also be integrated into effective service. Traditional healers need to be consulted. Accommodations must be made for the healing ceremonies. In acute care, tribal healers must consider the spiritual ramifications of assistive devices and treatment. Foreign objects have their own energy and spirit. They can disrupt Native American healing rituals, or be disrupted by them. Organ donations, transplants, and other surgical interventions that alter the body can be problematic. The spirit is obliged to return the body as complete as possible to the creator at the end of life. Self-destructive behaviors, such as alcohol abuse, are an affront to this obligation. Heroic life-saving efforts are not a priority in Native American healing. Healing is about balance. Respecting the spirits choice to leave this world is the balanced response; the body dies, the spirit lives on. "Dying with dignity" trumps "life at any cost."

Integration in rehabilitation and recovery is just as important. There is a chasm of distrust that must be recognized and confronted. Counseling and other "helping" organizations have consistently been in the service of assimilation into White culture and interpreting the needs of clients through the prism of Western values. "I'm from the government and I am here to help" is an especially hollow introduction on the reservation. Family members are reticent to approach service providers in issues with children and mental health because the historical consequence was often the removal of the person from the social network, creating disharmony in the person and tribe (Gone, 2008). For those who do come forward, there is an expectation for expert advice, but advice that is informed of the cultural and abides with it. Uncles, aunts, and elders may be actively engaged and expect to be consulted (Garrett & Carroll, 2000). Healing is collaborative and decision-making is deliberative. Words have power. Speaking about the person with a disability from a deficit perspective is counter-productive. Words are chosen carefully to match intent. Unkept promises of any kind are bad medicine. Thus planning is a slow process punctuated by silent contemplative intervals.

The most effective interventions are those that arise from the identity movement and empower the community (Archambault, 2001). For example, substance abuse has been a plague on the reservation since alcohol was introduced by Whites. The 12-step program, with its emphasis on a "higher power" has been effectively adapted to Native American culture (Garrett & Carroll, 2000). This required an interpretation of principles, the editing of a few steps, and a Native American view on alcoholism and its treatment. Native Americans prefer native healers approach to mental illness with or without Western medicine (Marbella, Harris, Diehr, Ignace, & Ignace, 1998).

Cultural competence is important to psychosocial rehabilitation counseling in a multicultural society (Lomay & Hinkebein, 2006). Native American VR is served through tribal VR programs, and is a family-centered affair, linked as they are to the extended family and more distant kinship bonds (Clark & Kelley, 2001). Embracing the customs and history of the tribe, understanding and living within your role, and becoming accepted within the community facilitates service delivery and communication with the tribe. Communication is key. Conflict can come in the simple pace of conversation or the imposition of Western values that derive status and identity out of accomplishment, rather than being valued for your own sake. Respect in communication requires spending time together, rather than being a task to be completed (Marshall, Johnson, & Lonetree, 2001). Problems are best approached indirectly and after appropriate social amenities. Humor is a subtle value and means of communicating among Native Americans; it provides an indirect path to subject matter, teaches through storytelling, and distances people from problems. Certain humorous exchanges (razzing) are part of the role played by extended family members and a sign of closeness played out in the community (Garrett, Garrett, Torres-Rivera, Wilbur, & Roberts-Wilbur, 2005). Rehabilitation efforts focus on the family to identify and marshal resources on behalf of the client (Sanderson, 2001).

CONCLUSION

Disability is experienced in the context of a life, of a family, and of a community. The person experiences disability not simply as an internal state, but in and through familial and community relationships. The culture in which the person is embedded creates the meaning of disability, creates the identity of the individual, and in very real ways, directs what is possible in terms of adjustment and adaptation. The meaning of and response to disability varies widely across cultures, but fundamental themes unite them: Family is the crucible; spirituality is the flame; and the only constant is change.

Family and the Social Support Network

Families are the core context in which the meaning of disability is coined. Although the operational definition of family changes across cultures, what families represent does not. The family is the first support network, from nuclear to extended. A strong support network is a bulwark against life stressors and a resource for the individual. Family is the frame for identity development in terms of the individual and the individual's relationship to the network (collective).

Individualism versus collectivism

Individualism is an orientation of emotional independence from the group, a sense of identity separate from the group, the primacy of personal goals over those of the group (Hofestede, 1983), and behavior directed by internal attitudes rather than group norms (Triandis, Chan, Bhawuk, Iwao, & Sinha, 1995). The "rugged individualism" that is a professed patriotic value is the arch example (Fowler & Wadsworth, 1991; Hofestede, 1983). The collectivist orientation draws its identity from group membership. The goals of the individual are the goals of the group or they are subordinate to the goals of the group. Behavior is governed by group norms. As we have shown, collectivist orientations are often represented in the cultural roots of immigrants and ethnic minorities in the United States. It is important to understand that the difference in these orientations has deep psychological and sociological implications. Collectivist self-esteem and identity are derived from a self-evaluation of one's worthiness as a member of the group and the value of the group to the community (Crocker, Luhtanen, Blaine, & Broadnax, 1994; Luhtanen & Crocker, 1992). The psychological issues that arise in this worldview and the appropriate therapeutic responses are substantively different than those issues arising from a worldview that promotes self-esteem through self-promotion (McCarthy, 2005). Mental illness manifests differently (see Katz et al., 1988; La Roche & Turner, 1997). Collectivist behaviors are less likely to be governed by personal states or traits (Church, 2000; Xie & Leong, 2008). Career choices are motivated by stability rather than self-actualization (Leong, 1991). The meaning of disability shifts in context as a function of the role perception of the person with a disability and the reciprocal expectations of the collective.

We have also seen that the collectivist value is expressed through family outward, and that there is a great deal of latitude in the definition of family across cultures. The nuclear family, with its limited connection to relatives, neighbors, and clan is actually the unusual model, and not a particularly resilient one at that. Extended families are a survival strategy, but they are also a healthy way to live. Extended families, as we have seen, are not necessarily blood and kin, but anyone who is committed to the role. We have seen that the boundary between person, family, and the world is not always clear and that experience with disability tests those boundaries.

Structures that have been created to serve the dominant culture are working off of process and outcome assumptions that may conflict with the collectivist worldview. Consider processes developing vocational goals from a client-centered perspective where "independent" living and "competitive" employment are pursued. At first glance, the language itself is loaded with individualistic meaning. How do we communicate independence in an interdependent world? What is competition in a cooperative? At what point is the family included in the planning process? Where is the community voice in the decision making? How does one generate employment options around stability rather than interest? Rehabilitation and career counseling need not work at cross-purposes or be misunderstood. In fact, counseling as a whole appears to be rather adaptable across settings (Lee & Kelly, 1996), as long as the counselor understands the collectivist perspective, recognizes its influence, and responds accordingly.

Spirituality and Religion

Spirituality is a uniquely human characteristic. We are unified in our need for organizing principles that bring order to the world. Religion and ritual are artifacts of fundamental spiritual beliefs that tell us who we are, what is required of us, and what shall become of us in the end. Religion interprets disability in the community according to its values and creates its own response. Where disability is God's will, the response is forbearance. Where disability is punishment for past sin, the response is atonement. Where disability is a gift, the response is celebration. Where disability disappears, the response is simply to live. Religious practices are the means by which individuals are included in community. The religious space is sanctifying and unifying. Out of faith comes teaching and sharing of values. Service to the community includes charity, support groups, and professional counseling or visionary healing.

History and Change

The only constant in the human condition is change. Tradition is the current interpretation of a history to which new events accrue everyday. As much as we try to preserve, everything evolves. At one point in time Korea did not have a written language. Feeling the need, one was engineered at the behest of the emperor, and a new tradition emerged. Trade among Native American tribes spanned the continent for thousands of years before the European invasion, and with trade came confluence. The Cultural Revolution in Communist China banned Confucianism, sought to supplant the traditional authority of family elders with the state, enforced "one child" families, and separated family members for years. The recent economic boom in China has brought westernized ideas and urbanization to the family structure. As a result, there is no "typical" Chinese family, even in China (Lee, 1996).

To understand the differences in ethnicity even within the group, you need to understand their shared history. Every ethnic group discussed, save one, migrated to this country in the relatively recent past, and the history of their immigration provides the narrative that describes their ethnicity and their ethnic heritage.

Becoming a minority

In reviewing the people's history, there is an unfortunate theme of ethnic oppression informing many minority cultural narratives, and a disturbing level of American culpability in what are at heart crimes against humanity. The history that creates minority experience does not go away, it simply folds into the next generation. Diabetes and alcoholism were not part of the Native American experience prior to contact with Europeans. Now they beget blindness, amputation, stroke, fetal alcohol syndrome, domestic violence, and suicide. As Native American culture defines itself in response to this legacy, their response becomes part of the new tradition. African American mistrust in the expertise of psychologists is well earned. The Civil Rights Movement has become part of the new tradition and the African American narrative. Self-determination is a theme in the ever-evolving definition of culture. The elephant in the room, as Horsman, Rodriguez, and Marini (2009) point out, is that a relatively new tradition and earmark of minority cultures is learned distrust of authority figures within the dominant culture and a general distrust of White people. The experience of disability within each culture is interpreted through the lens of this minority identity, this need to resist and affirm.

Acculturation/enculturation

The cultural roots we reviewed exist now in communion with each other and with the dominant popular culture . . . and through this communion, they are inevitably changing. There are two concepts to understand here. Acculturation is the adaptation of indigenous culture patterns to the norms of the dominant culture. Enculturation is the process by which people learn and maintain their indigenous culture (Cokely & Helm, 2007) within the framework of the dominant culture (Kim & Abreu, 2001). Thinking of these as dimensions of adjustment, we can imagine four developmental directions: (a) Assimilation (high acculturation, low enculturation) is complete identification with the dominant culture to the exclusion of the indigenous; (b) Integration (high acculturation, high enculturation) is the ability to "walk in two worlds" (Diemer, 2007) comfortably, to find a way to maintain the indigenous identity and values while often living in the other; (c) Separation (low acculturation, high enculturation) is an active rejection of the dominant, often by physically sequestering in enclaves or reservations, (d) Marginalization (low acculturation, low enculturation) is the loss of the traditional and failure to assimilate (Berry, 1980; Rudmin, 2003). How a person experiences disability in her life and how disability interfaces with the family and community depends upon the quality of the community response to these social dynamics. The issues of disability identity are different for Native Americans than they are for African Americans, Hispanics, or Asian Americans, and as we have shown they are different within groups as well. They are also different across generations even within immigrant families as they continue to evolve and adapt.

REFERENCES

Abraido-Lanza, A. F., Vasquez, E., & Echeverria, S. E. (2004). En las manos de Dios [in God's hands]: Religious and other forms of coping among Latinos with arthritis. *Journal of Consulting and Clinical Psychology, 72,* 91–102.

Allen, P. G. (1986). *The sacred hoop.* Boston, MA: Beacon Press.

Alvidrez, J. (1999). Ethnic variations in mental health attitudes and service use among low-income African American, Latina, and European American young women. *Community Mental Health Journal, 35,* 515–530.

Alvarez, L. R., & Ruiz, P. (2001). Substance abuse in the Mexican American population. In S. L. A. Straussner (Ed.), *Ethnocultural factors in substance abuse treatment* (pp. 111–139). New York, NY: Guilford Press.

Anderson, M. J., & Ellis, R. (1995). On the reservation. In N. A. Vace, S. B. DeVaney, & J. Wittmer (Eds.), *Experiencing and counseling multicultural and diverse populations* (3rd ed., pp. 179–198). Bristol, PA: Accelerated Development.

Archambault, J. (2001). Sun dance. In R. DeMallie (Ed.), *Handbook of North American Indians* (Vol. 13, pp. 983–995). Washington, DC: Smithsonian Institution.

Arthur, C. (2002). *In focus: Haiti.* New York: Interlink Books.

Atkinson, D. R. (2004). *Counseling American minorities* (6th ed.). Boston, MA: McGraw-Hill.

Atwood, M. D. (1991). *Spirit healing: Native American magic and medicine.* New York, NY: Sterling Publishing.

Batres, E. G. (2001). *Providing rehabilitation to persons from El Salvador* [Monograph]. Buffalo, NY: Center for International Rehabilitation Research Information & Exchange.

Berry, J. W. (1980). Acculturation as varieties of adaptation. In A. Padilla (Ed.), *Acculturation: Theory, models, and some new findings* (pp. 9–25). Boulder, CO: Westview.

Boff, L., & Boff, C. (1987). *Introducing liberation theology.* Maryknoll, NY: Orbis Books.

Boyd-Franklin, N. (2003). *Black families in therapy: Understanding the African-American experience.* New York, NY: Guilford Press.

Brandes, S. (1997). Sugar, colonialism, and death: On the origins of Mexico's day of the dead. *Comparative Studies in Sociology and History, 39,* 270–299.

Breeding, R. R., Rogers, J. B., Harley, D. A., & Crystal, R. M. (2005). The Kentucky migrant vocational rehabilitation program: A demonstration project for working with Hispanic farm workers. *Journal of Rehabilitation, 71*(1), 32–41.

Brice, A. (2002). *An introduction to Cuban culture for rehabilitation service providers* [Monograph]. Buffalo, NY: Center for International Rehabilitation Research Information & Exchange.

Chan, S. (1998). Families with Asian roots. In E. W. Lynch & M. J. Hanson (Eds.), *Developing cross-cultural competence* (pp. 251–355). Baltimore, MD: Paul H. Brookes.

Christopher, M. S., Skillman, G. D., Kirkhart, M. W., & D'Souza, J. B. (2006). The effect of normative and behavioral persuasion on help seeking in Thai and American college students. *Journal of Multicultural Counseling and Development, 34,* 80–93.

Church, A. T. (2000). Culture and personality: Toward an integrated cultural trait psychology. *Journal of Personality, 69,* 651–703.

Churchill, W. (1998). *A little matter of genocide: Holocaust and denial in the Americas, 1492 to the present.* San Francisco, CA: City Lights Books.

Clark, S., & Kelley, S. D. M. (2001). Traditional Native American values: Conflict or concordance in rehabilitation? *Journal of Rehabilitation, 58*(2), 23–27.

Cokely, K., & Helm, K. (2007). The relationship between African American enculturation and racial identity. *Journal of Multicultural Counseling and Development, 35,* 142–153.

Cooper, L. A., Gonzales, J. J., Gallo, J. J., Rost, K. M., Meredith, L. S., Rubenstein, L. V., et al. (2003). The acceptability of treatment for depression among African-American, Latino and White primary care physicians. *Medical Care, 41,* 479–489.

Crocker, J., Luhtanen, R., Blaine, B., & Broadnax, S. (1994). Collective self-esteem and psychological well-being among White, Black, and Asian college students. *Personality and Social Psychology Bulletin, 20,* 503–513.

De Paula, T., Lagana, K., & Gonzalez-Ramirez, L. (1996). Mexican Americans. In J. G. Lipson, S. L. Dibble, & P. A. Minarik (Eds.), *Culture & nursing care* (pp. 203–221). San Francisco, CA: UCSF Nursing Press.

De Torres, S. (2002). *Understanding persons of Philippine origins: A primer for rehabilitation service providers* [Monograph]. Buffalo, NY: Center for International Rehabilitation Research Information & Exchange.

Diemer, M. A. (2007). Two worlds: African American men's negotiation of predominatly White educational and occupational worlds. *Journal of Multicultural Counseling and Development, 35,* 2–14.

Dufrene, P. M. (1990). Exploring Native American symbolism. *Journal of Multicultural and Cross-Cultural Research in Art Education, 8,* 38–50.

Edwards, A., & Polite, C. K. (1992). *Children of the dream: The psychology of Black success.* New York, NY: Doubleday.

Falicov, C. J. (1998). *Latino families in therapy: A guide to multicultural practice.* New York, NY: Guilford Press.

Ferguson, T. M., Leach, M. M., Levy, J. J., Nicholson, B. C., & Johnson, J. D. (2008). Influences on counselors race preferences: Distinguishing Black racial attitudes from Black racial identity. *Journal of Multicultural Counseling and Development, 36,* 66–76.

Fowler, C. A., & Wadsworth, J. S. (1991). Individualism and equality: Critical values in North American culture and the impact on disability. *Journal of Applied Rehabilitation Counseling, 22,* 19–23.

Garrett, M. T. (1999). Understanding the "medicine" of American Indian traditional values: An integrative review. *Counseling and Values, 43,* 122–131.

Garrett, M. T., & Carroll, J. J. (2000). Mending the broken circle: Treatment of substance dependency among Native Americans. *Journal of Counseling & Development, 78,* 379–388.

Garrett, M. T., Garrett, J. T., Torres-Rivera, E., Wilbur, M., & Roberts-Wilbur, J. (2005). Laughing it up: Native American humor as spiritual tradition. *Journal of Multicultural Counseling and Development, 33,* 194–204.

Garrett, M. T., & Herring, R. D. (2001). Honoring the power of relation: Counseling native adults. *Journal of Humanistic Counseling, Education, and Development, 40,* 139–160.

Gilligan, C. (1993). *In a different voice.* Cambridge, MA: Harvard University Press.

Glover, N. M., & Blankenship, C. J. (2007). Mexican and Mexican Americans' beliefs about God in relation to disability. *Journal of Rehabilitation, 73*(4), 41–50.

Gone, J. P. (2008). 'So I can be like a whiteman': The cultural psychology of space and place in American Indian mental health. *Culture Psychology, 14,* 369–399.

Gordon, E., Minnes, P., & Holden, R. (1990). The structure of attitudes towards persons with a disability, when specific disability and context are considered. *Rehabilitation Psychology, 35,* 79–90.

Graf, N. M., Blankenship, C. J., Sanchez, G., & Carlson, R. (2007). Living on the line: Mexican and Mexican American attitudes towards disability. *Rehabilitation Counseling Bulletin, 50,* 153–165.

Hahn, H. (1988). The politics of physical differences: Disability and discrimination. *Journal of Social Issues, 44*(1), 39–47.

Hampton, N. Z., Yeung, T., & Nguyen, C. H. (2007). Perceptions of mental illness and rehabilitation services in Chinese and Vietnamese Americans. *Journal of Applied Rehabilitation Counseling, 38*(2), 14–23.

Hanline, M. F., & Daley, S. E. (1992). Family coping strategies and strengths in Hispanic, African-American, and Caucasian families of young children. *Topics in Early Childhood Special Education, 12,* 351–366.

Hays, P. A. (2008). *Addressing complexities in practice—Assessment, diagnosis, and therapy* (2nd ed.). Washington, DC: American Psychological Corporation.

Henderson, S. J., & Chan, A. (2005). Career happiness among Asian Americans: The interplay between individualism and interdependence. *Journal of Multicultural Counseling and Development, 33,* 180–192.

Hershenson, D. B. (2000). Toward a cultural anthropology of disability and rehabilitation. *Rehabilitation Counseling Bulletin, 43*(3), 150–157.

Ho, M. K. (1984). Social group work with Asian/Pacific Americans. *Ethnicity in Group Work Practice, 7,* 49–61.

Hoffstede, G. (1983). National cultures revisited. *Behavior Science Research, 18,* 285–305.

Horsman, E. N., Rodriguez, V. J., & Marini, I. (2009). The elephant in the room: Cultural distrust directed at white counselors. In I. Marini & M. A. Stebnicki (Eds.), *The Professional Counselor's Desk Reference* (pp. 185–198). New York, NY: Springer.

Hunt, P. C. (2002). *An introduction to Vietnamese culture for rehabilitation service providers in the U. S.* [Monograph]. Buffalo, NY: Center for International Rehabilitation Research Information & Exchange.

Jacobson, E. (2003). *An introduction to Haitian culture for rehabilitation service providers* [Monograph]. Buffalo, NY: Center for International Rehabilitation Research Information & Exchange.

Joe, R. E., & Miller, D. (Eds.). (1987). *American Indian cultural perspectives on disability* (pp. 3–23). Tucson, AZ: University of Arizona, Native American Research and Training Center.

John, R. (1988). The Native American family. In C. Mindel, R. Habenstein, & R. Wright, Jr. (Eds.), *Ethnic families in America: Patterns and variations* (pp. 325–363). Englewood Cliffs, NJ: Prentice-Hall.

Katz, M. M., Marsella, A., Dube, K. C., Olatawura, M., Takahashi, R., Nakane, Y. et al. (1988). On the expression of psychosis in different cultures: Schizophrenia in an Indian and in a Nigerian community (A report form the World Health Organization Project on determinants of outcome of severe mental health disorders). *Culture, Medicine, and Psychiatry, 12*, 331–355.

Kemp, C. (2005). *Mexican & Mexican-Americans: Health beliefs & practices.* Retrieved September 11, 2010, from http://bearspace.baylor.edu/Charles_Kemp/www/hispanic_health.htm

Kim, B. S. K., & Abreu, J. M. (2001). Acculturation measurement: Theory, current instruments, and future directions. In J. G. Ponterotto, J. M. Casas, L. A. Suzuki, & C. M. Alexander (Eds.), *Handbook of multicultural counseling* (2nd ed., pp. 394–424). Thousand Oaks, CA: Sage.

Kim, B. S. K., Atkinson, D. R., & Yang, P. H. (1999). The Asian values scale: Development, factor analysis, validation, and reliability. *Journal of Counseling Psychology, 46*, 342–352.

Kim-Rupnow, W. S. (2001). *An introduction to Korean culture for rehabilitation service providers.* [Monograph]. Buffalo, NY: Center for International Rehabilitation Research Information & Exchange.

La Roche, M. J., & Turner, C. (1997). Self-orientation and depression level among Dominicans in the United States. *Hispanic Journal of Behavioral Sciences, 19*, 479–488.

Lafitte, J. (1983). Counseling and the rehabilitation process. In *The special rehabilitation and research needs of disabled Hispanic persons* (pp. 51–58). Edinburg, TX: National Institute of Handicapped Research and President's Committee on Employment of the Handicapped.

Lam, C. S., Tsang, H., Chan, F., & Corrigan, P. W. (2006). Chinese and American perspectives on stigma. *Rehabilitation Education, 20*(4), 269–279.

Lee, E. (1996). Chinese families. In M. McGoldrick, J. Giordano, & J. Pearce (Eds.), *Ethnicity family therapy* (2nd ed., pp. 248–267). New York, NY: Guilford Press.

Lee, I. J., & Kelly, E. W., Jr. (1996). Individualistic and collective group counseling: Effects with Korean clients. *Journal of Multicultural Counseling & Development, 24*, 254–266.

Lee, W. M. L., Blando, J. A., Mizelle, N. D., & Orozco, G. L. (Eds.). (2007). *Introduction to multicultural counseling for helping professionals* (2nd ed.). New York, NY: Routledge.

Leavitt, R. L. (1992). *Disability and rehabilitation in rural Jamaica.* London, UK: Associated University Press.

Leong, F. T. L. (1991). Career development attributes and occupational values of Asian American and White American college students. *The Career Development Quarterly, 39*, 221–230.

Light, H. K., & Martin, R. E. (1996). American Indian families. *Journal of American Indian Education, 26*(1). Retrieved January 2, 2010, from http://jaie.asu.edu/v26/V26S1ame.htm

Liu, G. Z. (2001). *Chinese culture and disability: Information for U.S. service providers.* [Monograph]. Buffalo, NY: Center for International Rehabilitation Research Information & Exchange.

Livneh, H. (1988). A dimensional perspective on the origin of negative attitudes towards persons with disabilities. In H. E. Yuker (Ed.), *Attitudes towards persons with disabilities* (pp. 35–46). New York, NY: Springer.

Locust, C. S. (1985). *American Indian concepts concerning health and unwellness.* Monograph Series. Tucson, AZ: Native American Research and Training Center. NIDRR, USDOE (g00830094).

Locust, C. S. (1994). *The piki maker: Disabled American Indians, cultural beliefs, and traditional behaviors.* Monograph Series. Tucson, AZ: Native American Research and Training Center. NIDRR, USDOE (h133B30058).

Lomay, V. T., & Hinkebein, J. H. (2006). Cultural considerations when providing rehabilitation services to American Indians. *Rehabilitation Psychology, 51*(1), 36–42.

Lopez-De Fede, A., & Haeussler-Fiore, D. (2002). *An introduction to the culture of the Dominican Republic for rehabilitation service providers* [Monograph]. Buffalo, NY: Center for International Rehabilitation Research Information & Exchange.

Luhtanen, R., & Crocker, J. (1992). A collective self-esteem scale: Self-evaluation of one's social identity. *Personality and Social Bulletin, 18*, 302–318.

Marbella, A. M., Harris, M. C., Diehr, S., Ignace, G., & Ignace, G. (1998). Use of Native American healers among Native American Patients in an Urban Native American health center. *Archive of Family Medicine, 7*, 182–185.

Marinelli, R. P., & Dell Orto, A. E. (1999). *The psychological and social impact of disability.* New York, NY: Springer.

Marshall, C. A., Johnson, S., & Lonetree, G. (2001). Acknowledging our diversity: Vocational rehabilitation and American Indians. In C. A. Marshall (Ed.), *Rehabilitation and American Indians with disabilities: A handbook for administrators, practitioners, and researchers* (pp. 85–99). Athens, GA: Elliot & Fitzpatrick.

Matthews, A. K., Corrigan, P. W., Smith, B. M., & Aranda, F. (2006). A qualitative exploration of African-Americans' attitudes toward mental illness and mental illness treatment seeking. *Rehabilitation Education, 20*(4), 253–268.

McCarthy, J. (2005). Individualism and collectivism: What do they have to do with counseling? *Journal of Multicultural Counseling and Development, 33*, 108–117.

Melendy, H. B. (1972). *The Oriental Americans.* New York, NY: Hippocrene Books.

Michailakis, D. (2003). The system theory concept of disability: One is not born a disabled person, one is observed to be one. *Disability & Society, 18*(2), 209–229.

Miller, D. (2002). *An introduction to Jamaican culture for rehabilitation service providers.* [Monograph]. Buffalo, NY: Center for International Rehabilitation Research Information & Exchange.

Molina, C., Zambrana, R., & Aguirre-Molina, M. (1994). The influence of culture, class and environment on health care. In C. Molina & M. Aguirre-Molina (Eds.), *Latino health in the US: A growing challenge* (pp. 23–43). Washington, DC: American Public Health Association.

Monteith, M. J., & Spicer, V. C. (2000). Contents and correlates of Whites' and Blacks' racial attitudes. *Journal of Experimental Social Psychology, 36*, 125–154.

Phan, L. T., Rivera, E. T., & Roberts-Wilbur, J. (2005). Understanding Vietnamese refugee women's identity development from a sociopolitical and historical perspective. *Journal of Counseling & Development, 83*, 305–312.

Pichette, E. F., Garrett, M. T., Kosciulek, J. F., & Rosenthal, D. (1999). Cultural identification of American Indians and its impact on rehabilitation services. *Journal of Rehabilitation, 35*, 3–9.

Pinto, P. E., & Sahu, N. (2001). *Working with persons with disabilities: An Indian perspective.* [Monograph]. Buffalo, NY: Center for International Rehabilitation Research Information & Exchange.

Poole, S. (1996). *Our lady of Guadalupe: The origins and sources of a Mexican national symbol, 1531–1797.* Tucson, AZ: University of Arizona Press.

Rayle, A. D., Chee, C., & Sand, J. K. (2006). Honoring their way: Counseling American Indian women. *Journal of Multicultural Counseling and Development, 34*, 66–79.

Red Horse, J. (1983). Indian family values and experiences. In G. J. Powell (Ed.), *The psychosocial development of minority group children* (pp. 258–271). New York, NY: Brunner/Mazel.

Rivera, O. A. (1983). Vocational rehabilitation process and Hispanic culture. In *The special rehabilitation and research needs of disabled Hispanic persons* (pp. 39–41). Edinburg, TX: National Institute of Handicapped Research and President's Committee on Employment of the Handicapped.

Robinson, T. L., & Howard-Hamilton, M. (1994). An African-American paradigm: Foundation for a healthy self-image and healthy interpersonal relationships. *Journal of Mental Health Counseling, 16*(3), 327–339.

Rowley, D., & Rehfeldt, R. A. (2002). Delivering human services to native Americans with disabilities: Cultural variables & service recommendations. *North American Journal of Psychology, 4*(2), 309–316.

Rudmin, F. W. (2003). Critical history of the acculturation psychology of assimilation, separation, integration, and marginalization. *Review of General Psychology, 7*, 3–37.

Ruiz, R. A., & Padilla, A. M. (1977). Counseling Latinos. *The Personnel and Guidance Journal, 55*, 401–408.

Salas-Provance, M., Erickson, J. G., & Reed, J. (2002). Disability as viewed by four generations of one Hispanic family. *American Journal of Speech-Language Pathology, 11*, 151–162.

Sanderson, P. L. (2001). American Indians: An overview of factors influencing health care, disability, and service delivery. In C. A. Marshall (Ed.), *Rehabilitation and American Indians with disabilities: A handbook for administrators, practitioners, and researchers* (pp. 27–41). Athens, GA: Elliot & Fitzpatrick.

Schacht, R. M. (2001). Engaging anthropology in disability studies: American Indian issues. *Disability Studies Quarterly, 21*(3), 17–36.

Shakespeare, T., & Watson, N. (1997). Defending the social model. *Disability & Society, 12*(2), 293–300.

Shorris, E. (1992). *Latinos: A biography of the people.* New York, NY: W. W. Norris.

Smart, J. F. (2009). *Disability, society, and the individual* (2nd ed.). Austin, TX: ProEd.

Smart, J. F., & Smart, D. W. (1991). Acceptance of disability and the Mexican-American culture. *Rehabilitation Counseling Bulletin, 34*, 357–367.

Snowden, L. R. (2001). Barriers to effective mental health services for African Americans. *Mental Health Services Research, 3*(4), 181–187.

Sue, D. W., & Sue, D. (1999). *Counseling the culturally different: Theory and practice.* New York, NY: John Wiley & Sons.

Szymanski, E. M., & Trueba, H. T. (1994). Castification of people with disabilities: Potential disempowering aspects of classification in disability services. *Journal of Rehabilitation, 60*(3), 12–20.

Thomason, T. C. (2000). Counseling American Indians: An introduction for non-American Indian counselors. *Journal of Counseling & Development, 69*, 321–327.

Trevino, B., & Szymanski, E. M. (1996). A qualitative study of the career development of Hispanics with disabilities. *Journal of Rehabilitation, 62*(3), 5–13.

Triandis, H. C. (1971). *Attitude and attitude change.* New York, NY: John Wiley.

Triandis, H. C., Chan, D. K. S., Bhawuk, D. P. S., Iwao, S., & Sinha, J. B. P. (1995). Multimethod probes of allocentrism and idiocentrism. *International Journal of Psychology, 30*, 461–480.

Trimble, J. E., Fleming, C. M., Beauvais, F., & Jumper-Thurman, P. (1996). Essential cultural and social strategies for counseling Native American Indians. In P. B. Pedersen, J. G. Draguns, W. J. Lonner, & J. E. Trimble (Eds.), *Counseling across cultures* (4th ed., pp. 177–209). Thousand Oaks, CA: Sage Publications.

Turner, W. L., & Alston, R. J. (1994). The role of the family in psychosocial adaptation to physical disabilities for African Americans. *Journal of the National Medical Association, 86*(12), 915–921.

Vega, W. A., Kolody, B., & Aguilar-Gaxiola, S. (2001). Help seeking for mental health problems among Mexican Americans. *Journal of Immigrant Health, 3*, 133–140.

Vera, E. M., & Conner, W. (2007). Latina mothers' perceptions of mental health and mental health promotion. *Journal of Multicultural Counseling and Development, 35*, 230–242.

Wang, M. H., Chan, F., Thomas, K. R., Lin, S. H., & Larson, P. (1997). Coping style and personal responsibility as factors in the perception of individuals with physical disabilities by Chinese international students. *Rehabilitation Psychology, 42*(4), 302–316.

Weisman, A. G., (2000). Religion: A mediator of Anglo-American and Mexican attributional differences towards symptoms of schizophrenia? *Journal of Nervous & Mental Disease, 188*, 616–621.

Whaley, A. L. (2001). Cultural Mistrust: An important psychological construct for diagnosis and treatment of Black Americans. *Professional Psychology: Research and Practice, 32*, 555–562.

Wilson, K. B. (2005). Cultural characteristics of the African American community. In D. A. Harley, & J. M. Dillard (Eds.), *Contemporary mental health issues among African Americans* (pp. 32–52). Alexandria, VA: American Counseling Association.

Wong, F., & Halgin, R. (2006). The "model minority: Bane or blessing for Asian Americans? *Journal of Multicultural Counseling and Development, 34*, 38–49.

Wright, B. (1988). Attitudes and the fundamental negative bias: Conditions and corrections. In H. E. Yuker (Ed.), *Attitudes toward persons with disabilities* (pp. 3–21). New York, NY: Springer.

Xie, D., & Leong, F. T. L. (2008). A cross-cultural study of anxiety among Chinese and Caucasian American university students. *Journal of Multicultural Counseling and Development, 36*, 52–63.

Yip, A. (1997). Remembering Vincent Chin. *Asian Week, 18*(43). Retrieved September 25, 2010, from http://www.asianweek.com/061397/feature.html

Zavaleta, A. N. (2000). *Do cultural factors affect Hispanic health status?* Retrieved January 5, 2011, from http://vpea.utb.edu/elnino/researcharticles/doculturalfactorsaffect.html

Zhang, A. Y., Snowden, L. R., & Sue, S. (1998). Differences between Asian- and White-Americans' help-seeking and utilization patterns in the Los Angeles area. *Journal of Community Psychology, 26*, 317–326.

INSIDER PERSPECTIVE
The Story of Elvia Susana Prieto Armendariz

I was born on a hot Tuesday morning on May 20, 1986, in Gomez Palacio, Durango, Mexico, a small city about 5 minutes west of Torreon, Coahuila, Mexico, the city where all my family lives and where I grew up. I am the second child in the family, and at that time I was the first girl to be born on my dad's side of the family. My mom did not know she was having a girl, much less, that I was missing part of my left hand. At that time getting an ultrasound was not as common as it is now, so she only had regular checkups with the doctor. Being a nurse, and a mom for the second time, she knew what precautions to take. For that reason, the idea of having a child with a disability never occurred to her. Everybody was excited after I was born. The family was complete, with both a boy and a girl.

I remember asking my mom years later how she felt when she and my dad noticed that I was missing my left hand. She told me that they both cried, but at the same time thought that that was not a good reason to treat me differently than my brother. I was also born with eleven toes. The eleventh toe grew next to the small toe on my right foot but was surgically removed days after I was born. The doctors gave my parents the option of running some tests to find out what went wrong as I developed, but they chose not to do it. My mom spent much of the pregnancy in the operating room (OR) carrying out her nursing duties. One hypothesis the doctors stated was that the chemicals used in the OR had affected my development. My parents chose not to investigate further, so they are not sure whether or not this caused my birth defect. They already loved me as much as they loved my brother and did not see a point to having us go through the stress of such an investigation. My mom was depressed for some time and even felt guilty. Both of my parents spoke to a Priest and were told that they had to raise me just as my brother and teach me how to be independent. There was no reason why they should keep me at home and not expose me to the outside world because that would only create a heavy depression for me as well.

My family is a very traditional Mexican family, and I was raised to look up to my parents, grandparents, uncles, and any other older person. I was taught to obey them, be respectful to everyone in and out of the family, and to get along with my brother. My dad has a strong character, and sometimes I was even afraid of him. My mom is more laid back and of course very nurturing. There were times when I asked them why this happened to me. Of course, they did not have a medical explanation, but they always told me that that was how God wanted me to be and that it would serve a purpose within God's plan for my life. Fortunately, they tried to give both my brother and me the same opportunities, and I was put in the same school my brother was attending. It was a bilingual school where English is taught from preschool to 12th grade, and I got all my education from that school. My parents were worried that the administrators were going to reject me so they told the principal that my disability was not an impediment for me to be in the same school as my brother.

I don't remember if my classmates rejected me, although I am pretty sure it was the first time they had seen a girl who was physically different. I can say that I was one of the few students in the entire school with a physical difference, probably the only one. I was very outgoing, not shy at all, but I remember having only one good friend throughout preschool and the first years of elementary. As I started getting more involved and surrounded by other kids, I began to realize that things were not going to be as good as my young mind had envisioned. There were days when I would wait for my dad to pick me up from school, and several girls would stand in front of me saying things to each other about my missing hand. When I would attempt to hit a piñata or even just go to the park, other kids would stare and say things to each other about me. It sometimes made me feel like I was a stranger. Because I had not met another kid like me, I often thought that I was the only person in the world that was missing a hand. At other times when kids would say things, I would feel like going up to them and telling them that there was nothing wrong with me and that it was just how I was born. I would tell my parents that kids were saying things to me and they would say just to ignore them.

When I was in second grade I made a trip with my family to Houston, TX, where I was going to receive a prosthesis. I was really excited because for the first time I was going to experience what it felt like to have both complete arms, even though one would not be real. My parents were excited too because they knew it was going to allow me to do more things without depending too much on them, but at the same time it was going to be something new to which all of us would have to adapt. At the hospital, I was not given the opportunity to choose which prosthesis would be best for me. All I was able to tell the doctors was that I wanted one that would look like my right hand and never went to a psychologist for help in adapting to the prosthesis.

After several weeks in Houston learning how to use the prosthesis, I returned to Mexico happier than ever, unaware of the struggles that I was going to face. Other people would notice more that I had a fake hand, they would stare more, and a year later I lost the only "friend" I had. She abandoned me without any explanation aside from saying that she didn't want to be my friend anymore. Now I had to struggle to make new friends. From being an outgoing and confident girl I became shyer, more reserved, less outgoing, and I no longer wanted to wear the prosthesis. There were several occasions when I would fight with my parents because I didn't want to wear the prosthesis to school. I was more self-conscious of what others would say about my hand, so I would always try to cover it with my right hand. There were nights when I would cry until I fell asleep asking God why I was going through that. I would even ask him to allow me to wake up the next day with the part of my hand that I was missing. I later established a good friendship with another of my classmates, and until now I can say that she is my best friend. She didn't reject me and I never heard her say she felt embarrassed when we were together.

At home, my parents and grandparents gave me the same treatment as my brother and cousins. If I would get in trouble, there was no difference in my punishment. I never heard my parents tell me not to try something because my disability would impede it. I learned how to ride a bicycle with one hand, how to get on swings, I took swimming classes, I was in gymnastics and somehow I learned how to do the flips and turns with one hand. I was also in ballet and soccer. I learned how to drive, and the last thing I did was Hawaiian dance. I am grateful that I was given every opportunity to be a normal girl and experience a normal childhood. My parents never spoke about me as a person with a disability, and they certainly never treated me like one. This helped me understand that I had to give up saying that I could not do something I wanted to do before making the effort and trying it. Some activities were difficult to adapt to my needs, but in the end I knew nothing was impossible. My parents taught me to be the only one who set the limits as to what I wanted to do and never give up because they knew I would always find a way to accomplish what I wanted.

Even though I was able to participate in as many activities as I wanted and my parents were able to pay for them, there were occasions when I felt overprotected. I felt this way most during my adolescence. For example, I wanted to spend more time out at quinceañeras or get together with my friends. My dad would tell me he was worried that other people, guys and girls, would take advantage of me after seeing that I could probably not defend myself because of my disability. That is also the time when I felt like my brother was given more freedom, and I had to struggle more to get permission to go out. I think that in Mexican culture as how my parents were raised, it was not right or proper for a girl to be out partying late at night, and because of my disability they worried even more. My dad didn't even let me ask a guy to be my dance partner for my 15th birthday party because he said a girl should not ask a guy out, it's the guy who is supposed to do it. For that occasion and my high school graduation party, my brother was my dance partner, and I had no other choice. Through these years I felt that because my dad was not letting me meet guys, there was no one out there who would want to marry me because of the stigma people with disabilities have. Later I learned this was a misconception I had. Indeed, there would be someone who would see past my physical difference. I allowed this person to get close to me and to know me just as I am. He has been very accepting, but he has also helped me to see in what ways I can improve and grow as a person. He stayed by me in some of my toughest moments helping me to overcome my fears of failure and pushing me forward.

I have noticed that in Mexico people with disabilities are often portrayed as being unable to defend themselves. On TV, they are usually shown in such a way that the viewers see them with pity and feel sorry for them. Women with disabilities are seen as having fewer opportunities to move forward and succeed in life. I can say that women with a disability that live in small communities outside the city most likely stay home, remain uneducated, and do not receive the appropriate services. Families also feel shame about exposing them and do not allow them to integrate into society. Women with severe disabilities are neither seen on the streets nor receive an education. The families are scared to let them be part of society because they believe they are sick and should remain at home. Right now there is still much discrimination directed at people with disabilities in Mexico. They are seen as weaker people by the rest of society. There are places where therapy and other services are provided, but basically you need to prove that you don't have any resources to pay for them, otherwise you have to pay everything out of your pocket. For example, if I wanted to get a new prosthesis I would need to pay the full price because there is no such thing as Medicaid, Medicare, or services such as the ones provided by public vocational rehabilitation that would help cover all or even part of the cost.

As I was growing up, I was able to realize that missing a hand was not really a big problem. I am basically able to do as much as anybody else, and I always find some way to accomplish even those things that I struggle to do. Even now when I am doing something like, for example, opening a can, I don't feel comfortable asking someone for help, even though I struggle holding the can opener. My mom used to help me with my hair, too, but now I also feel uncomfortable when she helps me because I've learned to do it by myself. I know life is full of obstacles good and bad, but I cannot let myself down. I must keep moving forward because I always had my parents', grandparents', brothers', and friends' support, and I always knew I could achieve as highly as I wanted. They all somehow helped to provide me with the motivation I needed during hard times. Seeing them strong and not treating me with pity, I was, and still am inspired to work hard. Without their positive way of thinking, which was passed on to me, I don't think I could have made it through elementary, junior high, high school, and college.

It was difficult as everything in life is, but I always had a dream in my mind. I wanted to get to the day where I would walk to get my diploma with a good education in my hands. Because of the way I was born and raised, I felt that I wanted to be in a field where I could help others and be seen as an example of success. I want other people with disabilities to see that just because they are missing a part of their body or because they acquired a disability, they must not let themselves down. There is always a way to adapt our lives according to what we want to do. How much we will accomplish is ultimately up to us. Graduating with a bachelor's degree in rehabilitative services from the University of Texas Pan-American in Edinburg, TX, was my dream come true. At first, my parents were hesitant to let me move away from my country but realized and understood that at some point I had to leave the nest. They were happy to see me fulfilling my dream, but I knew that a bachelor's degree wasn't enough. Right after graduating I got accepted into the master's in rehabilitation counseling program at the same university. I am in the field I always dreamed to be in, and I am receiving much education and knowledge from my professors. I have faced many difficulties and in the past. There were days when I would call my parents crying because I felt like I couldn't make it. My family was always there for me providing unconditional support and always knew that college would not be an obstacle I could not overcome. My parents gave me and my brother as many tools as they could for us to be successful, and I will always be grateful for all the efforts they made. Without their support, I don't think I could have made it through college in the United States.

After graduating with my master's degree, I hope to work with people who have had amputations or who were born with conditions similar to mine. I want to assist them through the adaptation process and also work with them to accept their disability. I would also want to help them adjust if they are given a prosthesis or help them find resources to pay for one. I don't know if I can stay in the United States because of my student visa, but even if I return to Mexico, I can take that as an opportunity to give back to my people. As I have said, there is a great need for services for people with disabilities, especially those with physical disabilities. Wherever I decide to stay, I know that I am going to succeed. My parents raised me to be a strong woman and have given me the best tools to succeed in life. Because I do not know if my disability can be passed on, I sometimes worry that it can be when I have a child. If it does happen, I probably will do the same things my parents did for me. I would not blame it on anyone and would hope for the best for my child. For now, I am just enjoying what God has given me and taking every opportunity that I have to succeed in graduate school. Whatever comes in the next years, I know it is going to be the best for me. Just as I have done in the past, I will face all obstacles with courage and keep growing as a person every day.

DISCUSSION QUESTIONS

1. How does a history of struggle against injustice effect how people with disabilities from different cultural backgrounds see themselves, their families, and the state?
2. Where do the values, structures, and processes of rehabilitation counseling service conflict with the values, structures, and processes of ethnic communities? How do we negotiate the differences?
3. How will disability fare in the public discourse as the country becomes increasingly multicultural in demographics and all spheres of public influence?
4. How does one address spirituality and religion to best effect in rehabilitation counseling?
5. How does one speak to the issues of disability across faiths? Where might your own beliefs impair your ability to build a proper working alliance? Are there ways that spirituality transcends and unites the faithful across belief systems?
6. What is the significance of a healthy social support network in how disability is defined in a culture? What makes a culture, family, or individual resilient in the face of challenge? Do resilient communities cultivate better attitudes toward people with disabilities?
7. How do we derive useful knowledge out of the study of multicultural attitudes toward disabilities when the context is constantly evolving?

EXERCISE

A. Create a story-telling circle of between 6 and 8 people who you consider to be family or very good friends. Have them share their stories, any story, about their personal experiences with disability. Record, collect, review. What themes emerge?

FOUR

Attitudes Toward Disability by Special Interests and Occupational Groups

Irmo Marini

OVERVIEW

This chapter explores the impact that societal attitudes can have on persons with disabilities, both psychologically and socially. Affect, perceived self-esteem, and self-concept are largely influenced not only internally by our own thoughts and actions but also by input from our environment regarding how we perceive what others think of us and how we are treated by others (Charmaz, 1995; DiTomasso & Spinner, 1997; Graf, Marini, & Blankenship, 2009; Hopps, Pepin, Arseneau, Frechette, & Begin, 2001; Li & Moore, 1998; Marini, Bhakta, & Graf, 2009; Trieschmann, 1988). As such, although in Chapter 2 we discussed the origins of negative attitudes as well as strategies to change them, here we focus generally on empirical and conceptual studies pertaining to the views or perspectives of specific occupational and special interest groups. Stubbins (1991) advised the importance for rehabilitation psychologists and other counseling professionals to have an understanding of or insight into the motivations, perspectives, or paradigms with which other groups view, treat, and interact with persons with disabilities. These insights provide rehabilitation professionals with relevant others' perspectives as to how to better understand and work with these groups to facilitate better care for clients with disabilities.

Exploring the attitudes and resulting actions by various groups, be they medical, insurance, business, or political, has a distinct impact on the lives of people with disabilities. The global treatment of disability issues in the United States is arguably viewed by some as the proverbial "glass being half empty" and by others as half full. Indeed, the National Organization on Disability (NOD) reported to Congress in 2004 its commissioned 18-year Harris Poll survey results regarding the plight of Americans with disabilities finding that slow and modest progress had occurred during this period. Some of the 2004 conclusions, however, still showed many Americans with disabilities lagging behind those without disabilities in a number of key areas, including: (a) an overall 35% employment rate, (b) 22% reporting perceived job discrimination, (c) three times more people with disabilities living in poverty with household incomes of less than $15,000 a year compared with those without disabilities, (d) students with disabilities twice as likely to drop out of high school than those without a disability, (e) almost three times as many persons with disabilities had inadequate or no transportation, and (f) about 20% without health care compared with approximately 7% of those without disabilities.

These numbers would suggest continuing disparities for persons with disabilities in employment, community access, health care, quality of life, and socialization. But just how big an impact do discriminatory or ambivalent attitudes have on those with disabilities? The answers begin to emerge when exploring studies surveying these populations regarding their interactions within our society. Li and Moore (1998), for example, surveyed 1266 adults with disabilities by examining the relationship between accepting one's disability within the context of one's demographics and perceived lived experiences (e.g., life-space). They found that self-esteem and family/friend emotional support played a significant role in adjustment. Equally important to this sample was the perceived impact social discrimination had on their self-acceptance of disability. Participants who perceived being discriminated or devalued by society were less likely to adjust to their disability. The authors concluded that persons with disabilities are often segregated and feel isolated by society, and that re-formation of one's self-concept following an injury is intricately tied to one's perceptions regarding community attitudes and support. DiTomasso and Spinner (1997) similarly noted that poor physical community access and the negative attitudes of others are critical social integration obstacles, often leaving persons with disabilities experiencing greater levels of reported loneliness than those without disabilities.

Hopp et al. (2001) also found a high correlation between loneliness and social anxiety for 39 adults with physical disabilities who reported poor community access due to environmental barriers. Individual's who felt segregated or isolated reported poorer social skills from infrequent opportunities to interact with others. The authors concluded that reduced community access is linked to loneliness. Ironically, despite 20-year-old ADA legislation mandating civil rights and greater community public access to persons with disabilities, physical access barriers continue to be a frustration for many concerned. Marini et al. (2009) reviewed 160 letters to the editor of two popular physical disability magazines (*New Mobility* and *Paraplegia News*) between 2001 and 2007. They found that the most frequent type of letter written (34%) dealt with consumer anger and frustration over access barriers, including movie theaters, restaurants, wheelchair parking abuses, hotels, and taxis. Other highly ranked letter themes concerned adaptive aids, dealing with secondary health issues, financial concerns, and negative societal attitudes, where writers complained about being ignored and condescended to by others. Similarly, Graf et al. (2009) surveyed 78 persons with spinal cord dysfunction, requesting them to write, in 100 words or less, what experience(s) best exemplified their living with a disability. Although participants had no other restriction on their composition other than a word limit, the most frequent topical theme related to *physical access barriers* that once again generated anger and frustration among writers. These concerns rippled into the second-highest theme reported, which were *restricted community activities* that were forcefully imposed by environmental and employment barriers. This, in turn, created an impact on the *negative affect* some participants expressed, such as "it sucks" to have a disability. As with the Marini et al. (2009) study, the negative attitudes of others ranked fifth in themes of participants being ignored, condescended to, and treated like children.

Overall, as Lewin (1935) aptly hypothesized over 75 years ago with field theory, our self-concept is entwined and influenced by the reciprocal effect of an individual interacting with his or her environment. Although Lewin's field theory did not take into account the impact of disability, contemporary rehabilitation researchers have factored into the equation the concept of having one (Trieschmann, 1988; Wright, 1960, 1983). This interaction is conceptualized in the term "somatopsychology" that we discuss in greater detail later, but nevertheless propounds that our behavior (B) is a function (f) of psychosocial variables, such as self-esteem and coping skills (P), organic factors related to the disability, such as paralysis or blindness (O), and environmental or physical access and attitudinal factors (E), comprising the formula $B = f(\text{P} \times \text{O} \times \text{E})$. Although it appears from the above studies that many persons with disabilities experience anger and frustration on a regular basis due to environmental and attitudinal barriers, a number of differently focused studies suggest just the opposite, where those with disabilities report a relatively good quality of life and life satisfaction (Bishop, 2005b; Dijkers, 1997; Johnson, Amtmann, Yorkston, Klasner, & Kuehn, 2004; Schwartz & Sprangers, 2000; Smart, 2009; Wineman, 1990; Yerxa & Baum, 1986). Dijkers (1997) distinguishes between objective and subjective quality of life variables. He notes that persons with disabilities often do report a lower quality of life when considering objective factors such as pain, functional limitations, poor educational or vocational opportunities, community participation, and social contacts when compared with those without disabilities. However, despite these factors, persons with disabilities generally report their subjective well-being, life satisfaction, and quality of life as otherwise fairly stable, and in some cases ranked higher than those without disabilities. Keeping these initial findings in mind, we now begin exploring the general attitudes and perspectives of various occupational and special interest groups toward persons with disabilities, and the potential impact it can have on psychosocial adaptation.

ATTITUDE STUDIES PERTAINING TO OCCUPATIONAL GROUPS

Medical and Related Professions

Many of the recent psychology of disability texts describe the different models of conceptualizing disability (Chan et al., 2009; Mackelprang & Salsgiver, 2009; Olkin, 1999; Smart, 2009; Vash & Crewe, 2004). Smart (2009), for example, differentiates between the medical, environmental, functional, and the sociopolitical models. Other writers such as Olkin (1999) describe the moral model as well. As noted in Chapter 1, the *medical model* is perhaps the best established and is over 100 years old. Although the majority of the lay public subscribe to this model as well, this view of disability originated and is espoused by many in the medical profession, generally including, for example, physicians, nurses, physical therapists, occupational therapists, and related assistants. Its proponents view disability from a disease model, focusing on treating the diseased or damaged organ with the hope of curing it. When that is not possible, a chronic illness or disability is of course still treated by the medical profession, but arguably not with the same vigilance, enthusiasm, insurance funding, or accommodation (Longmore, 1993). Kroll, Jones, Kehn, and Neri (2006) found, for example, that the participants with spinal cord injuries whom they interviewed reported less frequent preventative care doctor visits due to inaccessible exam tables, rude treatment by staff, physicians having preconceived ideas as to what was ailing patients, denied services, and lack of physician knowledge about their disabilities. In the medical model, everyone is a patient, and this carries with it a number of unwritten rules or connotations, such as being compliant and never questioning your doctors (or related professionals) because they are always right (Mackelprang & Salsgiver, 2009). If you are not cured, it is somehow your fault and not the medical establishment's, and people with disabilities must otherwise learn to function in an able-bodied world (Longmore, 1993). Olkin (1999) believes it imperative that mental-health counselors first establish the paradigm model to which clients subscribe, because this then lays some of the foundation for working with clients. Knowing whether a disabled child's parents believe the disability to be a punishment for having sinned versus viewing their doctor as omnipotent and never to be questioned are two distinctly different issues that need to be addressed.

Another concern about the medical model perspective pertains to the pros and cons of current medical advances. On the one hand, advances in medical technology have extended the life and quality of life for millions of persons with disabilities; however, the ability to detect Down's syndrome and other genetic disabilities in the womb has resulted in some physicians presuming quality-of-life value judgments. Skotko (2005a, 2005b) reported research on more than 1000 mothers of children with Down's syndrome, citing that many mothers were either directly or indirectly advised by their physicians to abort their unborn children because their lives would not be worth living. Princeton bioethics professor Peter Singer has advocated for years that children born with severe disabilities should be euthanized primarily because their lives are not worth living and that the financial and psychological burden for parents is something parents should be spared from having to endure (Singer, 2000). He has proposed that parents be permitted up to 30 days after the birth of their child to make the decision of having a physician euthanize the child. Pro-life disability groups, such as Not Dead Yet, have vehemently criticized Singer for such stances, arguing that aside from making ignorant quality-of-life value judgments and assumptions about children born with severe disabilities, it becomes a slippery slope deciding who should live and who should die (Johnson, 2003). Bogdan and Taylor's (1989) study is one of several such findings that directly refutes Singer's contention. In interviewing over 100 parents of children who had profound or severe mental retardation, the authors noted that the parents had emerged through what was described as "sociology of acceptance." Essentially, despite the fact that their child could not verbally communicate with them, parents expressed that their child (a) could think and communicate with nonverbal cues; (b) displayed a distinct and unique personality; (c) could reciprocate companionship; and (d) had a distinct social place in the family and was included in family routines.

Attitudes toward persons with disabilities among medical professionals has met with mixed results, with variables such as the professional's occupation, his/her personality traits such as authoritarian beliefs, type of disability one works with, education and training level, and proximity to physically or directly working with persons with disabilities. Summarizing some of the older studies, Geskie and Salasek (1988) found that nurses and psychiatric aides, who have strong authoritarian beliefs, tend to hold more negative attitudes toward those with mental illness and/or mental retardation, believing that these populations should be socially restricted or segregated. One study found that psychiatric nurses and aides viewed patients with mental disorders as abnormal, dangerous, and unpredictable (Rosenbaum, Elizur, & Wijsenbeek, 1976). Staff members who have a lower education and work in closer proximity to persons with disabilities also tend to have more negative attitudes (Geskie & Salasek, 1988). Mental disorders are typically rated more negatively than physical or sensory impairments (Tringo, 1970). Yuker (1988) and others attribute some of this occurrence to the rehabilitation setting not allowing for "equal status" contact that is believed to be one of the necessary conditions for enhancing positive attitudes. Another commonly cited reason is that persons with chronic illness and disability represent people who remind medical professionals of their failures, or those who cannot be cured, which, in turn, causes feelings of helplessness for professionals. Sadlick and Penta (1975), however, found more positive attitude responses for a group of nurses who watched an educational video of persons with tetraplegia functioning independently in their home. The authors noted how the nurses basically felt more positive or optimistic of such patients' outcomes when viewing them doing better post-hospitalization.

More contemporary literature on medical professional attitudes suggests some similar trends. Gething, LaCour, and Wheeler (1994), for example, found that the nursing home administrator's attitudes toward people with disabilities as measured by the Interaction with Disabled Persons scale (Gething & Wheeler, 1992) were more positive than the nurses who had daily direct contact caring for the nursing home residents. The authors argue that the type of contact between nurse administrators and nursing staff were different in that the administrators had more of a "social contact" (e.g., "how are you?") role with the residents, whereas direct nursing staff had more of a caregiving role. Indeed, previous studies with nursing home staff reveal that nursing home jobs working with elderly patients were the least preferred among staff, with an expectation that the work is depressing, unpleasant, and tiresome (Armstrong-Esther, Sandilands, & Miller, 1989; Downe-Wamboldt & Melanson, 1990). Once again, type of contact and equal status interactions become the crux of whether negative or positive attitudes are formed. Yuker (1988) additionally argues that if the contact is one of providing assistance, it creates unequal status, and the individual is not perceived as competent.

Thomas (2001) interviewed 17 women with disabilities regarding their reproductive experience in the United Kingdom, combined with 68 other women's written narratives with regard to their experiences interacting with their physicians. Overall, although some women reported their physician experiences to be positive, many others perceived their physician as being indifferent, controlling, or hostile. Many participants expressed feeling gender oppressed and that their doctors could not see the patient behind their impairment. Some participants described their physician as not having the necessary training with respect to their disability.

Perhaps Garden (2009) best tackles one of the main problems of the medical model versus the social construct model paradigm regarding clinical empathy. Garden argues that although medical professionals acknowledge clinical empathy as important in their practice and medical training, there is often a hidden curriculum that suppresses the importance of empathy, and in fact highlights the burnout effects of becoming emotionally attached to one's patients (Hafferty & Franks, 1994; Marcus, 1999; Newton, Barber, Clardy, Cleveland, & O'Sullivan, 2008; Spickard, Gabbe, & Christensen, 2002). Some researchers argue, however, that physician empathy actually reduces burnout, and increases physician and patient satisfaction, while increasing patient well-being and trust (Kim, Kaplowitz, & Johnston, 2004).

Overall, it appears that medical professional attitudes toward disability continue to be complex and based on a number of factors. If both the medical professional and the patient have a higher education, it generally facilitates a more equal status and collaborative relationship; however, patients with lower education are perceived as less competent, and less likely to be included in joint decision making. Medical professionals with an authoritative personality are more likely to exclude patients from decision making as well. In addition, medical professionals such as direct care nursing staff may have more negative attitudes toward persons with disabilities because the nature of the contact is perceived as unequal, unpleasant, tiresome, and depressing (Armstrong-Esther et al., 1989; Downe-Wamboldt & Melanson, 1990). Teaching clinical empathy may help reduce negative attitudes toward disability however, more resistance to changing those with authoritarian personalities or those professionals who devalue or are prejudiced toward persons with disabilities is likely regardless.

Counseling and Related Professions

This area of attitude research includes rehabilitation counselors, social workers, and other mental health clinicians, excluding licensed psychologists, who are discussed later. Similar to the inconsistent results found among medical professionals' attitudes toward disability, counselor and related mental health clinician attitude studies also show mixed findings (Brodwin & Orange, 2002; Cook, 1998). Earlier studies, such as Byrd, Byrd, and Emener (1977), found that rehabilitation counselors had more negative attitudes about the potential employability regarding eight of 20 disabling conditions compared with employers who were only as negative about persons with alcoholism. Such findings unfortunately suggest that some rehabilitation counselors likely knowingly or unknowingly close their clients' cases as un-rehabilitated due to their preconceptions that certain clients are unemployable.

Similarly, Krauft, Rubin, Cook, and Bozarth (1976) rank ordered rehabilitation counselor attitudes pertaining to eight disabilities from most to least positive, finding that those counselors with the least positive attitudes in general had significantly fewer rehabilitated case closures than did counselors with more positive attitudes. This hierarchical preference toward having positive or negative attitudes toward some disability groups as opposed to others has some fairly consistent support empirically (Bowman, 1987; Byrd et al., 1977; Krauft et al., 1976; Tringo, 1970; Wilson, Alston, Harley, & Mitchell, 2002). One contributing factor studied by Bordieri (1993) found that rehabilitation counseling students rated persons with disabilities whom they perceived to have caused their own disability (e.g., attribution of blame) more negatively. Additionally, other researcher findings suggest that negative counselor beliefs and employability status decisions are even more prevalent for minority clients with disabilities (Rosenthal & Berven, 1999; Wilson et al., 2002). Wilson et al. (2002), for example, found that African American clients' cases were closed un-rehabilitated more often than Caucasian clients with similar disabilities, and those who did receive services were provided fewer services than Caucasian clients. Rosenthal, Chan, and Livneh (2006) did not find race to be a factor in their study of rehabilitation student attitudes in the context of hiring a counselor versus being a mentor or companion; however, they found age (more favorable attitudes toward younger persons) and disability type (paraplegia, epilepsy, multiple sclerosis, schizophrenia, and HIV-positive, respectively) to be significant attitude factors.

Snowden (2003) concedes that a history of mistreatment and discrimination against minority clients with mental health issues has created mistrust and fear among clients in seeking treatment, especially among the elderly. Choi and Gonzalez (2005) interviewed 18 mental health case workers regarding perceived barriers for older minority clients in accessing mental health services. The authors found that mistrust and fear concerns among elderly clients, as well as financial and transportation barriers, stigma, and lack of information regarding the referral process, posed obstacles as to why the elderly were reluctant to seek mental health services when they needed them.

Finally, other student college majors' attitude studies have shown some tendency toward more favorable attitudes held by rehabilitation counseling students when compared with other disciplines or practicing counselors (Carney & Cobia, 1994; Chan et al., 2009; Kaplan, 1982; Carney and Cobia (1994) administered the Attitudes Toward Disabled Persons scale (Yuker, Block, & Campbell, 1960) to 190 master's counselors in training students from rehabilitation counseling, school counseling, and community agency counselor programs. The rehabilitation counseling majors reported the most favorable attitudes, followed by school counselors, and finally the agency counselors. The authors did not find any differences in attitudes, regardless of what stage of training the students were in; however, they believed that student attitudes were largely formed prior to entering graduate school.

Overall, it appears that some of the major concerns from researchers regarding counselor attitudes pertain not only to whether attitudes are positive or negative toward different disability groups, but also whether negative counselor attitudes are carried over into bias and discrimination regarding who will receive services, fairness, and preconceived notions regarding client employability, intelligence, and emotional maturity (Cook, 1998). Although counselor attitude studies in general suggest that counselors hold more positive attitudes than the general public, counselors nevertheless are involved in decisions that may have a critical impact on their clients' independence, self-esteem, and quality of life (Cook, 1998; Garske & Thomas, 1990; Paris, 1993). The potential impact of counselor burnout or dissatisfaction in their job can amplify negative attitudes as well. In addition, specific counseling discipline, accurate education, and the paradigm model taught (e.g., medical model, social construct model, moral model) regarding disabilities appear to positively impact students' attitudes (Salih & Al-Kandari, 2007). Students' attitudes can be influenced depending on whether their academic faculty espouse the medical model paradigm of disability (possibly nursing, medical, social work, and psychology disciplines) or the social construct model of disability (possibly social psychology, rehabilitation counseling, and sociology). Although Olkin (1999) recommended that counselors establish their clients and family's disability paradigm beliefs, it is equally important for educators and counselors to assess their own views on the matter. With contemporary counseling approaches promoting client-counselor partnerships and empowering clients, it behooves educators, students, and practitioners alike to consider the value of the social construct model where appropriate.

Economists and Epidemiologists

Economists

Economists and epidemiologists share an overlapping similarity between their professions; they work with numbers. When it comes to discussing disability, economists have generally explored the topic in two divergent ways: the costs of disability in America with regard to the Gross National Product (GNP), and, the returns of disability in terms of business market revenue, jobs created, and collecting taxes (Rubin & Roessler, 2008). The economics of disability arguably dates back to fourth-century BC, when philosophers such as Plato and Aristotle espoused that infants born with a disability should be killed at birth because of the economic burden society would have to bear in caring for and feeding them. This argument has continued for some in the 21st century (Singer, 2000). In 2004, for example, the Congressional Budget Office reported that of the approximate $2.3 trillion or roughly 20% of the federal government spending budget, $492 billion went toward Social Security benefits, $473 billion toward Medicare and Medicaid, and an additional $136 billion toward retirement and disability programs (Congressional Budget Office, n.d.). Unquestionably, disability in America does carry a substantial cost in assisting persons with disability. On further inspection, however, one finds that a majority of these funds or approximately 81% go toward older recipients over age 62 and their survivors who will likely not reenter the workforce regardless of disability status (Social Security Beneficiaries

Statistics, 2009). As of 2009, there were just over 9.6 million workers with disabilities compared with the over 42 million collecting old-age and survivors benefits. Although on the surface, citing such projected numbers may suggest that persons with disabilities are perceived as consuming so much from the system, in reality, the majority of funds are utilized by older Americans at the end of their work lives. Indeed, statistics indicate that once persons are awarded Social Security benefits, less than 1% ever returns to competitive employment (Marini & Reid, 2001).

Various polls from time to time have shown an approximate 70% unemployment rate among persons with disabilities over the past several decades, despite the fact that approximately 70% of this population indicated that they would like to work if given the opportunity and under the right circumstances (Rubin & Roessler, 2008). Economists such as Yelin (1991) note that employment of persons with disabilities is largely linked to supply and demand, citing World War II as a period that evidenced the highest employment rate for persons with disabilities because many able-bodied Americans were involved in the war. Unfortunately, once the war was over, many disabled workers were displaced when their able-bodied counterparts returned home.

The flip side to economic reports that show disability in America to be an economic drain on society paints quite a different picture. Medical profession job creation and explosion in the areas of nursing, physical and occupational therapy, and speech language pathology, as well as related medical disciplines, are projected to continue to experience the fastest growth in the country (US Bureau of Labor Statistics, n.d.). In the public sector vocational rehabilitation arena, economists have reported a cost–benefit ratio of approximately $11 return (in paying taxes) for every $1 spent on rehabilitating someone, according to the Office of Management and Budget (Rehab Action, 1993). In addition, thousands of jobs and billions of dollars in profits are made each year with the sales of medical supplies and durable medical equipment. Whether such windfall profits are justified is sometimes questionable. For example, does a power wheelchair with a tilt/recline option really cost $35,000? Should 2 days in a hospital after a heart catheter procedure, including operating room rental, surgeon costs, and related medications, amount to $70,000? Some would argue that people with disabilities are a boon in a capitalist society as opposed to a financial drain, depending on who's paying the bill. Noble (1984) summed up the economic debate by contemplating whether the United States continues to aspire to embrace the moral philosophy of being a utilitarian society that advocates doing the greatest good for the greatest number. As health care costs continue to spiral out of control with no universal health care in sight, only time will tell whether we can strive toward utilitarianism, or continue to digress toward survival of the financially fittest.

Epidemiologists

Epidemiologists study the origin and spread of disease within populations, as well as specific characteristics and demographic numbers presented as group data regarding populations of persons with chronic illness and disability. Like economists, they often do not have a particular subjective agenda regarding disability, but generally present the statistics as they are. DeVivo and associates, for example, have spent much of their career exploring the group characteristics of persons with spinal cord injuries (SCI) (e.g., DeVivo, 1998; DeVivo, Black, & Stover, 1993; DeVivo, Hawkins, Richards, & Go, 1995). Their numerous studies have provided valuable information regarding life expectancy, employment rates, suicide rates, marriage rates, causes of death, and a host of other topics related to SCI. Unfortunately, because epidemiologists typically deal with large numbers of people and work with databases, sometimes critical information is often just gleaned over or not available for analysis because the information was never collected. An example might be studying life expectancy and finding out the top causes of death for persons with SCI, including respiratory problems, nonischemic heart disease, sepsis, ill-defined conditions, and genitourinary infections (DeVivo, Krause, & Lammertse, 1999). The limitation of such group number-crunching, however, is that there are often so many unexplained and unknown key extraneous variables. Unaddressed are questions such as, "What were the living conditions for these individuals? Did they have adequate health care? Did they have weight issues, smoke, or drink excessively?", and so on. This type of additional information becomes valuable for counselors in working for betterment of client living conditions, encouraging a healthier lifestyle, and pursuing available health care. Overall, although the statistics provide some useful global glimpse of disability issues, they may inadvertently lead some health professionals down a predetermined or misperceived path of assumptions about their clients or patients that is incorrect at best and discriminatory at worst. Such study findings should be applied cautiously.

Business and Employer Attitudes

Reviewing the history of business industry lobbying and employer attitudes reveals perhaps no greater adversary and liberator for persons with disabilities. The relationship with the disabled was adversarial in terms of lobbying against imposed federal regulations regarding not only having to hire qualified individuals with disabilities for jobs but also having to structurally make businesses physically accessible in compliance with public accommodations legislation (Peck & Kirkbride, 2001; West, 1991). Conversely, employers have also been liberators for persons with disabilities with regard to hiring them for jobs, thereby improving quality of life, self-concept, and life satisfaction (Krause, 1996; Szymanski & Parker, 1996). Szymanski and Parker (1996) noted that work defines a person's worth and place in society, but the very definition of work (being productive) and disability (being incapable) are antithetical. This contradiction regarding what skills employers expect from an ideal employee versus the perceived stigma regarding the capabilities of persons with disabilities, has, in part, led to the relatively consistent 70% unemployment rate among this population for the past several decades. This section may be best broken down by discussing businesses in having to conform to the Americans with Disabilities Act (ADA), and employer attitudes regarding hiring persons with disabilities.

   Business Conformity to the ADA: West (1991) discussed the immense opposition spearheaded by American business during the years leading up to the 1990 passage of the ADA. The ADA is commonly believed to be equivalent to the civil rights Movement for persons with disabilities. With its five titles, the ADA opened the door for those with disabilities to enjoy full participation in society. It reinforces the 1973 Reha-bilitation Act regarding employment and includes access to public places, transpor-tation, and telecommunications. The disparities in participation rates in public accommodations were evident in the 1986 Harris Poll (Lou Harris and Associates, 1986) indicating that in the past year, almost two-thirds of disabled Americans had not been to the movies, 75% had not seen a live theater or musical, almost two-thirds had not been to a sporting event, and persons with disabilities were three times more likely to have never eaten in restaurants.

The primary reason persons with disabilities back then did not frequent these establishments was because many perceived not feeling welcome, and many businesses in the 1980s were not accessible. Inaccessibility rivaled that of African Americans' seg-regation before the Civil Rights Movement. Small and big businesses argued that making their businesses physically accessible would be cost prohibitive, and many pro-pagandized that making expensive accommodations would put small businesses out of business (West, 1991). Prior to the ADA passing, one businessman sent a letter to a U.S. senator stating that the law was so vague that "it is a horror story for American employers . . . the law constitutes a hunting license for lawyers and for unscrupulous persons with fictitious or questionable disabilities" (West, 1991, p. xvii). Of course, none of the horror of an explosion of frivolous lawsuits ever materialized, and, as we know today, the majority of business modifications were nowhere near cost prohi-bitive to businesses. Indeed, research on physical accommodation has consistently shown that about 70% of modifications cost less than $500, an estimated 12% cost between $501 and $1,000, and less than 10% of all accommodations cost more than $2,000 (Samuelson, 1999; West, 1991). In addition, by 2002, more than 250,000 ADA Title I administrative charges had been filed, of which approximately 15% saw favorable verdicts or mediation for claimants. Persons filing with an attorney had median outcomes of approximately $19,750, whereas persons filing with the Equal Employment Opportunity Commission (EEOC) resolved their complaints for a median of $4,482. In the vast majority of instances, employers were, and continue to be, proved not guilty of discrimination (Moss, 2002). Not only is employment dis-crimination difficult to prove but also the potential settlement amounts are miniscule and often not worth the time and effort of most attorneys.

Employer Attitudes: There have been a plethora of studies regarding employer attitudes toward hiring persons with disabilities (e.g., Harris & Associates, 1987; Robert & Harlan, 2006; Schneider & Dutton, 2002). The 1987 Harris Poll and subsequent studies have shown that persons with disabilities are not only largely unem-ployed but also underemployed in the secondary labor market performing minimum or near-minimum-wage jobs (Lou Harris and Associates, 1987; McCarthy, 1988; Schneider & Dutton, 2002; West, 1991). McCarthy (1988) attributed some of these inequities to negative employer attitudes and posited several explanations based on the clinical services model, social systems model, and career development model. In the clinical services model, unemployment and underemployment are due to an indi-vidual's functional limitations, occupational and social skill deficits, poor motivation, and job search skill deficits. This model, similar to the medical model, attributes blame to the individual. The social systems model attributes unemployment and underemployment to lack of physical access, work disincentives, employer prejudice, and poor labor market conditions. Finally, the career development model attributes shortcomings of employment for persons with disabilities to individual deficits as well as the vocational rehabilitation system's focus on getting any job as opposed to planning out someone's career.

When it comes to employer attitudes, it has generally been shown that employers who hire employees with disabilities typically rate the hirings as positive experiences (DuPont Corp., 1990; Lou Harris and Associates, 1987). The 1987 Harris Poll of first-line managers, small-business managers, department heads, and equal employment opportunity personnel overall rated employees with disabilities as hard working, punctual, productive, and reliable when compared with employees without disabilities. The main reason cited for not hiring applicants with disabilities was because they lacked qualifications. Conversely, employers who have no experience hiring persons with disabilities generally have had unfounded concerns about presumable problems with higher absenteeism, increased insurance premiums, low productivity, safety, and ability to perform (Honey, Meager, & Williams, 1998; Pati & Adkins, 1981; Peck & Kirkbride, 2001). It appears overall that larger employers, employers having past experience hiring workers with disabilities, hiring decision makers who are female, decision makers with college degrees, and government sector employers are all favorable indicators of hiring persons with disabilities (J. Levy, Jessop, Rimmerman, Francis, & Levy, 1993).

A study by Schneider and Dutton (2002), with 55 employers of persons with disabilities and 47 disability employment advisers (DEA, equivalent to rehabilitation counselors) in England regarding attitudes toward workers with disabilities, found several divergent beliefs between groups. Some of the primary beliefs expressed by employers were that assistive technology modifications were very expensive, whereas the DEAs thought otherwise, and employers also perceived filing excessive paperwork in taking on disabled employees. Finally, Gilbride and associates studied 123 employer attitudes in hiring persons with disabilities in relation to vocational rehabilitation services (Gilbride, Stensrud, Ehlers, Evans, & Peterson, 2000). Employers unanimously indicated that they were glad to have hired someone with a disability, but it would be more difficult hiring persons with moderate or severe disabilities, such as blindness or mental retardation, as opposed to persons with heart disease, cancer, and HIV. Conversely, an Australian study of 656 employers regarding their satisfaction with the work performance of employees with disabilities indicated that the majority were less satisfied with disabled employees when compared with able-bodied employees in terms of quality, accuracy, and speed. The authors highlight, however, that speed and accuracy were not predictors of employer satisfaction with the nondisabled workers, suggesting that employers do not unilaterally evaluate all employees in the same way (Smith, Webber, Graffam, & Wilson, 2004).

The flip side to employer attitudes is exploring the attitudes of workers with disabilities. In Robert and Harlan's interviews with 243 government workers re: disability discrimination in the workplace, the author's cite employers' "strong and unrelenting" opposition to the ADA continues to plague potential job applicants with disabilities (Harlan, 2006, p. 600). Interview findings centered around three kinds of discrimination: *marginalization* or feeling like an outsider where coworkers and/or supervisors socially isolated employees with disabilities; *harassment*, both blatant and subtle consisting of jokes, rumors, sabotage, inappropriate questioning, and insensitive remarks; and, *fictitious identities*, whereby employees with disabilities were ascribed characteristics such as being treated as incompetent and helpless. In all instances, employees with disabilities reported feeling unwelcome working for the government. In Hernandez et al.'s (2007) study of 74 working age adults, participants indicated major barriers to employment being negative employer attitudes in hiring, lack of reliable transportation, and lack of education required to perform the jobs. Participants expressed concerns about rehabilitation counselors whom they perceived as nonresponsive and noncollaborative. Although many of the participants expressed an awareness of the Ticket to Work program, approximately one-third feared losing their cash and medical benefits and believed that persons with disabilities still faced significant barriers to employment.

Overall, persons with disabilities continue to perceive employer discrimination in hiring, maintaining, and promoting workers with disabilities. Larger companies with hiring personnel who tend to be female and educated, and companies with positive past experiences hiring persons with disabilities are all positive attitude indicators. Although only touched upon here, it also appears that there is a hierarchy of hiring, with the less severely disabled and those with certain types of disabilities, who, with the proper qualifications, are statistically more likely to be hired than those with more severe disabilities. The public views of employing persons with disabilities have become more positive over the past several decades, with a majority now believing that it is the right thing to do, and that persons with disabilities make capable employees (Burge, Kuntz, & Lysaght, 2007). Those employers who have hired persons with disabilities have experienced positive outcomes, and those typically smaller employers with no past experience hiring this population continue to discriminate based on unfounded fears of higher insurance premiums, lower productivity, greater safety concerns, and anticipated higher absenteeism rates.

Teacher Attitudes

An intense debate over the past several decades pertains to mainstreaming and full inclusion of students with disabilities into the least restrictive environment or regular education classroom (Hannah, 1988; Rao, 2004). At one end of the continuum are teachers who believe that with the right resources, students with various disabilities should be mainstreamed as much as feasible. At the other end are teachers who believe that students with disabilities slow down teaching and are a distraction to regular education students, ultimately believing that students with disabilities should be segregated (Hannah, 1988). There are also long-held beliefs and findings that teachers' preconceptions about the poor academic abilities of certain types of students with disabilities lead to a self-fulfilling prophecy whereby teachers expect less from, devote less time to, and administer lower grades to students with disabilities (Good & Brophy, 1972; Hannah, 1988; Rist, 1970; Rosenthal & Jacobsen, 1968). Kavale and Forness (2000), in their historical analysis of mainstreaming and integration, cite the 1980s

Regular Education Initiative (REI) push for full inclusion in regular education class-rooms and the fierce debate that has since ensued. With little empirical evidence to support REI, the argument among teachers and academics became an ideological one with highly emotional rhetoric from both sides comparing segregation, slavery, and apartheid with special education.

Some of the earlier research regarding teachers' attitudes suggests that similar to other attitude research, certain types of student disabilities sparked different preconceptions about such students. For example, children with mental retardation were thought to be low academic achievers, docile, and dependent; however, students diagnosed with an emotional disturbance were described as unhappy, aggressive, unmotivated to learn, impolite, dishonest, and unfriendly (Boucher & Dino, 1979; Moore & Fine, 1978). In addition, students with learning disabilities were described as aggressive, disruptive, angry, hostile, low academic achievers, socially distant, and frustrated (Boucher & Dino, 1979; Bryan & McGrady, 1972). Williams and Algozzine (1977) found that teachers were more willing to spend time working with students with physical and learning disabilities than with those who were mentally retarded or emotionally disabled. Overall, however, somewhat consistent findings suggest that although children with emotional and learning disabilities elicit negative feelings, teachers largely prefer to work with this population as opposed to students who are deaf or blind, rated low by teachers on teaching preference, but high on positive feelings (Panda & Bartel, 1972). Without the laws or available technology in the 1970s, communication with students who were deaf or blind was likely marginal at best. Hannah (1988) additionally cited other factors regarding teacher attitudes, including female teachers possess more positive attitudes, those with specialized training in disability possess more positive attitudes, previous contact had mixed results depending on the experiences, disruptive student behavior had a more negative impact on teachers' attitudes, and perceived or real student academic achievement corresponded to willingness to teach them.

More contemporary research on teachers' attitudes has shown a greater willingness to integrate certain students with disabilities who do not require additional time and responsibilities on the teacher's part (Houck & Rogers, 1994). Principals' attitudes have suggested that they lack specific knowledge about students with disabilities, perceive that such students would not be successful in regular education, and that such students would benefit from a mixture of regular education and one-on-one resource room education (Barnett & Monde-Amaya, 1998). Principals and education administrators did believe, however, that full-time general education placements offered students with disabilities more social and academic benefits, despite the fact that the support services would not be available. Interestingly, attitudinal differences between teachers and principals are similar to the nurse versus nursing home administrators noted earlier. Specifically, nursing administrators and principals who have less direct contact appear to have more positive attitudes, because their contact with disabled persons tends to be more of a social nature as opposed to caregiving or the day-to-day teaching.

In their quantitative analysis of 28 studies surveying the perceptions of over 10,000 general education teachers, Scruggs and Mastropieri (1996) found that although over two-thirds of the teachers approved the concept of inclusion of students with disabilities, only a small majority expressed a desire to actually do so. Less than a third of teachers believed that students with disabilities would benefit from full inclusion, and that students with more severe disabilities would negatively impact the general education class. These views in reality appear to be consistent with those of students with disabilities themselves. Although many students describe feelings of embarrassment, frustration, and anger being pulled out into resource special-education rooms, many have reported receiving the assistance they need in the resource room, as well as it being a quiet and supportive environment for them (Klingner, Vaughn, Schumm, Cohen, & Forgan, 1998; Lovitt, Plavins, & Cushing, 1999; Padeliadu & Zigmond, 1996). In addition, although Banerji and Dailey (1995) found that students with disabilities in regular education experience more positive social outcomes regarding tolerance and social support, there are also negative consequences, such as poor self-confidence, poor self-perceptions, and inadequate social skills (Tapasak & Walther-Thomas, 1999).

Attorneys in Personal Injury Litigation

The specialized field of forensic rehabilitation consulting deals primarily with tort litigation involving cases where individuals have sustained a disability due to alleged medical malpractice, product liability (e.g., seatbelt failure), or workers' compensation injuries. In an overly simplistic and broad brush explanation, the interests of plaintiff attorneys (who represent the injured party) are to highlight their client's injuries to emphasize its overall disabling impact, both physically and psychologically. Conversely, it is the defense attorney's job in representing the defendant (e.g., employer, insurance company, physician), to attempt to deflect blame from the client and/or marginalize the extent of monetary damages related to the disability when deemed excessive or unreasonable. Vocational and life care planning expert witnesses, as well as all other expert witnesses, are supposed to provide impartial, objective testimony. Unfortunately, this is sometimes more of an ideology as opposed to what occurs in reality (Binder & Rohling, 1996; Field, Choppa, & Weed, 2009; Robinson, Young, & Pomeranz, 2009).

In Wood and Rutterford's review of litigated long-term cognitive and psychosocial outcomes for persons with severe brain injuries, several conclusions have been found in a majority of litigated versus nonlitigated cases, including (a) more postconcussion symptoms are reported by litigants, (b) litigant symptoms last longer and are more debilitating in terms of returning to work, and (c) litigants demonstrate higher levels of psychological distress (Wood & Rutterford, 2006, p. 239). Unquestionably, the concept of malingering or secondary gain of litigants can come in to play in any lawsuit, and ideally plaintiff and defense attorneys alike should impartially seek out the truth no matter who they represent. In an effort to minimize frivolous lawsuits, Williams (2001) describes the impact of attorney fee shifting laws whereby if the litigant attorney loses at trial, he or she must pay the defendant's attorney fees.

Overall, it is important for rehabilitation consultants to know the intentions and perceptions of plaintiff and defense attorneys. Ethical plaintiff and defense attorneys will simply refer an expert in the case, provide a little background, and allow the expert to draw his or her own conclusions. Sometimes, however, attorneys for either side may attempt to unduly influence the expert's opinion. Again, many plaintiff attorneys typically want to maximize their clients' disabilities and resulting damages, while defense attorneys generally attempt to minimize or question the injured party's disability in an effort to reduce monetary damages. This is discussed later in the chapter regarding injured workers.

Sociologists' Versus Psychologists' Perspectives

The attitudes of sociologists and psychologists, like all other group attitudes, are not exclusively the same, noting that within-group differences are always present. Unlike attorney perspectives, which are often guided by the financial gain of their work and the side they represent, sociologists' and psychologists' frame of reference begins with their academic studies. With the noted exceptions of rehabilitation and social psychology, other psychology specializations dealing with human behavior have traditionally focused on psychopathology of the individual, giving little or no attention to external or environmental contributors to behavior (Forshaw, 2007; Olkin, 1999; Olkin & Pledger, 2003). This view stems from the medical model paradigm that psychologists adopted over a century ago, asserting that the individual is broken and must be fixed or cured, without considering environmental influences (Rothman, 2003; Tate & Pledger, 2003). Olkin (1999) noted that persons with disabilities must be viewed holistically and propounds *disability affirmative therapy*, which explores and acknowledges the potential psychological impact of social injustices and lack of access. To work almost exclusively with individuals with disabilities and ignore the myriad of external influences impacting their lives, Olkin believes, is tantamount to not competently performing one's job.

Conversely, social psychologists, much like sociologists, explore the external environment and how societal attitudes, politics, social justice, and so on can affect our lives (Forshaw, 2007). The Division of Rehabilitation Psychology of the American Psychological Association has also acknowledged the fact that persons with disabilities are psychologically affected by interacting with their environment, referred to as somatopsychology (Tate & Pledger, 2003; Vash & Crewe, 2004). Schultz (2009) indicates that although the rehabilitation model also stems from the medical model, it is not as stigmatizing, but does, however, still largely focus on a deficit- or pathology-based view of disability in which persons with disabilities must accept, adapt, or adjust to their situation.

Most promising to psychology and counseling in the past decade, however, is the introduction of the *International Classification of Functioning* (ICF) (Peterson, 2005, 2010; WHO, 2001). The *ICF* moves away from the traditional pathology-focused resources, such as the *International Classification of Diseases* and the *Diagnostic and Statistical Manual of Mental Disorders*, which focus almost entirely on individual deficits, and instead acknowledges and incorporates the individual-environmental interface. The *ICF* was developed around three broad categories, including body functions and structure, functional abilities related to specific tasks and participation in life situations, and severity of the disability and environmental factors (Peterson, 2010; WHO, 2001).

There remains some debate regarding what constitutes community participation. Hammel et al. (2008) conducted a focus group of persons with disabilities, noting their concerns that community participation is individualized and should not be prescribed by societal norms. Nevertheless, environmental factors include assistive technology, societal attitudes, environmental access, support and relationships, services, systems, and policies. As noted earlier, for example, if an individual is frustrated and angry over disabled-parking violators, rude hospital staff, and inaccessible medical examination tables, a thorough ICF evaluation would give credence to how these factors can affect an individual.

Sociologists', and the study of sociology, largely take a 180-degree turn away from psychology's focus on individual pathology, and instead look outward at how society has socially constructed or defined disability. Indeed, some sociologists argue that persons with disabilities are oppressed, excluded, and treated unequally by society, which further inhibits their adaptation in the community (Schultz, 2009; Thomas, 2004). Finkelstein (2001) noted that although it is a tragedy to have an impairment, it is societal oppression that prevents persons with disabilities from full and equal participation, and this in itself is tantamount to a crime (Finkelstein, 2001, p. 2). A similar model is reported elsewhere as the minority model of disability (Olkin, 1999), whereas the more centrist and emerging socio-environmental model (Tate & Pledger, 2003) reasserts the earlier works of Wright and Trieschmann, citing the interaction between an individual and his or her environment (Trieschmann, 1988; Wright, 1983).

In concluding this section, it is apparent that becoming familiar with how disability is perceived by various occupational groups can assist counseling professionals by providing insight regarding the paradigm framework others may be viewing as disability and why. Although these professionals are educated or indoctrinated that way, are financially motivated, or simply view disability in these terms, these group generalizations do not necessarily or exclusively imply that all such professionals hold these attitudes. We next turn to the perceptual paradigms driven by special interest groups, organizations, or agencies.

PARADIGM PERSPECTIVES OF SPECIAL INTEREST GROUPS, ORGANIZATIONS, AND AGENCIES TOWARD DISABILITY

In this section, the general beliefs and practices of various groups in relation to disability are explored. The health insurance industry, workers' compensation, nonprofit disability organizations, political groups, and disability groups are discussed, again cautioning that there are always individual differences, opinions, and beliefs within groups.

Health Insurance Industry

Despite the United States being an industrialized and technologically advanced society where many believe that its health care ranks among the best in the world, the reality is that the United States ranks 37 in health care and 24 in life expectancy according to the World Health Organization. The United States does, however, rank second overall in health care spending, and 14 overall in preventable deaths, which is largely attributed to the millions of citizens who are uninsured (WHO, 2000).

Traditionally, the federal and state governments have arguably medically provided for a disproportionate number of persons with disabilities, costing hundreds of billions of dollars annually (Centers for Disease Control and Prevention 2001). People with disabilities are generally either denied private insurance coverage or charged outrageous premiums, most often making health coverage unaffordable. Drainoni et al. (2006) notes that persons with disabilities are among the poorest in the nation, with statistics indicating them to be in poorer health and having greater risk of secondary complications compared with the general population (Kaiser Family Foundation, 2004). Steinberg, Wiggins, Barmada, and Sullivan (2002) found that persons with disabilities often underutilize preventative health care services, but frequently use high-cost emergency room services when in crisis. When queried, many persons with disabilities cite ongoing access barriers, including transportation problems, inaccessible examination tables and diagnostic equipment, insurance coverage restrictions, an uncoordinated and fragmented gauntlet of medical services, and negative attitudes and misperceptions about disability among the medical providers (Bingham & Beatty, 2003; DeJong & Frieden, 2002; Marini et al., 2009). Drainoni et al. (2006) found in their focus groups of 64 persons with disabilities and 23 proxies, similar concerns, including significant waiting periods due to authorization clearance, transportation barriers, spend-down policies of Medicaid for eligibility, inaccessible equipment, poor office communication between medical providers, lack of physician knowledge, and assumptions made about the disability by professionals to be major concerns.

Perhaps the most disturbing fact about the U.S. health insurance industry is its presumed focus on profits over quality of care (Rosenbaum, 2009). Insurance discrimination on the basis of health status, often excluding the most disabled citizens, has been a standard practice for decades. Recent health care reform signed by President Obama in 2010 promises to provide insurance coverage to an estimated 30 of the 45 million currently uninsured Americans, as well as eliminate preexisting conditions discrimination in the health insurance industry. In Rosenbaum's analysis of various health insurance discrimination practices, she cites various strategies the insurance industry uses to increase profits. Social solidarity and actuarial fairness are two concepts used in analyzing and underwriting risk in group coverage contracts. Companies consider factors such as weighing actuarial odds of the younger enrollees not becoming sick and not having to use health care services, versus older workers who may utilize the system more. Risk shielding is a concept whereby underwriters exclude certain preexisting conditions or limit coverage in an effort to shield profits. Risk shielding exclusions, and/or higher-risk premiums, have traditionally been underwritten for women and minorities. When high-risk individuals are admitted, they may later face coverage limits or be dropped from coverage altogether (Rosenbaum, 2009). Although the Healthcare Reform Act of 2010 is yet to be tested, federal legislation has traditionally been thwarted in curbing health care discrimination, with the health insurance industry continually finding ways to skirt new laws. The other major barrier to health care reform has been considerable lobbying efforts to influence political decisions by the health care industry. Attkisson (2009) reported there were 3000 health care lobbyists on Capitol Hill in 2009, equating to a six-to-one ratio of lobbyists to members of Congress, citing that many lobbyists were actually former members of Congress and staffers.

Finally, beyond the underwriting tactics of the health insurance industry re: minimizing their risk or profit loss by signing up too many persons with disabilities, there are the actions of hospitals themselves in maximizing profits. Although private hospitals are obligated by the Emergency Medical Treatment and Active Labor Act to treat those needing urgent care, statistics suggest otherwise. Shen, Cochran, and Moseley (2008) studied market factors and admission rates for 255,615 persons with serious mental illness (SMI) across five states, finding that 64% were treated in private, not-for-profit hospitals, 19% in investor-owned hospitals, and 16% went to public hospitals. Schlesinger, Dorwart, Hoover, and Epstein (1997) note how the effect of competition has led to what is known in the industry as "patient dumping," whereby persons with SMI are sent or dumped to public hospitals, especially in areas where more private hospitals are found.

Overall, one of the many unfortunate downsides to corporatist profit-making in the U.S. health care system is risk shielding of underwriting insurance contracts for group plans that target older, minority, female, and persons with chronic health conditions. In order to avoid paying out too much to hospitals and health care providers, insurance companies have traditionally excluded or limited coverage for those with serious disabilities. In certain instances, previous coverage may be canceled with few if any appeal options. It remains to be seen as to whether health care reform has any significant impact toward obtaining more equitable health coverage for all Americans.

Nursing Lobby and the Nursing Home Industry

One of the most powerful lobbying groups in Washington, DC is the nursing lobby; and one of the most coveted issues for the industry is the protection and continued government funding for nursing homes. Disability advocates such as American Disabled for Attendant Programs Today (ADAPT), a grassroots effort led by persons with disabilities, fight for various civil rights causes. Their 1980s wheelchair lockdowns brought access to subways in Atlanta and elsewhere, followed by protests to place wheelchair lifts on Greyhound and local route buses, and most recently, have advocated the motto "free our people from nursing homes." The primary argument has been that most persons with disabilities and the elderly would rather live at home with personal assistance than in a nursing home. The issue is at least 20 years old and continues to be fought on many battlefronts, arguing the cheaper economics of assisting someone at home as opposed to in a nursing home (http://www.adapt.org).

Statistics indicate that the average nursing home costs per resident in 2001 was $60,000 per year (Walker, 2006), and that between 1987 and 1996, total annual expenditures for nursing home care increased from $28 billion to $70 billion for an increase of 150% (Agency for Healthcare Research and Quality, 2001). Disability advocates argue that having a personal care attendant in the home costs approximately one-third of nursing home costs (Lafleur, 2009). The nursing lobby, however, continues to successfully advocate for Congress to steer approximately two-thirds of all Medicaid and Medicare long-term care funding to nursing homes as opposed to community living care. Different states are lobbied more heavily than others for the state share of Medicaid dollars. For example, in 2008, Tennessee spent 98% of its long-term care dollars on nursing homes, citing the very powerful nursing home industry's campaign donation and lobbyists (Nashville City Paper, 2008). Marini (2008) noted how the Memphis Center for Independent Living (CIL) and Denver, Colorado's Atlantis CIL have codeveloped a literal 21st-century disabled underground railroad for Tennessee nursing home residents who want to leave or "escape" the nursing home, then provide travel assistance to Denver and set up personal care assistance in a community apartment.

Lafleur (2009) noted the latest political effort to free up more community-based dollars with the 2007 then Senator Barack Obama's cosponsored Senate Bill 683—Community Choice Act, essentially allotting more funding toward community-based home care. This legislation was dropped, however, from the 2010 Healthcare Reform Act and currently is in a state of limbo. Several years ago, the U.S. Department of Health and Human Services recommended state Medicaid directors draft plans to help persons who wanted to move out of institutions or remain in their homes. Only 29 states submitted plans, and as of 2007, approximately 331,000 Americans were on waiting lists for government-funded community services assistance. Although the majority of Americans indicate that they do not want to live in a nursing home, there is yet to be enough advocacy by groups such as ADAPT and support from the American Association of Retired Persons (AARP), which have begun to realize the dignity and freedom of being cared for at home. There are also waiting lists for the more than 36,000 assisted living residences in the United States where persons can live independently in their apartments and have personal attendants available in the building for assistance. But Medicaid in most states currently does not cover assisted living facilities, despite the fact that it costs approximately one-half ($35,000 per year in 2005) of what a nursing home costs (Opdyke, 2006). Among one of the nursing home lobby strategies to maintain their Medicaid and Medicare funding levels is the argument of putting consumers with disabilities at medical risk for not having the best quality of care. Disability advocates argue, however, that most persons are medically stable and require basic assistance in dressing, bathing, cooking, and cleaning. In addition, there continues to be increased reports of nursing home abuses, including, neglect, overmedication, malnutrition, starvation, dehydration, and physical abuse, and subsequent lawsuits (Moody, n.d.).

Workers' Compensation

Workers' compensation was the first form of social insurance in the United States, introduced in 1908 to cover federal civilian employees engaged in hazardous work. By 1921, only six states were yet to implement workers' compensation, and today, all 50 states, the District of Columbia, Puerto Rico, and the U.S. Virgin Islands have their own variation of workers' compensation insurance (Sengupta & Reno, 2007).

By 2004, employers' costs for workers' compensation was up to 7% from a year earlier, totaling over $87 billion annually in medical care and cash benefits.

The basic concept behind workers' compensation is simple; employers agree to cover an employee injured at the worksite regardless of fault. Depending on what state one lives in, injured workers are covered for between 66% and 75% of their gross wage and all medical expenses if injured. In return, the employees give up the right to sue their employers. Prior to workers' compensation coverage, employees had to prove that employers was negligent in a tort lawsuit. Employees rarely won these cases, however, because employers generally could use one of three common defenses: (a) the employee either contributed to the injury, (b) a fellow employee caused the injury, or (c) employees assumed the risks of performing the job (Bevan, 2003). At the same time, many employers risked going bankrupt if they had to pay a substantial settlement to a seriously injured employee, and therefore workers' compensation was an amicable solution to both sides.

Although a chapter on the psychosocial aspects of work injuries is discussed more thoroughly later, the rapid growth and related issues in workers' compensation during the past century has had implications for injured workers and the industry. For injured workers, Scherzer and Wolfe (2008) cite the barriers that injured workers have typically encountered in accessing workers' compensation, including fear of being laid off, frustration dealing with the red tape bureaucracy of the insurance industry, not knowing about reporting procedures, and dealing with inconsiderate workers' compensation board (WCB) staff. Calvey and Jansz (2005) found similar concerns having interviewed 11 women who had gone through the system. Respondents expressed their perception that the WCB was on the employer's side, lacked empathy, sympathy, or care. This perceived distrust of the system is a reciprocal one, in that the WCB each year spends millions of dollars on special investigation units (SIU) to investigate fraudulent claims of workers they believe to be malingerers who are claiming they are too disabled to work and continue to receive benefits. The SIU industry membership exploded 850% by 1990, forming the International Association of Special Investigation Units, designed to police fraudulent claims for the insurance industry (Blakely, 1998). The industry estimates that for every one dollar spent on an investigation, seven to $10 in savings is returned through deterrence or restitution.

Injured workers, however, are not the only ones under surveillance. The last decade saw an alarming increase of fraud on behalf of health providers. Blakely (1998) cited a 1996 Conning Insurance Research study indicating that fraudulent workers' compensation claims comprise about 25% of all claims. Four types of fraud can be committed. The first is *claimant fraud* that involves the injured worker feigning or exaggerating an injury. Statistically, this is most common with disgruntled workers, workers who are about to be laid off, older workers, and blue-collar workers who have physically demanding jobs. The second type of fraud is *insurer fraud*, where an insurance company sells workers' compensation policies but then scams the employer by not paying on claims or simply vanishing. The third type of fraud is *premium fraud*, where business owners cheat the insurers to save on premiums. An example would be giving an underestimate on the number of employees in the company, or misclassifying more dangerous jobs as less risky. Finally, *provider fraud* refers to health provider's who may charge for procedures that are not performed, make up fictitious injured claimants, and bill the worker's comp carrier, or diagnose worthless treatment regimens for claimants that do nothing to improve their condition (Blakely). These white-collar criminals are often doctors, chiropractors, lawyers, and health care providers. The National Insurance Crime Bureau in 2000 estimated that workers' compensation insurance fraud was the fastest-growing crime in the country, with an estimated cost of $5 billion annually (California Department of Insurance, n.d.).

Overall, it becomes necessary for counselors to see both sides of the workers' compensation equation. As rehabilitation counselors working for private medical and vocational case management companies, counselors are responsible for assisting injured workers in their recovery, and to do so in a medically safe, but cost-efficient, manner. A central question debated in this industry, however, has been who is the client? The insurer pays the case management company in effect to expedite a claimant's return to work. The rehabilitation counselor case manager is paid by the insurer, but works with the injured worker and reports back to the insurance adjuster. Ethical dilemmas can arise for the rehabilitation counselor if the insurance adjuster attempts to dictate the injured worker's treatment, contrary to the rehabilitation counselors or medical provider's recommendations. For injured workers, distrust in the system is as common as the workers' compensation system's distrust is for claimant honesty. The rehabilitation counselor working in this industry is in a unique position to be an ambassador and intermediary between the insurer and the injured worker.

Nonprofit Disability Charity Organizations

The 1991 Harris Poll regarding attitudes nondisabled Americans had toward those with disabilities asked one particular question regarding the most popular sentiment or emotion that persons with disabilities evoked (Lou Harris & Associates, 1991). Oddly enough, the two most popular sentiments reported were pity and admiration. How could the general public be at such diverse ends on the emotional spectrum about these perceptions? The answer it appears comes from the media and how disability is portrayed or covered in various venues. The sentiment of admiration comes from heart-warming inspirational stories Zola (1991) describes as those about Olympic gold medalist runner Wilma Rudolph who had polio as a child, and Franklin Delano Roosevelt, America's 32nd President who hid his polio from the public but was arguably one of the greatest presidents in American history.

The concept of pity, however, largely stems from media coverage of disability in charity telethons (Smart, 2009). Smart noted how Franklin Roosevelt began the March of Dimes charity to raise money for polio, and that the Salk's vaccine was funded by the March of Dimes proceeds. Unquestionably, there are positive benefits of fundraising as in this case, and instances where funding may go directly to the disabled group for which the money is being raised, for such purposes as purchasing wheelchairs, offsetting surgical costs, research and development, and so on; however, at what cost? Many disability groups and individuals with disabilities have weighed in on the topic by protesting the telethons, arguing the portrayal of those with disabilities insinuates that they are poor, helpless, less than whole, and perpetually waiting to be cured (Barnett & Hammond, 1999; Smart, 2009; Smit, 2003). The demeaning portrayal of "Jerry's Kids" in the Muscular Dystrophy Telethon perpetuates the helpless, childlike image society has of persons with disabilities, and this pity approach is believed to be what is needed to solicit donations. Shapiro (1992) noted how Jerry Lewis and telethon supporters believed that tapping into the public's ability to pity and sympathize with the children was the best strategy to raise money for the cause. National Easter Seals Society founder James William's noted, however, that their telethon actually raised twice the amount of money when they stopped using the pity approach. Overall, although most charities have learned to listen to the complaints by disability advocates regarding the demeaning public perceptions that are conveyed with the pity approach, continual monitoring needs to occur.

PREPARING COUNSELORS TO WORK WITH OTHER GROUPS' PARADIGM PERSPECTIVES

Clearly, depending on the pedagogy of one's academic discipline's dogma, occupational job duties, economic rewards or losses, and personal philosophy regarding disability, a number of different paradigm perspectives can evolve. The insight gained from exploring these perspectives can assist counselors in knowing how to work with those who subscribe to these views, and either work with them, around them, or through them as necessary to provide what is best for clients with disabilities. Statistics continue to show persons with disabilities globally lagging behind the general population in areas of education, income, health care, and socialization. It behooves counselors and related professionals to continue advocating for equal status and the best possible services for disenfranchised groups. We explore how to do this in later chapters.

REFERENCES

Agency for Healthcare Research and Quality. (2001). *Annual nursing home expenses increased by 150 percent from 1987–1996.* Press Release, September 5, 2001. Retrieved from http://www.ahrq.gov/news/press/pr2001/inhexppr.htm

Armstrong-Esther, C. A., Sandilands, M. L., & Miller, D. (1989). Attitudes and behaviors of nurses toward the elderly in an acute care setting. *Journal of Advanced Nursing, 14*(1), 34–41.

Attkisson, S. (2009, October 20). *Health-care lobbyists' rise to power.* Retrieved from http://www.cbsnews.com/stories/2009/10/20/cbsnews_investigates/main5403220.shtml

Banerji, M., & Dailey, R. A. (1995). A study of the effects of an inclusion model on students with specific learning disabilities. *Journal of Learning Disabilities, 28,* 511–522.

Barnett, C., & Monde-Amaya, L. E. (1998). Principals' knowledge of and attitudes toward inclusion. *Remedial and Special Education, 19,* 181–192.

Barnett, J., & Hammond, S. (1999). Representing disability in charity promotions. *Journal of Community & Applied Social Psychology, 9,* 309–314.

Bevan, T. W. (2003). State workers' compensation programs. In S. L. Demeter & G. B. J. Andersson (Eds.), *Disability evaluation* (pp. 36–43). St. Louis, MO: Mosby.

Binder, R. L., & Rohling, M. L. (1996). Money matters: A meta-analytic review of the effects of financial incentives on recovery after closed head injury. *American Journal of Psychiatry, 153*(1), 7–10.

Bingham, S. C., & Beatty, P. W. (2003). Rates of access to assistive equipment and medical rehabilitation services among people with disabilities. *Disability and Rehabilitation, 25*(9), 487–490.

Bishop, M. (2005b). Quality of life and psychosocial adaptation to chronic illness and acquired disability: A conceptual and theoretical synthesis. *Journal of Rehabilitation, 71*(2), 5–13.

Blakely, S. (1998). Fighting fraud in workers' comp. *Nation's Business, 86*(4), 1–17.

Bogdan, R., & Taylor, S. (1989). Relationships with severely disabled people: The social construction of humanness. *Social Problems, 36*, 135–148.

Bordieri, J. E. (1993). Self blame attributions for disability and perceived client involvement in the vocational rehabilitation process. *Journal of Applied Rehabilitation Counseling, 24*(2), 3–7.

Boucher, C. R., & Dino, S. L. (1979). Learning disabled and emotionally disturbed: Will the labels affect teacher planning? *Psychology in the Schools, 16*, 395–402.

Bowman, J. T. (1987). Attitudes toward disabled persons: Social distance and work competence. *Journal of Rehabilitation, 53*(1), 41–44.

Brodwin, M. G., & Orange, L. M. (2002). In J. D. Andrew & C. W. Faubion (Eds.), *Rehabilitation services: An introduction for the human service professional* (pp. 174–197). Osage Beach, MO: Aspen Professional Services.

Bryan, T., & McGrady, H. J. (1972). Use of a teacher rating scale. *Journal of Learning Disabilities, 5*, 100–206.

Burge, P., Kuntz, H. O., & Lysaght, R. (2007). Public views on employment of people with intellectual disabilities. *Journal of Vocational Rehabilitation, 26*, 29–37.

Byrd, E. K., Byrd, P. D., & Emener, W. G. (1977). Students, counselors, and employer perceptions of severely retarded. *Rehabilitation Literature, 38*, 42–44.

California Department of Insurance. (n.d.). *Fraud: Workers' compensation fraud and convictions.* Retrieved from http://www.insurance.ca.gov/0300-fraud/0100-fraud-division-overview/0500-fraud-division-programs/workers-comp-fraud/index.cfm

Calvey, J., & Jansz, J. (2005). Womens experience of the workers compensation system. *Australian Journal of Social Issues, 40*(5), 285–311.

Carney, J., & Cobia, D. C. (1994). Relationship of characteristics of counselors in training to their attitudes toward persons with disabilities. *Rehabilitation Counseling Bulletin, 38*(1), 26–30.

Centers for Disease Control and Prevention. (2001). Prevalence of disabilities and associated health conditions among adults-United States, 1999. *Journal of the American Medical Association, 285*(12), 1571–1572.

Chan, F., De Silva Cardoso, E., & Chronister, J. A. (Eds.) (2009). *Understanding psychosocial adjustment to chronic illness and disability: A handbook for evidence-based practitioners in rehabilitation* (pp. 333–367). New York: Springer.

Charmaz, N. (1995). The body, identity, and self: Adapting to impairment. *The Sociological Quarterly, 36*, 657–680.

Choi, N. G., & Gonzalez, J. M. (2005). Barriers and contributors to minority older adults access to mental health treatment: Perceptions of geriatric mental health clinicians. *Journal of Gerontological Social Work, 44*(3/4), 115–134.

Congressional Budget Office. (n.d.). *The budget and economic outlook: Fiscal years 2000 to 2010.* Retrieved from http://www.cbo.gov/budget/historical.shtml

Cook, D. (1998). Psychosocial impact of disability. In R. M. Parker & E. M. Szymanski (Eds.), *Rehabilitation counseling: Basics and beyond* (3rd ed., pp. 303–326). Austin, TX: Pro-Ed.

DeJong, G., & Frieden, L. (2002). It's not just managed care; it's the larger health care system say researchers. *National Rehabilitation Hospital Research Update*, Spring (Suppl.), *1*, 4–7.

DeVivo, M. J. (1998). *Research update: Reader hospitalization costs of individuals with spinal cord injury.* Birmingham, AL: UAB-Spain Rehabilitation Center.

DeVivo, M. J., Black, K. J., & Stover, S. L. (1993). Causes of death during the first 12 years after spinal cord injury. *Archives of Physical Medicine and Rehabilitation, 74*, 248–254.

DeVivo, M. J., Hawkins, L. N., Richards, J. S., & Go, B. K. (1995). Outcomes of post-spinal cord injury marriages. *Archives of Physical Medicine and Rehabilitation, 76*, 130–138.

DeVivo, M. J., Krause, J. S., & Lammertse, D. P. (1999). Recent trends in mortality and causes of death among persons with spinal cord injury. *Archives of Physical Medicine and Rehabilitation, 80*, 1411–1419.

Dijkers, M. (1997). Measuring quality of life. In M. J. Fuhrer (Ed.), *Assessing medical rehabilitation practices: The promise of outcome research* (pp. 153–180). Baltimore, MD: Paul H. Brooks.

DiTomasso, E., & Spinner, B. (1997). Social and emotional loneliness: A re-examination of Weiss' typology of loneliness. *Personality and Individual Differences, 22*, 417–427.

Downe-Wamboldt, B. L., & Melanson, P. M. (1990). Attitudes of baccalaureate students nurses toward aging and the aged. *Educational Gerontology, 16*, 49–59.

Drainoni, M. L., Lee-Hood, E., Tobias, C., Bachman, S. S., Andrew, L., & Maisels, L. (2006). Cross-Disability experience of barriers to health-care access. *Journal of Disability Policy Studies, 17*(2), 101–115.

DuPont Corp. (1990). *Equal to the task II.* Wilmington, DE: Author.

Field, T. F., Choppa, A. J., & Weed, R. O. (2009). Clinical judgment: A working definition for the rehabilitation professional. *The Rehabilitation Professional, 17*(4), 185–194.

Finkelstein, V. (2001). *The social model repossessed.* The Disability Studies Archive UK, Centre for Disability Studies, University of Leeds. Retrieved from www.leeds.ac.uk/disability-studies/archiveuk/archframe.htm

Forshaw, M. (2007). In defense of psychology: A reply to Goodley and Lawthom (2005). *Disability & Society, 22*(6), 655–658.

Garden, R. (2009). Expanding clinical empathy: An activist perspective. *Journal of General Internal Medicine, 24*(1), 122–125.

Garske, G. G., & Thomas, K. R. (1990). The relationship of self-esteem and contact to attitudes of students in rehabilitation counseling toward people with disabilities. *Rehabilitation Counseling Bulletin, 34*, 67–71.

Geskie, M. A., & Salasek, J. L. (1988). Attitudes of health-care personnel toward persons with disabilities. In H. E. Yuker (Ed.), *Attitudes toward persons with disabilities* (pp. 187–200). New York, NY: Springer.

Gething, L., LaCour, J., & Wheeler, B. (1994). Attitudes of nursing home administrators and nurses towards people with disabilities. *Journal of Rehabilitation, 60*(4), 66–70.

Gething, L., & Wheeler, B. (1992). The interaction with Disabled Persons scale: A new Australian instrument to measure attitudes towards people with disabilities. *Australian Journal of Psychology, 44*(2), 75–82.

Gilbride, D., Stensrud, R., Ehlers, C., Evans, E., & Peterson, C. (2000). Employers attitudes toward hiring persons with disabilities and vocational rehabilitation services. *Journal of Rehabilitation, 66*(4), 17–23.

Good, T., & Brophy, J. (1972). Behavioral expression of teacher attitudes. *Journal of Educational Psychology, 63*, 617–624.

Graf, N. M., Marini, I., & Blankenship, C. (2009). 100 words about disability. *Journal of Rehabilitation, 75*(2), 25–34.

Hafferty, F. W., & Franks, R. (1994). The hidden curriculum, ethics teaching, and the structure of medical education. *Academic Medicine, 69*, 861–871.

Hammel, J., Jones, R., Smith, J., Sandford, J., Bodine, C., & Johnson, M. (2008). Environmental barriers and supports to the health, function, and participation of people with developmental and intellectual disabilities. Report from the state of the science in aging with developmental disabilities conference. *Disability and Health Journal, 1*, 143–149.

Hannah, M. E. (1988). Teacher attitudes toward children with disabilities: An ecological analysis. In H. E. Yuker (Ed.), *Attitudes toward persons with disabilities* (pp. 154–170). New York, NY: Springer.

Hernandez, B., Cometa, M. J., Velcoff, J., Rosen, J., Schober, D., & Luna, R. D. (2007). Perspectives of people with disabilities on employment, vocational rehabilitation, and the Ticket to Work program. *Journal of Vocational Rehabilitation, 27*, 191–201.

Honey, S., Meager, N., & Williams, M. (1998). *Employers' attitudes towards people with disabilities.* Grantham, England: Institute for Employment Studies.

Hopps, S., Pepin, M., Arseneau, I., Frechette, M., & Begin, G. (2001). Disability related variables associated with loneliness among people with disabilities. *Journal of Rehabilitation, 67*(3), 42–48.

Houck, C. K., & Rogers, C. J. (1994). The special/general education integration initiative for students with specific learning disabilities: A "snapshot" of program change. *Journal of Learning Disabilities, 27,* 58–62.

Johnson, H. M. (2003, February 16). Should I have been killed at birth? A case for my life. *The New York Times Magazine,* pp. 50–55.

Johnson, K. L., Amtmann, D., Yorkston, K., Klasner, E. R., & Kuehn, C. M. (2004). Medical, psychological, social, and programmatic barriers to employment for people with multiple sclerosis. *Journal of Rehabilitation, 70,* 38–49.

Kaiser Family Foundation. (2004). Health care priorities. In *Kaiser Health Poll Report.* Retrieved from http//www.kff.org/healthpollreport/CurrentEdition/about.cfm.

Kaplan, S. P. (1982). Rehabilitation counselors attitudes toward their clients. *Journal of Rehabilitation, 48,* 28–29.

Kavale, K. A., & Forness, S. R. (2000). History, rhetoric, and reality: Analysis of the inclusion debate. *Remedial and Special-Education, 21*(5), 279–296.

Kim, S. S., Kaplowitz, S., & Johnston, M. V. (2004). The effects of physician empathy on patient satisfaction and compliance. *Evaluation & the Health Professions, 27,* 237–251.

Klingner, J. K., Vaughn, S., Schumm, J. S., Cohen, P., & Forgan, J. W. (1998). Inclusion or pull-out: Which do students prefer? *Journal of Learning Disabilities, 31,* 148–158.

Krauft, C. C., Rubin, S. E., Cook, D. W., & Bozarth, J. D. (1976). Counselor attitudes toward disabled persons and client program completion: A pilot study. *Journal of Applied Rehabilitation Counseling, 7,* 50–54.

Krause, J. S. (1996). Employment after spinal cord injury: Transition in life adjustment. *Rehabilitation Counseling Bulletin, 39,* 244–255.

Kroll, T., Jones, G. C., Kehn, M. E., & Neri, M. T. (2006). Barriers and strategies affecting the utilization of primary preventive service for people with physical disabilities: A qualitative inquiry. *Health and Social Care within the Community, 14,* 284–293.

LaFleur, J. (2009, June 21). Nursing homes get old for many with disabilities. *Pro Publica.* Retrieved from http://www.propublica.org/feature/nursing-homes-get-old-for-many-with-disabilities-621

Levy, J., Jessop, D., Rimmerman, A., Francis, F., & Levy, P. (1993). Determinants of attitudes of New York State employers towards the employment of persons with severe handicaps. *Journal of Rehabilitation, 59*(1), 49–54.

Lewin, K. (1935). *A dynamic theory of personality.* New York, NY: McGraw-Hill.

Li, L., & Moore, D. , 1998. Acceptance of disability and its correlates. *Journal of Social Psychology, 138*(1), 13–25.

Longmore, P. K. (1993, October). *History of the disability rights movement and disability culture.* Address delivered to the California Disability Leadership Summit. Anaheim, CA.

Lou Harris and Associates. (1986). *The ICD survey of disabled Americans: Bringing disabled Americans into the mainstream.* New York, NY: International Center for the Disabled.

Lou Harris and Associates. (1987). *The ICD survey II: Employing disabled Americans.* New York, NY: International Center for the Disabled.

Lou Harris and Associates. (1991). *Public attitudes toward persons with disabilities.* New York, NY: International Center for the Disabled.

Lovitt, T. C., Plavins, M., & Cushing, S. (1999). What do pupils with disabilities have to say about their experiences in high school? *Remedial and Special Education, 20,* 67–76, 83.

Mackelprang, R., & Salsgiver, R. (2009). *Disability: A diversity model approach in human service practice.* Pacific Grove, CA: Brooks/Cole.

Marcus, E. R. (1999). Empathy, humanism, and the professionalism process of medical education. *Academic Medicine, 74,* 1211–1215.

Marini, I. (2008). Underground railroad of the 21st century. *SCI Psychosocial Process, 21*(1), 38–39.

Marini, I., Bhakta, M. V., & Graf, N. (2009). A content analysis of common concerns of persons with physical disabilities. *Journal of Applied Rehabilitation Counseling, 40*(1), 44–49.

Marini, I., & Reid, C. (2001). A survey of rehabilitation professionals or alternative provider contractors with Social Security: Problems and solutions. *Journal of Rehabilitation, 67*(2), 36–41.

McCarthy, H. (1988). Attitudes that affect employment opportunities for persons with disabilities. In H. E. Yuker (Ed.), *Attitudes toward persons with disabilities* (pp. 246–261). New York, NY: Springer.

Moody, E. F. (n.d.). *Nursing home statistics.* Retrieved from http://www.efmoody.com/longterm/nursingstatistics.html

Moore, L., & Fine, M. J. (1978). Regular and special class teachers' perceptions of normal and exceptional children and their attitudes toward mainstreaming. *Psychology in the Schools, 15*, 253–259.

Moss, K. (2002). *Overview: Enforcing Title I of the ADA—An unfunded mandate.* Retrieved from http://www.adaenforcementproject.unc.edu/press.html#overview

Nashville City Paper. (2008, March 17). *Powerful nursing home lobby helped craft advantageous system, officials say.* Retrieved from http://nashvillecitypaper.com/content/city-news

National Organization on Disability. (June 24, 2004). *Press Release. "Landmark survey finds pervasive disadvantages."* Washington, DC: NOD.

Newton, B. W., Barber, L., Clardy, J., Cleveland, E., & O'Sullivan, P. (2008). Is there hardening of the heart during medical school? *Academic Medicine, 83*, 244–249.

Noble, J. H. (1984). *Ethical considerations facing society in rehabilitating severely disabled persons* (Action Paper No. 5). Washington, DC: National Rehabilitation Association, Ninth Mary Schweitzer Memorial Seminar.

Olkin, R. (1999). *What psychotherapists should know about disability.* New York, NY: The Guilford Press.

Olkin, R., & Pledger, C. (2003). Can disability studies and psychology join hands? *American Psychologist, 58*(4), 296–304.

Opdyke, J. (2006). Coverage and access: Higher demand for assisted-living creates waiting lists, higher prices for care. *Wall Street Journal, 248*(54), B1–B4.

Padeliadu, S., & Zigmond, N. (1996). Perspectives of students with learning disabilities about special education placement. *Learning Disabilities Research & Practice, 11*, 15–23.

Panda, K. C., & Bartel, N. R. (1972). Teacher perception of exceptional children. *Journal of Special Education, 6*, 261–266.

Paris, M. J. (1993). Attitudes of medical students and health care professionals toward people with disabilities. *Archives of Physical Medicine and Rehabilitation, 74*, 818–825.

Pati, G., & Adkins, J. (1981). *Managing and employing the handicapped: The untapped potential.* Lake Forest, IL: Human Resource Press.

Peck, B., & Kirkbride, L. T. (2001). Why businesses don't employ people with disabilities. *Journal of Rehabilitation, 16*, 71–75.

Peterson, D. B. (2005). International classification of functioning disability, and health: An introduction for rehabilitation psychologists. *Rehabilitation Psychology, 50*, 105–112.

Peterson, D. B. (2010). *Psychological aspects of functioning, disability, and health.* New York: Springer.

"Powerful" nursing home lobby helped craft advantageous system, officials say. (2008, June). *News @ The City Paper.* Retrieved from http://nashvillecitypaper.com

Rao, S. (2004). Faculty attitudes and students with disabilities in higher education: A literature review. *College Student Journal, 38*(2), 191–198.

Rehab Action. (1993). Important points to emphasize. *In the Public Interest, 2*(3), 2.

Rist, R. (1970). Students social class and teacher expectations: The self-fulfilling prophecy in ghetto education. *Harvard Educational Review, 40*, 411–451.

Robert, P. M., & Harlan, S. L. (2006). Mechanisms of disability discrimination in large bureaucratic organizations: Ascriptive inequalities in the workplace. *The Sociological Quarterly, 47*, 599–630.

Robinson, R., Young, M. E., & Pomeranz, J. (2009). Content analysis of factors identified in vocational evaluation analysis reports. *The Rehabilitation Professional, 17*(4), 163–174.

Rosenbaum, M., Elizur, A., & Wijsenbeek, H. (1976). Attitudes toward mental illness and the role conceptions of psychiatric patients and staff. *Journal of Clinical Psychology, 32*, 167–173.

Rosenbaum, S. (2009). Insurance discrimination on the basis of health status: An overview of discrimination practices, federal law, and federal reform options. *Journal of Law, Medicine & Ethics, 37*(3), 103–120.

Rosenthal, D., & Berven, N. (1999). Effects of client race on clinical judgment. *Rehabilitation Counseling Bulletin, 42*, 243–264.

Rosenthal, D., Chan, F., & Livneh, H. (2006). Rehabilitation students' attitudes toward persons with disabilities in high and low stakes social contexts: A conjoint analysis. *Disability and Rehabilitation, 28*(24), 1517–1527.

Rosenthal, R., & Jacobsen, L. (1968). Teachers' expectancies: Determiners of pupils' IQ gains. *Psychological Reports, 19*, 113–118.

Rothman, J. C. (2003). *Social work practice across disability.* Boston, MA: Pearson Education, Inc.

Rubin, S. E., & Roessler, R. T. (2008). *Foundations of the vocational rehabilitation process.* Austin, TX: Pro-Ed.

Sadlick, M., & Penta, F. B. (1975). Changing nurse attitudes toward quadriplegics through the use of television. *Rehabilitation Literature, 36*, 274–278.

Salih, F. A., & Al-Kandari, H. Y. (2007). The effect of a disability course on prospective educators attitudes toward individuals with mental retardation. *Digest of Middle East Studies, 16*(1), 12–29.

Samuelson, R. (1999). Dilemmas of disability. *The Washington Post Weekly Edition*, p. 27.

Scherzer, T., & Wolfe, N. (2008). Barriers to workers' compensation and medical care for injured personal assistance services workers. *Home Health Care Services Quarterly, 27*(1), 37–58.

Schlesinger, M., Dorwart, R., Hoover, C., & Epstein, S. (1997). The determinants of dumping: A national study of economically motivated transfers involving mental health care. *Health Services Research, 32*(5), 561–590.

Schneider, J., & Dutton, J. (2002). Attitudes towards disabled staff and the effect of the national minimum wage. A Delphi survey of employers and disability employment advisers. *Disability & Society, 17*(3), 283–306.

Schulz, S. L. (2009). Psychological theories of disability and sexuality: A literature review. *Journal of Human Behavior in the Social Environment, 19*, 58–69.

Schwartz, C. E., & Sprangers, M. A. G. (2000). *Adaptation to changing health: Response shift in quality of life research.* Washington, DC: American Psychological Association.

Scruggs, T. E., & Mastropieri, M. A. (1996). Teacher perceptions of mainstreaming/inclusion, 1958–1995: A research synthesis. *Exceptional Children, 63*, 59–74.

Sengupta, I., & Reno, V. (2007). Recent trends in workers' compensation. *Social Security Bulletin, 67*(1), 17–26.

Sharpio, J. P. (1992). How the star and the muscular dystrophy association courted trouble. *U.S. New & World Report, 113*(10), 1–4.

Shen, J. J., Cochran, C. R., & Moseley, C. B. (2008). From the emergency department to the general hospital: Hospital ownership and market factors in the admission of the seriously mentally ill. *Journal of Healthcare Management, 53*(4), 268–280.

Singer, P. (2000). *Writings on an ethical life.* New York, NY: Ecco/Harper Collins.

Skotko, B. (2005a). Mothers of children with Down syndrome reflect on their postnatal support. *Pediatrics, 115*, 64–77.

Skotko, B. (2005b). Prenatally diagnosed Down's syndrome: Mothers who continued their pregnancies evaluate their healthcare providers. *American Journal of Obstetrics and Gynecology, 192*, 670–677.

Smart, J. (2009). *Disability, society, and the individual.* Austin, TX: Pro-Ed.

Smit, C. R. (2003). "Please call now, before it's too late": Spectacle discourse in the Jerry Lewis muscular dystrophy telethon. *Journal of Popular Culture, 15*(3), 687–703.

Smith, K., Webber, L., Graffam, J., & Wilson, C. (2004). Employer satisfaction with employees with a disability: Comparisons with other employees. *Journal of Vocational Rehabilitation, 21*, 61–69.

Snowden, L. R. (2003). Bias in mental health assessment and intervention: Theory and evidence. *American Journal of Public Health, 93*(2), 239–243.

Social Security Beneficiaries Statistics. (2009). Retrieved from http://www.ssa.gov/OACT/STATS/OASDIbenies.html

Spickard, A., Gabbe, S. G., & Christensen, J. F. (2002). Midcareer burnout and generalist and specialist physicians. *Journal of the American Medical Association, 288*, 1447–1450.

Steinberg, A. G., Wiggins, E. A., Barmada, C. H., & Sullivan, V. I. (2002). Deaf women: Experiences and perceptions of healthcare system access. *Journal of Women's Health, 11*(8), 729–741.

Stubbins, J. (1991). The interdisciplinary status of rehabilitation psychology. In R. P. Marinelli & A. E. Dell Orto (Eds.), *The psychological & social impact of disability* (pp. 9–17). New York, NY: Springer.

Szymanski, E. M., & Parker, R. M. (1996). Work and disability: Introduction. In E. M. Szymanski & R. M. Parker (Eds.), *Work and disability: Issues and strategies in career development and job placement* (pp. 1–8). Austin, TX: Pro-Ed.

Tapasak, R. C., & Walther-Thomas, C. S. (1999). Evaluation of a first-year inclusion program: Student perceptions and classroom performance. *Remedial and Special Education, 20,* 216–225.

Tate, D. G., & Pledger, C. (2003). An integrative conceptual framework of disability: New directions for research. *American Psychologist, 58*(4), 289–295.

Thomas, C. (2001). Medicine, gender, and disability: Disabled women's health care encounters. *Health Care for Women International, 22,* 245–262.

Thomas, C. (2004). How is disability understood? An examination of sociological approaches. *Disability & Society, 19*(6), 569–583.

Trieschmann, R. (1988). *Spinal cord injuries: Psychological, social, and vocational rehabilitation* (2nd ed.). New York, NY: Demos.

Tringo, J. L. (1970). The hierarchy of preference toward disability groups. *Journal of Special Education, 4,* 295–306.

U.S. Bureau of Labor Statistics. (n.d.). *Occupational Outlook Handbook 2010 edition.* Retrieved from http://www.bls.gov/oco/ooh_index.htm

Vash, C. L., & Crewe, N. M. (2004). *Psychology of disability* (pp. 288–299). New York, NY: Springer.

Walker, L. (2006). *Private savings, Medicaid and uncertain nursing home expenses, Working Paper Series.* Washington, DC: Congressional Budget Office.

West, J. (1991). *The Americans with Disabilities Act: From policy to practice.* New York, NY: Milbank Memorial Fund.

Williams, J. (2001). Effects of attorney fee shifting laws on claiming behavior. *Policy Sciences, 34*(3/4), 347–356.

Williams, R. J., & Algozzine, B. (1977). Differential attitudes toward mainstreaming: An investigation. *Alberta Journal of Educational Research, 23,* 207–212.

Wilson, K. B., Alston, R. J., Harley, D. A., & Mitchell, N. A. (2002). Predicting VR acceptance based on race, gender, education, work status at application, and primary source of supported application. *Rehabilitation Counseling Bulletin, 45*(3), 132–142.

Wineman, N. M. (1990). Adaptation to multiple sclerosis: The role of social support, functional disability, and perceived uncertainty. *Nursing Research, 39*(5), 294–229.

Wood, R. L., & Rutterford, N. A. (2006). The effects of litigation on long-term cognitive and psychosocial outcome after severe brain injury. *Archives of Clinical Neuropsychology, 21,* 239–246.

World Health Organization. (2000). *The World Health Report 2000-Health Systems: Improving Performance.* Press release WHO/44. Retrieved on May 5, 2010 from http://www.whoint/inf-pr-2000/en/pr2000-44.html.

World Health Organization. (2001). *International classification of functioning disability and health: ICF.* Geneva: World Health Organization. Retrieved from http/www.who.int/classification/icf

Wright, B. (1960). *Physical disability: A psychological approach.* New York, NY: Harper & Row.

Wright, B. (1983). *Physical disability: A psychosocial approach* (2nd ed.). New York, NY: Harper & Row.

Yelin, E. H. (1991). The recent history in immediate future of employment among persons with disabilities. *Milbank Quarterly, 69* (Suppls. 1–2), 129–149.

Yerxa, E. J., & Baum, S. (1986). Engagement in daily occupations and life satisfaction among people with spinal cord injuries. *Occupational Therapy Journal of Research, 6,* 272–283.

Yuker, H. E. (1988). *Attitudes toward persons with disabilities.* New York, NY: Springer.

Yuker, H. E., Block, J. R., & Campbell, W. J. (1960). *The scale to measure attitudes toward disabled persons. Human Resources Study Number 5.* Albertson, NY: Human Resources Center.

Zola, I. K. (1991). Communication barriers between "the able-bodied" and "the handicapped." In R. P. Marinelli & A. E. Dell Orto (Eds.), *The psychological and social impact of disability* (3rd ed., pp. 157–180). New York, NY: Springer.

INSIDER PERSPECTIVE
The Story of Miriam Kimmelman

When I was in the 5th grade, we began to study about the Civil War in history. Little did I know that my body was also beginning its own civil war, as I exhibited early symptoms of dystonia. My arm kept jerking up and down uncontrollably, causing embarrassment, confusion, and some notoriety among my classmates, some of whom tried to sit on my arm to keep it from moving. The arm movements stopped of their own accord, after some months, and then I began to have difficulty walking. By 6th grade, I could barely walk at all and used to crawl at home. My parents insisted that I continue in school, in between medical appointments, and finally I was diagnosed by two independent sources as having dystonia.

Dystonia is a chronic neurological disorder characterized by involuntary muscle contractions (extensor and flexor muscles contract at the same time), which force certain parts of the body into abnormal, sometimes painful, movements or positions. This is the official definition today, and it is still evolving with research, but 41 years ago when I was in the 6th grade, it was a hopeless diagnosis with no treatment. Despite all this, I managed to get symptom relief when I was in the 8th grade via neurosurgery from an innovative doctor who promised me some hope, with no guarantees, and I held on. I completed high school and went away to college, looking more or less normal.

Many symptoms returned, for reasons unknown, when I was about to complete my Junior year in college, but I managed to graduate with honors and decided to go on to graduate school in rehabilitation counseling. Another neurosurgical procedure was tried, with less success than the first two, but I got my M.A. and soon after, a job in a psychiatric hospital. I worked there for about 24 years, until, with the help of the ADA, a good lawyer who asked for an injunction from an intolerable commute, and the support of my husband and friends, I transferred to another New York State job as a vocational rehabilitation counselor for the State Rehab Agency (VESID). Ironically, DVR (VESID's name in 1966) had financially helped me go to college, along with a National Merit Scholarship and a NY Regents Scholarship.

I'm a native New Yorker (the hospital I was born in was converted to luxury housing some years back) and except for my four years at The University of Rochester, I have always lived in Manhattan. My husband and I met some 15 years ago in a yoga class and were married in 1991. Real estate, a big issue in New York, had us living an hour apart for about a year. Then we moved to Battery Park City in 1992, where we garden and enjoy living in a "suburban" Manhattan, in the shadow of the World Trade Center.

While I've always lived in Manhattan, I have always worked in downtown Brooklyn (and/or Staten Island, the main campus of the psychiatric hospital). I worked in a series of outpatient rehab programs, until the outpatient rehab component of the hospital was "cutback" and I was officially transferred to Staten Island. As I am a true New Yorker, I don't drive, and had to hook up with a series of carpools to travel to

Staten Island. The most "reliable" required me to meet the driver about 5 blocks from my home, at 6:55 a.m., along a busy highway where there was no shelter from rain or snow. This was the hospital's "reasonable accommodation" to my difficulty commuting. Had I gone by public transit, the trip would have taken $1\frac{1}{2}$ hours with good connections and involved walking (not a strength of mine), subway, ferry, and bus. I had to be ready to leave work at a specific time or be left to public transit to go home. My husband, my neurologist, and I began to see deterioration in my condition from stress and strain, but I really enjoyed working. However, a call from my father's home attendant at a morning staff meeting "broke the camel's back." She called me (interrupting the meeting) and told me I had to go to the hospital, no she didn't know exactly what was wrong (EMS didn't tell her in the ambulance) and I had to come quickly to sign something. My supervisor asked me to call the Express Bus Company (which doesn't schedule routes to Staten Island from Manhattan early in the AM) and find out their schedule, but she couldn't drive me to the stop for at least an hour! I begged someone else to drive me to the stop and cried all the way to the hospital. My father had broken his hip and I had to sign for the surgery. In 2 or 3 days I went to see my lawyer and she felt that my ADA case should be pursued. The rest is legal history.

Dystonia has had an impact on nearly every aspect of my life since its onset. In order to go to 6th grade, a 3-block (it could have been 3 miles) walk from our apartment house, my mother had to take me by taxi or when there was no taxi, stop a car on the street and ask for a ride. I was accepted into an exclusive high school for the 7th through the 12th grade. You had to take an exam. My parents and 6th-grade teacher were very proud, especially the 6th-grade teacher who knew that my only alternative was a health conservation class at a local junior high. The high school had no problem with me as long as I was just a name on a paper. But that first day, my mother was told that I had to leave. I always thought she had made it up, along with her threats of suing the school. But at my 25th High School Class Reunion there was the gym teacher, who, when she was reintroduced to me, said "you're the girl we didn't want" and it all came flooding back. Another teacher who I'd been in contact with over the years quickly said "but we were wrong, Miriam has done very well as you can see". It didn't matter anymore to me. I didn't want to hear about the "liability" the school might have incurred if I had fallen in 7th grade. At that time I could barely walk, always needed support, and "walked" backward. The school wouldn't let me use my wheelchair to get around safely. They did give me an elevator pass and allowed my classmates to take turns helping me go from class to class. At the reunion I returned in tears to my friends and tried to explain why I was crying. I had just gone from an independent and successful alumna to a dependent and useless child, at least in my mind.

In a big city like New York, I can never be "invisible," even at times I would like to feel that I could just blend into the crowd like other commuters, workers, etc. When I walk down the street on a New Year's Eve afternoon, strangers can ask whether I started celebrating early, because my gait is so unsteady. Children and adults will stare at me, sometimes it disturbs me and I make some nasty comments, such as, "would you like it if I stared at you because you look different, you idiots." In my neighborhood, everyone knows who I am and can start a conversation, for example, saying "I've seen you from my window every morning and think you are so courageous." There are days when I don't feel "courageous" and don't appreciate the intrusion. At my current job, I interview many consumers who apply for services, knowing that I likely won't be the assigned counselor. However, when these consumers call the receptionist for an update on their case, I am the only counselor "who walks funny and has white hair," and so calls are directed to me.

There are some pluses to dystonia. When I worked in the psychiatric center, I noticed that patients who were about to decompensate often changed their attitude about me—a useful diagnostic tool. And now, although I *do not* encourage this, consumers will say to me, "if you can do this, maybe I can too." At times, I probably take advantage of my disability by demanding a seat on the bus or subway, quite rudely if no one listens to me.

After much time, I realize that I am not dystonia. I can ignore my gait, until I catch sight of myself in a store window or a mirror. I have a number of supportive friends, and I got married to a terrific man. I am involved in the local dystonia chapter, have served as president and support group leader, and met some interesting people through this route. I am also involved in our local community garden and surprised my husband, who grew up gardening and not in a tenement as I did, by learning quickly how to tell the difference between weeds and flowers and how to effectively apply compost or mulch to enrich the soil. My husband introduced me to moderate hiking in Vermont, and we were able to share this interest. He even once acknowledged that I had a "good sense of direction" when we met up with hikers who said that we were headed to Canada, and I kept on saying that the trail blazes were not the same as the ones we had seen climbing up to that lovely vista.

But there are other times, usually stressful, which exacerbate my symptoms to the point that I can't ignore the gait, the hand problems, the twisted back, the difficulty breathing, the problems swallowing, or the slurred speech. Usually, it is negative stress—the difficulty with the long commute to work, the anniversary of my mother's death, my father's various illnesses and hospitalizations, and his final death. Then 2 weeks after my father died, my husband was suddenly hospitalized with a mysterious pneumonia that didn't get better. After nearly 2 years, he was still not well and our roles were reversed. My husband was such a good help and support to me and now I have to refill his oxygen humidifier and push his wheelchair, in addition to shopping, cooking, light cleaning, and working. Even my doctor can't factor out the role of stress and figure out how to reduce some spasms.

Maybe that is the key! The civil war that started when I was 10 is ongoing and there will also be conflicts between hopefulness and hopelessness, between independence and dependence, and between self-hate and self-worth. I am a person with generalized torsion dystonia, who happens to have white hair now, who happens to have arthritis and pain secondary to the dystonia, who happens to love quilting and gardening, who happens to be married to a terrific person (who is quite ill now), who happens to have very supportive friends and very intrusive encounters with strangers, who chose not to have children because intuitively I "knew" that dystonia was genetic, who has dimples and a nice smile, and who can curse like a sailor when I'm crossed.

There are many facets to every person you come across. Don't latch on to one label or even the most prominent facet your client presents to you. Learn about the person, at the rate tolerable to your client. Maybe that will enable you to grow as a counselor and your client to increase his/her independence from you and other "helpers" in his/her life. Coping with a chronic disability is a process that often follows an uneven path.

Ten years have passed since I wrote this chapter and many things have happened—both good and bad. It's always easier to begin with the bad things. My husband died and 9/11 happened. My world was shattered, my garden vacuumed of toxic dust, my arthritis worsened so that I could no longer quilt, my spine weakened from years of twisting, and my spinal cord became compressed endangering the lower half of my body. But, oh, so many good things! Friends saw to it that I wasn't alone, old friends got in touch and reconnected, crocuses bloomed in the spring of 2002, and now there is a new garden where a parking lot used to be. I have to accept help more often and it isn't so bad. With two spinal surgeries on my record, I have learned to walk again for the fourth time. Slowly I am relearning how to crochet. And most important of all, some of the genes that cause dystonia have been identified and there is some understanding of the proteins involved. And I'm still working. As I said previously, coping with a chronic disability follows an uneven path.

DISCUSSION QUESTIONS

1. Discuss hospital or physician contact experiences of students and/or family members re: medical staff empathy, time and effort with their case, and overall helpfulness.
2. Discuss anyone's experience with health insurance claims and itemized costs of hospital bills for services rendered.
3. Solicit any student's visits to relatives at nursing homes in terms of atmosphere, services, resident's demeanor, and staff interactions.
4. Solicit students' and/or family member's encounters with work injuries and/or attorneys in personal injury lawsuits and the outcome.
5. Solicit student stories for anyone they know who has a disability and has been discriminated against in attending a public function (e.g., restaurant, concert, sporting event, etc.).

EXERCISES

A. For a class activity, have students in groups monitor who parks in disabled parking spots at major grocery stores, movie theaters, and shopping malls.
B. Have students call various physician, dentist, and chiropractor's offices to see if they will pay to have an interpreter available to interpret for a patient who is deaf? Conversely, call several tour busline services and tell them you are enquiring about booking a bus trip for someone in a wheelchair who needs a bus with a lift.
C. Have students ask for a braille restaurant menu the next time they are at a restaurant.

PART TWO

The Psychology of Disability Surrounding the Individual and Family

FIVE

Theories of Adjustment and Adaptation to Disability

Irmo Marini

OVERVIEW

This chapter explores perhaps the most profound and important empirical question researchers have regarding the psychological and sociological impact of disability. How do persons with disabilities react to their situations, and why do some actually excel, whereas others become indefinitely incapacitated both mentally and physically? To begin with, there is some debate regarding appropriate terminology. Some experts, such as Olkin (1999), do not agree with the term "adjustment" to disability. Olkin argues that the concept of adjusting is a pathological term presuming something is wrong and implies persons with disabilities must successfully negotiate or transition through a series of stages to finally accept their situations (Olkin, 1999, p. 45). Olkin is not a proponent of the stage model of disability, but rather believes that individuals "respond" to their disabilities throughout their lives, and that final adjustment or acceptance does not exist. Other experts, such as Livneh (1991), do support a stage-like model and believe persons with later onset or adventitious disabilities often do transition through stages and often do reach a level of final adjustment or acceptance; however, may experience setbacks. Still other experts, such as Vash and Crewe (2004), describe how some persons with disabilities may actually "transcend" beyond their disabilities once they acknowledge or come to terms with their situations, accept the implications, and embrace the experience.

In this chapter, the terms "adjustment, adaptation, reaction, and response" are used interchangeably despite the fact that they may be different concepts but have overlapping definitions. When used, they will essentially refer to individuals with disabilities in their attempts to come to terms with their disabilities. The terms adjustment and adaptation also have a temporal or time component to them (Livneh & Antonak, 1997). In other words, one would typically need to be adapting before reaching final adjustment. Livneh and Antonak describe psychosocial adaptation as:

> an evolving, dynamic, general process through which the individual gradually approaches an optimal state of person-environment congruence manifested by;

(1) active participation in social, vocational, and avocational pursuits; (2) successful negotiation of the physical environment; and (3) awareness of remaining strengths and assets as well as existing functional limitations. (Livneh & Antonak, 1997, p. 8)

The concept of adjustment, however, is defined as:

a particular phase (e.g., set of experiences and reactions) of the psychosocial adaptation process. As such, adjustment is the clinically and phenomenologically hypothesized final phase—elusive as it may be—of the unfolding process of adaptation to crisis situations, including the onset of chronic illness and disability. It is alternatively expressed by terms such as (1) reaching and maintaining psychosocial equilibrium; (2) achieving a state of reintegration; (3) positively striving to reach life goals; (4) demonstrating positive self-esteem, self-concept, self-regard, and the like; and, (5) experiencing positive attitudes toward one's self, others, and the disability. (Livneh & Antonak, 1997, p. 8)

Also, as discussed in Chapter 2, each and every day we experience thoughts, emotions, and behaviors that may or may not be in congruence with each other (e.g., we can be emotionally upset about something, but behaviorally smile and pretend nothing is wrong). Each of the above concepts involves an emotional, cognitive, and behavioral response. When Olkin (1999) states that individuals respond to their disabilities, they actually feel and think something while they are responding. Likewise, when individuals accept their circumstances, this again involves certain cognitions, behaviors, and emotions that accompany successful adaptation. Therefore, persons who are believed to have genuinely adapted to their disabilities, should otherwise experience congruent feelings of contentment, thoughts of self-confidence with their disability identities, and some type of overt accompanying measurable behaviors, such as socializing more, assertiveness, being employed, volunteering, or attending school, and should have the desire and confidence to date if relevant.

Overall, seven common theories of adaptation to a traumatic physical disability are explored in this section. Some proposed theories have stronger evidence-based empirical support, whereas others are more qualitative and case study accounts as well as clinical observation. This chapter first explores persons born with a congenital disability, and questions whether such individuals actually experience any type of adjustment process since they have no pre-injury, nondisabled experience with which to compare their situations. Olkin (1999) shares her life experience as an individual born with polio, and prefers to describe her experience as "in response" to life circumstances she interfaces with in her external environment. Yet, other's born with a disability report different developmental experiences. Since this phenomenon of adaptation to a congenital disability is less understood or written about in the literature, we lead off with this investigation. The remaining chapter explores the following seven theories of adjustment, including stage models (Livneh, 1991), somatopsychology (Lewin, 1935; Trieschmann, 1988; Wright, 1983), the disability centrality model (Bishop, 2005), ecological models (Livneh & Antonak, 1997;

Trieschmann, 1988; Vash & Crewe, 2004), recurrent or integrated model (Kendall & Buys, 1998), transactional model of coping (Lazarus & Folkman, 1984), and chaos theory (Parker, Schaller, & Hansmann, 2003).

RESPONSE TO DISABILITY FOR PERSONS WITH CONGENITAL DISABILITIES

Although there is a plethora of conceptual and empirical literature regarding the adjustment or adaptation to an acquired disability, far less attention has been directed toward the psychosocial impact of a congenital disability, or those disabilities people have at birth (Varni, Rubenfeld, Talbot, & Setoguchi, 1989). Some researchers anecdotally believe that since individuals born with a disability have no predisability background to compare with or loss of function to grieve, they generally do not have any apparent difficulties adjusting (Olkin, 1999). In actuality, the available literature is inconsistent in these findings (Cadman, Boyle, Szatmari, & Offord, 1987; Olkin, 1999; Trask et al., 2003; Varni et al., 1989; Wallander, Varni, Babani, Banis, & Wilcox, 1988; Witt, Riley, & Jo Coiro, 2003).

From a psychosocial development standpoint, we theoretically all generally pass through a number of critical life cycle stages of development (Erikson, Erikson, & Kivnick, 1986). Erikson et al. unfortunately did not take into account when a disability occurs; however, he as a former student of psychodynamics, would likely view the individual as experiencing some pathology at various stages. Statistically, data from the 1994 to 1995 National Health Interview Surveys, Disability Supplement population study (Witt et al., 2003) indicate that psychological maladjustment was 10%–15% higher among children with CID as opposed to otherwise healthy children in the early 1970s (Pless, Roghmann, & Haggerty, 1972). As previously indicated, however, level of severity of disability has little impact on response (Wallander & Varni, 1998). In the 1994–1995 national health survey of biological mothers, the psychosocial status of 3362 disabled and nondisabled children and adolescents ages six to 17 were assessed. Children with psychiatric disabilities were excluded. Poor maternal health or mental health, child perceived family burden (scored by answering yes to one or more of three questions asking whether family disruptions in work status, sleep patterns, or financial problems occurred), and living in poverty were all positively associated with reported maladjustment of the children. Mothers of children with disabilities were more likely to be divorced, separated, or never married as well as in poorer health and depressed as opposed to mothers with a nondisabled child. In addition, children with communication or learning limitations also were positively associated with poor adjustment. Conversely, Varni et al. (1989) found that family cohesion, organization, and moral-religious emphasis, were all predictors of positive psychological and social adaptation in 42 children with congenital or acquired limb disabilities. Researchers also found that increased parental distress, such as wishful thinking and self-blame, were associated with increased distress among children and adolescents with cancer. It appears that environmental or external influences, such as emotionally stable family support and cohesion, are key factors that predict child adaptation.

Olkin (1999) notes that even among well-meaning or well-intended parents, children with disabilities can still run into adjustment problems. Specifically, Olkin discusses the "conspiracy of silence," where well-meaning parents intentionally withhold information or ignore discussing important topics with their child regarding his or her prognosis, sexuality, and so on, because the parents perceive it will upset their child. Similarly, some parents overprotect them by not allowing opportunities for their child to compete, or attempt new experiences for fear of him or her failing. This undermines the child's ability to handle stress and be exposed to new experiences, ultimately hurting the child as he or she becomes an adult (Hogansen, Powers, Geenen, Gil-Kashiwabara, & Powers, 2008). By being sheltered, some children with disabilities are often less physically independent, having had everything done for them, and as a result may experience low self-esteem and greater social anxiety and immaturity (Holmbeck et al., 2002; Levy, 1966; Thomasgard, 1998). Seligman (1975) describes the concept "learned helplessness" to describe instances where individuals repeatedly have things done for them over time, essentially learning to be helpless and unable to perform tasks or activities they could otherwise be capable of performing had they been taught or empowered to learn.

In referring back to the Erikson et al. (1986) theory of psychosocial development, some children with congenital disabilities might otherwise experience psychosocial difficulties with shame or self-doubt (Erikson's *autonomy versus shame*) at an early age as a result of not being allowed, or physically able, to explore their environment (Kivnick, 1991). This can carry over during school-age years (Erikson's *industry versus inferiority* stage), where children with severe disabilities are unable to master their environment and, at times, come under ridicule from fellow students (Connors & Stalker, 2007; Kivnick, 1991). Adolescents with disabilities can experience a particularly awkward and difficult time (Erikson's *identity versus identity confusion*). Generally believed to be a time when they develop a sense of identity, Kivnick (1991) notes how adolescents' general acceptance of their disabilities and mastery over their environment dictates the strength of their identities. If adolescents have been unable to master and/or explore their environment, they may theoretically succumb to societal expectations about disabilities. Other potentially problematic areas during teenage years include body changes due to puberty, body image, peer relations, sexuality, and rejection (Davis, Anderson, Linkowski, Berger, & Feinstein, 1991; Hofman, 1975; Gordon, Tschopp, & Feldman, 2004; Rousso, 1996). Livneh and Antonak (2007) cite the importance of body image on self-esteem, and note how persons with disabilities may be particularly vulnerable to poor body image perceptions. Not being viewed as "different" becomes critically important to the psychosocial well-being of adolescents; as the alternative, rejection and ridicule, can be devastating to self-esteem (Bramble, 1995; Connors & Stalker, 2007; Davis et al., 1991; Howland & Rintala, 2001; Gordon et al., 2004; Rousso, 1996).

Despite what appears to be a number of societal attitude barriers for persons growing up with an acquired or congenital disability, overall reports of happiness, contentment, and life satisfaction are mixed, but generally positive (Albrecht & Devlieger, 1999; Allman, 1990; Cohen & Napolitano, 2007; Connors & Stalker, 2007; Freedman, 1978; Lucas, 2007; Marinic & Brkljacic, 2008). Connors and Stalker (2007), for example, in interviewing 26 children aged 7–15, found that despite the children citing public reactions of sometimes being stared at, condescended, harassed, and being pitied; they otherwise reported seeing themselves in a positive way and basically similar to nondisabled children. As Thomasgard (1998) and others have found, however, parental perceptions and projections of their child's psychosocial well-being is frequently viewed much more negatively than the child views his or her own circumstances (Holmbeck et al., 2002; Trask et al., 2003), sometimes leading to parental guilt.

Marinic and Brkljacic (2008) surveyed 397 persons with varying types of disabilities compared with 913 nondisabled Croatians regarding levels of happiness and well-being. Of the group with disabilities, approximately 22% were either born with their disabilities or acquired them before age seven. The authors correlated happiness between both groups with life satisfaction by measuring *Happiness* with the Fordyce scale (1988), and subjective well-being (SWB) using the *Personal Wellbeing Index* (Cummins, 2006), which measures satisfaction with life domains. Results indicated both groups showed positive happiness and satisfaction with the majority of life domains; however, happiness levels of persons with disabilities were lower than the control group in several areas. Less than 15% of persons with disabilities rated themselves as "extremely happy" compared with 40% of the nondisabled control group. Overall happiness score means on a 10-point scale with 10 being extremely happy, showed the disability group ($M = 6.14$) scored slightly lower compared with the control group ($M = 7.8$). In contrast, Myers and Diener (1996) conducted a meta-analysis of 916 research projects from 45 countries with over one million participants, finding that people on average are moderately happy and scored a mean of 6.75/10 on the same scale. Participants in the Marinic and Brkljacic (2008) study also scored moderately satisfied regardless of disability. The disabled group, however, scored significantly different in the areas of happiness and physical safety and community acceptance. The authors opine that safety of the physical environment and positive or negative societal attitudes had an impact on their happiness, whereas this generally is not a consideration for persons without disabilities.

Overall, persons born with a disability are statistically at greater risk for substance abuse problems, twice as likely to drop out of school, and more likely to be living in poverty than children without disabilities (Helwig & Holicky, 1994; Olkin, 1999). Research indicates that family and community support are critical in the positive psychosocial development of children and adolescents. When family cohesion, stability, and nurturing are dysfunctional, the likelihood increases for children to grow up with greater levels of adjustment problems. In addition, the person–environment interaction has time and again in numerous studies proved to be critical regarding individual self-concept and adaptation to disability. There is, however, what Freedman (1978) describes as the "disability paradox," whereby persons with disabilities who otherwise perceive themselves as having successfully coped with environmental and societal barriers, and believe they have emerged even stronger than others, will generally report a very high quality of life and level of happiness (Weinberg, 1988).

THEORIES OF ADJUSTMENT AND ADAPTATION TO ACQUIRED DISABILITIES

A Brief History of Adjustment Theories

This section addresses seven various models of adjustment, adaptation, or reaction to an acquired disability that occurs sometime later in life. Again, some models have stronger evidence-based empirical support, whereas others are supported by clinical observation or qualitative self-report methods. As this line of academic study has evolved, some of the earliest theories on adjustment to disability were postulated by Dembo, Leviton, and Wright (1956), and later expanded upon by Wright (1960, 1983). Successful versus unsuccessful adjustment was initially conceptualized within a "coping" versus "succumbing" framework. Essentially, Dembo et al. (1956) theorized that successful coping involved assisting clients to recognize what they functionally could do as opposed to dwelling on what they no longer could do, emphasizing personal accomplishments, taking direct control of one's life, successfully negotiating physical and social access barriers, enjoying and expanding upon social activities and appropriately dealing with negative life experiences. Conversely, poor adjustment was described as succumbing to one's disability by dwelling on the past, focusing on one's limitations rather than assets, and passively accepting the disabled role as defined by society (e.g., helpless, pitied, incapable).

Wright (1983) refined her earlier theory by equating adjustment or acceptance to disability by emphasizing the values and beliefs individuals' ascribe of their conditions. Wright distinguished between successfully reevaluating one's disabling circumstances as opposed to devaluing or denigrating oneself with the onset of a physical disability. She proposed four reevaluation changes that must occur for successful adaptation. Specifically, (a) subordination of physique or placing less self-worth emphasis on one's physical appearance, (b) containing or minimizing the "spread" affect of the disability to other nonaffected functions and activities, (c) enlarging one's scope of values and interests consistent with one's abilities, and (d) transformation from comparative to asset values. In other words, instead of comparing oneself to those without disabilities, focusing more on remaining abilities and qualities one can engage in rather than the functions one can no longer engage in. Wright's thinking on adjustment to disability went through a transformation as well. In her 1983 classic, *Physical Disability: A Psychosocial Approach*, Wright affirms the significance of the social environment and interpersonal relationships on adjustment; whereas, in her 1960 book titled *Physical Disability: A Psychological Approach*, she focused mostly on the psychodynamics of adjustment and the individual. Although psychologists have been criticized for ignoring the impact of environmental barriers and negative societal attitudes on an individual's adjustment, Wright and others began to acknowledge this relationship early on (Forshaw, 2007).

Stage Models

Livneh (1986, 1991) provides a succinct summary and synthesis of more than 40 explicit and implicit stage models of adjustment, described as a reaction to a sudden and unexpected permanent physically disabling condition. The variations of this model range in theory from three to 10 stages, but most commonly four to six stages. Livneh cites several authors regarding a number of shared assumptions or rules of thumb applicable to these models. Several of the more pertinent assumptions are: (a) adjustment is not a static, but rather dynamic ongoing process, despite the concept that adaptation is considered to be the final outcome (Kahana, Fairchild, & Kahana, 1982); (b) the initial insult causes a psychological disequilibrium that typically restabilizes over time; (c) most individuals sequentially transition through time-limited stages by coming to terms psychologically with whatever trauma has occurred to them;

(d) although most individuals will experience most stages, others may not; (e) not everyone will transition through all stages sequentially; some individuals skip stages, some regress backwards to a previous stage, some can become stuck in a stage for long periods, whereas others may never reach the final adjustment stage (Gunther, 1969, 1971); (f) experiencing different stages separately and sequentially does not always occur, as some individuals may be observed to be in overlapping stages (Dunn, 1975) without any particular timeline, and often fluctuate based on individual circumstances and coping mechanisms; (g) observations at each stage can be correlated with certain cognitions, emotions, and behaviors; and (h) although stages are self-triggered, appropriate behavioral, psychosocial, and environmental interventions (counseling) can positively affect coping strategies to successfully transition toward adaptation (Livneh, 1991, pp. 113–114).

The five stages of adjustment to a sudden-onset physical disability postulated by Livneh (1991) are formulated as follows:

Initial impact
This first stage generally involves individual and often family reaction during the initial hours and days following a sudden and severe bodily trauma, such as a spinal cord injury, limb amputation, heart attack or sudden onset of a life-threatening disease. Two sub-stages are commonly identified; *shock* and *anxiety.* Shock is characterized as surreal with a described numbing-like affect (Gunther, 1971). Thought processes are disorganized, disoriented, and confused, and many individuals have difficulty concentrating and are unable to make simple decisions (Livneh & Antonak, 1997; Shands, 1955). Anxiety is described as overwhelming and can trigger a panic attack or hysteria-like behavior in extreme reaction cases. Some empirical support for these two reactions exists in the cross-sectional study by Livneh and Antonak (1991) with 214 rehabilitation facility inpatient and outpatient participants with various conditions, including spinal cord injury, cerebrovascular accidents, and multiple sclerosis. Participant's distinguished between past and present reactions to their disabilities, indicating earlier adaptation phases were reported significantly more frequently in the past than present, including shock, anxiety, depression, internalized anger, and externalized hostility.

Defense mobilization
This stage is characterized by two sub-stages as well: *bargaining* and *denial.* Bargaining is described as a religious or spiritual attempt to negotiate with God or higher power to be cured with the expectation of full recovery. In essence, the individual (and often the family) pray for survival and/or recovery with a promise to pay penance for any past wrongdoing (Livneh, 1991). Also, in return for a cure or recovery, individuals may promise to donate to the church, do charitable work, and so on. Livneh describes bargaining as being short-term in nature, whereas denial is seen as lasting longer. Although bargaining and denial are seen as overlapping, denial is viewed as a more "extensive level of suppression or negation of the disability and its ramifications in order to maintain self integrity." (Livneh, 1991, p. 119). Related to this is the extensively studied and debated coping dimensions of problem versus emotion focused coping (Carver, Scheier, & Weintraub, 1989; Folkman & Moskowitz, 2004).

Problem focused coping is described as a more task oriented, constructive, and positive way of dealing with stressful events, whereby an individual recognizes the problem, thinks of strategies to solve it, weighs the pros and cons of the decision, decides, and implements the chosen strategy (Cheng, Kuan, Li, & Ken, 2010; Endler & Parker, 1990). *Emotion focused coping* is described as a coping strategy to minimize or reduce the negative emotions associated with the stressor by denying, avoiding, or engaging in distracting activities (Folkman & Lazarus, 1980, 1985). The debate has centered around which coping strategy is more appropriate for alleviating an individual's distress. Typically, problem focused coping has received greater support; however, emotion focused coping appears best in instances where an individual experiences some emotionally overwhelming and extreme trauma that he or she has little control over, and the problem cannot be solved. More recently, researchers suggest that both coping domains cannot be clearly distinguished from one another, and may overlap and represent variations of one another (Endler & Parker, 1990; Folkman & Moscowitz, 2004). Cheng et al. (2010) in their study of 180 undergraduate students regarding problem and emotion focused coping strategies, found that "certainty emotions" (such as anger, disgust, happiness and contentment) elicited problem focused coping because the students perceived being in control of the situation. "Uncertainty emotions" (hope, surprise, worry, fear, and sadness) most often elicited emotion focused coping when the event was perceived as uncontrollable. These findings were originally supported by Folkman and Lazarus (1980) and have since been affirmed by Nabi (2003) and Smith and Ellsworth (1985).

Denial is the other major sub-stage cited during this period (Livneh, 1991; Livneh & Antonak, 1997). Denial is a defense mechanism to protect the self from overwhelming fear and sadness, by optimistically hoping things will get better, and temporarily escaping the immense emotional sadness and fear of the unknown. Smart notes that denial can take three forms: denying the presence of the disability, denying the implications of the disability, or denying the permanency of the disability (Smart, 2009, p. 393). Livneh (1991) cites additional cognitions, behaviors, and emotions during this stage, including distorting facts and selective attention to good news, repressing unacceptable realities, constantly seeking information, setting unrealistic goals, having unrealistic expectations, refusing to modify the home or talk to persons with similar disabilities, and evading future planning with the belief that it won't be necessary (Dunn, 1975; Falek & Britton, 1974; Gunther, 1971; Naugle, 1991). Ironically, persons in denial have been observed with a range of emotions, including cheerfulness and happiness at one end as they unrealistically hope for recovery (Parker, 1979), to despair and anger during moments of realizing the permanency of their disabilities (Weller & Miller, 1977). Meyerowitz (1980), however, noted that denial can be adaptive as well, protecting the individual from overwhelming life-altering news. As Livneh and Antonak (1997) cite, denial continues to be debated by researchers regarding its relative value or hindrance in adjusting to a disability. Specifically, Livneh and Antonak (1997) cite denial in the literature as either a stage or phase of adaptation in dealing with traumatic loss, or a defense mechanism that protects our ego to minimize or escape overwhelming anxiety. In this latter instance, denial is part of an emotion focused response, which has arguably been viewed as temporarily helpful soon after injury, especially where the circumstances cannot be controlled (Meyerowitz, 1980). Theoretically, and for practical application purposes, should counselors confront patients and their families regarding the seriousness and/or grim permanency of the disability, or should these individuals be allowed to "hope?" This is debatable. The practical application may indeed be to assist individuals by never taking their hope away, but to encourage them to continue with their rehabilitation programs, therapy programs, and so on, in the event that the disabilities may be with them for awhile. This tangible compromise could then be viewed as "healthy denial," where the individuals and their families continue to move forward, while not being denied their hope that a miracle or medical advances may exist in the near or distant future (I. Marini, pers. comm., September 14, 2009).

Initial realization

The third stage is again also characterized by two major sub-stages: *mourning and depression* and *internalized anger.* Mourning or grief is typically of shorter duration where the individual grieves the loss of body function and past way of life. Depression is generally longer and future oriented, where cognitions involve fear of an often uncertain and perceived grim future. Suicidal ideation is sometimes present during this stage as well as asking "why me" of God or higher power (Kubler-Ross, 1981). The theory of mourning and depression has encountered some debate among researchers as to whether or not all individuals actually go through a diagnosable clinical depression, and whether going through a depression is mandatory to move on to acceptance (Trieschmann, 1988). Wortman and Silver (1989) reviewed the existing empirical evidence regarding bereavement following a physical disability and found that not all individuals report experiencing a depression. Recently, Maciejewski, Zhang, Block, and Prigerson's (2007) brief study with 233 individuals who had suffered the death of a loved one from natural causes, found participants mourned the loss of a loved one more so than they reported becoming depressed. The temporal sequence reported by grieving loved ones included disbelief, which peaked at 1 month, yearning at 4 months, anger at 5 months, and a depression plateau at about 6 months postloss. Acceptance of the loss was observed to gradually occur as time went on over a 24-month observation period. Livneh (1991) and Livneh & Antonak (1997) cite common reactive depression observations during this stage as including feelings of hopelessness, despair, anxiety, intense sadness, withdrawal, and despondency as well.

Alternatively, Worden's task of mourning concept identifies four tasks that mourners can actively work through to adapt to their loss (Worden, 2009, p. 38). The first task involves accepting the reality that the loved one has died and will not return. Some mourner's see their loved one in a crowd, deny he or she is dead, keep their possessions ready for them to return, and so on. The second task Worden identifies is the process of experiencing the emotional and behavioral pain. Some mourner's repress painful emotions and do not allow themselves to feel the pain. Burying or avoiding such emotions can eventually lead to clinical depression. The third task involves adjusting to a world without the loved one. External adjustments include taking on the activities (e.g., paying bills, shopping, house chores) the loved one performed, while internal adjustments involve being an independent person from your loved one, concerning self-esteem, self-identity, and the like. Spiritual adjustments during this task involve making sense of the world and testing one's faith and beliefs as to why this happened. The final task is that of maintaining an enduring, healthy connection with the deceased loved one while moving on with a new life. Worden indicates that these tasks are not fixed stages and can be experienced and worked on simultaneously because grieving is a fluid and not a static process.

Smart (2009) differentiated between how the individual mourns and/or possibly becomes depressed following a disabling injury, and the societal expectation "requirement to mourn" as hypothesized by Wright (1983). It is expected that persons with disabilities should feel bad and constantly grieve their losses indefinitely because it is the presumed normal response to their misfortune. This societal belief that an individual must mourn and will continually grieve a loss is a common misconception, but a projected value judgment by others nonetheless regarding how they think they would feel if they became disabled. Despite studies showing that most persons with a traumatic onset disability gradually adjust to their situations over time, the societal requirement to mourn continues to be perpetuated (Livneh & Antonak, 1991; Marini, Rogers, Slate, & Vines, 1995; Silver, 1982; Wright, 1983).

Internalized anger essentially involves self-blame, guilt, and shame. The individual blames him or herself and often views the disability as punishment from God for some alleged wrongdoing (Hohmann, 1975; Marini & Graf, 2010). This self-blame can be amplified if the individual was indeed the cause of his or her injuries (e.g., drunk driving), which can make adjustment much more difficult (Livneh & Antonak, 1997). Suicidal ideation, risk-taking, and self-injurious behavior can occur at this stage as well. Janoff-Bulman (1979) differentiate between behavioral and characterological self-blame attributions and their perceived impact on adjustment. Behavioral self-blame refers to individuals who believe their behavior caused their injuries; and in such cases, individuals can adjust more readily knowing that they were, and are, in control of events. Conversely, characterological self-blame refers to individuals who attribute blame to flaws in their characters or personalities, and hence, believe their fate was unavoidable and deserving. Overall, research is mixed regarding self-blame attributions of disability, with some finding a positive relationship between coping and self-blame attributions (Janoff-Bulman, 1979) and others a negative relationship where individuals with spinal cord injury were perceived as coping less well (Bordieri, Comninel, & Drehmer, 1989; Westbrook & Nordholm, 1986). Bordieri and Kilbury (1991) surveyed 84 rehabilitation counseling graduates using observer simulation regarding self-blame attributions. They found that characterological self-blamers were rated as coping less well, more depressed, and having perceived less control of future life events than individuals who attributed blame to behavior.

Retaliation

In Livneh's (1991) conceptualization of the five-stage model of adjustment, retaliation is the fourth stand-alone stage with no sub-stages. In their 1997 description of this concept, Livneh and Antonak refer to retaliation as externalized hostility. This stage essentially involves "rebelling against a perceived dependency fate ... anger is now projected onto the external world in the form of hostility toward other people, objects, or environmental conditions" (Livneh, 1991, p. 124). During this stage, individuals may blame and lash out at perceived incompetent medical professionals for not doing enough, and/or significant others for no apparent reason due to frustration and anger. Behaviorally, individuals may become noncompliant with hospital rules, use profanity, make accusations, attempt to manipulate hospital staff and significant others, or physically strike others (Krueger, 1981–1982; Livneh & Antonak, 1997). Smart (2009) notes how some individuals may initially be angry with God about being unfairly punished. Marini and Graf (2010) surveyed 157 persons with spinal cord injury regarding their spiritual or religious beliefs and practices, and found that whereas some respondents were initially angry with God postinjury, this tended to subside over time in the majority, but not all cases.

Final adjustment or reintegration

This final stage delineates a cognitive, affective, and behavioral component. Livneh and Antonak note how acknowledgment is a cognitive reconciliation or acceptance of the disability and its permanency. A new disability self-concept is formed, and individuals seek to master their environment by problem-solving. Persons who reach this stage are able to "accept him or herself as a person with a disability, gain a new sense of self-concept, reappraise life values, and seek new meanings and goals" (Livneh and Antonak, 1997, p. 22). Emotionally, individuals are "okay" with their disabilities, and can talk about it without becoming upset. Behaviorally, persons in this stage will begin to actively pursue social, academic and/or vocational goals, and learn to successfully navigate physical and social environmental barriers. Livneh and Antonak (1991) found correlational support for acceptance among 214 rehabilitation patients during the temporal later phase of disability onset. Similarly, Marini et al. (1995) surveyed 63 persons with spinal cord injury during their first, second, or fifth year postinjury, finding that self-esteem increased over time, as respondents became more comfortable and confident with their disability status.

Despite all the caveats to the stage model of adjustment, a number of criticisms have been cited (Kendall & Buys, 1998; Olkin, 1999; Parker et al., 2003). Some concerns relate to the dangers of counselors expecting and anticipating persons with sudden onset physical disabilities to go through specific stages (Kendall & Buys, 1998). Others cite the complexity of human behavior and the attempt to fit everyone through these stages when there are so many complex individual differences regarding people's coping mechanisms, environmental factors, and extenuating circumstances (Parker et al., 2003). Related, some researchers argue that there exists little empirical support for the stage model of adjustment (Chan, Da Silva Cardoso, & Chronister, 2009; Olkin, 1999).

Although many injured persons have been found to progress from initially experiencing higher to lower levels of distress over time, others do not show any signs of intense distress, and some remain in a heightened level of distress for longer periods (Wortman & Silver, 1989). As discussed later with the recurrent model, some researchers argue that persons with physical disabilities do grieve the loss of bodily function and preinjury lifestyle, and that the permanency of the loss leads to recurrent and unpredictable periods of chronic sorrow (Burke, Hainsworth, Eakes, & Lindgren, 1992; Davis, 1987; Kendall & Buys, 1998; Teel, 1991).

Somatopsychology

As briefly introduced in Chapter 4, field theory postulated by Kurt Lewin (1935, 1936) centers around the belief that our self-concept or self-worth, can, and is affected by the feedback we perceive from interacting with others in our environment referred to as our "life space." Although Lewin's original theory did not include the impact a disability has on this reciprocal interaction, researchers since then have refined the hypothesis to include impact of disability (Barker, Wright, Meyerson, & Gonick, 1953; Dembo et al., 1956; Trieschmann, 1988; Wright, 1960, 1983). The revised theory has been encompassed as *Behavior* (B) is a function (*f*) of *Psychosocial* variables, such as self-esteem and coping skills (P), *Organic* factors related to the disability, such as paralysis or blindness (O), and *Environmental* or physical access and attitudinal factors (E), comprising the formula $B = f(P \times O \times E)$ summarized by Trieschmann (1988). Lewin's somatopsychology theory was the first to take a more social psychological view of human behavior as opposed to focusing exclusively on individual behavior in isolation.

Specific to this theory then, becomes the central question with regards to how do persons with disabilities perceive themselves in Western society's mirror? A synopsis of historical attitudes in general would suggest many persons with disabilities have been stigmatized, discriminated against, persecuted, devalued, dehumanized, and essentially treated as minorities (Chubon, 1994; Olkin, 1999; Smart, 2009; Mackelprang & Salsgiver, 2009). Arguably, for individuals who possess a more *internal locus of control*, many of these negative experiences would potentially not have as demoralizing emotional effect as for persons who have a more *external locus of control* (Elfstrom & Kreuter, 2006; Frank & Elliott, 1989). Past research indicates that the link between locus of control and emotional well-being is mediated by coping strategies (Elfstrom & Kreuter, 2006; Frank & Elliott, 1989). These authors found that persons with spinal cord injuries who perceived they were more in control of their life circumstances (internal locus) possessed greater levels of acceptance and emotional well-being than the group who believed their destinies were not in their hands (external locus). As Maltby, Day, and Macaskill (2007) note regarding clinical depression and various illnesses and disabilities, persons who are internally located tend to attribute their self-worth to their own efforts and internal evaluation, whereas persons who are externally located are more likely to evaluate their self-worth based on how others respond to them, and believe their circumstances are controlled more by environmental influences and not themselves. Wright (1983) would otherwise view those externally located individuals who regularly experience discriminating and demoralizing attitudes of others as more susceptible to "succumbing" to the societal limitations imposed by society, thereby adjusting less well.

Some of the empirical support for this theory centers around assessing the attitudes of persons with disabilities in relation to their lived experiences in the community. As earlier noted, Li and Moore's (1998) surveyed 1266 adults with disabilities re: acceptance of disability in relation to their experiences in the community. Aside from friends and family emotional support playing a significant role in adjustment, perceived societal discrimination had a negative impact on accepting one's disability. DiTomasso and Spinner (1997) additionally found their respondents with disabilities reported greater levels of loneliness when confronted by the negative attitudes of others. Similarly, Hopp Pepin, Arseneau, Frechette, and Begin's (2001) sample of 39 adults with physical disabilities showed a high correlation between feelings of loneliness, social anxiety, and poorer social skills they attributed to poor physical access in their communities. Finally, Graf, Marini, and Blankenship's (2009) qualitative survey of 78 persons with spinal cord dysfunction to compose in 100 words or less what experience(s) best exemplified their living with disabilities, most frequently reported anger and frustration from encountering physical access barriers in the community. Clearly, repeated negative experiences with others in society can, over time, impact how well someone adjusts to their disabilities.

Disability Centrality Model

The most recent adaptation model to chronic illness and disability (CID) has shown to have great promise theoretically, empirically, and with tangible clinical implications (Bishop, 2005). Drawing upon Devins' illness intrusiveness approach (Devins et al., 1983; Devins, 1994), Livneh's (2001) conceptual framework, and the value change concepts of Dembo et al. (1956; Wright, 1960, 1983), Bishop proposes the disability centrality model (DCM). Bishop (2005) describes six tenets as the theoretical underpinnings for DCM that factor in subjective and objective quality-of-life (QOL) satisfaction, and control over one's medical and environmental circumstances. These are summarized as follows: (a) the impact of a CID can be measured by a multidimensional subjective QOL measure; (b) QOL is an individual's overall perceived subjective satisfaction of life domains that are disproportional due to individual differences regarding which domains are more important (central) to us; (c) the onset of a CID results in an initial reduction in overall QOL and centrally important satisfying activities as well as feelings of personal control; (d) the degree of QOL reduced is dependent upon how many central domains are affected; (e) individuals seek to maintain and maximize overall QOL by minimizing gaps (distress) caused by the CID; and, (f) people strive to close these gaps by either changing their values and interests commensurate with their disabled abilities, employ strategies to increase perceived control over their health and environment, or alternatively do nothing to improve control or change their values (He, 2005a, p. 223; Bishop & Feist-Price, 2002; Devins et al., 1983).

Bishop (2005) incorporates the concept of domain satisfaction and importance described by Devins et al. (1983) and others (Frisch, 1999; Pavot & Diener, 1993) regarding the relative significance various QOL domains may have for each individual. For example, a construction worker with a grade 9 education who sustains a tetraplegia and has derived great satisfaction from work and playing sports preinjury will likely experience a poorer adjustment if he or she can no longer engage in either domain. In contrast, a professor with the same injury will likely be able to retain employment and try to compensate (develop new interests) for being unable to play sports. In both instances, the former individual would likely experience a greater reduction in satisfaction and perceived control than the professor, and hence a greater reduction in overall QOL (Frisch, 1999). Although Bishop (2005) concedes there will never be a universal agreement on what all the QOL life domains should include, there has been increased agreement over the years on certain domains, including physical and mental health, social support, employment or a satisfying or avocational activity, and economic or material well-being (Bishop & Allen, 2003; Jalowiec, 1990). Cummins (2002) differentiated between objective and subjective QOL domains. Objective indicators include more tangible domains, such as employment, wage earnings, marital status, and so on, whereas a more subjective assessment of one's QOL, which Roessler (1990) describes, is an individual's private assessment or feeling about his or her life situation. As Cummins (2005) has noted, however, there is a weak relationship between objective and subjective measures of QOL. In other words, people can have what others may think is a great job, income, marriage, and so on, and yet those that seem to have it all score poorly on life satisfaction, subjective well-being, and happiness (Dijkers, 1997; Myers & Diener, 1995).

In addition, incorporating Devins' illness intrusiveness model (Devins et al., 1983; Devins & Shnek, 2000) proposes that when individuals sustain a CID, the impact compromises psychological well-being by temporarily or permanently reducing positive or meaningful activities as well as reducing real or perceived control to regain the positive activities or outcomes and avoid negative ones. The central question then becomes whether or not individuals can compensate for lost interests that once brought them enjoyment but they no longer can engage in? With Bishop's DCM, the counselor must be able to assess what are the "central" or most important life satisfaction domains for clients, and how these can be compensated for or replaced (Groot & Van Den Brink, 2000; Misajon, 2002). This concept is similar to Wright's (1960, 1983) "value change" theory, whereby individuals who perceive a loss in one area of their lives, attempt to develop new interests within their capabilities (i.e., transitioning from enjoying jogging to reading for persons with a mobility impairment). This has also been termed "preference drift" (Groot & Van Den Brink, 2000) and "response shift" by Schwartz and Sprangers (2000).

Empirical support for DCM is building. Bishop (2005) assessed 72 college students with disabilities using the *Delighted-Terrible Scale* (Andrews & Withey, 1976), the *Ladder of Adjustment Scale* (Crewe & Krause, 1990), and what Bishop (2005) describes as the *Domain Scale*, which assessed 10 domains re: QOL. Overall, results indicated a positive correlation between QOL and psychosocial adaptation to CID. A second correlation was found between satisfaction and perceived control in relation to the impact of CID and QOL. Bishop describes counseling interventions that empowers clients to assert more control over their circumstances, developing new interests or response shift, and working through the loss of satisfying activities no longer accessible.

Bishop, Shepard, and Stenhoff (2007) conducted a follow-up DCM study with 98 persons with multiple sclerosis. In this study, Bishop et al. discuss subjective quality of life (SQOL) or subjective well-being relating to the previously described QOL domains (Johnson, Amtmann, Yorkston, Klasner, & Kuehn, 2004) and psychosocial adaptation. The assessments used were the *Delighted-Terrible Scale, Ladder of Adjustment Scale*, and the *Disability Centrality Scale* (DCS, Bishop & Allen, 2003); the last of which measures 10 life domains, including physical health, mental health (emotional well-being, happiness, enjoyment), work/studies, leisure activities, financial situation, relationship with significant other, family relations, other social relations, autonomy/independence, and religious or spiritual expression (Bishop & Allen, 2003, p. 7). Results indicated a positive correlation between scores on the self-management scale and both perceived control and QOL. The second positive correlation was found between scores on the Ladder of Adjustment Scale and overall QOL satisfaction across domains. Bishop et al. (2007) again cite similar tangible counselor intervention strategies involving assisting clients in developing new interests and asserting more control over their situations. Livneh and Antonak (1997) view the DCM as an ecological model; however, it is treated separately here due its emphasis on perceived control and satisfaction of life domains.

Ecological Models

Chan et al. (2009) make the observation that even within the ecological models of adjustment to disability, there is overlap representing the stage or phase theory of adjustment including early reactions of shock, anxiety, and denial; intermediate reactions of depression, internalized anger, and externalized anger; and later reactions involving acknowledgment, acceptance and adjustment (Chan et al., 2009, p. 58). As we conclude later, all of these proposed theories have overlapping and similar concepts.

Two theorists who summarize the complexity of ecological models best are arguably Trieschmann (1988) and Vash and Crewe (2004). These models involve a foundation of three major determining factors that consider: (a) nature of the disability, (b) characteristics of the person, and (c) environmental influences. Within each of these determining factors are subsets that require exploration by the counselor to assess what, if any, bearing each of these factors have on psychosocial adjustment. It is important to note that none of these factors may negatively influence poor adjustment, or conversely, any one of these factors in and of themselves if deemed important by the individual may delay or prolong adjustment. A brief summary of each is provided.

Nature of the disability

This factor explores aspects of the disability itself and the implications of each. The first sub-factor considers the *time of onset* regarding whether an individual was born with a disability or acquires it sometime later in life. Vash and Crewe (2004) discuss some potential implications for someone who is born with a disability, including being treated as an infinite child, isolated and overprotected, unable to engage in many childhood activities, and as (Olkin, 1999) describes, sometimes subjected to a "conspiracy of silence" where parents do not discuss their child's prognosis or treatment with him or her at the risk of upsetting their child. Conversely, as we explore in detail regarding the psychosocial aspects of an acquired disability, one can succumb to a whole host of other adjustment issues (Kendall & Buys, 1998; Livneh, 1991). The next sub-factor, *type of onset* concerns whether or not the disability had a sudden impact (spinal cord injury from a car accident) versus a prolonged onset (more gradual, such as multiple sclerosis) and the implications of each. In the case of sudden onset, perceived attribu-tion of blame becomes a factor that influences adjustment. Specifically, research is mixed regarding the implications of self-induced versus other-induced attribution of blame on adjustment. Although on the one hand, findings indicate those who accept the responsibility of their injuries may possess a more internal locus of control and therefore may adjust better, they also may be more self-critical and angry at the fact that they could have possibly prevented their accidents (Athelstan & Crewe, 1979; Bulman & Wortman, 1977; Reidy & Caplan, 1994). *Functions impaired* addresses the relative importance each of us place on our functional abilities. For example, some individuals are most terrified to lose their sight, whereas others fear becoming paral-yzed or losing their hearing the most. Related to this factor is the significance these abilities play in our lives. An academic whose livelihood and intrinsic interests revolve around reading may be devastated by vision loss. Wright (1983), however, reminds us of the "insider" perspective, whereby those persons who have lived and adapted to their disabilities emphatically disagree that it is the worst thing (bodily func-tion) they could lose. Unfortunately, many in the lay public perceive most any disability as a tragedy, and one that they are not certain they could live with (Olkin, 1999). *Severity of the disability* essentially considers how severe the disability is, with the once assumed belief that those with more severe disabilities were likely more maladjusted (Livneh & Antonak, 1991). Although some literature finds that this may indeed be the case, it is more commonly believed now that the severity of a disability has little or no impact on how someone will adjust (Livneh & Antonak, 1997; Shontz, 1991; Wallander & Varni, 1998). *Visibility of the disability* considers the reactions individuals with visible dis-abilities sometimes experience (wheelchair users), such as discrimination, devaluation, and being ignored (Graf et al., 2009; Marini, Bhakta, & Graf, 2009). Conversely, con-sider the plight of those with invisible disabilities unknown to the public (low back inju-ries) who may be thought of as lazy or unmotivated if unable to participate in certain activities, such as not wanting to find a job due to ongoing chronic pain. *Stability of the disability* addresses whether the disability is stable and will generally not become worse (spinal cord injury) versus those that have an uncertain prognosis, but become pro-gressively worse over time (Parkinson's disease) (Cheng et al., 2010; Elfstrom & Kreuter, 2006; Folkman & Lazarus, 1980; Frank & Elliott, 1989). The uncertainty of waking up each morning not knowing whether one will still be able to walk or see, not only leaves an individual with no control over their situation but also compro-mises making any future plans. Finally, the concept of *pain* deserves a category unto itself in addressing psychosocial adjustment. As Vash and Crewe (2004) emphasize, unlike many of the other disabilities, chronic pain is a primary or secondary debilitating condition that can have a significant negative impact on an individual's thoughts, emotions, and behaviors. Cognitively, individuals can exhibit poor concentration and attention, suicidal ideation, and reduced problem solving abilities. Emotions often include depression, feelings of hopelessness and helplessness, and despair (Banks & Kerns, 1996; Fishbain, Cutler, & Rosomoff, 1997). Behaviors have been defined as social isolation, withdrawal from activities, and in worst case scenarios, addiction to pain prescription medications and other substances and drug abuse (Lewinsohn, Clarke, & Hops, 1990; Waters, Campbell, Keefe, & Carson, 2004).

Personal characteristics

These determining factors involve individualized traits or characteristics. *Gender* largely considers gender differences in coping with disability as well as societal expectations of males and females (Hwang, 1997; Livneh, 1991; Marini, 2007; Tepper, 1997). There are mixed findings regarding which gender adjusts to a disability better; however, Western societal expectations of each gender are quite clear (Charmaz, 1995a, 1995b; Hwang, 1997). Men are supposed to be rugged, independent, breadwinners, stoic, athletic, dominant, and tough (Charmaz, 1995a, 1995b; Marini, 2007; Zilbergeld, 1992), whereas women are expected to be beautiful in physical appearance, passive, homemakers, and good nurturers (Hwang, 1997). Males and females with severe disabilities may not be able to live up to some or any of these expectations and may have difficulty adjusting if they rely on external cues (societal expectations) for affirmation of their self-concept/self-esteem (Charmaz, 1995a, 1995b; Marini, 2007; Nosek & Hughes, 2007). *Activities affected* relates to the significance individuals place on their activities. A hockey player who becomes paralyzed and is no longer able to play sports may experience greater difficulty adjusting than a professor who has the same injury but still can perform academic activities. Similarly, *interests/values/goals* pertain to the differing passions people have in their lives. Those who proverbially "put all their eggs in one basket" or have few if any interests, and lose the ability to engage in them, will likely find adjustment more stressful than those persons who have multiple interests and are still able to return to some of them (Massimini & Delle Fave, 2000; Schafer, 1996). Lewinsohn et al. (1990) indicate that when people experience a loss and withdraw from engaging in what once was pleasurable activities, there is a greater likelihood of lengthening or exacerbating a reactive depression. *Remaining resources* are described by Vash and Crewe (2004) as the abilities and traits an individual retains regardless of disability. These include intelligence, motivation, sense of humor, extroversion, social poise, resilience, emotional stability, and coping strategies; all of which have been implicated in positive adjustment (see Livneh, 1991). Finally, *spiritual and philosophical base* refers to one's spiritual or religious beliefs, particularly as to whether some people believe their disabilities are punishment from God or higher power, with the assumption that those who believe they are being punished will have a more difficult time adjusting (Byrd, 1990; Gallagher, 1995; Graf, Marini, Baker, & Buck, 2007). Conversely, individuals who believe their disability to be divine intervention or calling for them to serve a higher purpose for God will experience lesser adjustment difficulties (Eareckson, 2001; Graf et al., 2007).

Environmental influences

As extensively detailed earlier, environmental influences may have a significant impact on adaptation to disability (DiTomasso & Spinner, 1997; Graf et al., 2009; Hopps, 2001; Lewin, 1936; Li & Moore, 1998; Wright, 1983). In this determining factor, Vash and Crewe (2004) as well as Trieschmann (1988) describe several contributing factors. *Family acceptance and support* becomes significant in that if a disabled loved one is viewed as a contributing family member and not devalued, this generally correlates with a more positive adjustment to the disability (Li & Moore, 1998). In addition, those families that have been shown to possess positive coping strategies and support one-another, typically adapt well to the disability (Trask et al., 2003). *Income* plays an important role not so much in overall happiness, but rather overall QOL (Diener & Seligman, 2004; Inglehart, 1990; Lykken, 1999). Once people have their basic needs met, there is relatively little difference in happiness ratings between those who are extremely wealthy versus those of more modest means (Diener & Seligman, 2004); however, a higher income and adequate health care positively impacts ability to remain healthy as well as purchase necessary accommodations and equipment/ devices (modified van, accessible home) for a better QOL. *Available community resources* refers to support from local agencies, which could include Centers for Independent Living (CILs), Veterans Affairs services, Client Assistance Programs (CAPs), access to modernized hospitals, and so on. Individuals with severe disabilities who live in rural settings with no resources may not only have to travel long distances for appointments but also be required to be away from home and family at times, having to remain in the city for several days (Smith, Thorngren, & Christopher, 2009). *Social support* is also critical for positive adjustment and fostering self-esteem in most, but not all, instances (Buunk & Verhoeven, 1991; Li & Moore, 1998). Schwarzer and Leppin (1992) define functional support by differentiating between instrumental support (offering financial aid), informational support (giving information and advice), and emotional support (caring, empathy and reassurance). Functional support is further delineated by individuals' perceptions of the support they received (retrospective evaluation) and the perception of available support if needed (anticipation of getting the support) (Lakey & Cassady, 1990; Symister & Friend, 2003). Much like Yuker's (1988) extensive review of the impact of contact regarding positive and a regulator attitudes toward disability, empirical findings are somewhat mixed regarding the benefits of social support (Barrera, 1981; Cohen, 2004; Heller & Rook, 2001; Hupcey, 1998; Lazarus & Folkman, 1984a; Li & Moore, 1998). On the positive side, social support is believed to be a buffer against stress, an appropriate coping strategy, and a regulator negative emotions (Cohen, Gottlieb, & Underwood, 2000). For example, persons who sustain a severe disability may have friends who give or lend them money, help them in finding community resources, and provide emotional support by empathizing and genuinely listening to their concerns. Conversely, having a social support system who are themselves dysfunctional, have promised to help but always have excuses, or in the worst-case scenario take advantage of the person with the disability by neglecting, abusing, or stealing from him or her, are all clear examples of a potentially poorer adjustment process for the disabled individual. Finally, *institutionalization* becomes a concern for those persons with severe disabilities who are unable to physically take care for themselves, do not have the funding to hire an attendant, or have no family or friends who can perform a caregiving function. In such cases, individuals are faced with temporarily or permanently having to reside in a nursing home. Aside from most Americans not wanting to live in a nursing home, the U.S. General Accounting Office (2002) published a study indicating an approximate 25% abuse rate that either resulted in death or serious injury of nursing home residents nationwide. Forms of abuse include neglect, physical abuse, sexual abuse, and malnourishment. Clearly, individuals who have no choice but to live in a nursing home may, in the worse case scenario, be subjected to such abuse or minimally deprived of the freedom to control their environment and thus experience a resulting reduction in QOL (Bishop, 2005). In a best case scenario of well-run nursing homes, persons with severe disabilities may be medically well cared for as well as having a support network that residents would not otherwise have living alone.

Recurrent or Integrated Model of Adjustment

The recurrent or integrated model of adjustment following an acquired disability was essentially hypothesized due to perceived shortcomings of the stage or linear model of disability (Davis, 1987; Wikler, Wasow, & Hatfield, 1981; Wortman & Silver, 1989). One of the several criticisms of the stage model was its theoretical emphasis likening the stages of grief over a deceased loved one (Kubler Ross, 1981) to that of acquiring a disability. The main argument is that persons with acquired disabilities continue to live with their disabilities. Everyday therefore, although the emotional upheaval subsides over time, those with acquired disabilities will continue to periodically experience chronic sorrow throughout their lives. In this sense, there is never a final adjustment or adaptation stage where the disability no longer affects the individual (Davis, 1987; Kendall & Buys, 1998; Wortman & Silver, 1989).

Pertinent to this model are several key concepts. Beck's (1967) cognitive theory defines *cognitive schema* as our ingrained beliefs and assumptions regarding ourselves, others, and how the environment works (Beck & Weishaar, 1989). When a sudden and traumatic disability occurs, many individuals attempt to cling on to comfortable, old schemas due to the overwhelming anxiety and uncertainty the disability brings. Wright (1983) refers to this as "as if" behavior, whereby individuals attempt to minimize anxiety by denying or distorting reality and pretending as if nothing (the disability) has happened. As the old schema no longer adequately works and the individual begins to realize the implications of the disability, depression may set in (Kendall & Buys, 1998). Yoshida (1993) uses the analogy of a wildly swinging pendulum to describe the initial injury phase of anxiety, fear, and grief. Over time, however, the pendulum gradually slows to a middle set-point where individuals will either develop new positive or negative schema of life with a disability (Yoshida, 1993). Positive new schema are formed when individuals with traumatic disabilities can: (a) search and find meaning in the disability and in postdisability life; (b) learn to master or control their environment, their disabilities, and their futures; and (c) protect and enhance the self by incorporating the new disability identity (Barnard, 1990; Kendall & Buys, 1998, p. 17). Conversely, negative schema can also be formed about the disability, allowing stereotypical societal expectations about disability (helpless, incapable) to influence one's self-worth (Charmaz, 1983; Stewart, 1996). Wright (1983) would describe those who develop negative schema as otherwise having succumbed to their disabilities.

Undoubtedly, individuals with acquired disabilities who develop a more negative schema postinjury will in all likelihood be more susceptible to self-pity, low self-esteem and likely more frequent episodes of chronic sorrow. Regardless, according to the theory of recurrent periods of sadness, even individuals who have developed positive schema and have otherwise been successful in their lives will still experience the sorrow or sadness from time to time (Kendall & Buys, 1998). As some research has shown, it is quite likely that these periods of sorrow may be facilitated by environmental influences, such as a relationship rejection, job rejection, or discrimination perceived by the individual as due to his or her disability (Graf et al., 2009; Li & Moore, 1998; Marini et al., 2009). Overall, response to the disability varies for everyone, depending on one's coping mechanisms (Lazarus, 1993; Lazarus & Folkman, 1984a).

Transactional Model of Coping

The most frequently cited and empirically supported theory of coping with stressful events is that of Lazarus and Folkman's transactional theory (1984a, 1984b, 1984c). The author's define coping as "constantly changing cognitive and behavioral alternatives to manage specific external and/or internal demands that are appraised as taxing or exceeding the resources of the person" (Lazarus & Folkman, 1984, p. 141). These appraisal efforts are constantly changing as the individual interacts with his or her environment back and forth, like watching a tennis match. Central to transactional theory are two major components of a sequential appraisal process salient to when people encounter a stress inducing event. The first component referred to as *primary appraisal* is an individual's assessment as to whether a situation is stressful or not. Key to this appraisal is the motivational strength attributed to various personal goals (goal relevance) the stressor may pose, otherwise called goal congruence or incongruence. Individuals will assess whether the stressful event is deemed beneficial or harmful/threatening to the goal. Specifically in the case of disability, will the goal of maintaining optimal health be compromised by the stressful event. If not, no coping mechanisms are required and the individual returns to a state of emotional equilibrium. If however, the situation is deemed as harmful or threatening, the individual moves into the *secondary appraisal* component. At this level, individuals assess their options for coping and expectations about what will happen (Lazarus, 1993). Three sub-components are involved, including blame or who is the event attributable to; coping potential as to whether the individual has any control to change the circumstances of the event and whether they can influence the person–environment relationship; and future expectations regarding perceptions as to how the situation will play out. At both levels of appraisal, Lazarus and Folkman (1984a) discuss problem focused versus emotion focused coping strategies defined earlier. The authors suggest that emotion focused coping is more likely when individual's perceive they have no control over the situation, and that the stressful event (e.g., disability) is indeed harmful or threatening to achieving or blocking one's goals. Positive focused coping has previously been shown to be more effective in the long run as far as adaptive coping strategies, particularly in situations where individuals can insert some control over their situations to minimize or eliminate the stressor (Carver et al., 1989; Cheng et al., 2010; Folkman & Lazarus, 1991; Folkman & Moskowitz, 2004; Groomes & Leahy, 2002; Nilsson, 2002; Provencher, 2007).

Overall, the transactional model of coping has excellent application in understanding how persons with CID react and cope with a catastrophic injury resulting in significant functional loss and reduction in critical QOL domains (Bishop, 2005). In many such injuries, most individuals indeed do not have control over the situation, have initially little or no control over their health status, and in the case of permanently disabling injuries, such as a spinal cord injury or traumatic brain injury, are unable to perceive a positive future. Similarly, in cases where parents learn that their child is born with cerebral palsy, muscular dystrophy, or some other disabling condition, they too are likely to experience very similar emotions, cognitions, and behaviors as those with the disability (e.g., shock, anxiety, denial, anger, acceptance) (Livneh & Antonak, 2005).

Chaos Theory of Adjustment

Chaos and complexity theory (CCT) of adjustment is essentially the human application response of a phenomenon originally hypothesized from the disciplines of mathematics, meteorology, engineering, physics, biology, geography, astronomy, and chemistry (Livneh & Parker, 2005, p. 19). Its origination appears to lie with the mathematician and meteorologist Edward Lorenz back in the 1960s, when he famously coined the term "butterfly effect," essentially explaining how a butterfly flapping its wings in Brazil could ultimately end up causing a tornado in Texas a month later (Gleick, 1987). This theory, in addition to Rene Thom's (1975) multidimensional and nonlinear catastrophe theory, form the basis for its eventual application to human behavior.

An intriguing major concept about CCT is that despite its complexity and initial perceptions of random, nonorganized sets of behavior, is the notion that there is indeed an ordered and deterministic set of rules (Chamberlain, 1998). Several concepts must first be understood and are briefly defined here. *Nonlinearitis*, often referred to as "sensitive dependence on initial conditions" (Butz, 1997, p. 36). Nonlinear behavior is described as a nonrepetitive, unpredictable, aperiodic, and unstable phase that experiences critical junctions of instability called *bifurcation points* (Capra, 1996). These bifurcation points might otherwise be analogous to watching ice crack on a lake. Specifically, there is no order to when the ice will cease in one direction and fork off to another. Bifurcation of behavior after an acute injury is representative of the anxiety, fear and shock, and individual experiences during crisis, but with each critical bifurcation point (fork), it allows for growth, stability, and new behavior to result (Chamberlain, 1998). *Fixed point attractors* are stable and predictable set points that Livneh and Parker (2005, p. 20) describe as synonymous with watching water approaching a drain. *Limited cycle or periodic attractors* are predictable open and closed loops, with donut-shaped trajectories where the system approaches two separate points periodically but is unable to escape the cycle (Livneh & Parker, 2005, p. 20). *Strange attractors* are indicative of the unpredictable and unstable chaotic trajectories, which demonstrate the sensitive dependence on initial conditions and bifurcates over time (Capra, 1996). The fixed point attractors, limited cycle attractors, and strange attractors all constitute the first-, second-, and third-order changes, respectively.

Dynamic systems are neither random nor determined systems interconnected with one another that depend on the system itself (the individual), the environment, and the interaction between the two (similar to somatopsychology). Complex systems are open systems in that they exchange and lose energy, information, and material interacting with their environment (Cambel, 1993). In order to survive, the system must reduce internal disorder or entropy (decay), while drawing energy from the environment.

The level of entropy (minimal versus extreme) represents the degree of chaos occurring within the system or individual in human application. There are, however, also closed systems where the entropy cannot be dissipated, and new energy cannot enter from the environment. In closed systems that are isolated from renewable environmental energy, maximum entropy will continue (Kossmann & Bullrich, 1997). This may otherwise be a representation of what Livneh (1991) describes as "getting stuck" in a certain stage of psychosocial adjustment. *Self organization* is defined by Livneh and Parker (2005) as open systems with nonlinear trajectories that experience dramatic changes following a stressor (injury), spontaneously develops new structures and behaviors (schema), and experience internal feedback loops that ultimately self-organize, stabilize, and develop new ways of adaptation (Capra, 1996; Livneh & Parker, 2005, p. 21). *Self similarity* is similar patterns within chaotic systems, such as the fact that no two snowflakes are alike; however, they all have six sides. Self-similar patterns are called "fractals," which are determined patterns essentially fixed inside of the chaos (Mandelbrot, 1977).

In aligning the hard science of chaos theory with human behavior, Livneh and Parker (2005) indicate that under everyday conditions, most persons without disabilities essentially function under a state of cognitive and behavioral equilibrium. When a crisis occurs, however, we generally react in a more complex and unpredictable manner. Chaos is described as an indication of this overwhelming anxiety, capable of facilitating emotions such as depression and anger (Butz, 1997). As a result of these distressing emotions, adaptation involves a series of bifurcation points that are unpredictable and may be observed with varying degrees of maladjustment in different people (Francis, 1995). There are, however, some "self-similar" observations (e.g., shock, anxiety, denial, anger) that can be observed in most individuals. As time goes on, the individual generally reorganizes their cognitions, emotions, and behaviors to restore preinjury equilibrium. Interactions with the environment (others) can have a positive or negative affect on the individual's adjustment that may either slow, stall, or facilitate adaptation. Livneh and Parker suggests that counselors can assist persons with acquired CID to shift their focus and energy from past and present thinking, to the future, with goal directed and community oriented participation. Clients can be encouraged to look past their health and survival mentality, and begin thinking about social, vocational, and environmental mastery activities. Finally, knowing that many individuals instinctively retrench (withdraw, succumb) following a traumatic injury, counselors can encourage clients to recognize their spontaneity and creativeness and begin taking risks again (Livneh & Parker, 2005, p. 24).

Additional Adjustment Concepts

Value change system

Although indirectly addressed previously, there are several additional concepts and/or theories regarding acceptance of loss and disability worthy of noting. The first stems from Dembo et al. (1956) and later Wright's (1960) theory of value system changes that are necessary regarding acceptance of loss. In her later conceptualization, Wright (1983) cites four value changes that may or may not occur in any particular order for the individual. The first is *enlargement of the scope of values*. This pertains to individuals needing to refocus or let go of preinjury activities or values they are no longer able to perform, and instead expanding activities and interests to match their new abilities (e.g., an athlete who enjoyed playing sports becomes paralyzed and expands their values consistent with the limitations from their disabilities to enjoy reading). The second value change is *subordination of physique*, essentially cognitively reframing the significance of what is beautiful about oneself. Person's who place great importance on their physical appearance and abilities must be able to redefine remaining attributes (e.g., intelligence, personality) as becoming most important. The third value change, *containment of disability effects*, pertains to persons with disabilities not allowing the disabilities to "spread" to other parts of their beings and assertively correcting those without disabilities who assume this to be so. For example, someone with a physical disability may be presumed as also being mentally retarded. Numerous personal reports exist regarding a waitress asking a nondisabled companion what his or her wheelchair using partner would like to eat, based on the assumption that the individual is incapable of ordering for him or herself. The fourth value change needing to occur for successful adjustment is *transformation from comparative to asset values*, involving cognitive reframing as well. Asset values are more intrinsic and personal regarding what the individual finds to be valuable and needs to change in his or her life to sustain asset values. Comparative values, however, are evaluations we make on comparing what we have with what is supposedly normal and in relation to what others have. Therefore, refocusing on one's own assets without comparing to what other nondisabled persons perceived as normal or standard, needs to occur. Dembo et al. (1956) hypothesized in their coping with disability framework, that in order for persons with disabilities to successfully adapt and not ultimately succumb to the disability, they must be able to focus on the things they can do, take control of shaping their lives recognize personal accomplishments, manage negative life experiences, minimize physical and social barriers, and participate in activities that are pleasurable.

Good fortune comparison

This concept refers to some sense of relief persons with CID experience when they meet and/or perceive other persons with severe disabilities are much worse off than they. This is referred to as the "downward comparison," whereby one's perceived good fortune is from the belief that he or she could have sustained a more severe disability (Shotton, Simpson, & Smith, 2007). In the Shotton et al. (2007) study of psychosocial adjustment, appraisal, and coping strategies of nine persons with traumatic brain injuries (TBI), one of the significant findings was the comfort participants expressed in knowing their injuries could have been much worse. Psychologically, this realization allowed these individuals to enjoy what abilities they had remaining as opposed to what abilities they had lost.

Conceptualized Synthesis of the Seven Theories of Adjustment to an Acquired Disability

Having explored both the old and contemporary theories and concepts of psychosocial adjustment (adaptation, response, or reaction) to disability, what then are the major overlapping areas that appear to be consistently supported empirically? In other words, what cognitions, behaviors, and emotions do most persons who acquire a CID go through immediately following, then long after, a disability? We attempt to synthesize the areas of agreement various authors have conceptualized in essentially explaining the same process. The references for these conclusions are found within this chapter and therefore not all are repeated here.

First, following a traumatic, acquired injury with permanent long-term functional implications, all humans will experience some type of reaction. They may or may not experience Livneh's (1991) five stages of adjustment in the exact sequential order initially proposed; however, the caveats Livneh noted with the stage theory make these cognitions, behaviors, and emotions more probable since he indicated some people skip stages, regress back to a previous stage, overlap stages, and can become stuck in a stage. In analyzing this initial time period following injury, most people are overwhelmed with shock and anxiety, synonymous with the Parker et al. (2003) chaos theory in describing bifurcation points. This also overlaps with Yoshida's (1993) analogy of a wildly swinging pendulum initially following a trauma to explain the response to overwhelming anxiety and shock as part of the recurrent model (Kendall & Buys, 1998). This type of response lasts differing lengths of time for different people, based on personality traits and strengths of coping strategies, family stability and support, and type of interactions with the environment or community.

Second, as Lazarus and Folkman (1984a) have hypothesized, in appraising whether an event (injury) is considered harmful or a threat; unquestionably in such instances, it is. The disabling injury is largely not under an individual's direct control, and as Cheng et al. (2010) found, we tend to gravitate towards using emotion focused coping, because this is a situation we are unable to problem-solve our way out by self-repairing our bodily injuries. We therefore, must rely upon our physicians, and sometimes pray or bargain with God in the meantime, for a full recovery with or without medical intervention. Interestingly, Levin's (2001) analysis of over 200 epidemiological studies regarding religion/spirituality and its impact on mental and physical health, found positive relationships between religious participation and beliefs in relation to dealing with CID more positively.

Third, is whether or not some or most individuals experience a clinical reactive depression of a mild, moderate, or severe nature from the loss of perceived and/or real preinjury functioning and quality of life. Unquestionably, the majority of people will grieve the loss of bodily function and previous way of life, however, whether or not these same people will fall under the clinical diagnosis for depression varies from person to person. Again, synonymous with the Parker et al. (2003) bifurcation points (which way do the cracks in the ice go), how one adjusts depends on the personality traits and strengths in coping, family stability and support, and types of interactions with the environment. The person–environment interaction is essentially the theoretical framework for somatopsychology as well as the "dynamic systems" concept of Parker and colleagues' explanation of chaos theory. The ecological model is a more complex model, but essentially similar to somatopsychology, noting the interplay between aspects of the disability involving the person, personal characteristics and resources to cope, and the interplay with environmental forces (Trieschmann, 1988; Vash & Crewe, 2004). Basically then, whatever is considered a normal grief response (generally three to six months), beyond that may otherwise be classified as noteworthy to address in counseling (Livneh & Antonak, 1991; Silver, 1982). Suicidal ideation and suicide completion is statistically higher for persons with disabilities, so although not everyone will become depressed, some disability groups are more likely to think about suicide as an option compared with the general public (e.g., spinal cord injury vs deafness).

Fourth, is the occurrence of anger, be it internal or external. Do most people with acquired disabilities at some point after their injuries become angry? Olkin (1999) discusses the contradictory societal perception of persons with disabilities as expected to be happy and grateful for the charitable crumbs thrown their way but, conversely, are also required to indefinitely mourn their losses as well. She further asserts that society does not tolerate, accept, or understand anger from people with disabilities, but that whatever negative emotion is displayed, it is somehow always thought to be related or salient to the disability. Clinical observation and empirical studies suggest anger is a response, whether a short-term transitional occurrence or long-term periodic state (Graf et al., 2009; Livneh & Antonak, 1991; Marini et al., 2009). Livneh (1991) initially described self-blame and anger at God or higher power for causing the injury or not being able to prevent it. When the higher entity or medical profession is unable to cure impairments from the disability, the anger is redirected outwardly toward medical staff, family, and God or the higher power (Graf et al., 2007; Marini & Graf, 2011). What few researchers have addressed, however, is not so much anger, but the combination of sheer boredom and frustration persons with acquired disabilities feel during their first weeks and months of recovery, and later when they encounter environmental barriers and negative societal attitudes (Graf et al., 2009; Marini et al., 2009). Initially, the boredom and frustration persons with an acute injury experience waiting for the few minutes every day to see the doctor can be aggravating for many. Once out in the community, people with disabilities periodically become angry and frustrated in their interactions with others in the community regarding wheelchair parking violators, inaccessible washrooms, rude or condescending medical staff, long waiting times to see a doctor, and so on (Graf et al., 2009; Marini et al., 2009).

Fifth, and perhaps the most controversial, is whether persons with acquired or congenital disability eventually experience some type of final adjustment, adaptation, or transcendence to their disabilities (Livneh, 1991; Vash & Crewe, 2004). In defense of stage theory, Livneh (1991) noted the caveat that some individuals can regress back to an earlier stage. This is otherwise understood to mean that periodic setbacks can occur. Indeed, this is essentially very similar to the concept of periodic "chronic sorrow" that Kendall and Buys (1998) maintain in the recurrent model of adjustment. It is also synonymous with Parker and colleagues' (2003) chaos theory concept of "self organization," where individuals encounter bad events and adapt or change what is necessary and within their control to adjust to the situations. The larger question becomes, what causes these periodic instances of chronic sorrow? Only two answers are plausible: (a) the individual experiences additional or recurrent health problems (e.g., loss of sight with diabetes, severe pressure sore requiring surgery for spinal cord injury); or (b) someone or something in the person's "life space," interacting with the environment, upsets the individual. In the first instance, this potential health setback and subsequent sadness is an otherwise normal reaction. If these setbacks do not occur, it has already been demonstrated in various empirical studies that persons with disabilities revert to preinjury levels of emotions after roughly 2 months (Brickman & Campbell, 1971; Silver, 1982). The second instance regarding a negative experience with others or from encountering an environmental barrier; these causes are both socially constructed. A prejudicial or discriminatory attitude reminds the person with a disability that he or she not only has a disability but also is devalued by some people because of it (Li & Moore, 1998). Such interactions may well hurt the individual and can cause temporary sadness and/or anger as well. Similarly, when individuals with disabilities encounter an inaccessible restaurant or public place, it reminds them of their disability and the environmental barriers imposed on them that deny their civil rights (Graf et al., 2009; Marini et al., 2009). Regardless, many persons without disabilities in society will automatically assume that when someone with a disability appears upset, it is somehow salient to the disability, and this may indirectly be so (e.g., requirement of mourning) (Wright, 1983).

Finally, how do persons with disabilities reach any type of successful adjustment, adaptation, response or reaction to their disability? For stage theory proponents, it is by successfully transitioning through the various stages over time and coming to terms with the disability. As with the grieving process, time heals. For somatopsychology proponents, it is that critical person–environment interaction, where the individual possesses the personal characteristics and coping skills to succeed, and learns to control and master his or her environment. Disability centrality proponents also postulate mastering one's environment and substituting new and interesting activities that are central for sustaining satisfaction and quality of life in place of those once pleasurable activities no longer accessible due to the limitations imposed by the disability. Ecological models, are more complex, but again similar to somatopsychology in that psychosocial adjustment depends on the interplay of an individual's personal characteristics and coping abilities, aspects of the disability itself, and environmental influences, including family and community support.

Overall, all models arguably converge into one at some point, or certainly overlap enough to provide counselors with some good insights as to what persons with disabilities may experience. For those with congenital disabilities, there does not appear to be transitional stage of adjustment. It is more likely that this population will experience periodic sorrow if they allow themselves to sometimes wish they could do all the activities someone without a disability supposedly can do. Such cognitions, however, from the literature appear to be rare (Connors & Stalker, 2007). In addition, it appears emotional upsets may otherwise have an external cause, such as being ridiculed or reminded of one's minority status. Again, this would hopefully be a rare occurrence, and the literature suggests that persons with congenital disabilities are otherwise generally happy and satisfied with their quality of life. For those with acquired disabilities, there is for a time, an emotional instability in grieving the loss of bodily function and preinjury lifestyle. This does appear to stabilize in most cases over time, and it does so when individuals can cognitively reframe (adapt new cognitive schema) about their situations and what is important in life. This is accomplished by letting go of, and not dwelling on, what one used to be able to do, but instead focusing on new interests, values, and goals commensurate with remaining disability assets. The perception of being in control and mastering one's environment is central to reestablishing self-esteem. And, as discussed in the "disability paradox" theory (Freedman, 1978) and later in this text on positive psychology, persons who have not only survived their disabilities but also become very successful in spite of them, otherwise perceive themselves as stronger than most nondisabled persons. It therefore seems appropriate to end this chapter with Nietzsche's (1888) classic quote, "what does not kill me, makes me stronger," otherwise experienced as posttraumatic growth.

REFERENCES

Albrecht, G. L., & Devlieger, P. J. (1999). The disability paradox: High quality of life against all odds. *Social Science & Medicine, 48,* 977–988.

Allman, A. (1990). *Subjective well-being of people with disabilities: Measurement issues.* Unpublished master's thesis. University of Illinois.

Andrews, F., & Withey, S. (1976). Developing measures of perceived life quality: Results from several national surveys. *Social Indicators Research, 1,* 1–26.

Athelstan, G. T., & Crewe, N. M. (1979). Psychological adjustment to spinal cord injury as related to manner of onset of disability. *Rehabilitation Counseling Bulletin, 22,* 311–319.

Banks, S. M., & Kerns, R. D. (1996). Explaining high rates of depression in chronic pain: A diathesis-stress framework. *Psychological Bulletin, 119,* 95–110.

Barker, R. G., Wright, B. A., Meyerson, L., & Gonick, M. R. (1953). *Adjustment to physical handicap: A survey of the social psychology of physique and disability* (2nd ed.). New York, NY: Social Science Research Council.

Barnard, D. (1990). Healing the damaged self: Identity, intimacy, and meaning in the lives of the chronically ill. *Perspectives in Biology and Medicine, 33,* 535–546.

Barrera, M. (1981). Social support in adjustment of pregnant adolescents: Assessment issues. In B. H. Gottlieb (Ed.), *Social networks and social support* (pp. 69–96). Beverly Hills, CA: Sage Publications.

Beck, A. T. (1967). *Depression: Causes and treatment.* Philadelphia, PA: University of Pennsylvania Press.

Beck, A. T., & Weishaar, M. (1989). Cognitive therapy. In A. Freeman, K. M. Simon, L. E. Beutler, & H. Arkowitz (Eds.), *Comprehensive handbook of cognitive therapy* (pp. 21–36). New York, NY: Plenum.

Bishop, M. (2005). Quality of life and psychosocial adaptation to chronic illness and acquired disability: A conceptual and theoretical synthesis. *Journal of Rehabilitation, 71*(2), 5–13.

Bishop, M., & Allen, C. A. (2003). Epilepsy's impact on quality of life: A qualitative analysis. *Epilepsy & Behavior, 4*(3), 226–233.

Bishop, M., & Feist-Price, S. (2002). Quality if life assessment in the rehabilitation counseling relationship: Strategies and measures. *Journal of Applied Rehabilitation Counseling, 33*(1), 35–41.

Bishop, M., Shepard, L., & Stenhoff, D. M. (2007). Psychosocial adaptation and quality of life in multiple sclerosis: Assessment of the disability centrality model. *Journal of Rehabilitation, 73*(1), 3–12.

Bordieri, J. E., & Kilbury, R. (1991). Self-blame attributions for disability and perceived rehabilitation outcomes. *Rehabilitation Bulletin, 34*(4), 1–12.

Bordieri, L., Comninel, M., & Drehmer, D. (1989). Client attributions for disability: Perceived adjustment, coping and accuracy. *Rehabilitation Psychology, 34,* 271–278.

Bramble, K. (1995). Body image. In I. M. Lubkin (Ed.), *Chronic illness: Impact and interventions* (pp. 285–299). Boston, MA: Jones and Bartlett Publishers.

Brickman, P., & Campbell, D. T. (1971). Hedonic relativism and planning the good society. In M. H. Appley (Ed.), *Adaptation-level theory* (pp. 287–305). New York, NY: Academic Press.

Bulman, R., & Wortman, C. B. (1977). Attributions of blame and coping in the "real world": Severe accident victims respond to their lot. *Journal of Personality and Social Psychology, 35,* 351–363.

Burke, M. L., Hainsworth, M. A., Eakes, G. G., & Lindgren, C. L. (1992). Current knowledge and research on chronic sorrow: A foundation for injury. *Death Studies, 16,* 231–245.

Butz, M. (1997). *Chaos and complexity: Implications for psychological theory and practice.* Washington, DC: Taylor & Francis.

Buunk, B. P., & Verhoeven, K. (1991). Companionship and support at work: A microanalysis of the stress-reducing features of social interaction. *Basic and Applied Social Psychology, 12,* 243–258.

Byrd, E. K. (1990). A study of biblical depiction of disability. *Journal of Applied Rehabilitation Counseling, 21*(4), 52–53.

Cadman, D., Boyle, M., Szatmari, P., & Offord, D. R. (1987). Chronic illness, disability, and mental health and social well-being: Findings of the Ontario child health study. *Pediatrics, 79,* 805–813.

Cambel, A. B. (1993). *Applied chaos theory.* New York, NY: Academic Press.

Capra, F. (1996). *The web of life.* New York, NY: Anchor Books.

Carver, C. S., Scheier, M. F., & Weintraub, J. K. (1989). Assessing coping strategies: A theoretically based approach. *Journal of Personality and Social Psychology, 56,* 267–283.

Chamberlain, L. (1998). An introduction to nonlinear dynamics. In L. Chamberlain & M. Butz (Eds.), *Clinical chaos: A therapist's guide to nonlinear dynamics and therapeutic change* (pp. 3–14). Philadelphia, PA: Brunner/Mazel.

Chan, F., Da Silva Cardoso, E., & Chronister, J. A. (2009). *Understanding psychosocial adjustment to chronic illness and disability.* New York, NY: Springer.

Charmaz, K. (1983). Loss of self: A fundamental form of suffering in the chronically ill. *Sociology of Health and Illness, 5,* 168–195.

Charmaz, K. (1995a). The body, identity and self: Adapting to impairment. *Sociological Quarterly, 36,* 657–680.

Charmaz, K. (1995b). Identity dilemmas of chronically ill men. In D. Sabo & D. Gordon (Eds.), *Men's health and illness: Gender, power, and the body* (pp. 266–291). Thousand Oaks, CA: Sage.

Cheng, Y., Kuan, F., Li, C., & Ken, Y. (2010). A comparison between the effect of emotional certainty and uncertainty on coping strategies. *Social Behavior and Personality, 38*(1), 53–60.

Chubon, R. A. (1994). *Social and psychological foundations of rehabilitation.* Springfield, IL: Charles C. Thomas.

Cohen, C. B., & Napolitano, D. (2007). Adjustment to disability. *Disability and Social Work Education: Practice and Policy Issues, 6*(1/2), 135–155.

Cohen, S. (2004). Social relationships and health. *American Psychologist, 59,* 676–684.

Cohen, S., Gottlieb, B. H., & Underwood, L. G. (2000). In S. Cohen, L. Underwood, & B. Gottlieb (Eds.), *Social support measurement and intervention* (pp. 3–25). New York, NY: Oxford University Press.

Connors, C., & Stalker, K. (2007). Children's experiences of disability: Pointers to a model of childhood disability. *Disability & Society, 22*(1), 19–33.

Crewe, N. M., & Krause, J. S. (1990). An eleven-year follow-up of adjustment to spinal cord injury. *Rehabilitation Psychology, 35*(4), 205–210.

Cummins, R. A. (2002). *Caveats on the comprehensive quality of life scale (and a suggested alternative).* Melbourne, Australia: Deakin University School of Psychology.

Cummins, R. A. (2005). Moving from the quality of life concept to a theory. *Journal of Intellectual Disability Research, 49*(10), 699–706.

Cummins, R. A. (2006). *Personal Well-being Index* (4th ed.). Melbourne, Australia: Deakin University.

Davis, B. H. (1987). Disability and grief. *Social Casework, 68,* 352–357.

Davis, S. E., Anderson, C., Linkowski, D. C., Berger, K., & Feinstein, C. F. (1991). In R. P. Marinelli & A. E. Dell Orto (Eds.), *The psychological & social impact of disability* (pp. 70–80). New York, NY: Springer.

Dembo, T., Leviton, G., & Wright, B. A. (1956). Adjustment to misfortune: A problem in social psychological rehabilitation. *Artificial Limbs, 3,* 4–62.

Devins, G. M. (1994). Illness intrusiveness and the psychosocial impact of lifestyle disruptions in chronic life-threatening disease. *Advances in Renal Replacement Therapy, 1,* 251–263.

Devins, G. M., Blinik, Y. M., Hutchinson, T. A., Hollomby, D. J., Barre, P. E., & Guttmann, R. D. (1983). The emotional impact of end-stage renal disease: Importance of patients' perceptions of intrusiveness and control. *International Journal of Psychiatry in Medicine, 13,* 327–343.

Devins, G. M., & Shnek, Z. M. (2000). Multiple sclerosis. In R. G. Frank & T. R. Elliott (Eds.), *Handbook of rehabilitation psychology* (pp. 163–184). Washington, DC: American Psychological Association.

Diener, E., & Seligman, M. E. (2004). Beyond money: Toward an economy of well-being. *Psychological Science in the Public Interest, 5*, 1–31.

Dijkers, M. (1997). Measuring quality of life. In M. J. Fuhrer (Ed.), *Assessing medical rehabilitation practices: The promise of outcome research* (pp. 153–180). Baltimore, MD: Paul H. Brooks.

DiTomasso, E., & Spinner, B. (1997). Social and emotional loneliness: A re-examination of Weiss' typology of loneliness. *Personality and Individual Differences, 22*, 417–427.

Dunn, M. E. (1975). Psychological intervention in a spinal cord injury center: An introduction. *Rehabilitation Psychology, 22*(4), 165–178.

Eareckson, J. (2001). *An unforgettable story. Grand Rapids.* MI: Zondervan.

Elfstrom, M. L., & Kreuter, M. (2006). Relationships between locus of control, coping strategies and emotional well-being in persons with spinal cord lesion. *Journal of Clinical Psychology in Medical Settings, 13*(1), 93–104.

Endler, N. S., & Parker, J. D. A. (1990). Multidimensional assessment of coping: A critical evaluation. *Journal of Personality and Social Psychology, 58*, 844–854.

Erikson, E. H., Erikson, J. M., & Kivnick, H. Q. (1986). *Vital involvement in old age.* New York, NY: Norton.

Falek, A., & Britton, S. (1974). Phases in coping: The hypothesis and its implications. *Social Biology, 21*(1), 1–7.

Fishbain, D. D., Cutler, R. B., Rosomoff, H. L., Khalil, T., Gbdel-Moty, E., Sakek, S., Zaki, A., Saltzman, A., Jarrett, J., Martinez, G., & Steele-Rosomoff, R. (1997). Chronic pain associated depression: Antecedent or consequences of chronic pain? A review. *Clinical Journal of Pain, 13*, 116–137.

Folkman, S., & Lazarus, R. S. (1980). An analysis of coping in a middle-aged community sample. *Journal of Health and Social Behavior, 21*, 219–239.

Folkman, S., & Lazarus, R. S. (1985). If it changes it must be a process: Study of emotion and coping during three stages of a college examination. *Journal of Personality and Social Psychology, 48*, 150–170.

Folkman, S., & Lazarus, R. S. (1991). Coping and emotions. In A. Monet & R. S. Lazarus (Eds.), *Stress and coping* (pp. 207–227). New York, NY: Columbia University Press.

Folkman, S., & Moskowitz, J. T. (2004). Coping: Pitfalls and promise. *Annual Review of Psychology, 55*, 745–774.

Fordyce, M. (1988). A review of results on the happiness measures: A 60-second index of happiness and mental health. *Social Indicators Research, 20*, 355–381.

Forshaw, M. (2007). In defense of psychology: A reply to Goodley and Lawthom (2005). *Disability and Society, 22*(6), 655–658.

Francis, S. E. (1995). Chaotic phenomena in psychophysiological self-regulation. In R. Robertson & A. Combs (Eds.), *Chaos theory in psychology and the life sciences* (pp. 253–265). Mahwah, NJ: Erlbaum.

Frank, R. G., & Elliott, T. R. (1989). Spinal cord injury and health locus of control beliefs. *Paraplegia, 27*, 250–256.

Freedman, J. (1978). *Happy people.* New York, NY: Harcourt Brace Jovanovich.

Frisch, M. B. (1999). Quality of life assessment/intervention and the quality of life inventory (QOLI). In M. R. Maruish (Ed.), *The use of psychological testing for treatment planning and outcome assessment* (2nd ed., pp. 1227–1331). Hillsdale, NJ: Lawerence-Erlbaum.

Gallagher, H. G. (1995). *By trust betrayed: Patients, physicians, and the license to kill in the Third Reich* (Rev. ed.). Arlington, VA: Vandamere.

Gleick, J. (1987). *Chaos: Making a new science.* New York, NY: Viking.

Gordon, P. A., Tschopp, M. K., & Feldman, D. (2004). Addressing issues of sexuality with adolescents with disabilities. *Child and Adolescent Social Work Journal, 21*(5), 513–527.

Graf, N. M., Marini, I., Baker, J., & Buck, T. (2007). The perceived impact of religious and spiritual beliefs for persons with chronic pain. *Rehabilitation Counseling Bulletin, 51*, 21–33.

Graf, N. M., Marini, I., & Blankenship, C. J. (2009). 100 words about disability. *Journal of Rehabilitation, 75*(2), 25–34.

Groomes, D. A. G., & Leahy, M. J. (2002). The relationships among the stress appraisal process, coping disposition and level of acceptance of disability. *Rehabilitation Counseling Bulletin, 46*, 14–23.

Groot, W., & Van Den Brink, H. M. (2000). Life satisfaction and preference drift. *Social Indicators Research*, *50*, 315–328.

Gunther, M. S. (1969). Emotional aspects. In D. Ruge (Ed.), *Spinal cord injuries* (chap. 12, pp. 93–108). Springfield, IL: Charles C. Thomas.

Gunther, M. S. (1971). Psychiatric consultation in a rehabilitation hospital: A regression hypothesis. *Comprehensive Psychiatry, 12*(6), 572–585.

Heller, K., & Rook, K. S. (2001). Distinguishing the theoretical functional of social ties: Implications for support interventions. In B. R. Sarason & S. Duck (Eds.), *Personal relationships: Implications for clinical and community psychology* (pp. 119–139). New York, NY: John Wiley & Sons.

Helwig, A. A., & Holicky, R. (1994). Substance abuse in persons with disabilities: Treatment considerations. *Journal of Counseling and Development, 72*, 227–233.

Hofman, A. D. (1975). The impact of illness in adolescence and coping behavior. *Acta Paediatrica Scandinavica Supplement, 256*, 29–33.

Hogansen, J. M., Powers, K., Geenen, S., Gil-Kashiwbara, E., & Powers, L. (2008). Transition goals and experiences of females with disabilities: Youth, parents, and professionals. *Exceptional Children, 74*(2), 215–234.

Hohmann, G. W. (1975). Psychological aspects of treatment and rehabilitation of the spinal cord injured person. *Clinical Orthopedics, 112*, 81–88.

Holmbeck, G. N., Johnson, S. Z., Wills, K. E., McKernon, W., Rose, B., Erklin, S. et al. (2002). *Journal of Consulting & Clinical Psychology, 70*(1), 96–111.

Hopps, S., Pepin, M., Arseneau, I., Frechette, M., & Begin, G. (2001). Disability related variables associated with loneliness among people with disabilities. *Journal of Rehabilitation, 67*(3), 42–48.

Howland, C. A., & Rintala, D. H. (2001). Dating behaviors of women with physical disabilities. *Sexuality and Disability, 19*, 41–70.

Hupcey, J. E. (1998). Clarifying the social support theory–research linkage. *Journal of Advanced Nursing, 27*, 1231–1241.

Hwang, K. (1997). Living with a disability: A woman's perspective. In M. L. Sipski & C. J. Alexander (Eds.), *Sexual function in people with disability and chronic illness* (pp. 119–130). Gaithersburg: Aspen.

Inglehart, R. (1990). *Modernization and postmodernization: Cultural, economic, and political change in societies.* Princeton, NJ: Princeton University Press.

Jalowiec, A. (1990). Issues in using multiple measures of quality of life. *Seminars in Onocology Nursing, 6*, 271–277.

Janoff-Bulman, R. (1979). Characterological versus behavioral self-blame: Injuries into depression and rape. *Journal of Personality and Social Psychology, 37*, 1798–1809.

Johnson, K. L., Amtmann, D., Yorkston, K., Klasner, E. R., & Kuehn, C. M. (2004). Medical, psychological, social, and programmatic barriers to employment for people with multiple sclerosis. *Journal of Rehabilitation, 70*, 38–49.

Kahana, E., Fairchild, T., & Kahana, B. (1982). Adaptation. In D. J. Mangen & W. A. Peterson (Eds.), *Research instruments in clinical gerontology: Vol 1. Clinical and social psychology* (pp. 145–193). Minneapolis, MN: University of Minnesota Press.

Kendall, E., & Buys, N. (1998). An integrated model of psychosocial adjustment following acquired disability. *Journal of Rehabilitation, 64*, 16–20.

Kivnick, H. Q. (1991). Disability and psychosocial development in old age. In R. P. Marinelli & A. E. Dell Orto (Eds.), *The psychological & social impact of disability* (pp. 92–102). New York, NY: Springer.

Kossmann, M. R., & Bullrich, S. (1997). Systematic chaos: Self-organizing systems and the process of change. In F. Masterpasqua & P. A. Pena (Eds.), *The psychological meaning of chaos: Translating theory into practice* (pp. 199–224). Washington, DC: American Psychological Association.

Krueger, D. W. (1981–1982). Emotional rehabilitation of the physical rehabilitation patient. *International Journal of Psychiatry in Medicine, 11*(2), 183–191.

Kubler-Ross, E. (1981). *Living with death and dying.* New York, NY: Macmillan.

Lakey, B., & Cassady, P. B. (1990). Cognitive processes in perceived social support. *Journal of Personality and Social Psychology, 59*, 337–343.

Lazarus, R. (1993). Coping theory and research: Past, present, and future. *Psychosomatic Medicine, 55*, 234–247.

Lazarus, R. S., & Folkman, S. (1984a). *Stress, appraisal, and coping.* New York, NY: Springer.

Lazarus, R. S., & Folkman, S. (1984b). Coping and adaptation. In W. D. Gentry (Ed.), *Handbook of behavioral medicine* (pp. 282–325). New York, NY: Guilford Press.

Lazarus, R. S., & Folkman, S. (1984c). *Stress, appraisal, and coping.* New York, NY: Springer.

Levin, J. (2001). *God, faith, and health: Exploring the spirituality healing connection.* Hoboken, NJ: Wiley & Sons.

Levy, D. (1966). *Maternal overprotection.* New York, NY: W. W. Norton & Company, Inc.

Lewin, K. (1935). *A dynamic theory of personality.* New York, NY: McGraw-Hill.

Lewin, K. (1936). *Principles of topological psychology.* New York, NY: McGraw-Hill.

Lewinsohn, P. M., Clarke, G. N., & Hops, H. (1990). Cognitive-behavioral treatment for depressed adolescents. *Behavior Therapy, 21,* 385–401.

Li, L., & Moore, D. (1998). Acceptance of disability and its correlates. *Journal of Social Psychology, 138*(1), 13–25.

Livneh, H. (1986). A unified approach to existing models of adaptation to disability: Part I-A model adaptation. *Journal of Applied Rehabilitation Counseling, 17,* 5–16.

Livneh, H. (1991). On the origins of negative attitudes toward people with disabilities. In R. P. Marinelli, & A. E. Dell Orto (Eds.), *The Psychological & Social Impact of Disability.* New York, NY: Springer.

Livneh, H. (2001). Psychosocial adaptation to chronic illness and disability: A conceptual framework. *Rehabilitation Counseling Bulletin, 44*(3), 151–160.

Livneh, H., & Antonak, R. F. (1991). Temporal structure of adaptation to disability. *Rehabilitation Counseling Bulletin, 34*(4), 298–320.

Livneh, H., & Antonak, R. F. (1997). *Psychosocial adaptation to chronic illness and disability.* Gaithersburg, MD: Aspen.

Livneh, H., & Antonak, R. F. (2005). Psychosocial adaptation to chronic illness and disability: A primer for counselors. *Journal of Counseling & Development, 83,* 12–20.

Livneh, H., & Antonak, R. F. (2007). Psychological adaptation to chronic illness and disability: A primer for counselors. In A. E. Dell Orto & P. W. Power, *The psychological and social impact of illness and disability* (5th ed., pp. 125–144). New York, NY: Springer.

Livneh, H., & Parker, R. M. (2005). Psychological adaptation to disability: Perspectives from chaos and complexity theory. *Rehabilitation Counseling Bulletin, 49*(1), 17–28.

Lucas, R. E. (2007). Adaptation and the set-point model of subjective well-being: Does happiness change after major life events? *Current Directions in Psychological Science, 16,* 75–79.

Lykken, D. (1999). *Happiness.* New York, NY: Golden Books.

Maciejewski, P. K., Zhang, B., Block, S., & Prigerson, H. G. (2007). An empirical examination of the stage theory of grief. *Journal of the American Medical Association, 297,* 716–723.

Mackelprang, R., & Salsgiver, R. (2009). *Disability: A diversity model approach in human service practice.* Pacific Grove, CA: Brooks/Cole.

Maltby, J., Day, L., & Macaskill, A. (2007). *Personality individual differences and intelligence.* Harlow: Pearson Prentice-Hall.

Mandelbrot, B. (1977). *The fractal geometry of nature.* New York, NY: W. H. Freeman.

Marini, I. (2007). Cross-cultural counseling issues of males who sustain a disability. In A. E. Dell Orto & P. W. Power (5th ed.), *The psychological and social impact of illness and disability* (pp. 194–213). New York, NY: Springer.

Marini, I., Bhakta, M. V., & Graf, N. (2009). A content analysis of common concerns of persons with physical disabilities. *Journal of Applied Rehabilitation Counseling, 40*(1), 44–49.

Marini, I., & Graf, N. M. (2011). Spirituality and SCI: Attitudes, beliefs, and practices. *Rehabilitation Counseling Bulletin, 54*(2), 82–92.

Marini, I., Rogers, L., Slate, J. R., & Vines, C. (1995). Self-esteem differences among persons with spinal cord injury. *Rehabilitation Counseling Bulletin, 38*(3), 198–205.

Marinic, M., & Brkljacic, T. (2008). Love over gold—The correlation of happiness level with some life satisfaction factors between persons with and without physical disability. *Journal of Developmental Physical Disability, 20,* 527–540.

Massimini, F., & Delle Fave, A. (2000). Individual development in a bio-cultural perspective. *American Psychologist, 55,* 24–33.

Meyerowitz, B. E. (1980). Psychosocial correlates of breast cancer and its treatments. *Psychological Bulletin, 87,* 108–131.

Misajon, R. A. (2002). *The homeostatic mechanism: Subjective quality of life and chronic pain.* Unpublished doctoral dissertation, Melbourne, Australia: Deakin University.

Myers, D. D., & Diener, E. (1996). The pursuit of happiness: New research uncovers some anti-intuitive insights into how many people are happy- and why. *Scientific American, 27*(4), 70–72.

Myers, D. G., & Diener, E. (1995). Who is happy? *Psychological Science, 6,* 10–19.

Nabi, R. L. (2003). Exploring the framing effects of emotion. *Communication Research, 30,* 224–247.

Naugle, R. I. (1991). Denial in rehabilitation: Its genesis, consequences, and clinical management. In R. P. Marinelli & A. E. Dell Otto (Eds.), *The psychological and social impact of disability* (pp. 139–151). New York, NY: Springer.

Nietzsche, F. (1888). *Twilight of the idols.* 2003 reprint. New York, NY: Penguin Books.

Nilsson, D. H. (2002). *What's the problem?": A conceptual and empirical exploration adjustment to health condition and adjustment to hospitalization as indicators for intervention for social workers in health-care settings.* Unpublished DSW thesis. Melbourne, Australia: La Trobe University.

Nosek, M. A., & Hughes, R. B. (2007). Psychosocial issues of women with physical disabilities. In A. E. Dell Orto, & P. W. Power (5th ed.), *The psychological and social impact of illness and disability* (pp. 156–175). New York, NY: Springer.

Olkin, R. (1999). *What psychotherapists should know about disability.* New York, NY: Guilford Press.

Parker, R. M. (1979). *Assessing adjustment to disability through determining predominant feeling states.* Paper presented at the American Rehabilitation Counseling Association Meeting, Las Vegas, Nevada.

Parker, R. M., Schaller, J., & Hansmann, S. (2003). Castastrophe, chaos, and complexity models and psychosocial adjustment to disability. *Rehabilitation Counseling Bulletin, 46*(4), 234–241.

Pavot, W., & Diener, E. (1993). Review of the satisfaction with life scale. *Psychological Assessment, 5,* 164–172.

Pless, I. B., Roghmann, K., & Haggerty, R. J. (1972). Chronic illness, family functioning, and psychological adjustment: A model for the allocation of preventive mental health services. *International Journal of Epidemiology, 1,* 271–277.

Provencher, H. L. (2007). Role of psychological factors in studying recovery from a transactional stress-coping approach: Implications for mental health nursing practices. *International Journal of Mental Health Nursing, 16,* 188–197.

Reidy, K., & Caplan, B. (1994). Causal factors in spinal cord injury: Patients' evolving perceptions and associations with depression. *Archives of Physical Medicine & Rehabilitation, 75*(8), 837–842.

Roessler, R. T. (1990). A quality of life perspective on rehabilitation counseling. *Rehabilitation Counseling Bulletin, 34,* 82–90.

Rousso, H. (1996). Sexuality and positive sense of self. In D. M. Krotoski, M. A. Nosek, & M. A. Turk (Eds.), *Women with physical disabilities: Achieving and maintaining health and well-being* (pp. 109–116). Baltimore, MD: Paul H. Brookes.

Schafer, W. (1996). *Stress management for wellness.* Orlando, FL: Harcourt Brace.

Schwartz, C. E., & Sprangers, M. A. (2000). *Adaptation to changing health: Response shift in quality of life research.* Washington, DC: American Psychological Association.

Schwarzer, R., & Leppin, A. (1992). Social supports and mental health: A conceptual and empirical overview. In L. Montada, S. Filipp, & M. J. Lerner (Eds.), *Life crises and experiences of loss in adulthood* (pp. 435–458). Hillsdale, NJ: Erlbaum.

Seligman, M. E. P. (1975). *Helplessness.* San Francisco, CA: W. H. Freeman.

Shands, H. C. (1955). An outline of the process of recovery from severe trauma. *Archives of Neurology and Psychiatry, 73,* 403–409.

Shontz, F. C. (1991). Six principles relating disability and psychological adjustment. In R. P. Marinelli & A. E. Dell Orto (Eds.), *The psychological and social impact of disability* (pp. 107–110). New York: Springer.

Shotton, L., Simpson, J., & Smith, M. (2007). The experience of appraisal, coping and adaptive psychosocial adjustment following traumatic brain injury: A qualitative investigation. *Brain Injury, 21*(8), 857–869.

Silver, R. L. (1982). *Coping with an undesirable life event: A study of early reactions to physical disability.* Unpublished doctoral dissertation. Evanston, IL: Northwestern University.

Smart, J. (2009). *Disability, society, and the individual.* Austin, TX: Pro-Ed.

Smith, A. J., Thorngren, J., & Christopher, J. C. (2009). Rural mental health counseling. In I. Marini & M. Stebnicki (Eds.), *The professional counselor's desk reference* (pp. 263–273). New York, NY: Springer.

Smith, C. A., & Ellsworth, P. C. (1985). Patterns of cognitive appraisal in emotions. *Journal of Personality and Social Psychology, 48,* 813–838.

Stewart, J. R. (1996). Applying Beck's cognitive therapy to Livneh's model of adaptation to disability. *Journal of Applied Rehabilitation Counseling, 27,* 40–45.

Symister, P., & Friend, R. (2003). The influence of social support and problematic support on optimism and depression in chronic illness: A prospective study evaluating self-esteem as a mediator. *Health Psychology, 22,* 123–129.

Trask, P. C., Paterson, A. G., Trask, C. L., Bares, C. B., Birt, J., & Maan, C. (2003). Parent and adolescent adjustment to pediatric cancer: Associations with coping, social support, and family function. *Journal of Pediatric Oncology Nursing, 20*(1), 36–47.

Teel, C. S. (1991). Chronic sorrow: Analysis of the concept. *Journal of Advanced Nursing, 16,* 1311–1319.

Tepper, M. S. (1997). Living with a disability: A man's perspective. In M. L. Sipski & C. J. Alexander (Eds.), *Sexual function in people with disability and chronic illness* (pp. 119–130), Gaithersburg: Aspen.

Thom, R. (1975). *Structural stability and morphogenesis:* An outline of a general theory of model (Fowler, H., Trans.). Reading, PA: Benjamin.

Thomasgard, M. (1998). Parental perceptions of child vulnerability, overprotection, and parental psychological characteristics. *Child Psychiatry & Human Development, 28*(4), 223–240.

Trieschmann, R. (1988). *Spinal cord injuries: Psychological, social, and vocational rehabilitation* (2nd ed.). New York, NY: Demos.

U.S. General Accounting Office. (2002). *Nursing homes: More can be done to protect residents from abuse.* GAO/HEHS02-312, Washington, DC.

Varni, J. W., Rubenfeld, L. A., Talbot, D., & Setoguchi, Y. (1989). Family functioning, temperament, and psychologic adaptation in children with congenital or acquired limb deficiencies. *Pediatrics, 84*(2), 323–330.

Vash, C. L., & Crewe, N. M. (2004). *Psychology of disability* (pp. 288–299). New York, NY: Springer.

Wallander, J. L., & Varni, J. W. (1998). Effects of pediatric chronic physical disorders on child and family adjustment. *Journal of Child Psychology and Psychiatry, 39,* 29–46.

Wallander, J. L., Varni, J. W., Babani, L., DeHaan, C. B., Wilcox, K. T., & Banis, H. T. (1988). Family resources as resistance factors for psychological maladjustment in chronically ill and handicapped children. *Journal of Pediatric Psychology, 14,* 157–173.

Waters, S. J., Campbell, L. C., Keefe, F. J., & Carson, J. W. (2004). The essence of cognitive-behavioral pain management. In R. H. Dworkin & W. S. Breitbart (Eds.), *Psychosocial aspects of pain: A handbook for health care providers* (pp. 261–283). Seattle, WA: IASP Press.

Weinberg, N. (1988). Another perspective: Attitudes of people with disabilities. In H. E. Yuker (Ed.), *Attitudes toward persons with disabilities* (pp. 141–153). New York, NY: Springer.

Weller, D. J., & Miller, P. M. (1977). Emotional reactions of patient, family, and staff in acute-care period of spinal cord injury: Part 1. *Social Work in Health Care, 24*(4), 369–377.

Westbrook, M., & Nordholm, L. (1986). Reactions to patient's self or chance-blaming attributions for illnesses having life-style involvement. *Journal of Applied Social Psychology, 16,* 428–446.

Wikler, L., Wasow, M., & Hatfield, E. (1981). Chronic sorrow revisited: Parent versus professional depiction of the adjustment of mentally retarded children. *American Journal of Orthopsychiatry, 51,* 63–70.

Witt, W. P., Riley, A. W., & Coiro, M. J. (2003). Childhood functional status, family stressors, and psychosocial adjustment among school-aged children with disabilities in the United States. *Archives of Pediatrics and Adolescent Medicine, 157*(7), 687–695.

Worden, J. W. (2009). *Grief counseling and grief therapy: A handbook for the mental health practitioner* (4th ed.). New York, NY: Springer.

Wortman, C. B., & Silver, R. C. (1989). The myths of coping with loss. *Journal of Consulting and Clinical Psychology, 57*(3), 349–357.

Wright, B. (1983). *Physical disability: A psychosocial approach* (2nd ed.). New York, NY: Harper & Row.

Wright, B. A. (1960). *Physical disability: A psychological approach.* New York, NY: Harper & Row.

Yoshida, K. K. (1993). Reshaping of self: A pendular reconstruction of self identity among adults with traumatic spinal cord injury. *Sociology of Health and Illness, 15*, 217–245.

Yuker, H. E. (1988). *Attitudes toward persons with disabilities*. New York, NY: Springer.

Zilbergeld, B. (1992). *The new male sexuality*. New York, NY: Bantam Books.

INSIDER PERSPECTIVE
The Story of Michael Hoenig

"We're getting home just in time for my reader," I said to my friend Hugh as we pulled into the driveway of my Davenport, Iowa home. "Medicaid pays for her time, right?" he responded. The statement puzzled me. Hugh was a fellow Center for Independent Living board member, who should know better than to assume that all persons with disabilities receive public assistance.

Blind since birth, I was raised in a family with a very strong work ethic. Though my parents were not immune to preconceived notions about blindness, college and a full-time job were a part of my life plan since my earliest memory. Having attained my B.A. in psychology from Central College, Pella, Iowa, in 1984, I entered the University of Iowa's graduate program in rehabilitation counseling during the fall semester of that year. My 1985 internship at the Iowa Department for the Blind led to a position as a rehabilitation teacher, and I have enjoyed full-time employment since. After much prodding from a rehabilitation counseling professor turned colleague, I completed my M.A. in 1987.

Take away the blindness, and this sounds like a pretty normal scenario. One prone to generalities would assume that someone in my situation would own my own home and have a busy, active life. As a blind person, though, I frequently hear an astonished "You own your own home?" from new acquaintances. In the United States, one often hears of the dominance of the White male in our culture. I find it ironic, then, when a 70-something, well-intentioned woman runs in front of me to open the door, warning me: "It's heavy!"

As I pass through middle age, I find myself evaluating my life more and more frequently. By and large, this is a very pleasant exercise. My career has been very successful, and I am quite content with my present position at the University of Iowa as a manager of projects that serve individuals with disabilities. I am well-established financially, owning my own home and having enough money left over to take frequent trips, which have included 11 Caribbean cruises and jaunts to England, Mexico, the former Soviet Union, New Zealand, and Costa Rica. I am able to enjoy my passion for sports, music, dancing, and the theater, having realized a lifelong dream by attending a 2006 World Series game in St. Louis. I've been blessed with an eclectic mix of friends, and very rarely have to spend time alone when I choose not to do so.

I am a realist, however. Blindness has imposed some additional challenges. I have not, for instance, found a marriage partner. I am a very outgoing person by nature, but find situations that have the potential to lead to relationships awkward and sometimes intimidating. I've convinced myself that because I miss out on body language and need to rely on my potential partner for transportation, I may always experience great difficulty in finding a partner. I do not experience the same freedom that sighted persons enjoy in traveling. I can't decide to jump in the car for a spur of the moment weekend trip. When flying, I'm often asked to board a flight early or to wait until everyone has deplaned before I do so. When I walk into a new social setting, I am keenly aware that others notice my blindness. A quick scan of the local newspaper is not possible in the conventional manner. Recreation presents some challenges as well. With no adapted sports, such as beep baseball, goalball or a blind bowling league in our community, I have found participation in group sports to be almost impossible.

Do these barriers keep me from enjoying life? Absolutely not! I've come to realize that should I meet a suitable marriage partner, blindness will not keep us apart. I utilize several modes of transportation, including buses, cabs, paid drivers, walking, and most importantly, friends. By introducing myself in new social situations and striking up a conversation, I address the hesitancy so typical of someone who has just met their first real live person with a disability. By making computers and the Internet accessible to blind persons, assistive technology has opened the information superhighway, making that scan of the morning paper possible. To compensate for the lack of physical recreation opportunities, I've taken up dancing, which in turn has opened up an entirely new social network. My theater-going and cruise experiences are enhanced by friends who share my interests and have convinced me that my blindness is not a burden to them.

Ultimately, the key to my success and adaptability is an inner satisfaction. For me, that stems from a faith in an omnipresent God who governs every aspect of my life. I find that I am most challenged when I choose to abandon the belief that if God is for me, who can be against me. Though I turn to the Creator for inward strength, I turn outward to find joy in cultivating friendships. I truly believe that my blindness has resulted in friendships that otherwise would not have occurred. Take, for instance, the woman who observed my putting sour cream on a baked potato in a restaurant. She turned to her husband and said, "Just look at him. Isn't that wonderful!" I couldn't resist pointing out to her that I'd had lots of practice, and we soon fell into casual conversation that led to an extremely meaningful friendship. Then there is the middle school teacher who annually taught a disability awareness unit to her students. Appreciative of her work, I stopped by her school to say thanks, never dreaming that, several years later, I would count her among my closest friends. Yes, I must challenge stereotypes on an almost daily basis, but I find that doing so pays huge dividends.

My sense of humor has carried me through many situations that might have otherwise become stressful or embarrassing. I frequently slip in a pun during my daily 2-hour commute, putting new van pool passengers at ease. I'm the first to repeat the newest "blind joke," flying in the face of what many consider political correctness. If we can't laugh about our everyday experiences and share some of that humor with others, life gets boring rather quickly.

In the leadership training curriculum that one of our projects developed during the early portion of this decade, our consultant wrote: "We do not believe that a disability-free world is better." This statement has caused me to do a great deal of thinking. By now, it should be evident that I do not view blindness as a tragedy. Yet, I would not wish it on my child. I have to live with it, at least for now, and am going to do the very best I can. Yet, why would you want someone else to face the attitudinal and physical barriers that so frequently confront individuals with disabilities?

You are about to enter an extremely important profession. Unemployment among persons with severe disabilities is estimated at near 70%. You will have the opportunity to do something about that. If I impress nothing else upon you, I implore you to see the individuals you serve first as *persons*, not as clients. Yes, you do have to maintain a professional relationship, and yes, you will need to do assessments, but please do not form your opinions based on a test score. Your client has dreams, feelings, and aspirations, just as you do. Listen to them, and work with him/her to achieve them. I can tell you from personal experience that rehabilitation professional's who aren't willing to see their clients as capable human beings are doing them a disservice. My counselor did many good things for me, but the one thing that I best remember is a conversation during which he tried to persuade me to pursue a career in computer programming. I'd told him frequently that this field held no interest for me whatsoever. Though I now have very positive feelings and a great deal of respect for my lead professor in graduate school, I did not feel that way when he tried to exempt me from having to do a work sample as part of a class assignment.

As you reflect back on your life and career 15 years from now, perhaps you'll remember reading a small chapter written by a blind guy who knew how to put sour cream on his baked potato. Remember that this guy was once a rehabilitation client, and that he chose his career *with the assistance* of his counselor. As you do so, commit yourself once again to honoring the capabilities of each of your clients, and do the very best that you can to guide them as they exercise their right to chart their life course.

DISCUSSION QUESTIONS

1. Are there any real meaningful differences in the terms adjustment, reaction, adaptation and response? How might they be the same or different?
2. Of the seven proposed adaptation theories of adjustment to disability, which one(s) appear to have the greatest face validity and why?
3. Is the author correct in claiming that the theories are essentially describing the same phenomena?
4. Which functional abilities (e.g., sight, mobility, cognition, auditory) would be the most difficult to lose, and what abilities and subsequent enjoyable activities would you have left?
5. Which might be more difficult to experience; being born with a disability, or sustaining one later in life?

EXERCISES

A. Have students list what their top 5 most enjoyable activities are, then develop a list of 5 other potential substitute activities if they were no longer functionally able to enjoy the top 5 anymore due to a disability?
B. Ask students to outline what they perceive would be the single most difficult aspect of adjusting to any disability would be?

SIX

Family Adaptation Across Cultures Toward a Loved One Who Is Disabled

Noreen M. Glover-Graf

OVERVIEW

The first experiences of supportive and social units come, most often, from the family; a unit of persons united through blood, adoption, or marriage (U.S. Census Bureau, 2000). Here, parents are obligated to provide adequate basic care for their children by supplying food, shelter, medical care, and schooling. The onset of disability in the family creates challenges for them, sometimes even to basic care obligations, depending on the resources available to, and the unique characteristics of, the members. This chapter will discuss the impact of disability on family by examining the reactions of family members to disability, factors that influence adjustment to disability in the family, adjustment models, parenting reaction perspectives, effective family coping, the impact of disability based on the family role of the person with a disability, and cultural influence on family adaptation to disability.

DEFINING FAMILY

Much of the literature related to families and disability is written from the framework of the traditional family model, married parents living with children. But in fact only about 25% of American households are made up of a married man and woman with their children, and another 25% are persons living alone, many of them elderly and young unmarried persons. The remaining households are single-parent households, mixed families, same-sex parent households, extended family households, unmarried partners, and numerous other combinations of persons living together. In the United States, there is an average of 2.6 persons living in a household; the average income for the household is about $52,000. The percent of persons below poverty level is 14.3%. Compared with families without members with disabilities, families with members with disabilities are more likely to live in poverty and have a lower median income (U.S. Census Bureau, 2010). They are also more likely to have increased medical and childcare expenses, further taxing the financial resources of these families.

Because families are the primary support systems of persons with disabilities, it is important to understand the characteristics of healthy and well-functioning units. A healthy family depends less on the structure of the family, and more on particular characteristics of its members. With this in mind, families of any makeup, traditional, single-parent, extended family households, or otherwise, can be healthy families; however, a lack of financial, social, and personal resources will certainly make it more difficult to remain so. Lin (1994) described six characteristics that include:

1. Commitment that involves the prioritization of family over self, coordination of family roles and responsibilities, working together toward mutual goals, and supporting one another.
2. Togetherness, which refers to the family making arrangements for family time as in eating, playing, and celebrating together; it is less important as to what activities are shared as long as they are performed together.
3. Appreciation and admiration of an individual's strengths, talents, and interests. Encouragement of individual pursuits.
4. Good communication that establishes a sense of belonging, diminishes frustrations, and improves marital relations. This involves listening and conflict resolution rather than avoidance of a problem situation.
5. Spiritual well-being that involves the family sharing a common faith or spiritual beliefs that increases family cohesion.
6. Coping with crisis and stress that involves the family's willingness to face the reality of difficult situations and cope effectively, systematically, and rationally.

REACTIONS OF FAMILY TO DISABILITY

Emotional Reactions

In 1962, Olshansky described "chronic sorrow" as the regret and sorrow experienced by parents at the birth of a child with a disability due to the loss of the expected child. It was seen as an understandable sorrow that could last indefinitely as parents would reexperience sorrow at each of their child's developmental milestones. Twenty years later, Wolfensberger (1983) alternatively described *novelty shock crisis*, a state of confusion due to lack of information and societal reaction. This term illustrated the shift in thinking from disability as the problem in the family, to understanding that a lack of social supports was also a hindrance to caregivers. Today, the term "caregiver burden" is frequently used to assist in the understanding of the amount of responsibility placed on caregivers that can result in extraordinary stress (Zarit, Reever, & Bach-Peterson, 1980). Caregivers may need to provide assistance with daily activities even to the extent that they feel they are missing out on life that can lead to feelings of anger, resentment, and depression. They may become emotionally drained and physically exhausted due to increased financial responsibilities and may need to take over all or part of the disabled member's family responsibilities while maintaining their own.

Stress Reactions

Stress occurs when any demand placed on an individual or systems exceeds the coping capacity. Initially, stress is inevitable at the onset of significant changes of any type. The stress created by disability in the family can cause it to collapse and struggle, or it may lead the family to become stronger, closer, and a better-functioning system. Stress is more evident in families with disability than those without it (Hodapp & Krasner, 1995; Taanila, Syrjala, Kokkonen, & Jarvelin, 2002; Wallander & Noojin, 1995) and comes from a number of difficult family challenges, including repeated medical and emotional crises, financial hardships, difficult schedules, modification of activities and goals, societal isolation, difficulty in educational placements, and marital discord (Lavin, 2001; McCubbin & Patterson, 1983). Other factors that increase stress for parents include having a greater number of children and having difficulty accessing reliable childcare (Warfield, 2005). In a study to look at the everyday lives of families with children who have chronic illnesses, families reported daily stresses as including chronic preoccupation with making health decisions, restricted social lives, and overall low vitality (Martin, Brady, & Kotarba, 1992).

Due to the medical costs of chronic illness and disability, and the need for caretaking that can cause one family member to decrease or give up work, there can be considerable stress caused by the financial impact of disability to families. Park et al. (2003) determined that among children with disabilities who are 3–21 years old, 28% are living below poverty level, affecting their health, living environment, family interactions, productivity, and their emotional well-being. Additionally, mothers of children with disabilities tend to have lower incomes and work less hours than mothers of children without disabilities (Neely-Barnes & Dia, 2008). Higher family income has been found to allow for increases in parents' coping options and adaptability, and ability to spend time supporting and nurturing their children (McLeod & Shanahan, 1996; Yau & LiTsang, 1999).

Although stress has been noted as high in families, there is generally a decline in stress over time as the family adapts to their circumstances. In a longitudinal study that examined stress among parents of children with intellectual disabilities over a 7-year period, stress declined significantly over time in the areas of worry about speech deficits, intelligence deficits, behavior at home, behavior in public, and obtaining help. Parents in this study also had additional children without disabilities and rated the amount of stress due to the child with a disability as twice that of the amount of stress caused by a child in the home without a disability (Baxter, Cummins, & Yiolitis, 2000).

Marital Discord

Marital difficulties are frequently discussed in the literature as problematic when families experience disability. Taanila, Kokkonen, and Järvelin (1996) investigated the long-term effects of chronic illness, severe intellectual impairment, and physical disability on parents' marital relationships and found that 25% of the parents reported that their child's disability was a contributing factor to their marital impairment. Specifically, the intense demands of daily caretaking, unequal division of daily task labor, and insufficient available time for leisure activities were identified as contributing to marital discord.

While preexisting marital discord can serve to increase family stress, severe childhood disability may also contribute to the onset of marital difficulties and be responsible for the higher rates of divorce among couples. Divorce is more likely to occur in families where one of the parents acquires a disability or a child is born with or acquires a disability. In families with children with developmental disorders, this increase is generally small, with only a 5.35% greater chance of divorce (Hodapp & Krasner, 1995). In a study of children with a chronic illness and variety of disabilities, the percent increase in divorce was even lower at 2.9% (Witt, Riley, & Coiro, 2003). Contrarily, Singer and Farkas (1989) found that families with infants with disabilities reported greater closeness.

FACTORS THAT INFLUENCE ADJUSTMENT TO DISABILITY IN THE FAMILY

Families have great impact on the recovery/adjustment, well-being, and success of an individual with a disability (Degeneffe & Lynch, 2006; Kosciulek, 1994), and family competence is considered by many to be a key factor in adjustment to disability (Alston & McCowan, 1995). Power and Dell Orto (2004) noted seven family characteristics that will influence how a family reacts to disability, including:

1. *Risk factors* will contribute to poor functioning in a family; these include a lack of support systems, family compositions that may add to stress, such as single-parent households, stressed families, or families in conflict.
2. *Protective factors*, identified as strong family connections, effective communication, and problem solving, will increase the likelihood that families will successfully adapt.
3. *Belief systems* that are moderated by religious and cultural values impact how the family manages the demands of disability, makes sense of the disability, and communicates with health professionals.
4. *Access to coping resources*, including personality strengths, previous life experiences, positive attitudes, values and religious beliefs, extended family support, and community and financial resources.
5. *Family history* involves the previous experiences in dealing with illness and disability and managing losses.
6. *Family relationships and communication styles* involve the members' ability to be open and honest with one another, to nurture each other, and to function in a well-structured manner versus members acting in isolation.
7. *Who in the family is disabled* plays a role in that dreams and expectations are affected differently based on if the member is a caretaker or dependent. Caretaker impairment will have a more detrimental impact on the family.

ADJUSTMENT MODELS

A number of models have been used to describe the process of family adaptation to disability. The Family Stress Theory was propunded by Reuben Hill in 1949 after his work with families of soldiers. His ABCX model explained how a stressor event, the family's perception of that event, and the available resources interacted to avoid or create a crisis reaction. McCubbin and Patterson (1983) expanded this model in the Double ABCX model by incorporating the use of family coping mechanisms to deal with a crisis event, recognizing an accumulation of stress on families over time, and a need to use existing and new resources and coping skills to reach positive adaptation termed "bonadaptation."

The Family Resilience Model has also been utilized to examine family adjustment. Resiliency is the ability to adapt, adjust, and thrive in difficult times. In rehabilitation, resiliency refers to the ability to adapt and adjust to disability and then to achieve a successful outcome (Kosciulek, 1994; Lustig, 1997). Family resiliency refers to the family's ability to make successful adaptations. The Resiliency Model of Family Stress, Adjustment and Adaptation (McCubbin & McCubbin, 1993; McCubbin, Thompson, & McCubbin, 1996) focuses on how families can positively adjust and cope to maintain their quality of life. The model places emphasis on the functional capacity and strengths of the family rather than on deficits. It builds upon the positive assets of the family, specifically what the family is good at and then works toward increasing problem solving, coping, and adjustment. Thus, instead of assessing only the deficits and needs of the family, the counselor would assess family strengths in terms of existing resources to deal with family crisis, views and attitudes toward the crisis, and the family's coping and problem-solving skills.

Following this assessment, the counselor assists the family in building and utilizing resources and prepares the family to the extent possible for what to expect from the rehabilitation process and assists in developing realistic expectations for recovery. Counselors will also make efforts to help the family review and reframe the occurrence of disability in the family. Families are assisted in coming to understand that their reactions to disability and feelings of stress, being overwhelmed, or angry are all normal reactions to a crisis. By reframing the event as an opportunity to work as a family to overcome obstacles, the family can become stronger, more efficient, and closer. Finally, counselors build on existing coping skills, including communication skills and work history, moving toward open family communication so that fears, misconceptions, and apprehensions about family roles can be resolved and long-term goals can be established. With open communication, family members can make decisions about who will be a caretaker and what role changes will occur. If these issues are not dealt with openly, anger and resentment may result (Frain et al., 2007).

Stage models have been used to describe the adjustment of persons to disability (Livneh & Antonak, 1990) over time. Blacher (1984) described three stages of adjustment of parents, which include an initial emotional crisis in which parents experience feelings of denial and shock; a second stage of fluctuating emotions that include anger, depression, guilt, shame, rejection of the child, and overprotection of the child; and a final stage of acceptance. A revision of this model by Anderegg, Vergason, and Smith (1992) that emphasizes the grieving process consists of three stages: confronting, adjusting, and adapting.

More recently, a number of researchers have moved beyond the notion of adjustment and adaptation phases as being the final stages or end goal and have come to incorporate an additional growth phase, recognizing that families may grow closer as a unit due to the challenges and rewards brought on by disability (Bradley, Knoll, & Agosta, 1992; Naseef, 2001). While stage theories have the benefit of attempting to explain how people proceed toward adjustment, they have been criticized for insufficient attention to the unpredictable or recurrent and complex aspects of adjustment to disability (Kendall & Buys, 1998). Likewise, Snow (2001) and Esdaile (2009) found that mothers of children with disabilities find these theories condescending and meaningless because they do not take into account the variety of positive experiences, insights, and understandings gained from caring for a child with a disability.

PARENTING REACTION PERSPECTIVES

In reviewing the literature related to reactions of parents of children with disabilities, Ferguson (2002) described five approaches to conceptualizing parental reactions; *psychodynamic, functionalist, psychosocial, interactionist,* or *adaptational.* For a number of decades, a *psychodynamic approach* was the only lens used to describe parental reactions to disability. This led to viewing parental reactions from a pathological standpoint, viewed as either apathetic or involved and either angry or accepting. From this standpoint, parents' reactions were framed as unhealthy and neurotic. Even involvement with the child could be interpreted as resulting from underlying guilt. Justifiable anger at a lack of appropriate care could be seen as displaced anger and a lack of adjustment.

With a shift to behavioral treatment approaches in the 1960s, a *functionalist* approach frequently labeled parents' reactions as dysfunctional and children's parents were often seen as additionally disabling to the child. With the advent of the 1970s, the *psychosocial* approach to viewing disability focused on the interplay of the environment and the emotions of the parents. The emotions of shock, loneliness, stress, and grief became the focus. The work of Olshansky (1962) in the area of chronic sorrow, and Wolfensberger (1983) in the area of shock and grief are examples of using the psychosocial approach to conceptualize parental reactions. From this standpoint, parents are viewed as suffering from loss. The *interactionist* standpoint, which is an infrequent approach, views parental reactions as a function of societal stigma, fatigue, disempowerment, and poverty leading parents to feel powerless. Finally, a recent approach to viewing parental reaction is the *adaptational* approach that emphasizes supportive social policy and cultural values as essential components of parental reaction to disability. It emphasizes the adaptability and resiliency of families and recognizes coping skills, and positive aspects of raising a child with a disability, including the potential of marital and spiritual growth and family harmony. From this standpoint, families can be viewed as empowered, cohesive, and adapted.

EFFECTIVE FAMILY COPING WITH DISABILITY

The emotional, financial, and social impact of disability on the family will be largely determined by how the family responds to crisis and how effectively they manage and resolve conflict, make decisions, and meet role expectations. Families that avoid or seek to escape dealing with disability will likely experience greater disorganization and stress, whereas families that demonstrate competence in reorganizing and actively addressing issues by changing their behaviors and attitudes to meet new demands will likely have greater positive adjustment (Alston & McCowan, 1995).

In order to determine what family qualities are most helpful toward the effective adjustment of disability, McCubbin identified three family types, the Balanced, Midrange, and Extreme. The Balanced family possesses two characteristics that render them most resilient and functional: rhythm and regenerativity. Rhythm in a family refers to established rituals, rules, and routines that allow children to have a clear understanding of what is expected of them and allows for increased closeness and bonding among family members. These families also report greater flexibility and satisfaction. Regenerativity in families refers to family coherence and hardiness. Coherence involves the emphasis placed on caring for one another, respect, loyalty, trust, pride, and common values. Hardiness involves internal control of events, activity involvement, and willingness to explore and challenge themselves (McCubbin & McCubbin, 1988). Similarly, Walsh (2003) reflected this description of resilient families, listing three factors that assist them to succeed. First, families need to be able to make sense and meaning of the difficulties they face. Second, they need to affirm their strength and maintain a positive perspective. Finally, they need a shared spiritual belief system. In addition to these characteristics, families must also be flexible, connected, and resourceful to persevere.

In a recent study, Knestrict and Kuchey (2009) investigated resiliency among families who had children with severe disabilities and found a strong connection between socioeconomic status (SES) and family resiliency. Of the families they determined to be resilient, all were in the upper family income categories. Likewise, the lowest functioning families were in the low-income category. The effect of higher SES was that families were more likely to have health insurance benefits, additional income provided for a better level of care and allowed them to access information and services. They found that more money was available to provide for respite care, home remodeling, and additional activities, such as aquatic and equine therapy, and more leisure time. The authors acknowledge the potential for state and federal programs to equalize disability services across SES levels, but point to continued funding cutbacks that limit available services.

Families have expressed a number of other needs, which, if provided could assist in family functioning, including family and social support, medical information, financial information and assistance, help explaining the disability to others, childcare, and professional support and services (Sloper & Turner, 1992; Walker, Epstein, Taylor, Crocker, & Tuttle, 1989). In a study of needs for families with a child with CP, parents desired information on services, help planning for the future, help finding community activities, and more respite time. Parents whose children used wheeled mobility expressed needing help paying for home equipment and home modifications, and finding childcare workers, respite care providers, and community recreational activities (Palisano et al., 2010).

DISABILITY IMPACT AND THE FAMILY MEMBER WITH A DISABILITY

When a Child Has a Disability

The extent of the physical impairment, the predictability of the course of the illness, and whether or not it is life threatening affect the reactions of families and children to disability. The more severe and difficult the management of the disability is, the greater the family's susceptibility to stress reactions, frustration, and feelings of being overwhelmed (Lyons, Leon, Roecker Phelps, & Dunleavy, 2010). In examining the influence of predictability of symptoms in young children with chronic illnesses on parents' stress levels, Dogson et al. (2000) found that childhood illness with unpredictable symptoms caused significantly higher levels of distress.

In addition to severity and predictability, the child's age will have an impact on emotional adjustment. Children who are very dependent on their parents, who do not have opportunity to socialize with friends, or who are frequently absent from school due to medical conditions may be delayed in emotional and social development. If children are less socially mature, or if they have experienced rejection from peers, they may have difficulty making friends, feel rejected, and become isolated. Adolescents who are unable to achieve sufficient independence or explore friendships and intimate relationships, or whose body image is negative, may become frustrated and depressed (Falvo, 2005).

Other emotions that children and adolescents with disabilities may have are fear, grief, anger, and denial. Anger can be experienced as loud outbursts as well as moodiness, pouting, and silence. Grief may be experienced as sadness but can also be masked behind hostility and resentment toward others. Uncertainty related to medical procedures or returning to school or other social environments may trigger lingering fear and apprehension. Denial and unreasonable expectations may initially serve to protect the child from emotionally dealing with difficulties related to the disability, but they can also serve to keep the child from making efforts to adjust to the condition. (Power & Dell Orto, 2004).

As with other crises, parents' initial reactions to disability onset may present as shock and denial, a time of numbness, and disbelief. These reactions are productive in that they provide psychological protection until the family members work up to psychological coping but may also interfere with rational decision making if the parents refuse to accept the diagnosis or the permanency of a condition. Parents may then experience a number of emotions as a result of having a child with a disability, including being overwhelmed, confused, and profoundly sad (Power & Dell Orto, 2004). They may experience guilt, believing that something they did or failed to do may have caused the disability or may become depressed (Norton & Drew, 1994). Parental depression and feelings of helplessness and stress may then contribute to additional restrictions or limitations in the child with a disability (Tomasello, Manning, & Dulmus, 2010).

A number of studies have compared the impact of a birth of a child with a disability to a death in terms of adjustment because families have been noted to progress through the grief stages of shock, realization, defensive retreat, and acknowledgment (Norton & Drew, 1994; Wolfensberger, 1983). These studies suggest that parents grieve the death of the child that they anticipated and they grieve the loss of dreams they had for their child. Depending on the disability, parents may need to alter their physical, emotional, or cognitive expectations of their child. For example, for children with significant mobility impairments, parents who wished to play sports with their children may initially grieve that perception of a future loss. In addition, parents may experience anger or look to place blame on hereditary causes in themselves or their partners. If poor nutrition, drug use, or other controllable factors are suspected to have contributed to the child's disability, such as in fetal alcohol syndrome, intense guilt and societal scorn may also result (Vash & Crewe, 2004).

In a study of parents of children with intellectual disabilities, Gallagher, Phillips, Oliver, and Carroll (2008) found parents to have high levels of anxiety and depression that were most influenced by the amount of caregiver burden and their feelings of guilt. Another study by Norton and Drew (1994) identified the family hardships associated with raising a child with autism as difficulty with communication and bonding, sleep disruption, behavior problems, a need for consistent routine, respite care and problems, and future financial planning needs. The inability to effectively communicate and the child's rejection of physical contact and a seemingly noncaring attitude toward the family create difficulty in parental bonding. The child's behavior and need for consistency make traveling outside the home difficult. Children may sleep for only a few hours at night, causing sleep deprivation for parents. In addition, any disruption in routine may lead to screaming outbursts and prolonged crying. Due to the constant caregiving demands, respite is important, particularly for the primary caregiver, and siblings may be called upon to provide care that can either be seen as positive role modeling or, if used to excess, may have a negative impact.

In examining caregiving burdens of families with a member with intellectual and behavioral/psychiatric problems, Maes, Broekman, Dosen, and Nauts (2003) concluded:

> Psychiatric and behavioral problems are often incomprehensible and unpredictable, which causes the parents to feel dissatisfied, inadequate to cope, insecure and reticent to act. But feelings and motivations of parents on the other hand may also have profound effects on the behavioral difficulties of their child. Parents consider the psychiatric or behavioral problems of their child to be an extra burden and feel it more difficult to raise and manage such a child in the family situation. This forces them to change the situation and to call on the help of external services. (Maes et al., 2003, p. 454)

These authors conclude that families need more resources for respite, extended social support groups for emotional support specialized training, and recognition of negative feelings.

Not all parents react in the same way to having a child with a disability; whereas some report continued discomfort with their child, others find the child has strengthened their marriage and family life (Scorgie & Sobsey, 2000). In comparing differences in the mother's and father's reactions to a child with a disability, some studies have found that mothers' react with greater depression, express greater caregiver burden, and feel higher levels of stress than fathers do. They spend more hours caring for the child with a disability than fathers do. However, Hastings (2003) found that stress and depression levels were similar in mothers and fathers of children with autism but mothers exhibited higher levels of anxiety. In an additional study, Hastings et al. (2005) reported that despite race or ethnicity, mothers report experiencing both greater depression and greater positive effects from parenting a child with a disability than fathers do.

In addition to parents, grandparents are increasingly being called upon to care for their grandchildren with disabilities. This is especially true for African American and Latino families. Grandparents may have unique problems associated with caregiving because, unless they are the legal guardians, they have more difficulty accessing services and information (such as medical and school records) necessary for caretaking. In addition, they may have financial concerns, they may have difficulties due to aging and a need for respite, they may have problems associated with the child's parents, particularly if they have exited their child's life due to addictions or legal problems, and, they may have problems navigating social service, judicial, and educational systems (McCallion, Janicki, Grant-Griffin, & Kolomer, 2000). It is not surprising that grandparents have also been found to be susceptible to depression in some studies, but results vary and this remains unclear. What may be the most important to determining the amount of stress and caregiver burden experienced by grandparents may be strongly impacted by their beliefs and attitudes related to disability (Neely-Barnes & Dia, 2008). Positive effects of caretaking a grandchild with a disability have been noted as creating better relationships, and a greater sense of connectedness, meaning, and personal growth (Gardner, Scherman, Efthimiadis, & Shultz, 2004).

The decision to place a child outside of the home

The decision to place a child with a disability outside of the home is difficult for many parents. Several studies have demonstrated that increased stress is related to the extent of behavior problems (Maes et al., 2003) that may in turn affect the family's decision to place the child in residential care. This decision generally occurs at birth and in the transition out of high school. In a study to examine outside placement decisions of parents of young adults with severe intellectual disability, McIntyre, Blacher, and Baker (2002) found that outside home placement could be predicted by the extent of behavior problems and mental health problems of the young adult.

When a Partner Has a Disability

Because most of the caregiving falls upon the spouse, the impact of disability can be overwhelming for couples. Researchers have found that among couples in which one of the partners had spinal cord injury (SCI), the caregiving partner had equal or higher levels of stress, fatigue, resentment, and anger when compared with the partner with the disability (Chan, Lee, & Lieh-Mak, 2000; Weitzenkamp, Gerhart, Charlifue, Whiteneck, & Savic, 1997). Parker (1989) reviewed the impact of disability on the partner caregiver and concluded that they have higher levels of stress than any other caregiver due to the psychological and social effects of caring for their partner.

When a partner acquires a cognitive disability, such as traumatic brain injury (TBI), stroke, or Parkinson's, the caregiver loses the equitable relationship and assumes a parenting role for their spouse, and they often feel as if they have gained a child and lost a spouse. The spouse caregiver must take on many of the duties of the afflicted spouse and may need to assume all of the financial burden as well and is frequently forced to make difficult financial cuts that may involve liquidating assets. In order to provide sufficient care, the caregiver may need to reduce social time with friends and family, creating social isolation. Even if the caregiver finds time to socialize, socializing may be difficult because he or she will not fit well into either the couple's socializing world or the single world. Ultimately, the strain of caretaking, financial struggles, and social isolation may lead to a marital relationship that is void of sexual relations. For some, this overwhelming change in living conditions and relations leads to separation or divorce (Parker, 1989).

Multiple sclerosis (MS) is a progressive disorder that will involve increasing reliance on others for activities of daily living and social interactions. Hakim et al. (2000) identified a number issues related to living with MS that could affect partner relationships, including the reduction of social interactions and a shrinking number of friends, particularly as the disease progressed. Additionally, the partner with MS frequently retired early and many partners believed that their own careers were inhibited due to the spouse's illness. Partners also experienced higher levels of anxiety and depression associated with greater severity of MS. Even so, the authors did not find a greater incidence of divorce among couples with MS when compared with the general population.

For persons with SCI, the divorce rates are higher than the general population whether they marry before or after they are injured and the likelihood of marriage after injury is decreased (Brain and Spinal Cord.Org, 2010). Aside from the individual's adjustment to physical changes and pain, those in partner relationships will encounter a number of lifestyle changes that affect their relationships, such as changes to sexual intimacy, independence, raising children, job security, financial security, and recreational activity involvement. The emotional responses to these changes will also affect the relationship and may include depression and anxiety, suicide ideation (an initial suicide rate of four to five times that of the general population), and alcohol and drug abuse (Craig & Hancock, 1998). In a review of the literature on partner relationships and SCI, Kreuter (2000) found that divorce rates from 8% to 48% have been reported in the literature, depending on the time since injury for participants. In general, it appears that divorce rates are higher in the first 3 years and then decline to a normal rate. DeVivo and Richards (1992) noted a number of factors that put persons with SCI at greater risk for divorce, including being nonambulatory, being female, not having any children, being young, having a previous divorce, and having an injury less than 3 years old. In a study that interviewed 55 couples with preinjury or postinjury marriages, Crewe, Athelstan, and Krumberger (1979) and DeVivo, Hawkins, Richards, and Go (1995) found more stability and life satisfaction in postinjury marriages. Kreuter, Sullivan, and Siosteen (1994) studied marriage stability following SCI and found differences on based on the age of the couple; older couples had greater emotional attachment or relationship satisfaction than younger couples.

Despite the negative public perception that persons who date people with disabilities as being deviate or desperate (Olkin, 1999), in a qualitative study to examine females who were dating men with SCI, Milligan and Neufeldt (1998) found that maladaptive motivations were not present. They identified a number of factors related to the disability that influenced the development of the relationships. Nondisabled participants described their partners as well adjusted to their SCI and exhibiting autonomous attitudes. These elements in combination with individual personality traits were described as important features of their attraction. Attributes of the nondisabled female partners included open-mindedness about a relationship with a person with SCI, previous experiences with disability, role flexibility, acceptance of the partner's need for assistance, commitment to foster independence, and resiliency against social disapproval.

In relation to cognitive and mental health disabilities, studies have also shown high rates of divorce. Lefley (1989) identified problem behaviors in families of persons with severe mental illness, including persons with disabilities' abuse of family members, conflicts with neighbors, noncompliance with medications and other interventions, unpredictable reactions, and mood swings. Butterworth and Rodgers (2008) reported that a number of studies have demonstrated that divorce frequently follows the acquisition of mental illness in couples where one partner has a mental illness. Causes of marital termination have been attributed to relationship dissatisfaction, marital conflict, and social causes. In couples where both partners have a mental illness, divorce rates have been shown to be eight times that of the general population.

Studies related to couples in which one partner acquires a TBI have reported varying rates of divorce ranging from 15% to 54% and dependent on factors such as the length of the relationship preinjury and how much time has elapsed since the injury. In a study that examined 120 persons with TBI, people who were more likely to stay married had been in longer-term preinjury marital relationships, were older, had less severe TBI, and their injuries were not due to violent crimes (Kreuter, Marwitz, Hsu, Williams, & Riddick, 2007).

When a Parent Has a Disability

Early speculation related to children being raised by persons with disabilities suggested that children were in danger of negative emotions and behaviors, such as anxiety and depression, and developmental issues, such as dependency, helplessness, overcompliance, social alienation, and isolation. However, empirical literature presents no definitive evidence of these negative parenting effects. Buck and Hohmann (1983) reported that children raised by a father with SCI showed no difference from other children in terms of physical health measures, personality disturbance, body image or sexual orientation, or in interpersonal relationships. The differences noted in male children were that they were more conventional, practical, and tough-minded but less secure than other males. Female children were found to be more self-assured, imaginative, and unconventional but were less tough-minded and realistic than other females. Coles, Pakenham, and Leech (2007) studied children of parents with MS and noted that often these children assume caregiving roles by cleaning, cooking, shopping, budgeting, and giving emotional support. Children with a parent who has MS have also been shown to have higher levels of anxiety dysphoria, somatization, interpersonal difficulties, and hostility and less satisfaction with life (Pakenham & Bursnall, 2006). The fact that positive and negative affects are present is to be expected because children who have parents with disabilities have different growing-up experiences and challenges. However, negative differences may be directly related to a lack of financial and social supports to alleviate overburdening children.

Parents with mental retardation (MR) face problems such as poverty, lack of parenting models, isolation from families, lack of public resources, and limited experiences. For these parents, providing adequate parenting depends on long-term support (Whitman & Accardo, 1993). Incidences of neglect and abuse are due to a lack of support and resources more than cognitive deficit (Tymchuk & Andron, 1990). In a study of children whose parent/s had MR, two-thirds were diagnosed with MR or developmental delays. Most of the delays were corrected with intervention pointing to the need for additional resources and supports. In addition, a number of studies have demonstrated the need for and efficacy of parenting skills training for parents with MR (Feldman et al., 1992; Whitman & Accardo, 1993).

Parents with sensory impairments reported difficulty in assisting children with school work and a need to rely on children as interpreters (Strom, Daniels, & Jones, 1988), and hearing children of deaf adults (CODA) often grow up in the deaf culture, learning sign language and acting as interpreters for parents. These children grow up with distinct advantages but can also feel caught between two worlds and sometimes describe being raised as a deaf child (Harrington, 2001).

When a Sibling Has a Disability

Depending on the age of the child, siblings may have a number of reactions to a sister or brother with a disability. Young children may experience some fear that they may catch the disability, or they may believe they are responsible in some way for the disability due to wishful or magical thinking (Batshaw, 1991), or they may feel jealous or embarrassed of their sibling, causing abusive behaviors (Havens, 2005; Pearson & Sternberg, 1986). Poor adjustment of siblings has been attributed to high levels of family conflict, poor parent functioning, low family adaptability and cohesion, and deficit problem-solving skills and communication.

In a study of 49 siblings, Giallo and Gavidia-Payne (2006) found that they had significantly higher overall adjustment difficulties, emotional and peer problems, and lower levels of socialization compared with the normative sample. In order to investigate how family characteristics, family routines, and problem solving influence sibling adjustment, these authors determined that (1) sibling adjustment to disability was not significantly impacted by sibling level of daily stress and coping skills, (2) level of parent stress was a predictor of sibling adjustment, (3) siblings in households with regular and consistent family routines exhibited fewer adjustment problems, and (4) siblings had better adjustment in households that demonstrated great problem-solving strategies and more effective communication.

Research involving siblings has also described some positive benefits (Crossman, 1972; Hannah & Midlarsky, 1985), but siblings are often expected to assume additional responsibilities, such as providing for the inclusion, socialization, and physical care of their sibling with a disability (Skrtic, Summers, Brotherson, & Turnbull, 1984; Swenson-Pierce, Kohl, & Egel, 1987). Parents of nondisabled siblings who can provide care and socialization may benefit from the additional assistance, but some studies have determined that nondisabled siblings may be given too much responsibility for their maturity level. Charles, Stainton, and Marshall (2009) discussed the negative impact for young caregivers as including the loss of their childhood and increased stress. However, siblings report both positive and negative effects related to caregiving. In a study of school-aged siblings' stressors, siblings identified being the most stressed when they felt embarrassed in the presence of their friends, they felt the happiest when they played with their sibling, and the most uplifted when their sibling expressed affection through hugs and kisses (Orfus & Howe, 2008).

Most of the literature related to siblings of persons with disabilities focuses on the childhood relationships between the disabled and nondisabled siblings. However, as the person with a disability ages and parents become too old to care for their children, the sibling may be called upon to provide extensive care. While some persons with disabilities may move into group homes, the demand for residential care far exceeds availability and waiting lists for group homes may be prohibitively long. In a study of persons who provide care for their adult siblings with a disability, Altman and D'Ottavi (2005) noted that siblings who provide housing and care are more likely to be persons of color, and live in a low-income and female head-of-household family.

CULTURAL IMPACT ON FAMILY ADAPTATION

For a more detailed account of cultural differences historically in relation to disability, see Dr. Millington's Chapter 3. For the purposes of this section, I briefly address culture in relation to family dynamic and responses. Disability is defined differently across cultures in terms of the meaning of experience, family values, and interaction with social systems. Understanding cultural differences in family function is essential to understanding the adjustment process as well as understanding the strengths of family systems. Living as a minority family in the United States differs from living in the majority culture in a number of ways identified by Sue and Sue (1999). Families must frequently deal with racism and there is a greater likelihood of living in poverty. Family values, while not in conflict with the majority values, place greater emphasis on family and less emphasis on the individual. Values and dreams related to wealth, occupation, and status may differ in their meaning to minorities. They are also likely to be transitioning into assimilation and live juggling two cultures and come from histories that include slavery, immigration, and refugee status, and may have been forced from their countries or made difficult decisions to leave. They may also be in the process of learning or using English, which may not be a good substitute for expression.

African Americans

The African American (AA) family differs in that it utilizes extended family members as primary caretakers, has great flexibility in family roles, is intensely religious, and has developed coping skills to stressors brought on by racism, poverty, and unemployment

(Hines & Boyd-Franklin, 1982). Alston and Turner (1994) examined AA family strengths noting strong kinship bonds that include immediate, extended, and even fictive kin. They suggest that one reason AA families do not access rehabilitation service may be that they have the capacity to support a family member with a disability through the adjustment to the disability. Greater role flexibility is present in AA families for a number of reasons, including the fact that AA women frequently are in a head-of-household position by choice or because a disproportionate number of men in the AA community are incarcerated, unemployed, or living out of the home. When the mother is employed, extended family members or older children are enlisted to provide for childcare and household duties. Unlike families that adhere to ridged roles, the AA family has adapted to avoid overload through role flexibility. In the case of disability in the family, members may be accustomed to assuming a variety of family roles and duties.

Religious orientation has also been noted as strength for African Americans because it offers spiritual inspiration, social support, and an opportunity for ventilation of distress and other emotions. The church is viewed as a further extension of the family that emphasized positive outlook and increased self-esteem. It also assists in providing for basic needs, such as shelter, food, clothing, childcare, and assistance in locating work (Alston & Turner, 1994).

Other family strengths noted by Alston and Turner (1994) are education and work ethics. African Americans value education and encourage children to succeed academically because this is considered as one of the pathways to social and economic upward mobility. Despite the perception that African Americans lack work ethics, they actively seek job opportunities and support family members work efforts.

Alston and McCowan (1995) determined that African Americans who adjust well to disability have families that are close and supportive, have strong emotional support, and have members willing to assist with AODs. These authors suggested that AA families are not easily disrupted by disability and can accommodate disability while maintaining stability, humor, and generosity. They also suggest that AA families benefit from a lack of traditionally defined roles and are able to redefine and reassign family roles as needed to meet the needs of the family. Interestingly, and perhaps one of the obvious cultural differences is that conflict was not predictive of poor adjustment. AA families did not view the expression of family conflict as an obstacle to adjustment. Rather the expression of disagreement and emotions were seen as natural and acceptable.

Asian Americans

Significant differences exist in Asian American outlook related to disability. The core values of Asian families are family, duty to family, family welfare, family reputation, harmony, education, wisdom, knowledge, humility, work, and self-sacrifice (Lynch & Hanson, 2004). Depending on the level of acculturation, Asian parents may view children with disabilities as shameful or humiliating and may believe that they are to blame. As the family becomes more acculturated, negative attitudes are replaced with attitudes of hope and acceptance (Cho, Singer, Brennar, 2003). In a study of first-generation Chinese families with a child with a disability, Parette, Chuang, and Huer (2004) noted that parents were involved, valued education, were concerned about social stigma, and did not express shame about their child's disability.

In a study of Chinese families in New York, Ryan and Smith (1989) determined that language barriers caused almost half the parents not to understand their child's diagnosis. Parents were also inclined to view disability as a temporary condition and many exhibited reactions of denial, guilt, and only partial acceptance. Parents attributed disability to either natural, supernatural, and metaphysical causes. Supernatural cause resulted from a belief there had been a religious or ethical violation that caused a deity to become angry. A third of the parents surveyed believed in a metaphysical cause for their child's disability and attributed disability to a lack of balance between the Yin and Yang, considered essential for health. Imbalances were seen to produce fever and chills in children, which were seen as having the potential to lead to disability. These parents used alternative medicine that included incense to remove evil spirits, acupuncture, and wearing silver bracelets.

Latino Families

The Latino population of the United States has increased by 50% since 1990. Due to poor health care, exposure to violence, and work in settings that expose them to greater physical risks, disability is prevalent in Latino communities (World Institute on Disability, 2004). While every culture and every family is different, and they come to the United States from a number of Central American and South American countries, some common themes are present in Latino families, including religion, family, and gender roles. Religion is important to community and family life and most Latinos practice Catholicism, but many also have additional beliefs that are related to their countries of origin. Many Latinos believe that things that happen in their lives are beyond their control and are meant to be; they also may engage in magical thinking and have a strong belief in miracles and the power of prayer. They may believe in positive or negative spirits that can cause difficulties or bad luck in their families and marriages (de Rios, 2001; Falicov, 1998).

For Latinos, the purpose of marriage is to have children and there is little separation between the two. Family is frequently the top priority and couples tend to include children in nearly all activities and outings. Extensive interaction with large and extended families is common, and extended family is frequently relied upon for social, emotional, and financial support. Perhaps due to the high value placed on family interaction, Skinner, Bailey, Correa, and Rodriguez (1998) found that many of the 150 Latina mothers in their study believed that having a child with disabilities made them better mothers. Latino families with disabilities have long been credited with viewing disability as a punishment from God (Falicov, 1998; Vega, 1990), but in a study of Mexican and Mexican-American beliefs about God in relation to disability, Graf and Blankenship (2007) found that only a small minority of Mexicans and Mexican-Americans believed disability to be a punishment from God.

Disability that affects gender roles may be particularly difficult for Latinos because gender roles tend to be traditional, with the male expected to be the financial provider, to be physically and emotionally strong, and to be a protective authority figure. Women are expected to provide for the children and elderly family members and to be self-sacrificing; they are in charge of the home and children but are expected to defer to their husbands. While these traditional roles have begun to change for many Latinos, these traditional beliefs and roles are the foundation for current practices and beliefs (Vega, 1990).

SUMMARY

Understanding the role of the family and how it functions to enhance or to detract from the lives of people with disability is imperative because this basic social unit can provide a lifetime of love, support, encouragement, and care. It is important to assess family needs and support services so that the family does not become overwhelmed or feel isolated in their endeavors to assist their loved one and to integrate into the larger community. This involves understanding numerous differences in family reactions and functioning based on the resilience of the family, who in the family has the disability, the extent of the disability, the resources available, and cultural beliefs and practices.

REFERENCES

Alston, R. J., & McCowan, C. J. (1995). Perception of family competence and adaptation to illness among African Americans with disabilities. *Journal of Rehabilitation, 61*(1), 27–32.

Alston, R. J., & Turner, W. L. (1994). A family strengths model of adjustment to disability for African American clients. *Journal of Counseling and Development, 72*, 378–383.

Altman, R., & D'Ottavi, M. (2005). Siblingship, co-residence & adult disability: An exploratory family analysis. *Allacademic Research*. Retrieved from http://www.allacademic.com/meta/p_mla_apa_research_citation/0/2/1/2/8/pages21286/p21286-1.php

Anderegg, M. L., Vergason, G. A., & Smith, M. C. (1992). A visual representation of the grief cycle for use by teachers with families of children with disabilities. *Remedial and Special Education, 13*, 17–23.

Batshaw, M. L. (1991). *Your child has a disability: A complete sourcebook of daily and medical care*. Boston, MA : Little, Brown and Company.

Baxter, C., Cummins, R. A., & Yiolitis, L. (2000). Parental stress attributed to family members with and without disability: A longitudinal study. *Journal of Intellectual & Developmental Disability, 25*, 105–118.

Blacher, J. (1984). Sequential stages of parental adjustment to the birth of a child with handicaps: Fact or artifact. *Mental Retardation, 22*, 55–68.

Bradley, V., Knoll, J., & Agosta, J. (1993). *Emerging issues in family support (Monograph No. 18)*. Washington, DC: American Association on Mental Retardation.

Brain and Spinal Cord.Org. (2010). *Spinal cord injury statistics*. Retrieved from http://www.brainandspinalcord.org/spinal-cord-injury/statistics.htm

Buck, F., & Hohmann, G. (1983). Parental disability and children's adjustment. In E. Pan, T. Backer, & C. Vash (Eds.), *Annual review of rehabilitation* (pp. 203–241). New York, NY: Springer.

Butterworth, P., & Rodgers, B. (2008). Mental health problems and marital disruption: Is it the combination of husbands' and wives' mental health problems that predicts later divorce? *Social Psychiatry and Psychiatric Epidemiology, 43*, 758–763.

Chan, R. C., Lee, P. W., & Lieh-Mak, F. (2000). Coping with spinal cord injury: Personal and marital adjustment in the Hong Kong Chinese setting. *Spinal Cord, 38*, 687–696.

Charles, G., Stainton, T., & Marshall, S. (2009). Young careers: Mature before their time. *Reclaiming Children & Youth, 18*, 38–41.

Cho, S. J., Singer, H. S., & Brenner, B. M. (2003). A comparison of adaptation to childhood disability in Korean immigrant and Korean Mothers. *Focus on Autism and Other Developmental Disabilities, 18*(1), 9–19.

Coles, A. R., Pakenham, K. I., & Leech, C. (2007). Evaluation of an intensive psychosocial intervention for children of parents with multiple sclerosis. *Rehabilitation Psychology, 52,* 133–142.

Craig, A., & Hancock, K. (1998). Living with spinal cord injury: Longitudinal factors, interventions and outcomes. *Clinical Psychology and Psychotherapy, 5,* 102–108.

Crewe, N., Athelstan, G., & Krumberger, F. A. (1979). Spinal cord injury: A comparison of preinjury and postinjury marriages. *Archives of Physical Medicine and Rehabilitation, 60,* 252–266.

Degeneffe, C. E., & Lynch, R. T. (2006). Correlates of depression in adult siblings of persons with traumatic brain injury. *Rehabilitation Counseling Bulletin, 49,* 130–142.

de Rios, M. D. 2001. *Brief psychotherapy with the Latino immigrant client.* New York, NY: Haworth Press.

DeVivo, M. J., Hawkins, L. V. N., Richards, J. S., & Go, B. K. (1995). Outcomes of post-spinal cord injury marriages. *Archives of Physical Medicine and Rehabilitation, 76,* 130–138.

DeVivo, M. J., & Richards, J. S. (1992) Community reintegration and quality of life following spinal cord injury, *Paraplegia, 30,* 108–112.

Dogson, J. E., Garwick, A., Blozis, S. A., Patterson, J. M., Bennett, F. C., & Blum, R. W. (2000). Uncertainty in childhood chronic conditions and family distress in families of young children. *Journal of Family Nursing, 6,* 252–266.

Esdaile, S. A. (2009) Valuing difference: Caregiving by mothers of children with disabilities. *Occupational Therapy International, 16,* 122–133.

Feldman, M., Case, L., Garrick, M., MacIntyre-Grande, W., Carnwell, J., & Sparks, B. (1992). Teaching child care skills to mothers with developmental disabilities. *Journal of Applied Behavior Analysis, 25,* 205–215.

Falicov, C. J. 1998. *Latino families in therapy.* New York, NY: Guilford Press.

Falvo, D. (2005). *Medical and psychosocial aspects of chronic illness and disability.* Sudbury, MA: Jones and Barlett Inc.

Ferguson, P. M. (2002). A place in the family: An historical interpretation of research on parental reactions to having a child with a disability. *Journal of Special Education, 36,* 124–130.

Frain, M. P., Lee, G. K., Berven, N. L., Tansey, T., Tschopp, M., & Chronister, J. (2007). Effective use of the resiliency model of family adjustment for rehabilitation counselors. *Journal of Rehabilitation, 73*(3), 18–25.

Gallagher, S., Phillips, A. C., Oliver, C., & Carroll, D. (2008). Predictors of psychological morbidity in parents of children with intellectual disabilities. *Journal of Pediatric Psychology, 33,* 1129–1136.

Gardner, J. E., Scherman, A., Efthimiadis, M. S., & Shultz, S. K. (2004). Panamanian grandmothers' family relationships and adjustment to having a grandchild with a disability. *International Journal of Aging and Human Development, 59,* 305–320.

Giallo, R., & Gavidia-Payne, S. (2006). Child, parent and family factors as predictors of adjustment for siblings of children with a disability. *Journal of Intellectual Disability Research, 50,* 937–948.

Graf, N. M., & Blankenship, C. B. (2007). Mexican and Mexican Americans' beliefs about god in relation to disability. *Journal of Rehabilitation, 73*(4), 41–50.

Hakim, E. A., Bakheit, A. M. O., Bryant, T. N., Roberts, M. W. H., McIntosh-Michaelis, S. A., Spackman, A. J. et al. (2000). The social impact of multiple sclerosis: A study of 305 patients and their relatives. *Disability and Rehabilitation, 22,* 288–293.

Hannah, M. E., & Midlarsky, E. (1985). Siblings of the handicapped: A literature review for school psychologists. *School Psychology Review, 14,* 510–520.

Harrington, T. (2001). Hearing children of deaf parents. *Galludet University.* Retrieved from http://library.gallaudet.edu/Library/Deaf_Research_Help/Research_Guides_(Pathfinders)/Hearing_Children_of_Deaf_Parents.html

Hastings, R. P. (2003). Child behaviour problems and partner mental health as correlates of stress in mothers and fathers of children with autism. *Journal of Intellectual Disability Research, 47,* 231–237.

Hastings, R. P., Kovshoff, H., Ward, N. J., Espinosa, F., Brown, T., & Remington, B. (2005). Systems analysis of stress and positive perceptions in mothers and fathers of pre-school children with autism. *Journal of Autism and Developmental Disorders, 35,* 635–644.

Havens, C. A. (2005). Becoming a resilient family: Child disability and the family system. *National Center on Accessibility, 17*. Retrieved from http://www.indiana.edu/~nca/monographs/17family.shtml

Hines, P. M., & Boyd-Franklin, N. (1982). Black families. In M. McGoldrick, J. Pearce, & J. Giordano (Eds.), *Ethnicity and family therapy* (pp. 84–107). New York, NY: Guilford Press.

Hodapp, R. M., & Krasner, D. V. (1995). Families of children with disabilities: Findings from a national sample of eighth-grade students. *Exceptionality, 5*, 71–81.

Kendall, E., & Buys, N. (1998). An integrated model of psychosocial adjustment following acquired disability. *Journal of Rehabilitation, 64*, 16–20.

Knestrict, T., & Kuchey, D. (2009). Welcome to Holland: Characteristics of resilient families raising children with severe disabilities. *Journal of Family Studies, 15*, 227–244.

Kosciulek, J. (1994). Dimensions of family coping with head injury. *Rehabilitation Counseling Bulletin, 37*, 244–257.

Kreuter, J. S., Marwitz, J. H., Hsu, N., Williams, K., & Riddick, A. (2007). Marital stability after brain injury: An investigation and analysis. *NeuroRehabilitition, 22*, 53–59.

Kreuter, M. (2000). Spinal cord injury and partner relationships. *Spinal Cord, 38*, 2–6.

Kreuter, M., Sullivan, M., & Siosteen, A. (1994). Sexual adjustment after spinal cord injury comparison of partner experiences in pre- and post-injury relationships. *Paraplegia, 32*, 759–770.

Lavin, J. L. (2001). *Special kids need special parents: A resource for parents of children with special needs.* New York, NY: The Berkley Publishing Group.

Lefley, H. P. (1989). Family burden and family stigma in major mental illness. *American Psychologist, 44*, 556–560.

Lin, P. L. (1994). *Characteristics of a healthy family.* United States Department of Education. Retrieved from http://www.eric.ed.gov/PDFS/ED377097.pdf

Livneh, H., & Antonak, R. F. (1990). Reactions to disability: An empirical investigation of their nature and structure. *Journal of Applied Rehabilitation Counseling, 21*, 13–21.

Lyons, A., Leon, S., Roecker Phelps, C., & Dunleavy, A. (2010). The impact of child symptom severity on stress among parents of children with ASD: The moderating role of coping styles. *Journal of Child & Family Studies, 10*, 516–524.

Lustig, D. (1997). Families with an adult with mental retardation: Empirical family typologies. *Rehabilitation Counseling Bulletin, 41*, 138–156.

Lynch, E. W., & Hanson, M. J. (2004). *Developing cross cultural competence.* Baltimore, MD: Paul H. Brookes.

Maes, A., Broekman, T. G., Dosen, A., & Nauts, J. (2003). Caregiving burden of families looking after persons with intellectual disability and behavioural or psychiatric problems. *Journal of Intellectual Disability Research, 47*, 447–445.

McCallion, P., Janicki, M. P., Grant-Griffin, L., & Kolomer, S. (2000). Grandparent careers II: Service needs and service provision issues. *Journal of Gerontological Social Work, 33*, 57–84.

McCubbin, H., & McCubbin, M. (1988). Typologies of resilient families: Emerging roles of social class and ethnicity. *Family Relations, 37*, 247–254.

McCubbin, H. I., & Patterson, J. M. (1983). Family transitions: Adaptation to stress. In H. I. McCubbin & C. R. Figley (Eds.), *Stress and the family: Coping with normative transitions* (Vol. 2, pp. 5–25). New York: Brunner/Mazel.

McCubbin, H. I., Thompson, A. I., & McCubbin, M. (1996). *Family assessment: resiliency, coping, and adaptation.* Madison, WI: University of Wisconsin System.

McCubbin, M. A., & McCubbin, H. I. (1993). Family coping with health crises: The resiliency model of family stress, adjustment and adaptation. In C. Danielson, B. Hamel-Bissell, & P. Winstead-Fry (Eds.), *Families; health, and illness* (pp. 21–64). New York, NY: Mosby.

McIntyre, L. L., Blacher, J., & Baker, B. L. (2002). Behavior/mental health problems in young adults with intellectual disability: The impact on families. *Journal of Intellectual Disability Research, 46*, 232–249.

McLeod, J. D., & Shanahan, M. J. (1996). Trajectories of poverty and children's mental health. *Journal of Health and Social Behavior, 31*, 207–220.

Martin, S. S., Brady, M. P., & Kotarba, J. A. (1992). Families with chronically ill young children: The unsinkable family. *Remedial and Special Education, 13*, 6–15.

Milligan, M. S., & Neufeldt, A. H. (1998). Postinjury marriage to men with spinal cord injury: Women's perspectives on making a commitment. *Sexuality & Disability, 16,* 117–132.

Naseef, R. A. (2001). *Special children, challenged Parents: The struggles and rewards of raising a child with a disability (Revised Edition).* Baltimore: Paul H. Brooks: Publishing Co., Inc.

Neely-Barnes, S. L., & Dia, D. A. (2008). Families of children with disabilities: A review of literature and recommendations for interventions. *Journal of Early and Intensive Behavior Intervention, 5*(3), 93–107.

Norton, P., & Drew, C. (1994). Autism and potential family stressors. *The American Journal of Family Therapy, 22,* 67–76.

Olkin, R. (1999). *What psychotherapists should know about disability.* New York, NY: Guilford.

Olshansky, S. (1962). Chronic sorrow: A response to having a mentally defective child. *Social Casework, 43,* 190–193.

Orfus, M., & Howe, N. (2008). Stress appraisal and coping in siblings of children with special needs. *Exceptionality Education International, 18,* 166–181.

Palisano, R. J., Almarsi, N., Chiarello, A., Orlin, M. N., Bagley, A., & Maggs, J. (2010). Family needs of parents of children and youth with cerebral palsy. *Child Care, Health and Development, 36,* 85–92.

Parette, P., Chuang, S. L., & Huer, M. B. (2004). First-generation Chinese American families' attitudes regarding disabilities and educational interventions. *Focus on Autism and Other Developmental Disabilities, 19,* 114–123.

Pakenham, K. I., & Bursnall, S. (2006). Relationship between social support, appraisal, and coping and both positive and negative outcomes for children of a parent with MS and comparisons with children of healthy parents. *Clinical Rehabilitation, 20,* 709–723.

Park, J., Hoffman, J., Marquis, A., Turnbull, D., Turnbull, H. R., Poston, D. et al. (2003). Toward assessing family outcomes of service delivery: Validation of a family quality of life survey. *Journal of Intellectual Disability Research, 47,* 367–384.

Parker, G. (1989) Spouse carers—Whose quality of life? In S. M. Baldwin, C. Godfrey, & C. Propper (Eds.), *Quality of Life: Perspectives and Policies* (pp. 120–130). London, UK: Routledge and Kegan Paul.

Pearson, J. E., & Sternberg, A. (1986). A mutual-help project for families of handicapped children. *Journal of Counseling and Development, 65,* 213–215.

Power, P. W., & Dell Orto, A. E. (2004). *Families living with chronic illness and disability.* New York, NY: Springer.

Ryan, A. S., & Smith, M. J. (1989). Parental reactions to developmental disabilities in Chinese American families. *Child and Adolescent Social Work, 6,* 283–299.

Scorgie, K., & Sobsey, D. (2000). Transformational outcomes associated with parenting children with disabilities. *Mental Retardation, 38,* 195–206.

Singer, L., & Farkas, K. J. (1989). The impact of infant disability on maternal perception of stress. *Family Relations, 38,* 444–449.

Skinner, D., Bailey, D. B., Correa, V., & Rodriguez, P. (1999). Narrating self and disability: Latino mothers' construction of identities vis-a-vis their child with special needs. *Exceptional Children, 65,* 481–495.

Skrtic, T. M., Summers, J. A., Brotherson, M. J., & Turnbull, A. P. (1984). Severely handicapped children and their brothers and sisters. In J. Blancher (Ed.), *Severely Handicapped Young Children and Their Families: Research in Review* (pp. 215–246). New York: Academic Press.

Sloper, P., & Turner, S. (1992). Service needs of families of children with severe physical disability. *Child: Care, Health and Development, 18,* 259–282.

Snow, K. (2001). *Disability is natural.* Woodland Park, CO: Brave Heart Press.

Strom, R., Daniels, S., & Jones, E. (1988). Parent education for deaf families. *Educational and Psychological Research, 8*(2), 117–128.

Sue, D. W., & Sue, D. (1999). *Counseling the culturally different: Theory and practice.* New York, NY: John Wiley & Sons.

Swenson-Pierce, A., Kohl, F. L., & Egel, A. L. (1987). Siblings as home trainers: A strategy for teaching domestic skills to children. *Journal of the Association for Persons with Severe Handicaps, 12,* 53–60.

Taanila, A., Kokkonen, J., & Järvelin, M. R. (1996). The long-term effects of children's early-onset disability on marital relationships. *Developmental Medicine & Child Neurology, 38,* 567–577.

Taanila, A., Syrjala, L., Kokkonen, J., & Jarvelin, M. R. (2002). Coping of parents with physically and or intellectually disabled children. *Child: Care, Health & Development, 28*, 73–86.

Tomasello, N. M., Manning, A. R., & Dulmus, C. N. (2010). Family-centered early intervention for infants and toddlers with disabilities. *Journal of Family Social Work, 13*, 163–172.

Tymchuk, A., & Andron, L. (1990). Mothers with mental retardation who do or do not abuse or neglect their children. *Child Abuse & Neglect, 14*, 313–323.

U.S. Census Bureau. (2000). *Census 2000 profiles of general demographic characteristics, United States.* Retrieved from http://www.census.gov/prod/cen2000/doc/ProfilesTD.pdf

U.S. Census Bureau. (2010). *U.S. quick facts from the U.S. Census Bureau.* Retrieved from http://quickfacts.census.gov/qfd/states/00000.html

Vash, C. L., & Crewe, N. M. (2004). *Psychology of disability.* New York, NY: Springer.

Vega, W. A. 1990. Hispanic families in the 1980s: A decade of research. *Journal of Marriage and the Family, 52*, 1015–1024.

Wallander, J. L., & Noojin, A. B. (1995). Mothers' report of stressful experiences related to having a child with a physical disability. *Children's Health Care, 24*, 245–256.

Walker, D. K., Epstein, S. G., Taylor, A. B., Crocker, A. C., & Tuttle, G. A. (1989). Perceived needs of families with children who have chronic health conditions. *Children's Health Care, 18*, 196–201.

Walsh, F. (2003). Family resilience: A framework for clinical practice. *Family Process, 42*, 1–18.

Warfield, M. E. (2005). Family and work predictors of parenting role stress among two-earner families of children with disabilities. *Infant & Child Development, 14*, 155–176.

Weitzenkamp, D. A., Gerhart, K. A., Charlifue, S. W., Whiteneck, G. G., & Savic, G. (1997). Spouses of spinal cord injury survivors: The added impact of caregiving. *Archives of Physical Medicine and Rehabilitation, 78*, 822–827.

Whitman, Y. B., & Accardo, J. P. (1993). The parent with mental retardation: Rights, responsibilities and issues. *Journal of Social Work and Human Sexuality, 8*, 123–136.

Witt, W. P., Riley, A. W., & Coiro, M. J. (2003). Childhood functional status, family stressors, and psychological adjustment among school-aged children with disabilities in the United States. *Archives of Pediatric Adolescent Medicine, 157*, 687–695.

Wolfensberger, W. (1983). *Normalization based guidance, education and supports for families of handicapped people.* Downsview, Ontario, Canada: National Institute on Mental Retardation.

World Institute on Disability. (2004). *Reaching the Latino disability community.* Retrieved from http://www.wid.org/programs/access-to-assets/equity/equity-e-newsletter-june-2004/reaching-the-latino-disability-community/

Yau, M. K., & LiTsang, C. W. (1999). Adjustment and adaptation in parents of children with developmental disability in two parent families: A review of the characteristics and attributes. *British Journal of Developmental Disability, 45*(1), 38–51.

Zarit, S., Reever, K., & Bach-Peterson, J. (1980). Relatives of the impaired elderly: Correlates of feelings of burden. *Gerontologist, 20*, 649–655.

INSIDER PERSPECTIVE

The Story of Francia Malone

My name is Francia Malone. I am a 28-year-old (in 2002) single African American female with ocular albinism. I live in Flint, Michigan, where I attended high school and junior college. I obtained an associate's degree in liberal arts, with a concentration in gerontology. Other areas of study were business, human relations, multicultural studies, and psychology. At present, I am self-employed as a respite care provider.

A respite care provider offers assistance and companionship in the absence of the primary caregiver. This allows the caregiver to take a brief "time-off" during the day or overnight. I chose this type of work because I enjoy working with the elderly population. Older adults are a lot of fun to be around and very insightful about life. It makes me feel good to know that not only am I making a difference in someone else's life, but someone is contributing to my life as well. I have held several jobs in the human services field, but working with the elderly is the most rewarding. My long-term goal is to own and operate an adult day care for seniors. One of the most important things, as a person with a disability, is being self-sufficient. On September 21, 2000, President Bill Clinton came to Flint, Michigan, in what was probably one of his last addresses on disability issues. I had the opportunity to hear him speak at the college campus that I previously attended. Mr. Clinton and other representatives who attended with him spoke with regard to a "disability" not being the cause of a person contributing to society or the workforce. Mr. Clinton also spoke briefly on "bridging the digital divide" for persons with disabilities and others. This would allow anyone and especially the disabled to communicate through a computer simply by looking at the screen and giving commands.

I agreed that with proper assistance and training anyone with a disability should be able to receive reasonable accommodations on the job and rehabilitation services to make them employable. In this century, modern technology is advancing so rapidly that persons with disabilities will be able to run a business or work without leaving their home. The same is true for parents who have a child with a disability. In spite of the severity of the disability, children and parents will be able to benefit. Parents will have the option of home schooling their children using the computer and Internet. It is very important that children learn early that there are other options for a quality education other than the classroom. As a child with a visual disability, I understand how difficult school can be. The option of home schooling was unavailable for me as a child, but today it is a growing trend among families of children with severe disabilities. I know from experience, that teasing and name-calling can have a lasting affect on a child's self-esteem. Everyone, regardless of whether they choose to admit it, would like to fit in and be accepted by their peers. For this reason, I would like to share my own personal experiences with those of you who are not disabled. I hope that you will have a better understanding of how difficult living in a society can be when you are considered "different." I was in kindergarten when my parents were told that I had a permanent visual disability known as "congenital motor nystagmus." Congenital is from birth and nystagmus means eye movement. My parents took me to an eye specialist who said that nothing was wrong and I might need glasses later on. From this time on, I struggled in school. I would tell the teachers that I was unable to see what was written on the chalkboard. The teachers told me to sit as close to the board as I could and try to do the best that I can.

I was always prescribed glasses that never seemed to help me. I would accommodate for the nystagmus by tilting my head back and forth or closing one eye and looking with the other. I continued to do this process year after year. The system that I created did not seem to be working for me anymore, and it was eventually in college that I realized that something was not right.

In 1990, after a couple semesters of college, I started experiencing fatigue, headaches, and sharp pain in my eyes. I did research and found that my vision problems could be associated with a genetic condition called albinism. At this point, I went to my opthamologist and told him about the problems. His response was "well . . . there is nothing else I can do for you." I remember leaving his office in tears and with nowhere to turn. If he couldn't help, and he is a specialist . . . then maybe nothing could be done.

I was always told that my vision would not change for years, so I didn't really know what to do with some information I had found on the topic. I started having more headaches, lightheadedness, and photophobia (sensitivity to light and glare), and my vision was becoming worse. Unfortunately, I had to leave college at that time, but in 1994, I was able to finish part of my program to obtain my associate's degree. It wasn't until 1997 that I heard about a clinic that helps people with different low-vision conditions. I told the low-vision specialist the problems that I was experiencing. I told him that I believed for many years that I had albinism, but was never tested. The eye doctors that I previously saw told me that nothing could be done. The specialist, responded by saying "that is what most of them say because they were not trained in low vision."

I proceeded to tell him about the problems that I had since I was a child regarding seeing, feeling off balance, and dizziness. We talked for a while and I felt like he really understood what I had been feeling for years. He gave me the name of a rehabilitation specialist and recommended that I speak with her regarding services that are offered to individuals with low-vision problems. He recommended some low-vision devices to try for a while and see if I noticed any improvement after using them.

In early May 1999, I was sent some information on albinism. There was an article included regarding persons who had been underdiagnosed and misdiagnosed with congenital nystagmus. This conclusion was drawn after albinism had been ruled out. Albinism, I was never tested for albinism? The article ended by saying "if you have questions about your own inheritance of albinism or your children, seek genetic counseling." That September I decided to try a different eye specialist and he actually agreed that I could possibly have inherited albinism. He recommended that I seek genetic counseling.

In November, I went for genetic counseling. The counselor could not believe that I had never been tested for albinism and noted how I didn't fit the appearance of what people like to call "an albino" with white hair and skin, and so the proper diagnoses was overlooked. He also stated that in his research, some types of albinism are so identical that they are hard to separate.

Occulocutaneous affects the hair, eyes, and skin and ocular mainly affects the eyes. These two types of albinism are very closely related in physical appearance and the visual difficulties as well. He read the characteristics like freckles, pigmented moles, nystagmus, and photophobia, all of which were present in me. Then he asked, "Are there other family members who have the condition?" I said "Yes, but most of them are deceased now." He showed me that there were over 20 or more types of albinism, and that I had inherited a recessive type of albinism passed on from both my parents. For nearly all types of albinism, both parents must carry an albino gene (in order to have a child with the condition). When both parents carry the gene and neither parent has albinism, there is a 1 in 4 chance at each pregnancy that the baby will have some type of albinism. This type of inheritance is known as "autosomal recessive inheritance." Although, many people with albinism do have white hair, color ranges from white to brown depending on the ethnic background. The same is true with the skin and eyes.

A Web site dedicated to providing accurate and positive information about albinism stated that people with albinism have been depicted as being "devil worshippers," curses from God, and evil in movies. The movie that gained the most attention was *Me, Myself & Irene*. This movie made fun of people with albinism. The star of the movie, Jim Carrey, was on *Entertainment Tonight* and said that the movie was made in fun and was not meant to offend anyone. One thing I have learned about having this disorder is that people have a habit of assuming that I don't have a disability because I don't look like it. Society is misinformed about albinism and the visual problems that are present. People do not seem to understand the difference between visually impaired and total blindness.

In the course of a week I shop at Meijer and Kmart, going early in the morning because I discovered that the stores are less crowded and I am able to get more help from the customer service clerks. I ask the clerks to show me where something is in the store. They will respond by saying "if you look down the aisle you will see . . .." I used to respond by acting like I could see what the clerk was talking about. This led to spending a lot of unnecessary time wondering around trying to find things. Now when I go into one of these stores, if I am alone, I immediately start the conversation by saying "I don't see small print well . . . can you show me where the soap is located." When I start this way, I am "clearly" letting the clerks know that I am visually impaired in spite of not looking like it. Second, I ask the clerk to "show me" where the items are and not to tell me or point to the item. Last and most important, I let the clerk know that I need "help."

Living with any disability can be a challenge and often frustrating. I have made several adjustments in my daily life. The form of albinism that I inherited involves a visual disability that causes a reduced visual acuity, nystagmus, sensitivity to glare, and photophobia. Wearing photo chromic lenses over my regular glasses helps to cut down on light and glare. I turn the contrast on my television down darker so that the screen is not bright. My curtains are closed most of the time to block out the sun from the outside. I wear hats when I leave home to keep the brightness out of my eyes. I use a telescope to read distant signs and a small hand-held magnifier for reading labels on items at the store.

My family and friends have played a big role in my vision rehabilitation. They read menus, signs, newspapers, and so on. The fact that I have always been visually impaired and self-sufficient helps. They are also learning to adjust to my vision changes.

Community access like transportation where I live is sometimes unpredictable, and so I depend on family and friends to take me to places where I cannot reach by bus. The bus is often late or breaks down. I realize that others have to depend on the bus, but for me it is not an option. For a sighted person riding the bus, they also have the option of driving a car. The local "curb-to-curb" service is not exactly dependable, but the city has been working on ways to improve the service. The taxi service is the most dependable source of transportation. Local taxis have contracts with agencies to ensure that a blind or visually impaired person has a way to get back and forth to work. Transportation is one of the biggest issues faced by those of us with a disability and more importantly for those of us who are blind or visually impaired. So until the transportation gets better, I will continue to find ways to get around and get help from friends and family.

Sometimes, I think "Why would God allow me go through all this, what could be the purpose?" The purpose is to make a difference in society by using my experiences with albinism to educate others. I believe that my life has been, and will continue to be an example of how easy it is to judge someone based on the outer appearance.

After acceptance comes determination. I chose to go and pursue my goals and aspirations in spite of my disability. If I were to make a positive impact in the lives of others, it had to ultimately begin with me. If I had any hope of reaching my goals, I knew that I would need help. Albinism is a visual disability that qualifies me for services from the state and local government. I was informed that my visual disability was severe enough to receive rehabilitation service and financial assistance. I had an opportunity to work with a rehabilitation counselor who also had albinism. My counselor shared some of her own experiences and situations she had encountered in her life. This helped me because she was empathic and knew how I felt. Over the past 2 years, there were some stumbling blocks that kept me from getting the type of job that I desired. My counselor never gave up and in the end, all the work paid off. It was because of her determination and diligence that allowed me to become self-employed.

In addition to helping me become self-employed, she helped me to obtain low-vision aids, independent living training, keyboarding skills, and computer training for assistive technology. The most important things that happened to me were my level of confidence in my abilities and my self-esteem grew. My counselor helped me to see my "abilities" and not focus so much on the "disability."

A counselor should possess all of the above characteristics: caring, compassionate, patient, understanding, and willing to see the "potential" in a person with a disability and not the disability. A counselor should never assume that they know how it feels to be disabled (unless they are). It is important to make the client a part of their rehabilitation plan. This can be achieved by allowing them to hit and miss, even if the rehab plan has to be changed a few times a year. For example, I was interested in going back to college and pursuing my bachelor's degree. I wanted to go full time but because I also have rheumatoid arthritis, it was recommended that I go part-time. My plan had to be altered to fit my needs several times until we found something that actually worked.

Today, I am happy to say that I enjoy being a respite care provider. In spite of the obstacles that I have had to face in my life, I feel that the experiences that I went through contributed in making me a better person. Here is a passage that I now live by: "God always has more for you today, than what you went through yesterday" (Bishop T. D. Jakes).

DISCUSSION QUESTIONS

1. Discuss anyone's experience with a family member who has a disability and how that has impacted family life in positive and negative ways.
2. Ask students to identify advantages and disadvantages in using a stage model to explain family adjustment to disability.
3. Ask students to identify the traits of resilient families and compare these to their own families.
4. Solicit stories from students with disabilities about personal family experiences or feelings related to family life with a disability.
5. Have students debate the issue of placing a "disruptive" child with a mental illness outside of the home.

EXERCISES

A. For a class activity, have students review their own family characteristics using the 7 family characteristics identified by Power and Dell Orto (2004).
B. Have students make a list of cultural similarities and differences related to dealing with family members with disabilities in the African American, Asian, Caucasian, and Latino cultures.
C. For a homework assignment, have students interview the parent of a child with a disability about the hardships and family growth related to the disability.

SEVEN

Sexuality and Disability

Noreen M. Glover-Graf

OVERVIEW

Sexuality and disability is a topic that has been neglected for a long time by professionals. In their review of the literature, Kazukauskas and Lam (2010) identified the reasons for this neglect: inadequate supports, time constraints, no guiding policies in facilities, lack of training, negative attitudes, and discomfort on the part of counselors. Additionally, they noted recent studies that reported counselors' limited knowledge and discomfort in addressing body and sexual functioning topics such as bowel and bladder functions, body image, sexual acts and behaviors, sexual preference, and reproductive function and choice (Booth, Kendall, Fronek, Miller, & Geraghty, 2003; Haboubi & Lincoln, 2003). Kazukauskas and Lam (2010) contend that rehabilitation counselors may be the only professionals that remain with consumers throughout the process of rehabilitation and are ethically committed to addressing the full range of needs for persons with disabilities so that consumers can become as fully integrated and independent as possible. In order to accomplish this, they must be competent and knowledgeable about issues of sexuality:

... the sheer nature of some sexuality issues (e.g., dysinhibition, sexually inappropriate behavior, social skills issues) necessitates that all rehabilitation professionals regardless of specialization, be able to handle sexuality-related situations that may arise. (Kazukauskas & Lam, 2010, p.16)

Based on their study of 199 certified rehabilitation counselors related to knowledge, attitude, and comfort in addressing the sexuality and disability issues of consumers, the authors recommended enhancing training and education. This chapter focuses on (a) sexuality and related components; (b) disability and intimate relationships; (c) disability type and related sexual issues; (d) sexual orientation, sexual functioning, procreation, and parenting; (e) sex education, sex therapy, and sexual surrogates; and (f) sexual abuse.

SEXUALITY AND RELATED COMPONENTS

Defining Sexuality

Defining sexuality is complex because in involves all the factors that affect how individuals view themselves and behave in relation to their gender. They are influenced by their upbringing, the culture they associate themselves with, and society at large. The World Health Organization states, "The definition of sexuality is complex: it includes gender roles and sexual orientation and is influenced by the interaction of biological, psychological, cognitive, social, political, cultural, ethical, legal, historical, religious and spiritual factors" (World Health Organization, 2010a, p. 4). Daily (1984) views sexuality from a psychological, emotional, and functional perspective and describes sexuality as having five components: identity, intimacy, sensuality, sexualization, and reproductive aspects. *Identity* is the continual process of discovery of who we are in relation to our sexuality, *intimacy* refers to emotional closeness with others, *sensuality* is the experience of our body through our five senses, *sexualization* is the use of the body for the benefits of control, manipulation, and influencing others, and finally, *reproductive aspects* involve the functions of conceiving and child-rearing.

It is important to understand that these components are integrally connected and influenced by society and culture and by the rules set up to govern sexual behaviors, including the selection of a socially acceptable mate. Even though society seems to be allowing for greater flexibility regarding sexuality, it is more aptly described as increased tolerance for those who deviate from the expected norm. While persons who choose homosexual relationships are now considered somewhat socially acceptable, only a few countries, and only a few U.S. states, allow for same-sex marriage; and those that have, seem inclined to repeal their decisions. Hard-fought legal sanctions against discrimination based on race or ethnicity have created tolerance for marriages between persons of differing cultures, but tolerance of sexual relationships and sexual expression for persons with disabilities is yet to be achieved.

Sexual Stigmatization

Vash and Crewe (2004) discuss the historical sexual stigmatization of persons with disabilities as originating from biological and social sanctions that attempted to eliminate what was viewed as a "defective gene pool" because survival was based on physical abilities. As society has progressed, survival is no longer contingent on physical ability. Vash and Crewe (2004, p.85) point to a lessening of "the rejection of disabled mates." This is a far cry from "acceptance," which is apparent to those persons with disabilities seeking mates and may profoundly affect the self-esteem since finding a mate is often regarded as symbolic of one's desirability and worth.

Olkin (1999) discussed sexual myths about people with disabilities (PWDs), noting that much of society views PWDs as lacking sex drive, incapable of sexual performance, and lacking both the social skills and appropriate judgment to be sexually appropriate. Persons without disabilities (PWOD) who partner with PWDs are frequently viewed as either deviant or desperate. As well, a number of myths related to the sexuality of women with disabilities (WWDs) may negatively affect the behavior of individuals in society and the willingness to engage in romantic and intimate relationships with persons with disabilities. Morris (1993) describes some of these from an insider perspective:

> That we are naïve and lead sheltered lives
> That we are asexual or at best sexually inadequate
> That we cannot ovulate, menstruate, conceive or give birth, or have orgasms,
> That if we are not married or in a long-term relationship it is because no one wants us and not through our personal choice to remain single or live alone
> That our only true scale of merit and success is to judge ourselves by the standard of their world
> That we are sweet, deprived little souls who need to be compensated with treats, presents, and praise. (Morris, 1993, p. 16)

The impact of rigid social role expectations on persons with disabilities has been profound. As early as the 1980s the rehabilitation literature has discussed the psychosocial issues related to the stigmatization of WWDs as asexual and dependent. When women are viewed as unable to meet their obligations to have children or nurture children and when they are viewed as unable to be employed, society views them as both roleless and sexless (Danek, 1992; Thurer, 1991).

Social Construction of Gender Identity and Body Image

Clearly, persons with disabilities are deprived of sexual equality despite social advances. In order to further understand this disparity, it is necessary to examine the social construction of gender identity and body image. While gender usually refers to the biological makeup of a person, there is also a strong social component that contributes to how we define sex differences. Our gender expectations, roles, and interactions are also determined by the social distribution of sex-based power and resources (Gentile, 1993).

Gender-based roles influence how individuals think and feel about themselves and others as males and females. For example, in a traditional Northern American household, women are expected to have greater responsibility tending to the household and the children, and men are expected to take on greater responsibility in providing financial support for the family. These roles reinforce the woman as a psychological/emotional caretaker and the man as a physical/financial caretaker. If a woman is physically, psychologically, sensually, or developmentally impaired, how will she clean the house? How will she bath the children? Will she be able to engage in sexual activity with her husband? If a man is impaired, how will he make money to pay the bills? How will he be able to manage house repairs?

While these questions are still relevant today, it is clear that the lines that define the traditional role distribution have become increasingly blurred. It is frequently necessary for both partners to have full-time jobs to support the family, parenting roles and responsibilities are shifting, and there is an increase in single-parent households. Even so, traditional roles and attitudes appear resistant to change because they are deeply ingrained in today's social structure. Questions about being able to meet traditional roles and responsibilities continue to contribute to the reluctance to consider

PWDs as intimate and sexual partners and to recognize and normalize the sexual needs and desires of PWDs.

Sedikides, Oliver, and Campbell (1994) examined gender differences in relation to romantic relationships. In a study of the costs and benefits of romantic relationships, the authors noted that for both males and females, the most important benefits were described as companionship, feeling loved and loving, and happiness. However, females viewed intimacy, self-growth and understanding, and increased self-esteem as more beneficial, and males viewed sexual gratification as more beneficial. Females viewed a loss of identity and innocence as a greater cost and males viewed monetary loss as more consequential. In other words, females continued to believe they would be emotional caretakers at the risk of losing their identity and males continued to believe that they were less intimate and more responsible financially.

Impact of Gender-Based Values and Social Roles on People With Disabilities

In our society, even our values tend to have either a masculine or feminine orientation. For example, assertiveness is associated with males and compassion with females. Interestingly, many of the values that guide rehabilitation professionals are masculine based rather than feminine based. For example, Burns (1993) noted that independence is a masculine-oriented goal, whereas interdependence and the importance of relationships tend to be a feminine orientation. Yet, most rehabilitation counselors are quick to vocalize the importance of the greatest amount of independence possible as the ultimate outcome goal. This lack of taking gender into account can pose difficulties for consumers who have a strong female orientation. While *interdependence* is still not a focus of rehabilitation, some agencies have begun to write policy that reflects as much independence *as desired* by the consumer. In New York, the Vocational and Educational Services with Disabilities (VESID) Web site lists: "One major goal of the vocational rehabilitation process is to foster the greatest degree of independence and responsibility, as desired by an individual." (VESID, 2011, para. 3). While still not an acknowledgment of the feminine perspective as equally viable, it leaves open the possibility of accommodating potential gender differences.

Burns (1993) noted that in terms of sexuality, treatment discrepancies are apparent. For example, when male consumers exhibit inappropriate behaviors, they are more likely to be viewed as behaving "badly." Similar inappropriate behaviors from female consumers will be considered as "psychological problems." Similarly, Scotti, Evans, Meyer, and Walker (1991) noted that women are more likely to be punished or medicated for equivalent sexual behaviors that may be ignored or rationalized when exhibited by male clients. Clearly, much needs to be done to create equality in treatment that gives consideration to issues of gender in terms of values, expectations, and desires of consumers.

Self-Esteem and Body Image

The effect of social messages about sexual roles and expectations is profound. Messages from society, treatment professionals, caretakers, and the portrayal of sexuality by the media have had great impact on how PWDs feel about their bodies and themselves. The fact that beauty is socially dictated is historically evident. From the painting of Rubin, when larger sizes were an indication of beauty and prosperity, to the fashion photography of the present, where there have been recent bans against using severely underweight models in advertisements, there is always a clear message from society regarding physical beauty and sexual desirability.

Today the average person in the United States is exposed to 5,000 advertisements a day (Aufreiter, Elzinga, & Gordon, 2003). Billions of dollars are spent on making the body fit into whatever socially constructed image of beauty is currently accepted. People subject themselves to endless diets. They have surgeries to alter the face, to add and subtract from breasts, hips, and stomach size and shape, and recently, surgeries to increase height that involves cutting and lengthening of leg bones. They have injections to reduce lines on the face, have hair transplants, and spend billions of dollars on products that claim to make them appear younger. All this is for the sake of conforming to socially imposed standards that people hope will render them attractive to others and therefore more desirable and ultimately more lovable. What is the message in all this to persons with physical deformities, with losses of limbs or other body parts, and for those who need mobility aids?

In a study of sexual identity, body image, and life satisfaction among 134 women with and without physical disabilities, Moin, Duvdevany, and Mazor (2009) noted similar sexual desires and needs, but differences in lower levels of body image, sexual self-esteem, and sexual and life satisfaction for WWDs when compared with women without disabilities (WWODs). These differences were even more apparent in younger women. The study also found that about one-third of the WWDs did report sexual satisfaction, and that sexual satisfaction was also found to be strongly correlated to life satisfaction.

When physical appearance is altered as a result of disability, the body falls further away from the expectations of society and body image, and the attitude one has toward the physical self may decline and affect self-esteem. A low self-esteem affects a person's willingness and confidence to engage in social activities and to engage in relationships with others. Lack of socialization can further contribute to a person's isolation, lower quality of life, and lack of self-confidence to the point that the possibility of rejection appears so great that it may no longer seem worth the risk. Persons with physical anomalies may fear that others will laugh at them, reject them, or come to think of them as deviant. Even more than the body, the face plays an important role in a person's self-image and self-identity and is distinctly different from that of the rest of the body.

Callahan theorized that each body part holds a symbolic meaning as well as functional use; arms symbolize strength, hands symbolize creativity and the ability to provide, legs represent speed and vitality, and reproductive organs indicate pleasure, intimacy, and procreation. In her examination of facial disfigurement (one's self-presentation to others) in persons with head and neck cancer, Callahan described the "profound psychological trauma" (Callahan, 2004, p. 73) that can occur in terms of one's body integrity and sense of self. Similarly, 60 years ago, in reviewing psychosocial problems associated with facial deformities, MacGregor concluded that coupled with the adjustment problems of the person and societal negative attitudes, prejudice, and discrimination: "Wherever plastic surgery can correct or improve the facial injury or congenital malformation, it should be undertaken as early as possible in order to avoid not only the obvious disadvantages, but to prevent deep psychological wounds which may be incurred but not so easily eliminated." (MacGregor, 1951, p. 638).

In brief, accepting and loving one's body as it is in a society that does not endorse or support such a notion is challenging. A number of practices can assist in increasing body image, but much of it relies more on changing one's thinking more so than one's body, refusing to accept the media-portrayed image of the beautiful man or woman and giving up the practice of comparing oneself with those photo-altered images of often emaciated women or muscle-bound men. Yuen and Hanson (2002) concluded that physical activity could increase body image for persons with acquired mobility impairments. In their study, persons who were physically active evaluated both their physical appearance and their health as more positive; they showed more concern about their physical fitness and were more satisfied with their bodies than those with mobility impairment who were not active.

A number of studies also suggest that attention to making oneself as attractive as possible has positive affects on self-image and physical appearance for PWDs Kammerer-Quayle (2002). Elks noted that physical attractiveness has been shown to affect:

> ... heterosexual dating, peer acceptance, teacher behavior, attitude change, employment interviews, and jury decisions, and that attractive people are less likely to be judged to be mentally ill, are liked and helped more, and judged to have higher social skills and greater opportunities for social interaction than unattractive people. (Elks, 1990, p. 36)

A recent controversy over cosmetic surgery for children with Down syndrome (DS) brought to light the ethical dilemmas involved in such a practice when in 2008 the parents of a child with DS subjected the 5-year-old to a number of surgeries on the tongue, eyes, and ears to correct the facial indicators of DS. As parents, they sought to eliminate the future stigmatization their child would face, but a number of bioethicists argued that it was an unnecessary and elective surgery that should have waited for the child to reach the age of consent (Fox News, 2008). Adult protective services have also expressed concerns related to a growing increase in cosmetic surgery for persons with intellectual disabilities (Cambridge, 2002), and a number of cases have come before hospital ethics boards weighing the value of enhancement and restorative procedures in adults and children (Opel & Wilfond, 2009). The National Down Syndrome Society (NDSS, 2011) acknowledges cosmetic surgery for children with DS as a personal choice of parents but does not encourage cosmetic surgery, stating that:

> The goal of inclusion and acceptance is mutual respect based on who we are as individuals, not how we look. Altering a child's appearance as a means of encouraging acceptance does not change the reality of the disability. In fact, some education experts believe that the physical characteristics of Down syndrome may

offer visual cues to people about an individual's disability and thus foster an easier acceptance and understanding of that disability. Many families believe that to alter their child's facial features would be to disrespect his or her individuality and that an important part of that individuality is the condition of Down syndrome. (NDSS, para. 3)

For rehabilitation counselors, simply ignoring the importance of physical appearance or waiting for adjustment to occur is not appropriate, because appearance is clearly tied to how people feel about themselves and interact with others. Kleve, Rumsey, Wyn-Williams, and White (2002) demonstrated the importance of social supports and interactions in positive adjustment to disfigurement. But, interaction may depend on self-esteem, and self-esteem may be tied to body image. Thus, attention to physical appearance may need to move beyond basic hygiene concerns to application of cosmetics and, in some cases, cosmetic surgery. These considerations have historically been extended to persons with disabilities only on a limited basis, such as for those with facial burns. However, a person's level of adjustment to having an apparent physical difference also needs to be taken into consideration because those with poor adjustment may demonstrate feelings of depression, social avoidance and anxiety, fear of being evaluated negatively by others, and shame. Demographic variables, including age and sex, can also influence adjustment to physical differences. Overall, women reporting more difficulty than men with visible physical differences, and late adolescents and young adults also typically have greater concern for visible differences. Even hidden physical differences can interfere with adjustment because if the physical differences are typically concealed, distress may also be high due to fear of others finding out, suggesting that the secrecy and anticipated discovery by others can also increase distress (Moss & Rosser, 2008).

DISABILITY AND INTIMATE RELATIONSHIPS

Partnering Desires and People With Disabilities

In 1943, Abraham Maslow identified basic human needs as love, affection, and belonging that encompass both the need to love and the need to feel loved in order to overcome loneliness and feelings of alienation. While recognizing the need for love, Vash and Crewe (2004) discussed pairing as a part of a preprogrammed biological drive that is reinforced, if not required, by society. The state of being without a partner is viewed by society as an indication of one's inferior status, bringing humiliation and disgrace to the individual. The proof of one's worth often comes with the acquisition of a partner. Clearly, much of today's values are embedded in past survival needs that are no longer relevant; a time when a lack of medical sophistication led to numerous infant deaths and death of mothers during childbirth. Because successful procreation was far more contingent upon physical makeup, people with disabilities were generally excluded from consideration as life partners and dismissed as sexually responsive or desirable. Changes in survival rates and medical advances appear to have little effect on some attitudes as persons who do become partners of PWDs are frequently seen as being less intelligent, and less sociable, than partners of PWODs (Goldstein & Johnson, 1997).

People with disabilities are not excluded from experiencing partnering desires or, unfortunately, from the messages imposed by society. They look to attract partners for reasons of love, intimacy, and security, yet it is difficult to see role models with disabilities represented as sexually and physically attractive. For some persons with disabilities, values of physical beauty will become less meaningful to the fulfillment of their lives, yet the importance of relationships and pairing will not necessarily diminish (Wright, 1960). Vash and Crewe (2004) note that, like PWODs, not all PWDs will be interested in pairing or having children, but for most people partnering is a strong urge. Not only will they need to deal with the devices that indicate disability, such as wheelchairs, canes, and so on, which may cause people to reject them, but they will also need to overcome the negative or dismissive attitudes of others.

Attitudes of PWODs

Perhaps the greatest barrier to partnering is the attitudes of PWODs. A few studies have looked at how attractive PWODs will find PWDs (Man, Rojahn, Chrosniak, & Sanford, 2006; Marini, Feist, Chen, Torres-Flores, & Del Castillo, in review; Miller, Chen, Glover-Graf, & Kranz, 2009). Rojahn, Komelasky, and Man (2008) found that college students reported similar romantic attractiveness to people with and without disabilities but noted a clear preference shown for physical health, suggesting a disconnection between the explicit ratings and implicit attitudes. A number of researchers have also investigated attitudes toward having relationships with PWDs (Howland & Rintala, 2001; Kreuter, 2000; Snead & Davis, 2002; Wada et al., 2004). Wong, Chan, Da Silva Cardoso, Lam, and Miller (2004) concluded that the type and severity of the disability are major determinants in the choice to become involved with a person with a disability. Miller et al. (2009) found that college students were willing to have friendships and acquaintanceships with PWDs, and also willing to date PWDs; however, they were least willing to marry or have a partnership with PWDs, especially with those having severe disability. Additionally, PWODs were more willing to become involved with persons with physical disabilities and least willing to engage with persons with psychological disabilities.

The Impact of Type of Disability

Antonak (1981) noted a hierarchy of stigma attached to disability; those with physical disabilities receive the least social stigma, and those with psychiatric disabilities receive the greatest stigma. Gordon, Chariboga-Tantillo, Feldman, and Perrone (2004) assessed attitudes regarding friendship and marital relationships with PWDs and concluded that the majority of students were more willing to be friends with persons with medical, physical, and sensory impairments, but were less inclined to want friendships with persons with mental retardation and psychiatric illness; only 13% stated that they would marry someone with a psychiatric illness and 4% with mental retardation. In their study, Miller et al. (2009) found that college students were the least willing to marry or have a partnership with persons with cognitive or psychiatric disabilities.

The Impact of Severity of Disability

Taleporos and McCabe (2003) found that people who reported greater severity of disabilities as measured by level of independent functioning were less likely to have partners or to be married than those with less severe disabilities. Individuals with the most severe disabilities were also less likely to have partners and were less likely to be married than persons with less severe or no disabilities. Similarly, Miller et al. (2009) determined that the more severe the disability, the less willing PWODs was to engage in a relationship. While this finding is expected and distressing, they also found that the personal attributes of intelligence, kindness, and humor in PWDs were the most likely to overcome intimacy reluctance on the part of PWODs by increasing their reported willingness to enter into more intimate relationships with PWDs.

While not often seen in the rehabilitation literature, Vash and Crewe (2004, p. 97) noted that some persons are sexually attracted to amputees. While they term this as "unwholesome turns," they also note that there is some discussion regarding if such an attraction "empowers or exploits people with disabilities" (Vash & Crewe, 2004, p. 98). The notion of rejecting society's repulsion of a stump is powerful. Terming such an attraction as "sick" plays into the ever-present insistence that beauty is regulated by society. If, however, there is coercion, manipulation, or force used in the satisfaction of one person's desires, the health of the fantasy is a moot point because abuse is in place. In a 1998-documentary titled *My One-Legged Dream Lover*, Kath Duncan explores amputee fetishism (Duncan & Goggin, 2002) as having a limited number of researchers (Dixon, 1983; Kafer, 2000). The Web site ASCOT-World (http://www.ascotworld.com) is a disability and amputee support group and social club that contains a matchmaking online service that welcomes devotees (the term used for nondisabled persons who are attracted to persons with amputations).

The Impact of Types of Relationships

For a number of reasons, PWDs often have more difficulty forming friendships and finding partners for romantic relationships than people without disabilities (De Loach, 1994; Goldstein & Johnson, 1997; Howland & Rintala, 2001; Rintala et al., 1997). One reason revolves around the process of obtaining a mate, which generally progresses from an acquaintance relationship to friendship, courtship, romance, and finally to a long-term commitment. While most people seem willing to acknowledge and interact with people with disabilities on an acquaintance level, some studies have shown that many people are less willing to progress to dating and marriage.

A few studies have examined the attitudes of persons without disabilities in relation to engaging in intimate relationships with persons with disabilities. These studies have concluded that persons with disabilities may have difficulty making friends, forming romantic relationships, and finding partners. For the most part, these are discouraging in that PWODs express a willingness to have casual relationships but are less willing to date or marry PWDs (Miller et al., 2009).

In a survey of 1,013 students, Hergenrather and Rhodes (2007) found that females held more positive attitudes toward dating and marrying PWDs than did males. Measuring attitudes is important; however, attitudes do not necessarily translate into action. Despite more reported positive attitudes among females without disabilities, males with disabilities reported that WWODs were only interested in friendships. Likewise, WWDs believed that men made judgments not to date them based on devices such as wheelchairs and prosthetic devices.

Fear and discomfort may also play a role in persons decisions related to intimacy with PWDs. Milligan and Neufeldt (1998) found that women were more willing to date men with spinal cord injury (SCI) if they had previously been in relationships with PWDs, suggesting that initial discomfort may be overcome with exposure. Another important factor in this study was the level of independence and adjustment of the male as being relevant to female willingness to consider partnering; those perceived as more adjusted were more desirable partners. Thus, not only does the person without a disability need to work through discomfort and uncertainty, but the person with a disability is more desirable if viewed as adjusted and more self-sufficient. In this study, other concerns of females about dating persons with SCI were reported as care giving, health concerns, restriction of activities and physical limitations, financial issues, and sexuality/conception issues.

Similarly, in a study examining the attitudes of 395 college students, Marini et al. (in press) found that 66% of students surveyed indicated that they would not have a problem dating someone in a wheelchair after having seen a photograph and reading a brief bio of the individual. Of the 33% who indicated that they would not be willing to become intimately involved with people in wheelchairs, the top-rated reasons included the perception of caretaking as being too much work, feeling awkward in not knowing what to say or how to treat them, believing the person would be sick too often, and believing that the PWDs could not be sexually satisfying. Those students who had had a previous close relationship with someone with a disability, however, were more likely to be open to having a more intimate relationship. The authors concluded that students with a past close disability relationship, could separate societal myth and misconceptions regarding wheelchair users.

For many people, a committed and loving marriage is the ultimate goal. The ability of a relationship to withstand challenges will depend on the particular strengths of the couple both individually and as a pair. Couples who enter a relationship where disability is already a factor do so with at least some anticipation of the potential challenges they will face. However, when disability occurs after the establishment of a relationship, greater difficulties have statistically been supported, and divorce is more likely to occur (DeVivo & Richards, 1996).

Kreuter (2000) examined the relationships of 49 persons with SCI and concluded that those who were injured before the marriage had more stable marriages than those injured after marriage. Similarly, sexual satisfaction was reported as greater among couples where the marriage is postdisability (Crewe & Krause, 1988). In predisability marriage, when one partner became the caregiver of the other, there was a negative impact on the relationship; and, when the partner with the disability was female, there was a greater likelihood of divorce. Overall, divorce statistics for people with disabilities are high, and there is a lower rate of marriage among this population (DeVivo, Hawkins, Richards, & Go, 1995; Urey & Henggeler, 1987). DeVivo et al. (1995)

examined over 600 recorded marriages among persons with spinal cord injury and found almost twice as many divorces as would be expected among nondisabled persons of the same age and gender.

DISABILITY TYPE AND SEXUAL ISSUES AND CONCERNS

Sexuality and Physical Disabilities

In a study to examine sexuality and quality of life, McCabe, Cummins, and Deeks (2000) reported that persons with congenital physical disabilities had low levels of sexual experience and knowledge and had negative feelings related to sexuality, but they had high sexual needs and desired to increase their sexual knowledge. In terms of sexual experiences, 12% had never romantically kissed or hugged anyone, nearly 30% had never held someone while naked, almost 40% had never engaged in sexual intercourse, and 60% were not currently having intercourse in a relationship. Their study determined that while sexuality was associated with quality of life, it was not associated with life satisfaction, making the point that, at least for their sample, sexuality and sexual experiences add an important and desired dimension to life but are not necessary for achieving satisfaction in life.

Shakespeare (2000) noted the social and financial difficulties related to establishing a sexual relationship as follows:

> It also helps to have someone to have sex with. Most people meet potential partners at college, at work, or in social spaces. Unfortunately, disabled people often don't get to go to college, or to work, or achieve access to public spaces because of physical and social barriers. Being sexual costs money. You need to buy clothes, to feel good about, and go places to feel good in. If you are poor, as 50% of disabled Americans are, then it is correspondingly harder to be sexual. More than money, being sexual demands self-esteem. It demands confidence, and the ability to communicate . . . . (Shakespeare, 2000, p. 161)

Taleporos, Dip, and McCabe (2002) point to the positive connection between sexuality variables and psychological well-being. In a study of 748 PWDs and 448 PWODs, they found that persons with higher self-esteem were more likely to be sexually satisfied and feel good about their bodies and their sexuality. However, because WWDs are frequently viewed as asexual (Di Giulio, 2003), little attention has been paid to their sexual functioning, creating barriers to sexual fulfillment faced by women. Stinson, Christian, and Dotson (2002) found that due to negative stereotypes, women with developmental disabilities lacked access to gynecological health care, were given limited choices regarding reproductive issues, and had a lack of sex education. In addition, several social, psychological, and physical barriers prevent women from sexual expression and functioning (Christian, Stinson, & Dotson, 2001; Westgren & Levi, 1999).

Vash and Crewe (2004) point to a number of physical issues related to sexual activity, including the effects of paralysis, pain, amputations, neurological impairments, and bowel and bladder dysfunction upon the ability to experience erotic sensation. In a study of 504 WWDs and 442 WWODs, to compare sexual experiences, Nosek, Howland, Rintala, Young, and Chanpong (1997) reported that women with physical disabilities did not differ from WWOD in sexual desire but they did find significantly lower levels of sexual activity, satisfaction, and response. The level of sexual activity among WWDs was predicted by living with a significantly positive attitude. Women who had a more positive self-image and viewed themselves as approachable reported higher sexual activity. Interestingly, the severity of their disability was not a factor in the level of sexual activity. Factors related to positive sexual response included having a positive attitude toward using assistive devices, higher income level, and less stereotypical concern. Greater sexual satisfaction was predicted by sexual activity and a more positive attitude about assistive devices.

Problems related to sexual functioning after SCI are reported as arousal, frequency of sexual activity, initiation, and enjoyment (Klebine, 2007; Kreuter, Sullivan, & Siosteen, 1994). Two interesting qualitative studies conducted by Whipple, Richards, Tepper, and Komisaruk (1996) and Richards, Tepper, Whipple, and Komisaruk (1997) reported that women with SCI initially dissociate themselves from their sexuality, believing that they can no longer experience sexual pleasure. Over time they may become ready to reintegrate sexuality into their lives. Men with SCI are more likely to report limited opportunity for sexual expression and are often unsatisfied with their sexual lives.

In a study to examine issues that negatively impact sexuality for men with SCI, Sakellarious (2006) identified the topics of *dependency, spread, body beautiful, social disapproval, personal assistance, and impairment* as barriers. Participants revealed that the frustration that comes from societal views of independence is more closely related to body performance rather than self-direction. Participants stated that others were more likely to see the wheelchair than the person in it. Like women, participants believed that they were being held to a standard of the socially prescribed beautiful body, which they could not attain, leading to "aesthetic anxiety." Practically, the need for a personal assistant was also noted as a barrier to sexual expression because privacy was limited in that attendants needed to undress, empty the bladder, and position the individual for them to participate in sexual activity. Physical impairment of bodily sensation also was noted as a barrier for some as were financial resources and environmental barriers that limited accessibility.

Sexual Concerns and Learning Disability

Concerns related to the sexual function of persons with developmental disabilities differ greatly from those related to people with physical challenges and are frequently based on the capacity of the person to understand sexual functioning in terms of consequences and the rights of others. Szollos and McCabe (1995) noted that persons with intellectual disabilities frequently have misinformation related to sexual functioning. Staff members who care for persons with learning disabilities frequently experience discomfort with the sexual expression of such individuals. Double standards are commonplace in the beliefs related to sexuality and persons with learning disabilities. One study, for example, found that even persons opposed to abortion on moral grounds believe that it should be made available if the woman has a learning disability. Staff members were also found to frequently rely on personal judgments rather than facility policies when they felt a need to address sexual behaviors by residents. Many times this led to the cessation of normal sexual expression and interaction. At other times, staff members tolerated inappropriate behaviors or sexual harassment rather than deal appropriately with these behaviors (Parkes, 2006).

There are also concerns related to the sexual abuse of others that appears to occur with greater frequency among this population than the general population (Brown & Stein, 1997). In a study of mild and moderate learning disabilities to investigate how women experience their sexual lives, McCarthy (1998) reported that these women commonly find themselves engaged in sexual activity that is not to their liking and not of their choice and point to lack of preparation of social service providers on how to deal with behaviors and events related to sexual abuse by and to people with developmental impairments (Brown & Turk, 1992; Brown, Hunt, & Stein, 1994).

Men with learning disabilities may present caregivers with a number of challenging behaviors, including the use of pornographic material, cross-dressing, prostitution, and pedophile tendencies. When looking at the sexual encounters of men and women with learning disabilities, it is interesting to note that women without learning disabilities do not engage in sexual contact with learning-disabled men, but men without disabilities do engage in sexual activity with both men and women with learning disabilities. Pornography is often gained through those sexual encounters and intended to create sexual vulnerability. Cross-dressing is problematic when theft of women's clothing takes place, when embarrassment or ridicule results, or when it results in abuse of the PWDs. Prostitution also renders men, like WWDs, vulnerable to sexual assault, sexually transmitted diseases, and exploitation. Men with disabilities may be offered goods and money for sex in public parks and toilets. Whereas WWDs tend to be at greater exploitation risk in treatment facilities, men are at greater risk in public areas. This type of exposure may lead to sadomasochistic sexual activities that can be adopted by the PWDs and then perpetrated on others. Finally, there is concern that men with learning disabilities may have pedophile tendencies. Generally, while this may be an accurate representation of some males with developmental disabilities (DD), behaviors that indicate sexual interest in children seem to indicate developmental immaturity, identifying and relating to children may be due to the neglect of their sexuality (Cambridge & Mellan, 2000).

Sexuality and Cognitive Disabilities

Cognitive impairments, such as those that occur as a result of a cerebral vascular accident (stroke) or a traumatic brain injury (TBI), can include physical impairments but typically include behavioral, emotional, and intellectual problems. According to the Center for Disease Control, there are about 1.5 million TBIs per year, and most occur in young males with 85% occurring before the age of 25. Sexual dysfunction following brain injury is common and may include impotence, lack of ability to ejaculate, premature ejaculation, loss of sensation, and diminished sexual libido, body image and sexual identity problems, decreased self-esteem, disturbing exhibitionist behaviors, sexual preoccupation, and masturbation (Ducharme, n.d.; Ducharme & Gill, 1990; O'Carroll, Woodrow, & Maroun, 1991).

Because the ability to regulate behaviors is diminished in persons with head injury, other behaviors may also emerge that are detrimental to satisfying sexual experiences. For example, persons with head injuries may be distracted during sexual activity, may talk incessantly or aimlessly, or may experience fatigue and confusion. Emotionally, persons with TBI may be lacking in emotional connection or sensitivity toward their partners and may exhibit self-centered behaviors, showing little regard for their partners' needs or desires. Treatment for sexual and other behavioral problems includes medications and behavioral therapy (Ducharme, n.d.).

Sexual Concerns and Psychiatric Illness

Intimate relationships among persons with serious mental illness differ from people in the general population in that there is generally less intimacy and less commitment in these relationships. They tend to have sex sooner and the relationships are for a shorter term. They are also more likely to have concurrent sexual relationships and report being less sexually satisfied in their sexual encounters (Perry & Wright, 2006). Of all the types of disability, psychiatric disabilities are the most stigmatized, and that contributes, along with lower income and less social opportunities, to these persons pairing with other persons who are also less socially accepted. According to Perry and White (2006),

> People with serious mental illness are often forced to try to meet their sexual needs or forge a relationship with other "social undesirables." In short they seem to take what they can get in terms of where, when, and with whom to have sex. This not only results in relationships that are less satisfying, less intimate, and much shorter lived, but also increases HIV risk by concentrating sexual activity within high-risk populations like IV drug users, sex workers, and others with serious mental illness. (Perry & Wright, 2006, p. 180)

In general, people with mental illness do not use safe sex practices, report lack of satisfaction with their sexual and social lives, and lack a sense of intimacy in relationships. Consumers who live in residential care settings also lack privacy. A number of barriers exist to fulfilling sexual activity in residential settings, including policies that require shared rooms, no sexual activity, frequent histories of sexual abuse, social stigmatization, and low self-esteem, medications that interfere with desire and function, intrusive symptoms, social skill deficits, and a lack of support and education related to sexual expression and activity (Cook, 2000).

In an overview of sexuality and psychiatric disabilities, Knoepfler discusses differences in sexual functioning, noting that persons with depression are likely to show little sexual desire, as opposed to persons with manic disorders who may exhibit rapid transitions in desire and rapid escalation. Knoepfler states that persons with personality disorders are varied but "tend to act in impulsive ways disregarding consequences" (Knoepfler, 1991, p. 214) and that persons with schizophrenia, who experience an inability to distinguish between fantasy and reality, may imagine or engage in bizarre sexual behaviors (Knoepfler, 1991). As there are different types of schizophrenia, this characterization is likely true for only a small portion of individuals with the disorder; however, one contribution of this work is that it makes clear that it is important to consider the effects of specific diagnoses on sexuality to avoid the trap of stereotyping individuals in terms of sexual needs, desires, and behaviors.

In a study specific to understanding sexuality among persons with schizophrenia, Volman and Landeen (2007) studied five women and five men with schizophrenia. They found that participants did form and maintain intimate relationships. They viewed their sexuality as one of the factors that made them the same as persons without mental illness. They considered their sexuality as part of their well-being and essential in their lives. Sexuality was viewed as physical and emotional and more meaningful when sex was within the context of an intimate relationship. However, all the participants felt that the symptoms of their illnesses and effects of the medications had a strong impact on their sexuality and compromised their view of themselves, sexual functioning, and ability to have intimate relationships. They noted problems with hearing voices, weight gain, difficulty with achieving orgasm, and decline in libido. Participants also discussed the effects of social stigma that resulted in being judged and rejected, delaying the age of sexual knowledge and experience until much later in life. Finally, strategies that helped participants were identified as using counseling, medical compliance, positive self-talk, and engaging in a healthy lifestyle. However, talking about sex was identified as causing shame and embarrassment, often leading to not bringing up important concerns with clinicians.

Sexual Concerns and Chronic Health Conditions

For persons with chronic health conditions, physical limitations and pain as well as emotional state may affect sexuality. Persons need to be able to communicate changes in sexuality, including interest, a need for different types of sexual stimulation, and altered positioning and activities. Body pain may have a direct influence on sexual activity and persons may need to make adjustments, such as interrupting sexual activity multiple times to deal with pain or wait for it to subside. This may lead to avoidance of sex with a partner and feelings of grief over the loss and fear of impotency. Partners may feel unloved, angry, and resentful. They may also feel guilty for diminished empathy and causing pain to their partners. Pain management, sexual preferences, and alternatives that take into account religious, cultural, and personal beliefs may be assistive, along with couple's therapy (Claiborne & Rizzo, 2006).

Other chronic health conditions are HIV and AIDS. For this population, most of the literature focuses on the prevention of infecting others through abstinence or the use of condoms. In a study of over 2000 men who had sex with men, 40% were found to engage in unprotected anal sex with a person of unknown HIV status (Golden, Brewer, Kurth, Holmes, & Handsfield, 2004). While much of the sexuality literature for persons with other disabilities focuses on assisting persons engage in healthy sexual behaviors, little is written for persons who are HIV positive. Not only do they need to focus on not infecting others but also they must protect themselves from acquiring new strains of the virus or other sexually transmitted diseases (STDs), placing them at greater health risk. In addition, persons who are HIV positive will have concerns related to telling partners, anger if they believe their partners transmitted the disease to them, and fear or guilt if they have transmitted the disease to their partners (HIV InSite, 2005). For women who are HIV positive and become pregnant, the risk of the child contracting HIV is about 25% if precautions are taken and considerably less with appropriate use of medication. Because vaginal delivery and breastfeeding increase the risk of contraction, these are avoided for HIV-positive women. Couples who wish to have biological children risk infection of one another (if one partner is not seropositive) and the child. The risk may be reduced by minimizing the number of unprotected sexual interactions through only engaging in unprotected sex at the point of ovulation. Another method is to use intrauterine insemination after washing the sperm free of HIV (Gilling-Smith, 2000).

SEXUAL ORIENTATION, SEXUAL FUNCTIONING, PROCREATION, AND PARENTING

Sexual Orientation and People With Disabilities

Kline (1991) referred to sexual orientation as encompassing heterosexual, bisexual, and homosexual relations. Also, there are persons who do not engage in sexual activity who are referred to as nonsexual, and persons who have a lack of any sexual orientation referred to as asexual. Kline also distinguishes sexual orientation from gender identity that includes a psychological self-connection to a gender, to both genders, or to neither. *Transgendered* refers to persons who identify with the opposite gender. *Transsexuals* have received sexual reassignment procedures to physically change their biological identity and *transvestites* utilize clothing and makeup to identify with the opposite gender.

Homosexual and bisexual preference in the general population vary from 2% to 13%, with more males than females reporting homosexuality, but few studies have examined the sexual orientation of persons with disabilities, including one study by Axtell (1999) that interviewed bisexual and lesbian women and their partners who had disabilities. Nosek et al. (1997) examined sexual orientation of women with physical disabilities and found that 87% of the women with SCI were attracted to men, 4% were attracted to women, 7% to both men and women, and 2%t were not attracted to either gender. McCabe, Cummins, and Deeks (2000) found that 16% of their sample of persons with disabilities reported at least one same-sex experience and about 5% reported frequent same-sex activity.

Sexual Functioning

Overall, sexual functioning is important to PWDs, but sexual dysfunction is far more prevalent. In a study of 681 persons with SCI, return to sexual functioning was listed as the top personal priority for persons with paraplegia. It was the second priority for persons with tetraplegia, with only the desire for recovery of arm or hand function superseding sexual recovery desire (Anderson, 2004). For women with SCI, Jackson and Wadley (1999) found an overall substantial decrease in sexual activity following injury. However, over time, participation increased from 49% 1 year after injury to 76% after 10 years.

Sexual dysfunction among couples in the general population is about 13% compared with 40% of persons with chronic diseases and 73% for persons with Multiple Sclerosis (MS) (Zorzon et al., 1999). Sexual functioning for most WWDs is generally not physiologically impaired, but depending on the type and extent of the disability, a number of concerns may need attention. For women with injury in the spinal cord, sexual dysfunction is most often related to a lack of desire to engage in sexual activity and may be more of an emotional and psychological problem than a physiological one. Initial concerns may be related to sexual satisfaction, exploration, and arousal. Individuals and couples may or may not need to try different methods for achieving sexual pleasures. Sexual arousal is both an emotional and physical response that may occur through any of the senses. Arousal can be achieved through the stimulation of any body part, including not only the clitoris and vagina but also breasts, mouth, ears, and feet. A willingness to explore options and discuss body pleasure and sensations will be mutually beneficial.

A number of physiological issues are also of concern for women with SCI, including bladder management, bowel management, autonomic dysreflexia (AD), and spastic hypertonia. Bladder and bowel accidents can be minimized or avoided through management of food and fluid intake and establishing a consistent routine for emptying the bladder and bowel. For women with catheterization, the bladder can be emptied prior to sexual activity. Depending on the type of catheter, the catheter can be removed or partially removed and the tubing may be fastened down with tape to avoid kinking or accidental removal. Autonomic dysreflexia (AD) is a life-threatening condition that may be of concern for individuals with SCI. While laboratory studies have not shown AD to be induced by sexual activity, an onset of multiple symptoms (rise in blood pressure, irregular heart beat, fever, face flushing, chills, headaches, blurred vision, nasal congestion, and sweating) would require ceasing sexual activity and seeking medical assistance or advice (Spinal Cord Injury Information Network, 2007).

Males with SCI experience both emotional and physiological changes associated with their sexuality and sexual performance. In the general population, men experience psychogenic erection due to psychological arousal (sexual thoughts or visual or auditory stimuli) and reflex erections due to physical contact. For men with SCI, depending on the level and completeness of injury, impairment may occur to one or both of these functions. Men with low-level injuries may retain psychogenic arousal, but higher-level injuries will result in impairment of this function. However, most men with SCI can achieve reflex erections (unless the S2–S4 nerve pathways are damaged). Also, erectile dysfunction (ED) is not uncommon among men with SCI in that they may not be able to sustain an erection that is sufficient to meet couples' desires. ED can be treated through medication or a variety of alternative treatments. Oral medication consists of phosphodiesterase inhibitors, such as Viagra[®] (sildenafil) or Cialis[®] (tadalafil), that increase blood flow into the penis. Risks of engaging in sex can include priapism (prolonged erection) that can be very painful because the blood fails to drain from the penis and can lead to permanent damage to the ability to have erections and any onset of symptoms must be medically attended to immediately. Alternative treatments include injections directly into the side of the penis that produce erections that last several hours, placement of a pellet into the urethra (Medicated Urethral System Erection (MUSE), and the use of a hand- or battery-operated cylinder vacuum pump that pulls blood into the penis that is then constricted with a band. (Spinal Cord Injury Information Network, 2007) A number of sex and masturbation products are available through Disabilities-R-Us (http://disabilities-r-us.com), a support and resource Web site created by PWDs. Another type of assistive treatment involves surgical implantation of a penile prosthesis of variable firmnesses or inflatable devices.

Similar physiological concerns (altered libido, bladder and bowel dysfunction, and spasticity) are present for persons with MS that has an onset between 20 and 40 years of age and is twice as common in women as in men (van den Noort & Holland, 1999). For women, decreased vaginal lubrication, impaired ability to masturbate, genital numbness, fatigue, depression, and decreased self-esteem are also of concern (Foley & Sanders, 1997); physical symptoms may be reduced through the use of vibrators, lubricants, and medication to reduce nerve pain. Christopherson, Moore, Foley, and Warren (2006) reported that educational materials are also beneficial in diminishing sexual difficulties for partners but recommend additional counseling for relaxation and positioning as well as dealing with pain and depression. For all persons with neurological impairments, body mapping may be a useful technique because it involves discovery and mapping of the body parts that receive sensory pleasure, those that involve discomfort, and those that are neutral. This mapping identifies body areas that experience arousal and those that need to be avoided or protected (Matthews, 2009).

Fertility

Fertility issues for men deal primarily with issues of achieving ejaculation and collecting healthy sperm. Because the quality of sperm generally declines following SCI, the collection of sperm within a week of the injury may prove important for men who wish to father biological children. After that time sperm, quality may not be sufficient for the production of children. Additionally, most men with SCI are unable to reach ejaculation, and the collection of sperm may need to be assisted through the use of penile vibratory stimulation (PVS), which utilizes a vibrator designed to provoke ejaculation. Semen is collected and processed in a medical setting to reduce the risk of AD. Other methods of collecting semen include electroejaculation, which applies electrical stimulation through the anus and induces the release of semen, prostrate massage, which applies pressure and massage to the prostate gland, and surgical removal of sperm, which is both costly and the least effective method of viable sperm collection (Brackett, Lynne, Ibrahim, Ohl, & Sonksen, 2010).

For women with SCI, menstruation may cease at the onset of injury, but for the majority of women it resumes within 6 months. Becoming pregnant and giving birth are generally not impaired, and birth control is resumed for women who are sexually active. Jackson and Wadley (1999) found that sexually active women with SCI showed a decrease in the use of birth control pills and an increase in elected sterilization and condom use.

Reproductive Choice

"Reproductive health implies that people are able to have a responsible, satisfying, and safe sex life and that they have the capability to have children and the freedom to decide if, when, and how often to do so." (World Health Organization, 2010b, para. 2). Public controversy over the right of some persons with disabilities to marry stems largely from concerns related to the upbringing of children that may result from that union. Influenced by the Eugenics movement in the early 1900s, tens of thousands of persons with cognitive disabilities were institutionalized and prohibited from sexual relations until, in the 1920s, the cost of segregating and overseeing such large numbers became prohibitive, and sterilization was implemented as a means of ultimately extracting "feeble-mindedness" from society (Block, 2000). In order to control reproduction among persons with disabilities, nearly 30 US states passed laws that permitted involuntary sterilization of people with disabilities (Silver, 2004), resulting in the forced and indiscriminate sterilization of approximately 60,000 PWDs, in particular adolescents who reached the age of sexual maturation (Reilly, 1991).

Today, sterilization is far more restrictive and regulated by federal rules and state laws. Consideration is also given to a number of ethical issues and revolves around the rights of the individual to be sexually active, expressive, and to procreate that are weighed against the rights of the unborn child to receive adequate care (American Academy of Pediatrics, 2009). Although sterilization is still used as a parenting deterrent, fewer physicians are willing to conduct sterilization without a court mandate (Block, 2000).

Parenting

Historically, the right to reproduce and become a parent has been violated for persons with disabilities. According to Kirshbaum (2000), parenting is one of the last frontiers for people with disabilities. In her article, O'Toole (2002) states that although little research has explored parenting and persons with disabilities, many WWDs are successful parents despite societal barriers and a lack of sex education, expectations of celibacy, social views of PWDs as undesirable partners, sterilization, high rates of divorce at disability onset for married women, and removal of child custody from WWDs.

Societal concerns for parenting by PWDs are based on physical ability and cognitive capacity concerns. The decision to become a parent for a person who has physical impairment and limitations was examined by McNary (1999). Her interviews revealed that the parenting decision was influenced by a number of concerns related to physical considerations, such as having the stamina and energy to raise children and the emotional and financial effect of their disability on their children. Physically, they wondered about their ability to perform childcare tasks, particularly if they "...ended up in a wheelchair" (McNary, 1999, p. 99). They also worried about the safety of their children and their ability to sufficiently respond when necessary. Despite these concerns, participants revealed significant determination and belief in their ability to manage; as one participant stated, "I can conquer it .... I'm not going to let it stop me from doing something that I have wanted all my life" (McNary, 1999, p. 98).

In the United States, approximately 15% of all parents of children under the age of 18 have disabilities (U.S. Department of Health and Human Services, 2002). Among single parents, 24% have disabilities (McNeil, 1993). In the United States, there is significant variation across major categories of disability in terms of the proportion of disabled adults who are parents (Toms-Barker & Maralani, 1997): About 40% have sensory impairments, 26% are physically impaired, 24% are psychiatrically disabled, and 16% have cognitive disabilities. Differences between parents with and without disabilities include the following: parents with disabilities are slightly older, they are less likely to be married and more likely to be married to another person with a disability, and they have more children with disabilities. They are also more likely to be unemployed, 48% versus 22%, and living in households with income below the poverty level than are parents without disabilities (McNeil, 1993; Toms-Barker & Maralani, 1997).

In a study of 1,200 parents with disabilities, most (70%) of which were physical, participants indicated a number of parenting problems that included pressures to voluntarily become sterile (14%) and to have an abortion (13%). In addition to attitudinal barriers, other parenting problems were reported as

- Physical difficulty with chasing, carrying, and lifting their children, participation in recreational activities with their children, traveling with their children, and lack of space in the home and inaccessibility.
- Childcare access due to cost, lack of transportation, and lack of services and information about appropriate child care.
- Lack of knowledge, high cost, and low attainability of adaptive parenting equipment (such as wheelchair accessible cribs and baby lifters).
- Although over half of the parents reported using personal assistants for help with childcare, problems included difficulty with availability, reliability, and interference with parents role. (Toms-Barker & Maralani, 1997).

A number of relatively recent changes have taken place that give recognition to the idea that parenting problems for persons with disabilities are more likely related to lack of services and supports, low income, and knowledge deficits than to the abilities of persons with disabilities to raise a child who is physically, intellectually, and emotionally healthy. Legislative changes have included the removal of discriminatory language from legal proceedings related to child custody, parent rights, adoption, and divorce (Callow, Buckland, & Jones, 2008). In addition, a number of Web sites are now available to provide parents with disabilities with support and information, such as Parents with Disabilities Online (http://disabledparents.net/).

SEX EDUCATION, SEX THERAPY, AND SEXUAL SURROGATES

Sex education is not a one-time event that occurs in the early schooling years, but rather a continued process of learning about physical, emotional, and psychological sexual interactions and functions. When changes to the body and psyche occur due to disability, aging, or other significant events, there is frequently a need for additional learning related to sexuality issues. Unfortunately sex is an uncomfortable topic for many people, including health professionals and caregivers. Health providers may assume counselors are addressing the topic and counselors believe these needs are being addressed by health workers. Among cancer patients, only between 17% and 23% reported that sexuality concerns were addressed. However, 67% of men and 39% of women felt it was important to discuss sexuality. They wanted to be asked about their sex lives and wished for information on body image, libido, fertility, and general well-being (Southard & Keller, 2009).

Lack of knowledge about sexuality and sex has been reported about a number of disabilities and is reflective of the need for more sex education. Little sexual knowledge has been reported for persons with physical and intellectual disabilities (McCabe, 1999). For persons with intellectual disabilities, there are a number of concerns related to education. One fear is that talking about sexual issues will encourage inappropriate sexual behaviors. This has led parents and schools to avoid conversations related to sex. Another issue centers around the feelings of the person; it is anticipated that talk about sexual issues will lead to distress or embarrassment. Even researchers hesitate to conduct research to examine sexuality because they fear they may cause some type of emotional damage (McCarthy, 1998), or that the person may not be able to give consent, or that they may be accused of sexual abuse by the participant (Brown & Thompson, 1997). In their study to examine college students with learning disabilities reactions to sexuality research, Thomas and Kroese, (2005) found that while a few participants were embarrassed, the majority of participants showed no embarrassment or distress and no inappropriate behaviors were apparent. In fact, several students reported positive affects related to having the opportunity to talk about sex.

Probably one of the most controversial topics for PWDs is the use of sex therapy, sex coaches, and sex surrogates. Sex therapy is generally a short-term psychotherapy that centers around issues of sexual intimacy, feelings, and functioning provided by licensed therapists who may be certified through the American Association of Sexuality Educators, Counselors, and Therapists (ASSECT). Persons with disabilities might receive sex therapy for a number of issues related to sexual desire, arousal, functioning (anorgasmia, premature ejaculation, and dyspareunia), or intimacy problems associated with disability (Mayo Clinic, 2010).

From the standpoint that sexuality and sexual expression are human rights, Shapiro (2002) argues that sexual surrogacy is an appropriate means of sexual gratification for persons with disabilities and an opportunity not only to be sexual but also to reclaim their bodies.

> Simply put, sexual surrogacy is not prostitution nor is it simply gratification in its most vulgar meaning. Sexual surrogacy is a therapeutic process which attempts to have the patient begin a dialogue with their own body in an attempt to, in a meaningful way, transcend simple gratification. (Shapiro, 2002, New Thinking and Approaches, para. 1)

Shapiro further believes that surrogacy should be government supported as a "therapeutic mechanism in the on-going rehabilitation of persons with disabilities" (Shapiro, 2002, Introduction Section, para. 5).

In a brief description on Disaboom (www.disaboom.com), an information Web site for persons with disabilities, Fulbright (n.d.) lists the advantages of working with a sexual surrogate as overcoming a sexual disorder, gaining self-confidence, and skills and attitudes for healthy sexual functioning and well-being. According to the International Professional Surrogates Association (IPSA, n.d.):

> In this therapy, a client, a therapist and a surrogate partner form a three-person therapeutic team. The surrogate participates with the client in structured and unstructured experiences that are designed to build client self-awareness and skills in the areas of physical and emotional intimacy. These therapeutic experiences include partner work in relaxation, effective communication, sensual and sexual touching, and social skills training. Each program is designed to increase the client's knowledge, skills, and comfort. As the days pass, clients find themselves becoming more relaxed, more open to feelings, and more comfortable with physical and emotional intimacy. The involvement of the team therapist, a licensed and/or certified professional with an advanced degree, is a cornerstone of this therapy process (IPSA, para. 1).

A number of disadvantages exist, including access outside of the states of Florida, California, New York, and Pennsylvania. Due to legal and ethical concerns, many surrogates keep their practice secret. Also, sex workers may falsely present themselves as surrogates (Fulbright, n.d.). The cost of this service is prohibitive for many persons with disabilities. While individual session cost is said to mimic local therapist charges, the cost of intensive therapy for 1 or 2 weeks would range from $4000.00 to $8000.00 (IPSA, para. 6).

SEXUAL ABUSE OF PERSONS WITH DISABILITIES

Frequency of Sexual Abuse

A limited number of studies have attempted to estimate the prevalence of abuse against persons with disabilities. Sobsey (1994) estimated that WWDs are raped at least one-and-a-half times more often than women in the general population. WWDs, like WWODs, are most frequently assaulted by a familiar person, in a familiar place, such as at home or at work (Andrews & Veronen, 1993). In reviewing the prevalence of abuse, it is apparent that the less likely a person is to defend oneself, either physically or psychologically, greater is the chance of one's being abused. The less credible they are considered, such as those with cognitive or physiological impairments, the more they are likely to be abused and the less likely they are to prosecute. Several studies have found that prosecution of cases of sexual abuse for victims with cognitive impairment is only between 5% and 9% (Brown, Stein, & Turk, 1995; Mansell, 1995).

Among persons with developmental disabilities, sexual abuse is particularly high. Civjan (2000) found a rate of sexual abuse among women with developmental disabilities of 83% and Wilson and Brewer (1992) found that women with developmental disabilities were 10.7 times more likely to have been sexually assaulted than

WWODs. Brown et al. (1995) noted that victims ranged from profoundly to mildly disabled, but that most (61%) fell into the severe-to-moderate (IQ 21–50) categories. Interestingly, among this disability group, males and females were equally likely to be abused, but almost all of the perpetrators were male and known to the victim. Several studies have noted that only 2%–3% of perpetrations are committed by persons unknown to victims with mental retardation (Brown et al., 1995; Furey, 1994); 53% of identified perpetrators of sexual abuse against persons with developmental disabilities were other consumers, and 20% of perpetrators were identified as staff/volunteers (Brown et al., 1995).

Institutionalization also increases the risk of abuse. Sobsey and Mansell (1990) found that the risk of sexual abuse among persons living in institutional settings was two to four times higher than for those living in the community. Perpetrators who are staff members may use threats or bribes (Andrews & Veronen, 1993) or may sexually victimize persons while they are unconscious, medicated, or restrained (Musick, 1984), and the risk of exposure to multiple offenders is increased by high turnover rates due to low wages and minimal employee screening.

Persons who have sensory impairments are also sexually abused at high rates. Welbourne, Lipschitz, Selvin, and Green (1983) reported that among women who were blind from birth, 50% had been sexually abused. However, studies of persons with sensory impairment are scarce and tend to be limited to clinical populations that are not generalizable to the general population. Another study found that the overwhelming majority of deaf children and adolescents admitted to a psychiatric facility had histories of sexual abuse (Willis & Vernon, 2002).

The rate of sexual abuse of women with physical disabilities is similar to that of women without disabilities (Young, Nosek, Howland, Chanpong, & Rintala, 1997), but Nosek, Foley, Hughes, and Howland (2001) concluded that these abusive relationships tend to continue for longer durations. Unlike other disabilities, much of the research conducted with women with substance abuse disabilities examines abuse that occurred prior to the onset of the disability. Abusive histories have been found to be prevalent among the majority of women in treatment for chemical dependency (Glover, Janikowski, & Benshoff, 1996; Wadsworth, Spampneto, & Halbrook, 1995) and believed by many researchers to be a contribution to the onset of chemical dependence.

The Dynamics of Abuse Against WWDs

Sexual abuse is motivated by a need for feeling of power and control, and it is frequently maintained by manipulation, coercion, and threats. Most perpetrators share similar characteristics, including a need for immediate gratification, poor impulse control, and anger. Girls with disabilities may be particularly vulnerable to abuse because they are frequently unwelcome in social activities and have less exposure to social interaction. When they reach dating age, they may have confusion associated with their own needs and desires. Their desire to feel like "normal women" may lead to relationships that make them more susceptible to abuse. They may come to believe that their choices are limited to celibacy or sexually violent relationships, and that they should be grateful for any sexual attention (Womendez & Schneiderman, 1991). Cattalini (1993) noted additional factors that may increase vulnerability to abuse as physical and emotional isolation from others, feelings of powerlessness, low resistance to bribery and coercion, sexual repression, little understanding of abuse, and poor self-protection skills. In a qualitative study of 72 women with physical and cognitive disabilities, Saxton et al. (2001) identified difficulties with personal boundaries, imbalances of power, and a sense of loyalty and obligation to service providers as interfering with the willingness to end or report the abuse, particularly if the perpetrator was a family member.

It is also important to note especially for women that the disability may have been caused by abuse. Over 2 million women are seriously assaulted by their male partners every year (Coble et al., 1992). Sobsey (1994) estimated that violence was a contributing factor to the cause of 10%–25% of development disabilities. For women with violence-induced disability, it is important to consider who caused the disability and whether the perpetrator is now a caretaker (CALCASA, 2001).

Contributing Factors to Sexual Abuse

The sexual abuse of persons with disabilities must be viewed within the framework of societal attitudes and structure. Historically, WWDs have been sexually regulated by society through forced sterilization, forced contraception, and forced pregnancy termination, and some physicians continue to recommend sterilization for WWDs but rarely suggest the same for males with similar disabilities (Beck-Massey, 1999).

The societal view that WWDs are asexual and roleless has further served to devalue and dehumanize WWDs, making it easier for caregivers and perpetrators to excuse abusive behaviors with the rationalization that WWDs do not understand perpetrated sexual acts as negative or even that they are helping their victim in some way. Additional stereotypical assumptions and stereotypes that contribute to the vulnerability of WWDs were outlined by Chenoweth (1993) as promiscuity, unattractive and grateful for attention, childlike, compliant, maternally inept, and insensitive to sexual trauma. These perceptions have led to lack of sexual education, learned passivity, low reporting, exposure to multiple people without preventative measures, and low help-seeking.

The view that WWDs are asexual has also contributed to making WWDs with disabilities vulnerable because little to no attention is given to training women to recognizing potentially abusive situations, self-defense, or reporting abuse. Nosek (1996) found that vulnerability to abuse was increased through architectural barriers, inappropriate mobility aids, and exposure to medical and institutional settings because these limited the ability of people with disabilities to escape. Unfortunately, even exposure to disability services has been found to increase sexual abuse. Sobsey and Doe (1991) found that 44% of their sample of 162 persons with disabilities who were sexually abused had perpetrators who gained access to them by way of disability services, including paid service providers, psychiatrists, and residential staff. They estimated that exposure to the disability service system increased the risk of sexual victimization by 78%.

In a review of the literature, Andrews and Veronen (1993) identified eight areas that contribute to greater vulnerability to abuse for WWDs, including (1) dependency on others for care, (2) perceptions of powerlessness, (3) lower risk of perpetrator discovery, (4) lower believability, (5) lack of appropriate and comprehensive sexual education for persons with disabilities, (6) social isolation, (7) physical helplessness, and (8) mainstreaming without consideration for self-protection. They also concluded that sexual involvement with personal attendants was not uncommon. Other contributing factors to sexual vulnerability include the imbalance of power, difficulties in recognition and reporting of abuse, and the dynamics involved in using relatives and friends to provide services (Saxton et al., 2001).

When persons with disabilities are abused, crises intervention may include having an escape plan in place, a temporary stay at a confidential women's shelter, and making permanent plans to separate from the abuser (Nosek, Howland, & Young, 1997). Unfortunately, services such as those within the justice systems, women's shelters, and medical services can present barriers that inhibit access and participation. Barriers to acquiring assistance after violence is identified by the Center for Research on Women with Disabilities (CROWD) from WWD reports as including (1) they were not believed, (2) they were discriminated against, (3) transportation was not available, (4) referrals were inappropriate, and (5) services were inaccessible. Many existing programs and shelters frequently do not include alternative formats such as Braille, do not provide attendant care, and are not fully accessible.

Legislation and Trends

Originally enacted in 1994, the Violence Against Women Act (VEWA) was reauthorized in 1998 and again in 2000 with a new language that specifically includes WWDs, allocating millions of dollars for research and programming to enhance protection, strengthen education, and end violence and abuse (Whatley, 2000). Included in the Office funding stream are grant competitions related specifically to WWDs. In 1998, the Crime Victims with Disabilities Awareness Act was passed, which mandates that disability status needed to include information gathered from crime victims. Accurate data on the prevalence of crime and violence perpetrated against WWDs would strengthen calls for more services and supports.

For people with disabilities, current legislation issues related to sexuality are related to marriage penalties, child custody, and childcare. For persons with disabilities, the decision to marry and cohabitate may be a costly one that they simply cannot afford because funding decisions are based on combined income. Marrying can cause social security benefits to be reduced or lost and couples are at risk for losing Medicaid and personal assistant benefits. Couples who cannot afford to lose these benefits are put in the position of living together in secret, which will impact employer health benefit coverage (Fiduccia, 2000).

Issues of child rearing can be complicated by regulations related to personal assistance services. Only a few states include child care as an activity of daily living, and that has profound implications for child care when there are functions related to children that cannot be provided by a parent with a disability. Many states prohibit personal assistants from providing childcare activities, which has implications for both childcare and child custody should the couple divorce (Fiduccia, 2000).

Finally, until recently, little attention has been paid to providing persons with physical impairment alternative self-defense strategies. Recent training has emerged in self-defense from the seated position while in a wheelchair and self-defense utilizing the wheelchair and mobility aids as weapons against would-be perpetrators. In addition, specific weapons training is also emerging for persons with disabilities that takes into account the strength and mobility of PWDs (Madorsky, 1990; McNab, 2003). These trainings are available to people with disabilities through associations such as the International Disabled Self-Defense Association (http://www.defenseability.com/index.htm).

CONCLUSION

Issues related to sex and sexuality for persons with disabilities incorporate a number of important topics that can affect how people with disabilities view themselves and live their lives. This chapter discussed the social construction of gender identity and body image and the role that social construction plays in the sexual stigmatization and abuse of PWDs. Societal attitudes additionally play a role in self-esteem and body image for PWDs and affect their intimate partnering choices. Additionally, PWDs have a number of issues and concerns that are specific to the type and severity of their disability and may impact their sexual functioning, reproductive choices, and feeling about parenting.

REFERENCES

American Academy of Pediatrics. (2009). *Sterilization of minors with developmental disabilities*. Retrieved from http://aappolicy.aappublications.org/cgi/content/full/pediatrics;104/2/337

Anderson, K. D. (2004). Targeting recovery: Priorities of the spinal cord-injured population. *Journal of Neurotrauma, 21*, 1371–1383.

Andrews, A. B., & Veronen, L. J. (1993). Sexual assault and people with disabilities. Special issue: Sexuality and disabilities: A guide for human service practitioners. *Journal of Social Work and Human Sexuality, 8*, 137–159.

Antonak, R. F. (1981). Prediction of attitudes toward disabled persons: A multivariate analysis. *Journal of General Psychology, 104*, 119–123.

Aufreiter, N., Elzinga, D., & Gordon, J. (2003). Better branding. *The McKinzey Quarterly, 4*, 28–39.

Axtell, S. (1999). Disability identity: Interviews with lesbians and bisexual women and their partners. *Journal of Gay, Lesbian, and Bisexual Identity, 4*, 53–72.

Beck-Massey, D. (1999). Sanctioned war: Women, violence, and disabilities. *Sexuality and Disability, 17*, 269–276.

Block, P. (2000). Sexuality, fertility, and danger: Twentieth-century images of women with cognitive disabilities. *Sexuality and Disability, 18*(4), 239–254.

Booth, S., Kendall, M., Fronek, P., Miller, D., & Geraghty, T. (2003). Training the interdisciplinary team in sexuality rehabilitation following spinal cord injury: A needs assessment. *Sexuality and Disability, 21*, 249–261.

Brackett, N. L., Lynne, C. M., Ibrahim, E., Ohl, D. A., & Sonksen, J. (2010). Treatment of infertility in men with spinal cord injury: *Nature Reviews Urology, 7*, 162–172.

Brown, H., Hunt, N., & Stein, J. (1994). Alarming but very necessary: Working with staff groups around the sexual abuse of adults with learning disabilities. *Journal of Intellectual Disability Research, 38*, 393–412.

Brown, H., & Stein, J. (1997). Sexual abuse perpetrated by men with intellectual disabilities: A comparative study. *Child Abuse Review, 3*(1), 26–35.

Brown, H., Stein, J., & Turk, V. (1995). The sexual abuse of adults with learning disabilities: Report of a second two-year incidence survey. *Mental Handicap Research, 8*, 3–24.

Brown, H., & Thompson, D. (1997). The ethics of research with men who have learning disabilities and abusive sexual behavior: A minefield in a vacuum. *Disability and Society, 12*, 695–707.

Brown, H., & Turk, V. (1992). Defining sexual abuse as it affects adults with learning disabilities. *Mental Handicap, 20*, 44–55.

Burns, J. (1993). Invisible women–women who have learning disabilities. *The Psychologist, 6*, 102–105.

CALCASA. (2001). *Creating access, serving survivors of sexual assault with disabilities.* Sacramento, CA: California Coalition against Sexual Abuse (CALCASA).

Callahan, C. (2004). Facial disfigurement and sense of self in head and neck cancer. *Social Work Health Care, 40*(2), 73–87.

Callow, E., Buckland, K., & Jones, S. (2008). *The disability movement and a new focus on legislating protection for children in families with parental disability.* Berkeley, CA: Through the Looking Glass. Retrieved from http://www.lookingglass.org/publications

Cambridge, P. (2002). Cosmetic surgery for people with learning disabilities: Considerations for adult protection practice. *The Journal of Adult Protection, 4*(2), 9–20.

Cambridge, P., & Mellan, B. (2000). Reconstructing the sexuality of men with learning disabilities: Empirical evidence and theoretical interpretations of need. *Disability & Society, 15*, 293–311.

Cattalini, H. (1993). *Access to services for women with disabilities who are subjected to violence.* Canberra, Australian: Government Printing Service.

Chenoweth, L. (1993). Invisible acts: Violence against women with disabilities. *Australian Disability Review, 2*, 22–28.

Christian, L., Stinson, J., & Dotson, L. A. (2001). Staff values regarding the sexual expression of women with disabilities. *Sexuality and Disability, 19*, 283–291.

Christopherson, J. M., Moore, K., Foley, F. W., & Warren, K. G. (2006). A comparison of written materials vs. materials and counseling for women with sexual dysfunction and multiple sclerosis. *Journal of Clinical Nursing, 15*, 742–750.

Civjan, S. R. (2000). Making sexual assault and domestic violence services accessible. IMPACT, 13 [electronic version]. Retrieved May 15, 2011, from http://ici.umn.edu/products/impact/133/over6.html

Claiborne, N., & Rizzo, V. M. (2006). Addressing sexual issues in individuals with chronic health conditions. *Health and Social Work, 31*(3), 221–224.

Coble, Y. D., Eisenbrey, A. B., Estes, E. H., Karlan, M. S., Kennedy, W. R., Numann, P. J., et al. (1992). Violence against women: Relevance for medical practitioners. *Journal of the American Medical Association, 267*, 2184–2189.

Cook, J. A. (2000). Sexuality and people with disabilities. *Sexuality and Disability, 18*, 195–206.

Crewe, N. M., & Krause, J. S. (1988). Marital relationships and spinal cord injury. *Archives of Physical Medicine and Rehabilitation, 69*, 435–438.

Daily, D. (1984). Does renal failure mean sexual failure. *The Renal Family, 6*, 2–4.

Danek, M. M. (1992). The status of women with disabilities revisited. *Journal of Applied Rehabilitation Counseling, 23*(4), 7–13.

De Loach, C. P. (1994). Attitudes toward disability: Impact on sexual development and forging of intimate relationships. *Journal of Applied Rehabilitation Counseling, 25*(1), 18–25.

DeVivo, M. J., & Richards, J. S. (1996). Marriage rates among persons with spinal cord injury. *Rehabilitation Psychology, 41*(4), 321–339.

DeVivo, M. J., Hawkins, L. N., Richards, J. S., & Go, B. K. (1995). Outcomes of post-spinal cord injury marriages. *Archives of Physical Medicine and Rehabilitation, 76*, 130–138.

Di Giulio, G. (2003). Sexuality and people living with physical or developmental disabilities: A review of key issues. *Canadian Journal of Human Sexuality, 12*, 53–68.

Dixon, D. (1983). An erotic attraction to amputees. *Sexuality and Disability, 6*, 3–19.

Ducharme, S. (n.d.). *Brain trauma and sexuality.* Retrieved from http://www.stanleyducharme.com/resources/combin_injury.htm

Ducharme, S., & Gill, K. M. (1990). Sexual values, training, and professional roles. *Journal of Head Trauma Rehabilitation, 5*(2), 38–45.

Duncan, K., & Goggin, G. (2002). "Something in your belly" Fantasy, disability, and desire in my one-legged dream lover. *Disabilities Studies Quarterly, 22*(4), 127–144.

Elks, M. A. (1990). Another look at facial disfigurement. *The Journal of Rehabilitation, 56,* 36–40.

Fiduccia, B. W. (2000). Current issues in sexuality and the disability movement. *Sexuality and Disability, 18,* 167–174.

Foley, F. W., & Sanders, A. S. (1997). Sexuality, multiple sclerosis and women. *MS Management, 4,* 3–10.

Fox News. (2008, March 10). *Outrage over parents' decision to have Down syndrome child undergo cosmetic surgery.* Retrieved from http://www.foxnews.com/story/0,2933,336432,00.html

Fulbright, Y. K. (n.d.) Where to find a sex surrogate partner. *Disaboom.* Retrieved from http://www.disaboom.com/sexuality-and-disability/finding-a-sex-surrogate-partner

Furey, E. (1994). Sexual abuse of adults with mental retardation: Who and where. *Mental Retardation, 32,* 173–180.

Gentile, D. A. (1993). Just what are sex and gender, anyway? A call for new terminological standard. *Psychological Science, 4,* 120–122.

Gilling-Smith, C. (2000). Assisted reproduction in HIV-discordant couples: Reproductive options for HIV-positive men. *The AIDS Reader, 10,* 581–587.

Glover, N. M., Janikowski, T. P., & Benshoff, J. J. (1996). Substance abuse and past incest contact: A national perspective. *Journal of Substance Abuse Treatment, 13,* 185–193.

Golden, M. R., Brewer, D. D., Kurth, A., Holmes, K. K., & Handsfield, H. H. (2004). Importance of sex partner HIV status in HIV risk assessment among men who have sex with men. *Journal of Acquired Immune Deficiency Syndromes, 36,* 734–742.

Goldstein, S. B., & Johnson, V. A. (1997). Stigma by association: Perceptions of the dating partners of college students with physical disabilities. *Basic and Applied Social Psychology, 19,* 495–504.

Gordon, P. A., Chariboga-Tantillo, J., Feldman, D., & Perrone, K. (2004). Attitudes regarding interpersonal relationships with mental illness and mental retardation. *Journal of Rehabilitation, 70*(1), 50–56.

Haboubi, H. H., & Lincoln, N. (2003). Views of health professionals on discussing sexual issues with patients. *Disability and Rehabilitation, 25,* 291–296.

Hergenrather, K., & Rhodes, R. (2007). Exploring undergraduate student attitudes toward persons with disabilities: Application of the disability social relationship scale. *Rehabilitation Counseling Bulletin, 50,* 66–75.

HIV InSite (2005). *Sex and sexuality.* Retrieved from http://hivinsite.ucsf.edu/insite?page=pb-daily-sex

Howland, C. A., & Rintala, D. H. (2001). Dating behaviors of women with physical disabilities. *Sexuality and Disability, 19,* 41–70.

International Professional Surrogates Association. (IPSA). (n.d.). *What is surrogate partner therapy?* Retrieved from http://www.surrogatetherapy.org/SurrogatePartnerTherapy.html

International Professional Surrogates Association. (IPSA). (n.d.). *Intensive surrogate partner therapy.* Retrieved from http://www.surrogatetherapy.org/IntensiveTherapy.html

Jackson, A. B., & Wadley, V. A. (1999). Multicenter study of women's self-reported reproductive health after spinal cord injury. *Archives of Physical Medicine & Rehabilitation, 80,* 1420–1428.

Kafer, A. (2000). Amputated desire, resistant desire: Female amputees in the devotee community. *Disability World, 3, June/July.* Retrieved from http://www.disabilityworld.org/June-July2000/Women/SDS.htm

Kazukauskas, K. A., & Lam, C. S. (2010). Disability and sexuality: Knowledge, attitudes, and level of comfort among certified rehabilitation counselors. *Rehabilitation Counseling Bulletin, 54,* 15–25.

Kammerer-Quayle, B. (2002). Image and behavioral skills training for people with facial difference and disability. In M. G. Brodwin, F. Tellez, & S. K. Brodwin (Eds.), *Medical, psychosocial and vocational aspects of disability* (pp. 95–106). Athens, GA: Elliott & Fitzpatrick.

Kirshbaum, M. 2000. A disability culture perspective on early intervention with parents with physical or cognitive disabilities and their infants. *Infants and Young Children, 132*, 9–20.

Kleve, L., Rumsey, N., Wyn-Williams, M., & White, P. (2002). The effectiveness of cognitive-behavioural interventions provided at Outlook: A disfigurement support unit. *Journal of Evaluation in Clinical Practice, 8*, 387–395.

Klebine, P. (2007). Sexuality for women with spinal cord injury. InfoSheet #21, *Spinal Cord Injury Information Network*. Retrieved from http://www.spinalcord.uab.edu/show.asp?durki=51288&site=1021&return=21479

Kline, C. (1991). *Counseling our own: The lesbian/gay subculture meets the mental health system.* Seattle, WA: Consultant Services Northwest.

Knoepfler, P. T. (1991). Sexuality and psychiatric disability. In R. P. Marinelli & A. E. Dell Orto (Eds.), *The psychological & social impact of disability* (pp. 210–222). New York, NY: Springer.

Kreuter, M. (2000). Spinal cord injury and partner relationships. *Spinal Cord, 38*, 2–6.

Kreuter, M., Sullivan, M., & Siosteen, A. (1994). Sexual adjustment after spinal cord injury (SCI) focusing on partner experiences. *Paraplegia, 32*, 225–235.

McCabe, M. P. (1999). Sexual knowledge, experience and feelings among people with disability. *Sexuality & Disability, 17*, 157–170.

McCabe, M. P., Cummins, R. A., & Deeks, A. A. (2000). Sexuality and quality of life among people with physical disability. *Sexuality and Disability, 18*, 115–123.

McCarthy, M. (1998). Interviewing people with intellectual disabilities about sensitive issues: A discussion of ethical issues. *British Journal of Learning Disabilities, 26*, 140–145.

McNab, C. (2003). *Martial arts for people with disabilities.* Broomall, PA: Mason Crest Publishers.

McNary, M. E. (1999). Themes arising in the motherhood decision for women with multiple sclerosis: An exploratory study. *Journal of Vocational Rehabilitation, 12*, 93–102.

McNeil, J. (1993). *Americans with disabilities: 1991–92.* U.S. Bureau of the Census, Current Population Reports, P70–33. Washington, DC: U.S. Government Printing Office.

MacGregor, F. C. (1951) Some psycho-social problems associated with facial deformities. *American Sociological Review, 16*, 629–638.

Madorsky, J. G. (1990). Self defense for people with disabilities. *Western Journal of Medicine, 153*, 434–435.

Matthews, V. (2009). Sexual dysfunction in people with long-term neurological conditions. *Nursing Standard, 23*(50), 48–56.

Man, M., Rojahn, J., Chrosniak, L., & Sanford, J. (2006). College students' romantic attraction toward peers with physical disabilities. *Journal of Developmental and Physical Disabilities, 18*, 35–44.

Mansell, C. (1995). Researching the sexual abuse of adults with learning disability. *Journal of the Association for Practitioners in Learning Disability, 12*(2), 15–18.

Marini, I., Feist, A., Chen, R., Torres-Flores, L., & Del Castillo, A. (in press). Student attitudes toward intimacy with persons who are wheelchair users. *Rehabilitation Education.*

Maslow, A. H. (1943). A theory of human motivation, *Psychological Review, 50*, 370–396.

Mayo Clinic. (2010). *Sex therapy.* Retrieved from http://www.mayoclinic.com/health/sex-therapy/MY01349/rss=1

Miller, E., Chen, R., Glover-Graf, N. M., & Kranz, P. (2009) Willingness to engage in personal relationships with persons with disabilities. *Rehabilitation Counseling Bulletin, 20*, 1–14.

Milligan, M. S., & Neufeldt, A. H. (1998). Postinjury marriage to men with spinal cord injury: Women's perspectives on making a commitment. *Sexuality and Disability, 16*, 117–132.

Moin, V., Duvdevany, I., & Mazor, D. (2009). Sexual identity, body image, and life satisfaction among women with and without physical disability. *Sexuality and Disability, 27*, 83–95.

Morris, J. (1993). Gender and disability. In J. Swain, V. Finkelstein, S. French & M. Oliver (Eds.), *Disabling barriers – Enabling environments* (pp. 85–92). London: Sage.

Moss, T. P., & Rosser, B. (2008). Psychosocial adjustment to visible difference. *The Psychologist, 21*, 492–495.

Musick, J. L. (1984). Patterns of institutional sexual abuse. *Response to Violence in the Family and Sexual Assault, 7*(3), 1–11.

National Down Syndrome Society (NDSS). (2011). *Cosmetic surgery for children with Down syndrome.* Retrieved from http://www.ndss.org/index.php?option=com_content&view=article&id=153 %3Aposition-papers&catid=54%3Apublic-relations&Itemid=140&limitstart=6

Nosek, M. A. (1996). Sexual abuse of women with physical disabilities. In D. M. Krotoski, M. A. Nosek, & M. A. Turk (Eds.), *Women with physical disabilities: Achieving and maintaining health and well-being* (pp. 153–173). Baltimore, MD: Brooks.

Nosek, M. A., Howland, C. A., Rintala, D. H., Young, M. E., & Chanpong, G. F. (1997). *National study of women with disabilities: Final report.* Houston, TX: Center for Research on Women with Disabilities.

Nosek, M. A., Howland, C. A., & Young, M. E. (1997). Abuse of women with disabilities: Policy implications. *Journal of Disability Policy Studies, 8,* 157–176.

Nosek, M. A., Foley, C. C., Hughes, R. B., & Howland, C. A. (2001). Vulnerabilities for abuse among women with disabilities. *Sexuality and Disability, 19,* 177–189.

O'Carroll, R. E., Woodrow, J., & Maroun, F. (1991). Psychosexual and psychosocial sequelae of closed head injury. *Brain Injury, 5,* 303–313.

Olkin, R. (1999). *What psychotherapists should know about disability.* New York, NY: Guilford.

Opel, D. J., & Wilfond, B. S. (2009). Cosmetic surgery in children with cognitive disabilities: Who benefits? Who decides? *The Hastings Report, 39*(1), 19–21.

O'Toole, C. J. (2002). Sex, disability and motherhood: Access to sexuality for disabled mothers. *Disabilities Studies Quarterly, 22*(4), 81–101.

Parkes, N. (2006). Sexual issues and people with a learning disability. *Learning Disability Practice, 9*(3), 32–37.

Perry, B. L., & Wright, E. R. (2006). The sexual partnerships of people with serious mental illness. *The Journal of Sex Research, 43,* 174–181.

Reilly, P. (1991). *The surgical solution: A history of involuntary sterilization in the United States.* Baltimore, MD: Johns Hopkins University Press.

Richards, E., Tepper, M., Whipple, B., & Komisaruk, B. R. (1997). Women with complete spinal cord injury: A phenomenological study of sexuality and relationship experiences. *Sexuality and Disability, 15,* 271–283.

Rintala, D. H., Howland, C. A., Nosek, M. A., Bennett, J. L., Young, M. E., Foley, C. C. et al. (1997). Dating issues for women with physical disabilities. *Sexuality and Disability, 15,* 219–242.

Rojahn, J., Komelasky, K. G., & Man, M. (2008). Implicit attitudes and explicit ratings of romantic attraction of college students toward opposite-sex peers with physical disabilities. *Journal of Developmental and Physical Disabilities, 20,* 389–397.

Sakellarious, D. (2006). If not the disability, then what? Barriers to reclaiming sexuality following spinal cord injury. *Sexuality and Disability, 24,* 101–111.

Saxton, M., Curry, M. A., Powers, L. E., Maley, S., Eckels, K., & Gross, J. (2001). "Bring my scooter so I can leave you": A study of disabled women handling abuse by personal assistance providers. *Violence Against Women, 7,* 393–417.

Scotti, J. R., Evans, I. M., Meyer, L. H., & Walker, P. (1991). A meta-analysis of intervention research with problem behavior: Treatment validity and standards of practice. *American Journal on Mental Retardation, 96,* 233–256.

Sedikides, C., Oliver, M. B., & Campbell, W. K. (1994). Perceived benefits and costs of romantic relationships for women and men: Implications for exchange theory. *Personal Relationships, 1,* 5–21.

Shakespeare, T. (2000). Disabled sexuality: Towards rights and recognition. *Sexuality and Disability, 18,* 159–166.

Shapiro, L. (2002). Incorporating sexual surrogacy into the Ontario Direct Funding Program. *Disability Studies Quarterly, 22,* 72–81. Retrieved from http://www.dsq-sds.org/article/view/373/493

Silver, M. (2004). Eugenics and compulsory sterilization laws: Providing redress for the victims of a shameful era in United States History. *George Washington Law Review, 72,* 862–892.

Snead, S. L., & Davis, J. R. (2002). Attitudes of individuals with acquired brain injury towards disability. *Brain Injury, 16,* 947–953.

Sobsey, D. (1994). *Violence in the lives of people with disabilities: The end of silent acceptance?* Baltimore, MD: Paul H. Brookes.

Sobsey, D., & Doe, T. (1991). Patterns of sexual abuse and assault. *Sexuality and Disability, 9*, 243–259.

Sobsey, D., & Mansell, S. (1990). The prevention of sexual abuse of persons with developmental disabilities. *Developmental Disabilities Bulletin, 18*, 51–65.

Southard, N. Z., & Keller, J. (2009). The importance of assessing sexuality: A patient perspective. *Clinical Journal of Oncology Nursing, 13*, 213–217.

Spinal Cord Injury Information Network. (2007). *Sexual function for men with spinal cord injury.* Retrieved from http://www.spinalcord.uab.edu/show.asp?durki=22405

Stinson, J., Christian, L., & Dotson, L. (2002). Overcoming barriers to the sexual expression of women with developmental disabilities. *Research & Practice for Persons with Severe Disabilities, 27*, 18–26.

Szollos, A. A., & McCabe, M. P. (1995). The sexuality of people with mild intellectual disabilities, perceptions of clients and caregivers. *Australian and New Zealand Journal of Developmental Disabilities, 20*, 205–222.

Taleporos, G., Dip, G., & McCabe, M. P. (2002). The impact of sexual esteem, body esteem, and sexual satisfaction on psychological well-being in people with physical disability. *Sexuality and Disability, 20*, 177–183.

Taleporos, G., & McCabe, M. (2003). Relationships, sexuality and adjustment among people with physical disability. *Sexual and Relationship Therapy, 18*, 25–43.

Thomas, G., & Kroese, B. S. (2005). An investigation of students' with mild learning disabilities reactions to participating in sexuality research. *British Journal of Learning Disabilities, 33*, 113–119.

Thurer, S. L. (1991). Women and rehabilitation. In R. P. Marinelli & A. E. Dell Orto (Eds.), *The psychological & social impact of disability* (pp. 32–38). New York, NY: Springer.

Toms-Barker, L., & Maralani, V. (1997). *Challenges and strategies of disabled parents: Findings from a national survey of parents with disabilities.* Berkeley: Through the looking glass. Retrieved from http://www.lookingglass.org/publications

Urey, J. R., & Henggeler, S. W. (1987). Marital adjustment following spinal cord injury. *Archives of Physical Medicine and Rehabilitation, 68*, 69–74.

US Department of Health and Human Services, National Center for Health Statistics. National Health Interview Survey, 2000 (Computer file). 2nd ICPSR version. Hyattsville, MD: US Department of Health and Human Services, National Center for Health Statistics (producer), 2000. Ann Arbor, MI: Inter-university Consortium for Political and Social Research (distributor), 2002.

Van den Noort, S., & Holland, N. J (1999). *Multiple sclerosis in clinical practice.* New York, NY: Demos Medical Publishing, Inc.

Vash, C. L., & Crewe, N. M. (2004). *The psychology of disability.* New York, NY: Springer Publishing.

Vocational and Educational Services with Disabilities (VESID). (2011). *100.00 Consumer involvement policy.* NYSED.gov. Retrieved from http://www.vesid.nysed.gov/current_provider_information/vocational_rehabilitation/policies_procedures/0100_consumer_involvement/policy.htm

Volman, L., & Landeen, J. (2007). Uncovering the sexual self in people with schizophrenia. *Journal of Psychiatric and Mental Health Nursing, 14*, 411–417.

Wada, K., Iwasa, H., Okada, M., Murakami, T., Kamata, A., Zhu, G. et al. (2004). Marital status of patients with epilepsy with special reference to the influence of epileptic seizures on the patient's married life. *Epilepsia, 45*, 33–36.

Wadsworth, R., Spampneto, A. M., & Halbrook, B. M. (1995). The role of sexual trauma in the treatment of chemically dependent women: Addressing the relapse issue. *Journal of Counseling and Development, 73*, 401–406.

Welbourne, A., Lipschitz, S., Selvin, H., & Green, R. (1983). A comparison of the sexual learning experiences of visually impaired and sighted women. *Journal of Visual Impairment and Blindness, 77*, 256–259.

Westgren, N., & Levi, R. (1999). Sexuality after injury: Interviews with women after traumatic spinal cord injury. *Sexuality and Disability, 17*, 309–319.

Whatley, J. (2000). Violence against women with disabilities: Policy implications of what we don't know. *IMPACT, 13*(3), 4–5.

Whipple, B., Richards, E., Tepper, M., & Komisaruk, B. R. (1996). Sexual response in women with complete spinal cord injury. *Sexuality and Disability, 14*, 191–201.

Willis, R. G., & Vernon, M. (2002). Residential psychiatric treatment of emotionally disturbed deaf youth. *American Annuals of the Deaf, 147*, 31–37.

Wilson, C., & Brewer, N. (1992). The incidence of criminal victimization of individuals with an intellectual disability. *Australian Psychologist, 27*(2), 114–117.

Womendez, C., & Schneiderman, K. (1991). Escaping from abuse: Unique issues for women with disabilities. *Sexuality and Disability, 9*, 273–280.

Wong, D. W., Chan, F., Da Silva Cardoso, E., Lam, C. S., & Miller, S. M. (2004). Rehabilitation counseling students' attitudes toward people with disabilities in three social contexts: A conjoint analysis. *Rehabilitation Counseling Bulletin, 47*, 197–204.

World Health Organization. (2010a). *Measuring sexual health: Conceptual and practical considerations and related indicators.* Retrieved from http://whqlibdoc.who.int/hq/2010/who_rhr_10.12_eng.pdf

World Health Organization. (2010b). *Sexual and reproductive health.* Retrieved from http://www.euro.who.int/en/what-we-do/health-topics/Life-stages/sexual-and-reproductive-health

Wright, B. A. (1960). *Physical disability: A psychological approach.* New York, NY: Harper & Row.

Young, M. E., Nosek, M. A., Howland, C., Chanpong, G., & Rintala, D. H. (1997). Prevalence of abuse of women with physical disabilities. *Archives of Physical Medicine and Rehabilitation, 78*(5), 34–38.

Yuen, H. K., & Hanson, C. (2002). Body image and exercise in people with and without acquired mobility disability. *Disability & Rehabilitation, 24*, 289–296.

Zorzon, M., Zivadinov, R., Bosco, A., Monti Bragadin, L., Moretti, R., Bonfigli, L. et al. (1999). Sexual dysfunction in multiple sclerosis: A case-control study: Frequency and comparison of groups. *Multiple Sclerosis, 5*, 418–427.

INSIDER PERSPECTIVE

The Story of Jennifer L. Addis

When I woke up the morning of March 15, 1997, I had no idea that it would mark the last day of my independence. It was a typical Saturday morning for me other than the fact that I was having a bachelorette party for my future sister-in-law. I was the maid of honor, so I wanted things to be just right. That afternoon all the girls had gotten together and discussed who would be the designated drivers. I volunteered myself and was responsible for picking up the bride-to-be. Later she decided to drive herself, which left me driving alone and that was when my boyfriend/fiancé at the time had volunteered to be my designated driver. I knew we would be drinking and it seemed to be a responsible decision at the time, and so I agreed. He showed up later with two of his friends and we all piled in his single cab pickup truck and headed home.

We were only minutes away from home when I realized that my life was in jeopardy. My designated driver started driving erratically at a high speed. We approached a bend in the road when he made a critical decision that profoundly changed my life forever. He decided to pass another vehicle on the right side of the road, at approximately 80–85 miles per hour. We began to fishtail. He counter-steered, but the truck lost traction and we soon were out of control. The gravel consumed us and sucked the truck in. The last thing I remembered was seeing the gravel on the right side of the road. We went up and over the ditch, rolling several times before smashing into a tree. The truck landed upside down, and sometime during the impact I was thrown out of the vehicle. The truck was crushed like a tin can.

I woke up barely able to breathe. My body was numb and frozen. I heard people desperately calling out my name and scrambling all around me. I tried to call back, but my voice was just a whisper. Finally, I felt the warmth of someone's hand against my left cheek attempting to protect my face from the frost-bitten ground. I remember feeling a sense of security, but yet a little uncertainty, because at this point I wasn't sure whether I was imagining it all or not. I cautiously opened my eyes and sighed with relief . . . *I am alive.*

The fire and police departments arrived at the scene and were very cautious about moving me, due to a possible neck injury. They successfully stabilized me and transported me by Flight for Life to Froedtert Memorial Hospital in Milwaukee, Wisconsin.

My designated driver was arrested at the scene for driving under the influence of alcohol and later was charged with first-degree reckless endangerment and causing bodily harm while intoxicated. His blood alcohol level was .21, more than 2 times the legal limit. I was the only one injured and of course the designated driver, who irresponsibly put so many lives in danger, was completely unharmed.

In just mere seconds my life changed without any warnings, and I was now forced to live my life as a quadriplegic at the age of 24. Imagine somebody chopping your head off, putting you in bed, and turning the lights off. It was a very traumatic experience. I felt almost child-like.

The next time I woke up, I was in the hospital in the intensive care unit. That strange numbness continued to flow throughout my body. C3, C5, and C6 of my spinal cord were injured, which basically meant that I was paralyzed from the chest down, also known as quadriplegia. I spent the next 2 months in the hospital with a vigorous schedule everyday consisting of intense occupational, physical, and recreational therapy.

The capabilities I once took for granted, like brushing my teeth, writing, doing my hair and makeup, going to the bathroom on my own, and walking, all had new meaning to me. It was like starting my life all over again, only in a much harder sense. The main difference was that this time I knew what I was missing and it was a hard concept to grasp on to.

At such a young age it was hard to accept the fact that I would not be able to do any of these activities on my own, but I chose to keep fighting. I chose not to look back, not to change, and just be myself. I do not blame anyone for what has happened to me because my situation is not going to change if I did. I just look forward and move ahead. I am still that strong, determined individual that I was before, but I am in a wheelchair now. I have the same personality, attitude, and ambition. I keep my hope and faith and I do not let anyone take that hope away from me. I stay optimistic, because in my heart I know that the future holds something good for me. I truly believe that my faith has been the number one ingredient in getting through these difficult times for me.

Today, after many hard and painful days of therapy, I am at a C-6 level in my right arm and at a C-5 level in my left, which means that I have both wrist and biceps, but I am much stronger on my right side. With therapy and determination I have learned how to brush my teeth, apply my makeup, write, and work on my computer; all completely independently, just to name a few. It has not been easy and it has been a painful journey, but I stayed focused and I did not give up.

One very important piece of advice I would like to share with everyone is how critical therapy is in moving forward and learning how to simply live life again in this capacity; in a wheelchair. I think this issue needs to be strongly addressed to every patient. I had and continue to have a great support system between my friends and family, but most of all I had the most dedicated and qualified occupational therapist, Debbie, who gave me the motivation and encouragement I needed to persevere. Debbie reminded me everyday that no matter what had happened to me physically, I was still the same Jenny and my body may have changed, but my paralysis did not have to define me as an individual. She believed in me when I needed someone to believe in me the most and helped me to stay focused on what was important during the most critical time of my recovery. She reassured me that my life did not have to end just because I was now physically challenged. This was just a new chapter in my life and a new beginning.

One other very important aspect to a successful recovery is that I work hard at keeping relationships as much the same as before the accident as possible, for example, my relationship with my boyfriend at the time. This is not easy because of course there are always unexpected problems and obstacles when dealing with a spinal cord injury. I have caregivers come every morning and night to help me with my bowel program, catheterizing, showering, dressing, and whatever other personal cares I may need. My boyfriend and I were living together, and so it gave him the opportunity to go to work or go to the gym and personal space. This is so important for any personal relationship. Sometimes this type of situation is harder on the caregiver than it is for us, the ones being cared for. Of course, there were situations when I needed personal help and care from him, such as catheterizing, which I did every 4–6 hours, and when dealing with an injury of this magnitude, there is always the unexpected, such as your bowels working voluntarily. When something like this happens to a person, there is a loss of dignity and privacy. He never made a big scene about any personal situations and I needed that, especially in an intimate relationship. At the time, I didn't know what I would have done without him. He helped to give me the strength and confidence that I needed to keep going.

Over time, our lives became very strained and stressed, but I tried to make the best out of such an unfortunate situation. About 3 $\frac{1}{2}$ years after the accident my boyfriend, the designated driver on the night of my accident, and I broke up for many reasons. I was growing up and changing, but he was staying the same. Every promise he had made to me after the accident, from a wheelchair accessible home to practicing total sobriety or to never drink and drive again, kept going unanswered. I was so unhappy and knew that I needed to make some changes in order for happiness to exist in my life again. Of course, I had many concerns, such as where was I going to live, finances, and dating. Why would anyone want to choose me as a partner over an able-bodied woman? I felt like we were distant as a couple as well. I didn't see him look at me the same anymore and felt myself falling completely out of love with him. We didn't even kiss anymore. I knew that I deserved more than he was giving me. I felt like I was headed down a road of despair and depression. I could not go down that same road and watch him continue destroying my life or yet someone else's. It was very confusing to see him drink again, and it was even more confusing to hear that he had gotten behind the wheel drunk again. I was realizing qualities about this individual that I had never noticed before, such as his lack of care for me, and I needed to get out. So after he neglected me on many levels, I found the courage to leave. I left before he destroyed my life even more than he already had. Along with a disability comes significant financial needs, and from the moment this all began he promised that no matter what, he would always take on the financial responsibilities I had in the future due to the car accident, because he was the driver who was responsible for causing my injury. Plus, he did not want to be sued and he did have the means to help me financially. So I had no reason not to believe his promises. I was entirely wrong, though; he did not see that promise through. I shouldn't have put so much trust in him, should have sued him from the start, and should have looked after myself. If only I knew back then what I know now.

I think intimate relationships and dating are huge concerns for people in wheelchairs. Even though I may be paralyzed, it doesn't mean that I do not have the same needs and urges as every other individual, disabled or able-bodied, has. Everything on the inside works exactly the same as before. My menstrual cycle works the same, and I can still get pregnant. Believe it or not, I can still have an orgasm! People forget that sexual urges are controlled by your mind, and so if you are emotionally, as well as physically, invested in a partner it can be just as, if not more, rewarding being in a relationship with someone disabled.

I am currently dating someone who is one of the most sincere and genuine people I have ever met. A lot of people are intimidated by the wheelchair, but in my experience I have found that if the opposite sex approaches me, they are most likely very caring, sincere, and genuine people. It takes a lot of guts and a very special person to get involved with an individual who has a disability, and so when it happens to us we need to take advantage of the sincerity, open up, and let them in. I did and it is the best thing that has ever happened to me.

Before my accident I had worked at a bank for 6 years. I started there as a bank teller, received multiple promotions, and then 2 months prior to my accident I reached my goal and was promoted to an officer of the bank. Immediately after my accident my intentions were to go back to work at the bank, but when the time came after a year and a half, the home office wanted to send me to another location doing a totally different job. My job functions would consist of answering telephones in the basement with no face-to-face contact with the customers. My occupational therapist looked over my job functions and duties and found that everything could be adapted to qualify me to go back to my original position. There was only one duty, tearing a traveler's check out of a book, that they found to be a problem and the home office focused on that like a sore thumb. I was extremely upset, because before my accident I did above and beyond what was expected of me and I was a very dedicated employee. I felt that I earned and deserved more than they were giving. I was very disappointed and walked away without making an issue out of it. Now, I wish I would have pursued it legally and set an example for others in similar situations.

Through my experience I have found that it does not matter whether or not you have a disability, how old you are, your race, or sex. We are all equal. You should always treat others with the respect they deserve and the way you would like to be treated. No one should be discriminated against for any reason. I would not have decided to go back to work if I didn't think I could handle it. I want to succeed and I know it would have worked out. To this day after seeing how far I have come, I have realized that they are the ones missing out, not me. I am very disappointed in them, and I cannot believe how ignorant and insensitive they are. I realized that it is not a place that I want to work or even be associated with.

I sometimes become very sad over the loss of not only my job but also my dignity, control over everyday functions, and independence, and of many feelings and emotions that go along with everyday living. When these unfortunate feelings find their way out I realize how easy it is to give up, but I know that once I let these feelings take over, it could mean the end of my progress, happiness, and everything I have worked so hard for. I would eventually go down hill, and this injury would get the best of me, but I am not giving up that easily! I try to stay focused and I remember the goals I have promised myself.

On May 6, 1999, I was chosen to represent the state of Wisconsin as Ms. Wheelchair Wisconsin. That experience gave me the opportunity to become more involved in my community and the state as an advocate, not only for women in wheelchairs but also for the physically challenged in general. I also was given the opportunity to represent the state of Wisconsin in the national pageant, Ms. Wheelchair America, in Fort Lauderdale, Florida. My platform was simple, the consequences of drinking and driving.

Since the pageant, I highly promote and advocate for the Ms. Wheelchair Wisconsin's Association. I believe that we need to bring public awareness to this accomplishment and make the public aware of the meaning behind this pageant. It is not a beauty pageant and you are not judged on how you look in a bikini, but on your personal achievements since the onset of your disability, your attitude, and your inner beauty. We need to stress that having a disability is not the end of the world, but an opportunity to share the privilege of life and all it has to offer.

I have gone back and forth with my career, since I began this journey and struggled with whether I could have a purpose on this Earth again, in this capacity, in a wheelchair. I've always wanted to know that what I am doing with my life is working to the most of my potential and is making a difference in the world. Nothing will change the fact that I am paralyzed, and so I know that I have two choices, either to be angry confined to a wheelchair or to be happy confined to a wheelchair. I chose the latter.

Today, I am a motivational, inspirational, and educational speaker. I speak at a countless number of schools, colleges, universities, churches, conventions, and conferences on issues ranging from drinking and driving, abusive relationships, overcoming adversity, good decision making, and overall, the car accident itself, just to name a few. I want these young adults to see that this can happen to anyone. I did not think it would happen to me, but it did.

I have been a board member for the Bryon Riesch Paralysis Foundation for about 10 years. Our sole purposes are to raise money for spinal cord injury research and work to promote the quality of life for the physically challenged. I hold my faith and hope for a cure someday close to my heart, not necessarily for myself, but for my nieces, nephews, and future generations.

I am a model and committee member for the Fashion Show for All Abilities. The fashion show's purpose is a community awareness event, highlighting the reality that persons with disabilities are valuable customers and that businesses benefit by extending courtesy and respect to them. It focuses on issues such as too narrow aisles, inaccessible dressing rooms, and poorly trained salespeople. The mission is to educate and bring awareness to society on the concept that "fashion is for everyone."

I currently work with an online magazine for women in wheelchairs called mobileWOMEN.org, as an advice columnist. My column, "Hey Jen," is a safe, interactive forum, whether physically challenged or not, to discuss anything and everything that may be on your mind, such as fashion, dating, sex, or serious real-life issues. It's a site that gives you a boost of inspiration if needed or someone to listen to your personal struggles who truly understand. If you feel it, live it, hurt from it, are interested in it, or are just curious about it, I encourage people to share it and discuss it with me, because I've either felt it, have lived it, was hurt by it, am interested in it, or had the curiosity about it myself! Nothing is too personal in my book!

I am a volunteer member and Membership Coordinator for the Waushara County Chapter. Our goal is to help create, support, and protect just one small portion within our county of the Wisconsin Ice Age Trail. I came on board when the chapter asked me to help fundraise for the Bohn Lake Accessible Hiking Trail Project in Waushara County. I am proud to say that the accessible hiking trail is no longer just a vision; it is a reality! I am also a volunteer and member of the Ice Age Trail, Alliance (IATA). The IATA is a volunteer and member-based organization working to create, support, and protect the Ice Age National Scenic Trail. The 1200 mile trail, winding through Wisconsin, traces world-renowned Ice Age features. The trail serves as both a monument to the state's glacial heritage and a premier recreational resource. The IATA is a nonprofit organization dedicated to preserving Wisconsin's glacial heritage for the education and enjoyment of present and future generations.

I am the Founder of the Web site www.InspirationSpeaks.me and have been an advocate and volunteer for groups such as the National Spinal Cord Injury Association (NSCIA), Home Care Consumer Advisory Committee (HCCAC), and the Aging and Disability Resource Center (ADRC). My goals in the future include publishing my biography and a new piece called "A Note to God." I also hope to have a family and children of my own someday!

Some of my greatest assets include my positive attitude, outgoing personality, and a very optimistic outlook on the future. I am confident that medical research is close to finding cures for so many neurological diseases and disorders and optimistic that the quality of life will keep improving for so many deserving people. I truly believe that if a person has the hope, miracles can happen! I hold my faith close to my heart and I do not let anyone take it away. Therefore, no matter what, I wake up looking forward to a new and prosperous day.

One of the greatest barriers I face on a daily basis, as do others living with a physical challenge, is the lack of wheelchair accessibility all over the country. I love to travel, and more than once I have experienced problems with airports breaking my wheelchair, rude and insensitive employees, unaffordable prices, and delayed pickups. I have also had to call 24 hours in advance to reserve accessible transportation and even then it is sometimes impossible to find. I believe that education and public awareness are the keys to progress and making wheelchair accessibility consistent and successful. Stronger and more powerful legislation and new laws are the answer. We must demand that these laws be implemented and enforced in order to end discrimination and to provide equal opportunities. The disabled are contributing citizens and deserve ready access to all the promises of American life. Unfortunately, this will be an issue that will be around for a long time, so as an individual who is physically challenged, I understand that there may be situations I will have to work around, try to deal with them appropriately and effectively at that moment, and work on changing them. Some advice I would suggest is patience and understanding. With education lacking in this area, the best thing to do is to bring awareness to the issue within the community and demand that the necessary changes are made for the future.

One of the biggest messages I want to convey to society is that just because a person may be in a wheelchair or dealing with a physical challenge does not mean that they are different from anyone else. We have the exact same needs and wants as any other individual in society. I am a motivational speaker for many reasons: one being to change these misperceptions and stereotypes about others who may be living life with a physical or mental challenge. I personally do not want to be defined by my disability. Everyone is molded together differently, which makes us the unique individuals we are. Our individuality should not be judged as being normal or not normal. I believe that as a society, we need to get past the outer appearance of a person and look at their inner beauty. Inside everyone has similar feelings and deal with the same issues of everyday living. If you pay close attention you will find that we all have a lot in common and everyone is dealing with some type of handicap, mine happens to be physical, which is easy to connect with visually, but someone else may be struggling with depression, alcoholism, or obesity, just to name a few. This is something we, not only the disabled population but also the able-bodied as well, need to work on, educating and bringing awareness within our communities to the fact that people in wheelchairs or with any disability are their equals.

Overall, considering the obstacles and struggles I face each and every day, my life is headed in a positive direction. I think about how close I came to losing the opportunity to spend time being an auntie to my six nieces and nephews, another moment reminiscing with family and friends, developing a new healthy relationship with my boyfriend, cuddling with my puppies, or even just watching the sunset. We all take these things for granted, which is a natural response, but sometimes we need to step back and remember that these are God-given gifts, privileges, not rights. We all need to work on respecting the value of life and to understand that it can all be taken away faster than the blink of an eye. My goal is to help bring awareness to the community and remind every person I interact with just how precious life is. To most, I have lost everything to this tragic accident, but really God has blessed me with understanding something most people will never realize in a lifetime ... the significance of life.

DISCUSSION QUESTIONS

1. Have students make a list of the top personal attributes they find most desirable in a partner and then discuss the impact of personal values upon partner selection.

2. Discuss anyone's experience with a family member or friend with a disability related to dating attempts or experiences.

3. Ask students to discuss their own feelings about the impact of media on body image and how it has affected them personally.

4. Discuss the case of a person who chooses to raise a child without the use of arms. Then watch "Amazing Woman with No Arms" on You Tube at http://www. youtube.com/watch?v=__mo1JXmi7U

EXERCISES

A. For a class activity, have students role play an interview with a person who is disabled asking about sexual issues or concerns.

B. For a class group activity, have students debate the topic of parenting for persons who have severe disabilities, with one group supporting parenting and another group arguing against.

C. For a homework assignment, have students interview a person with a disability using an online support group about what is important in a long-term relationship with a partner.

EIGHT

The Psychosocial World of the Injured Worker

Irmo Marini

OVERVIEW

The chronically injured worker is perhaps one of the most fascinating psychosocial topics relating to disability. Work in Western society is a coveted way of life that often dictates on which side of the tracks one will live, who one's friends are, our social status, socioeconomic status, health care and mortality rate, and who our spouse or partner will be. In essence, for most Americans and especially males, work often defines who they are and their self-concept (Chubon, 1994; Newman, Perry, & Pan, 1985; Sager & James, 2005). Indeed, in Western society, one of the immediate questions we are asked by new acquaintances at social gatherings is, "So what do you do for a living?"

For the chronically injured worker, negotiating the often confusing and sometimes dehumanizing gauntlet of receiving workers' compensation benefits (WCB) for employees fortunate enough to have coverage may quickly turn into an injured worker's nightmare (Binder, 1992; Dodier, 1985; Fallenbaum, 2003; Gribich, McGartland, & Polgar, 1998; Willis, 1986). In this chapter, we explore a number of topics related to the world of work, the psychological impact of disability on the disabled worker, the impact of chronic pain, systemic problems in the WCB and Social Security Administration's (SSA) programs, key players in the gauntlet, the impact on the family of an injured worker, and the discipline of disability management (DM).

DISABILITY DEMOGRAPHICS

There are currently over 57.6 million Americans collecting some form of Social Security benefits, with 5.7 million awarded benefits in 2009 alone. Seventeen percent or 971,000 of these beneficiaries were workers with disabilities (Turpin, 2010). The SSA conceded several years ago that with the aging of America and fewer workers paying into the SSA trust fund, it is expected to exhaust its funds by 2037, and has already begun to pay out more disability insurance than it annually collects (Turpin). The average monthly wage supplement for males in 2009 was $1,189, and for females $925, both well under the poverty levels in the United States. Disability payments alone were made to approximately 11.7 million Americans aged 18–64, disabled children, and widowers.

Workers' compensation statistics are more difficult to come by since they are compiled separately by each state. Recent national statistic trends indicate that in 2004, federal programs paid workers' compensation medical and cash benefit expenditures of over $56 billion, while nonfederal employers paid out $87.4 billion, up over 7% from 2003, covering an estimated 125.9 million employees (Sengupta & Reno, 2007). A 5-year comprehensive study by California's Division of Workers' Compensation from 2000 to 2005 used a sample of over 91,000 injured workers and found that return-to-work rates were highest for those with elbow, grip, hands, and toe injuries at approximately 77% within 12 months. Conversely, the lowest return-to-work rates were for mental illness (52%), head injuries (57%), and low-back spine injuries, at 60% (DWC, 2007). The most common type of workers' compensation injury claims are low-back injuries at approximately 50% (Newman et al., 1985). A study by Webster and Snook (1989) found that for low-back injury claims, 25% of claimants accounted for 96% of the WCB costs for that year. Similarly, Hashemi, Webster, Clancy, and Volinn (1997) noted in 1992, of 100,000 low-back injury claims, 10% of the claims accounted for 86% of the total costs to the system.

Demographic information about injured workers is also interesting (see International Rehabilitation Associates, Inc. 1981, in Newman et al., 1985). Research suggests that over 66% of injured workers are male, and over 65% of all work injuries take place performing blue-collar, physical labor-type work where lifting, bending, and carrying heavy materials are required. Beals and Hickman (1972) found the average educational level of injured workers to be grade 9. The incidence of chronic low-back pain with or without surgery is evident in over 90% of cases. It appears that states with the highest level of reported disability cases, otherwise known as the "disability belt," are mostly those found in the southeastern part of the United States, where poorly educated workers engage in physically demanding and dangerous jobs, such as mining, fieldwork, factory work, and related manufacturing and processing jobs (Erickson, Lee, & Von Schrader, 2010).

WORKERS' COMPENSATION

Germany developed the first form of industrial accident insurance in 1884, and the United States began similar efforts in 1908 with congressional enactment of the Federal Employers' Liability Act designed to provide insurance to federal workers (Sengupta & Reno, 2007). By 1920, 42 of the 48 states had workers' compensation statutes. Workers' compensation insurance is essentially a promise, compromise, and contract between workers and employers. In essence, workers give up the right to sue an employer for a work injury in exchange of an employer-based promise covering full medical care and wage replacement benefits regardless of fault. This agreement has been beneficial for injured workers who previously used to lose over 95% of all lawsuits due to having the burden of proof that the employer was negligent. The three most common successful arguments employers used in their defense were: (a) *assumption of risk doctrine*—whereby the employee was aware or should have been aware of the job hazards; (b) *fellow-servant doctrine*—essentially claiming that if a coworker was negligent, the employer could not be held responsible; and the (c) *contributory negligence doctrine*—where the worker had to prove that he/she was not careless and essentially did not contribute to the injury (Bevan, 1996; Matkin, 1995).

Although workers' compensation has indeed dramatically decreased the number of lawsuits brought against employers by their injured employees, and the no-fault agreement has mainly been very successful, it has not been without its problems (Bevan, 1996; Fallenbaum, 2003; Gribich et al., 1998). Bevan (1996) describes gray areas where a presumed work injury is covered by defining injuries sustained "in the course of" and "arising out of" the worker's employment. Examples such as driving to/from work, stopping for personal reasons along the way, and engaging in social activities, such as work-related entertainment, may all end up being argued in court. In addition, occupational diseases, such as lead poisoning, asbestos, and other body deteriorating conditions, become more difficult to prove. Indeed, Bevan indicates that the workplace causes some 6%–10% of cancer cases, and 5%–10% of coronary heart disease and cerebrovascular disease.

When Trust Breaks Down in Workers' Compensation Claims

Statistically, over 66% of injured workers return to work (RTW) within 6 months post-injury, an additional 17% within a year, and the remaining 16% have not returned after 12 months (Shrey, 1995). Research suggests that for a variety of reasons, the longer an individual is off work, the less likely he/she will ever return (Pati, 1985; Waddell & Sawney, 2002). In many instances, employer and employee distrust becomes heightened with the passage of time. Employer-paid insurance adjusters and/or case managers may directly or indirectly insinuate that the injured worker is feigning or exaggerating the injury for secondary gain (e.g., medical and wage benefits, family sympathy and attention, avoiding grueling work or work conditions) (Hadler, Carey, & Garrett, 1995). On the other hand, the injured employee often views the employer and workers' compensation personnel as uncaring, and may seek out an attorney for representation, especially if the employee has been terminated after reaching maximum medical improvement (Rogers & Payne, 2006; Shrey, 1995; Tarasuk & Eakin, 1995). Once the employer/employee relationship and trust has deteriorated to this point, employers may resort to videotape surveillance of the injured worker with the hope of catching him performing heavy lifting work, and thus contradicting what he has indicated he is otherwise able to do. In being able to produce such evidence, employers hope to reduce or negate any settlement, or to stop paying WCB.

Prior to this point, however, the buildup of employee anger, confusion, and exasperation involves several factors and people (Rogers & Payne, 2006; Shrey, 1995). Since chronic pain is common in over 90% of cases, most of the injured workers often do not feel capable of returning. Unfortunately, there are no conclusive diagnostic tests that can validate a patient's pain complaints, and doctors otherwise are left with the patient's subjective experience, typically using a visual analog scale of 1–10 (10 signifying a need to go to the emergency room). The confusion starts when the workers' compensation physician and often the patient's family physician attempt to determine when the injured worker has reached maximum medical improvement, what the work restrictions are, and when the injured worker can RTW (Rogers & Payne, 2006; Shrey, 1995). Although supposedly objective medical opinions should be rendered, in most instances, the workers' compensation physician typically gives a more liberal prognosis indicating that the worker is able to RTW with few restrictions. The injured worker's family physician or one who has treated him at length, most often has almost completely opposite opinions (Bevan, 1996; Newman et al., 1985; Rogers & Payne, 2006; Sager & James, 2005).

Other key people involved may also give the injured worker conflicting messages. An initial supporting spouse postinjury may become resentful over time with mounting financial problems, family role changes, social and emotional withdrawal of the injured spouse, and perceived lack of effort to help out with any homemaking or child care (Newman et al., 1985; Sachs & Ellenberg, 1994). The case manager may be perceived as pushing too hard for the injured worker to attend therapy, appointments, and RTW, despite complaints of pain and fears of reinjury (Fallenbaum, 2003; Newman et al., 1985). Some injured workers feel the same way about insurance adjusters and a perceived unsympathetic employer (Gilbride et al., 2000; Sager & James, 2005). Once an attorney is consulted, he/she may advise the injured worker not to RTW for fear of it minimizing a potential settlement (Newman et al., 1985). Overall, many injured workers who have not encountered the system in this fashion before, often experience additional somatic pain complaints due to the added stress of litigation.

NEXT STOP, SOCIAL SECURITY BENEFITS

If an injured worker has been severely injured and is medically deemed not only unable to return to his or her former job but also unable to return to any type of work for 12 months or longer, he or she is permanently disabled from a vocational standpoint (Robles & Marini, 2005). Some injured workers may have what is called a "closed period" of disability, such as two broken legs, and are unable to work for 12 months or longer; however, those with more serious and permanent injuries will likely be off work indefinitely. Robles and Marini cite SSA statistics that indicate that less than 1% of all awarded beneficiaries ever return to gainful employment. Process-wise, an injured worker, if covered by workers' compensation, will first be placed on WCB for a limited time, depending on state workers' compensation laws, and then once those are exhausted and if the worker is still unable to RTW, he or she will file for Supplemental Security Disability Insurance (SSDI) and/or Social Security Income (SSI) with the SSA. The entire process may take several months to several years if there are multiple denials.

This process is once again more expedient for unquestionable medically severe injuries. Persons with spinal cord injuries or severe head injuries typically are awarded benefits as soon as they apply. For injured workers with less severe injuries, such as low-back herniated disc(s) or carpal tunnel syndrome, convincing others is often a much greater struggle (Bevan, 1996; Marini, 2003; Marini & Reid, 2001). In such cases, where the impact of a diskectomy or laminectomy surgery has no demonstrative effect on reducing subjective chronic pain complaints, injured workers must begin a long and stressful ordeal in trying to "prove" that they are totally disabled and cannot work (Hanson & Gerber, 1990, p. 6).

Applying for SSDI benefits and/or SSI has five levels of appeal (Robles & Marini, 2005). Persons applying with perceived lesser or questionable disabilities are often turned down when initially submitting their paperwork to the SSA (Scheer, 1995, p. 192). Statistics show varying levels of success for applicants with each appealed denial decision up to, and including, the U.S. District Court. Much like the vastly different medical opinions rendered by the workers' compensation physician and the injured worker's family doctor, Social Security-appointed physicians conducting independent medical evaluations (IMEs) once again are very different than the family physician (Bevan, 1996). The SSA physician often renders the claimant capable of working and performing heavier work than the family physician or one retained by the claimant's representative. The family or representative retained physician often opines that the injured worker is totally vocationally disabled (Rogers & Payne, 2006; Sager & James, 2005). Physician objectivity in these common decision differences call into question physician competence and/or ethics, once again leaving the injured worker confused and frustrated.

A PRIMER ON THE IMPLICATIONS OF CHRONIC PAIN

Chronic pain is generally described as pain that lasts longer than 6 months (Gatchel, 1996). Perhaps the most insidious culprit of diminished RTW efforts of injured workers is due to subjective complaints of chronic pain (Tait, 2004; Williams, 2004). In order to have a better understanding of the injured worker's world and RTW, the implications of chronic pain are often the elephant in the room. We briefly explore the anatomy, theory, and assessment of chronic pain, as well as later describing the psychosocial impact of chronic pain on the injured worker. As noted earlier, chronic pain costs the United States over $125 billion per year in treatment and lost work productivity (Arnoff, 1998). Despite advances in medical technology, surgery, therapy, and psychopharmacology, Feuerstein and Zastowny (1996) cite government statistics indicating that work-related musculoskeletal disorders and subsequent chronic pain account for 60% of all occupational illnesses (Bureau of Labor Statistics, 1991). These disorders often include repetitive motion damage involving the tendons, bones, muscles, and nerves related to the back, wrist, elbows, hands, arms, or legs. As such, pain complaints related to musculoskeletal disorders are the most frequent reason for primary care physician visits (Deyo & Tsui-Wi, 1987).

The most common International Classification of Disability (ICD-10-CM, 2010) diagnostic low-back pain conditions are herniated discs (most frequently L4–L5), degenerative changes such as spondylosis, spinal stenosis involving cord compression, lumbosacral joint instability, spondylolisthesis, lumbago, postlaminectomy syndrome, sciatica, and sprains and strains (Feuerstein & Zastowny, 1996). Nerve-related injuries include brachial plexus lesions, carpal tunnel syndrome, lesions of the ulnar nerve, and thoracic outlet syndrome. Common tendon- and muscle-related disorders are cervicalgia (neck pain), shoulder rotator cuff syndrome, bicipital tenosynovitis, and lateral epicondylitis (tennis elbow).

Interestingly, contrary to popular belief (Samra & Koch, 2002), many physicians estimate that fewer than 5% of all low-back pain patients are malingerers or exaggerate their symptoms for secondary gain (Fordyce, 1995; Hadjistavropoulos, 1999). Rogers and Payne (2006) noted how claimants complaints of pain are often disregarded, and how they become upset when physicians or others suggest that the pain may be psychological. Biddle, Roberts, Rosenman, and Welch (1998) report, however, that many workers may actually be underreporting their work-related injuries. Brooker, Frank, and Tarasuk (1997) noted that economic factors also play a role in pursuing disability claims. Specifically, the authors found that during economic booms, chronic low-back pain claims increased; however, in economic downturns when jobs were sparse, similar claims decreased.

Pain Models

Only two theories are briefly discussed here, and for a more comprehensive discussion on these topics, the reader is referred to *Psychological Approaches to Pain Management* by Gatchel and Turk (1996) as well as the *Psychosocial Aspects of Pain: A Handbook for Healthcare Providers* by Dworkin and Breitbart (2004). Briefly, the Gate Control Theory (GCT) of pain proposed by Melzack and Wall (1965) integrates both physical and psychological factors of three systems in processing nociceptive stimulation—sensory-discriminative, motivational-affective, and cognitive-evaluative subjective experience of pain. The GCT model incorporates somatic and psychogenic factors, noting acute pain responses to be primarily reflexive (dorsal horn nerve input of the spinal cord and processing in the brain), but later potentially exacerbated by psychological influences, such as mood, motivation, secondary gain, and so on.

The biopsychosocial model focuses less on the physiological or anatomical aspects of chronic pain and centers more on the behavioral and psychosocial factors, including symptom reporting, and the cognitive, emotional, and behavioral responses to treatment (Turk, 2004). For example, Deyo (1986) found that of approximately 80% of patients complaining of back pain, no physical basis for pain could be identified, and 30%–50% of patients who seek treatment for pain have no diagnosable disorder (Dworkin & Massoth, 1994). The biopsychosocial model focuses on chronic pain as an illness, not a disease. Turk differentiates the two by describing disease as "an objective biological event that involves disruption of specific body structures or organ systems caused by pathological, anatomical, or physiological changes" (Turk, 1996, p. 7). Conversely, illness is described as "a subjective experience or self-attribution that a disease is present; it yields physical discomfort, emotional distress, behavioral limitations, and psychosocial disruption" (Turk, 1996, p. 7). It is this inter-action between biological, social, and psychological variables that holistically describe the experience of chronic pain. Turk noted how these variables may influence one another. For example, an individual who does not engage in muscle strengthening exercise and as a result becomes physically deconditioned may exacerbate pain due to inactivity. This model also takes into consideration studies involving the placebo effect, and how in numerous instances, chronic pain can be reduced with a placebo (fake pain pill) and sympathetic understanding (Blanchard, 1987; Deyo, Walsh, & Martin, 1990; Greene & Laskin, 1974).

Psychosocial Impact of Disability and Pain on the Injured Worker

The end result for the injured worker in this perplexing gauntlet of often time-consuming opposing opinions in having to prove that he or she is totally disabled inevitably adds to psychological and somatic complaints of chronic pain. Prolonged litigation-added stress, with mounting litigation and medical costs as attorneys from each side retain experts whose opinions are frequently 180-degrees opposite one another, generally exacerbates the claimant's condition (Conte & Van Antwerp, 1995). Gribich et al. (1998) discuss the medicolegal implications in workers' compensation litigation and the conflicting roles of physicians as gatekeepers and service providers that ultimately contribute to the stigmatization of injured workers being perceived as malingerers. The authors conducted in-depth interviews with injured workers who complained about physician judgmental attitudes, lack of support from the workplace, hostile treatment from workers' compensation personnel, and having to repeatedly tell their stories to perceived unsympathetic audiences.

Sager and James (2005) similarly interviewed six formerly employed injured women regarding their perspectives going through the workers' compensation system. The women reported confusion and lack of knowledge of the rehabilitation process, perceived lack of support and feeling alone with a sense that no one was on their side, unsatisfying RTW options, and covert discrimination from coworkers, management, and the insurance company with threats of losing their jobs if they did not return. The authors noted the combination of these factors as primary reasons why many injured workers do not want to RTW.

Crook, Milner, Schultz, and Stringer (2002) cited over 2,000 published articles in which researchers had attempted to identify predictors of low-back disability, noting that previous attempts had failed due to being biomedical in nature. Schultz et al. (2004) attempted to develop an RTW predictive model based on psychosocial factors in the cases of 253 subacute and acute chronic pain injured workers. The authors' model was more successful in predicting who would RTW as opposed to who would not, with the two greatest predictors being perceived expectations of recovery and health change. In addition, but to a lesser extent, coworker support, positive versus negative interactions with workers' compensation and the employer, and occupational stability also predicted RTW. Although earlier studies have cited psychological distress such as depression, anxiety, and related pain emotions as being negative RTW factors, the Crook study did not find these factors to be significant (Asmundson & Norton, 1995; Linton, 2000; Turk, 2002).

Overall, hundreds of predictive RTW studies have rendered a number of fairly consistent findings as to the medicolegal-psychosocial reasons why some injured workers may never return to gainful employment. In the vast majority of cases, chronic pain is inevitably linked to the primary disability. Feuerstein, Menz, Zastowny, and Barron (1994) reviewed the literature and delineated five predictive RTW categories for 1 year postinjury work-related chronic pain patients. The predictive indices included medical history, demographics, physical findings, pain, and psychosocial factors. Implicated in poor RTW were higher reported pain severity (Polatin & Mayer, 1992); lower levels of satisfaction with treatment (Hazard, Haugh, Green, & Jones, 1994); lower levels of pain management cooperation (Barnes, Smith, Gatchel, & Mayer, 1989); and higher levels of reported hypochondrias, distrust, depression, and premorbid pessimism (Barnes et al., 1989). In addition, other predictors of RTW showing promise include passive coping, fear-avoidance beliefs, catastrophizing, and internal locus of control (Burton, Tilloston, Main, & Hollis, 1995; Cole, Mondlock, & Hogg-Johnson, 2002; Jensen, Romano, Turner, Good, & Wald, 1999).

Other predictors of injured worker RTW have explored the external or environmental factors involved. Feuerstein and Zastowny (1996) and others summarize external factors, including harsh work demands, job dissatisfaction, poor coworker and employer support, job stress, poor family support, ongoing litigation, and financial disincentives to RTW (Antoniazzi, Celinski, & Alcock, 2002; Marini, 2003; Newman et al., 1985; Rogers & Payne, 2006; Tait, 2004). As noted earlier, the longer workers are out of work, the less likely they are ever to return (Marini & Reid, 2001; Tait, 2004).

Cognitions

Injured workers with chronic pain sometimes have similar negative thinking patterns regarding beliefs about their circumstances and recovery (Chapman & Okifuji, 2004; Gatchel, 1996). Individual's who perceive that they will not recover, are distrustful of the medical system, and do not engage in therapeutic conditioning are less likely to recover (Williams & Keefe, 1991). Flor and Turk (1989) noted how individuals appraise their bodily functions and how these bodily functions impact their physiological responses, and vice versa. Some individuals catastrophize their situations and generally do not recover as well as those who are not as pessimistic. Drukteinis (2004) further describes the observation that for those individuals who believe that they will not recover, this often becomes a self-fulfilling prophecy and leads to learned helplessness. This is perhaps no more evident than when persons with disabilities are applying for Social Security benefits and must prove that they are totally disabled and cannot work (Marini, 2003; Marini & Reid, 2001). It is also evident in ongoing workers' compensation claims where workers are thought to be malingering (Bevan, 1996).

Beliefs, appraisals, and expectancies about the disability and related pain are central concepts in recovery (Turk, 1996). Many individuals differ in how they think about their disabilities and pain. Those who believe the pain to be beyond their control and do little to improve their situations are more likely to do nothing. Conversely, injured workers who trust the medical system believe that they can control or minimize the impact of their disabilities, and expect that positive outcomes tend to adapt better (Williams & Keefe, 1991).

Behavioral responses

Overlapping with one's cognitions is an individual's behavioral response to his or her beliefs, appraisals, and expectancies of disability and pain. Wiesenfeld-Hallin and Hallin (1984) describe the "vicious circle" of cognition and behavior in misinterpreting nociceptive pain responses. Specifically, the intense pain experienced during the acute injury itself is not soon forgotten. Injured workers often engage in fear-avoiding behaviors whereby they avoid any strenuous activity that may exacerbate their pain. They become hypervigilant to any stimuli that causes any discomfort, and thus begin the vicious circle of misinterpreting slight pain as potentially reinjuring themselves. This leads to ever-increasing sedentary activities, including afternoon naps, sitting in a recliner for long periods, and further deconditioning themselves. In this deconditioned state where weight gain is common, soon any discomfort from any activity is automatically stopped (Philips, 1987a).

Other common behavioral responses for injured workers with chronic pain involve social withdrawal from family and friends as well as outings (Newman et al., 1985). This withdrawal from what were once pleasurable activities may exacerbate depressive symptoms for the injured worker and/or his spouse and family (Lewinsohn, Clark, Hops, & Andrews, 1990; Newman et al., 1985). Sexual inactivity is also common not only because the act of intercourse itself may be painful but also because of low sex desire or negative side effects from medication (Ahern, Adams, & Follick, 1985; Maruta, Osborne, Swenson, & Holling, 1981; Polatin, 1996). Another potential poor coping problem is aberrant drug-seeking behavior for the injured worker who is addicted to pain medication, muscle relaxants, and/or antidepressants (Portnoy, 1994; Schoefferman, 1994). Some chronic pain patients go from doctor to doctor (aka hopping) looking for multiple prescription renewals and someone to validate their disabilities (Conte & Van Antwerp, 1995).

Emotional responses

The most common emotional responses of chronic pain patients are anxiety, depression, frustration, and anger (Gatchel, 1996; Newman et al., 1985). The Minnesota Multiphasic Personality Inventory (MMPI) has been used extensively to assess the psychological impact of chronic pain (Sternbach, 1974). Sternbach, Wolf, Murphy, and Akeson (1973) compared the MMPI profiles of patients with acute low-back pain against those patients with chronic low-back pain. What is commonly referred to as the "neurotic triad" from such profiles suggests that chronic pain sufferers abnormally spike on the scales of hysteria, depression, and hypochondria. With acute patients, the spikes are not evident; however, over time, the changes are believed to be attributable to financial worries, lack of sleep, constant discomfort, preoccupation with health, exhaustion, fewer friends, fewer interests, and despair (Gatchel, 1996; Sternbach, 1974). Turk (1996) has argued that the MMPI is an invalid assessment with this population because it is based on the medical model and does not take into consideration psychosocial factors.

Gatchel (1996) describes the mental deconditioning stages postinjury. During the initial stage, the individual experiences fear, anxiety, and worry regarding his or her situation and the future. With persisting pain after 2–4 months, Gatchel describes a second stage involving depression-learned helplessness, anxiety disorders and symptom magnification, and anger from distrust of the system and breakdown of perceived entitlement. Kerns, Rosenberg, and Jacob (1994) found that chronic pain patients had internalized anger regarding their pain intensity and frequency of pain behaviors, while Corbishley, Hendrickson, and Beutler (1990) found that 88% of patients they treated acknowledged feelings of anger and frustration over their circumstances. Finally, Gatchel (1996) describes stage three as patient acceptance of the sick role, with feelings of resignation and hopelessness. Beals (1984) noted how compensation issues can serve as disincentives for individuals in trying to get better. Fernandez and Turk (1995) further describe frustration related to ongoing symptoms, repeated treatment failures, and externally directed anger with the insurance provider, employer, health care system, and family members.

Finally, injured workers and others who experience chronic pain generally report co-occurring or reactive depression postinjury in 30%–54% of cases (Atkinson, Slater, Patterson, Grant, & Garfin, 1991; Banks & Kerns, 1996; Magni, Caldieron, Rigatti-Luchini, & Merskey, 1990). Rudy, Kerns, and Turk (1988) and others have found, however, that patients who appraised aspects of their pain as controllable and continue to function despite pain, generally reported less depression (Turk, Okifuji, & Scharff, 1995). Individuals with a preinjury history of depression or other psychiatric illness consistently show poorer recovery rates in chronic pain cases, and report higher levels of pain with more pain behaviors and perceived greater disability (Krause, Weiner, & Tait, 1994; Picus, Burton, Vogel, & Field, 2002).

Overall, the cognitions, behaviors, and emotions that injured workers transition through have been compared with stages of the grieving process (Newman et al., 1985). For those who are unable to RTW, the vast majority report chronic pain. Since the majority of injured workers have lower levels of education, little experience with the health care system, and little knowledge of their conditions, their reactions are often confusion, frustration, anxiety, and trepidation. With mixed messages coming from insurance adjusters, physicians, case managers, attorneys, and family members, injured workers with chronic pain becomes angered and distrusting of their employers and the medical system. An individual's beliefs, appraisal, and expectations often play a key role as to whether he or she will recover well enough to RTW (Gatchel, 1996; Turk, 1996). Injured workers who trust and believe in the medical system, who perceive that they have control over their situations, and who engage in rehabilitation with the expectation of recovery, statistically recover better.

Familial and Cultural Impact in the Lives of Injured Workers

As family and cultural differences have an impact on the adaptation of a family member with a disability, these factors are also critically important in the lives of injured workers. We have previously discussed the potential for financial and emotional stressors for family members as well as role changes, boundary problems, and intimacy difficulties (Rubin, 1979; Sachs & Ellenberg, 1994). An initially rallying, supportive family soon after a work injury occurs may become frustrated, overwhelmed, and resentful over time if the injured parent appears to be making little effort to help out with homemaking responsibilities or get better (Sachs & Ellenberg, 1994). However, in situations where resilient family members continue to reinforce pain behavior, research indicates that this can be counterproductive (Otis, Cardella, & Kerns, 2004). Specifically where pain is involved, studies show that when a spouse positively reinforces his or her injured partner (e.g., back rubs, taking away chores, making special meals), the injured partner displays a higher frequency of pain behaviors (e.g., facial grimaces, sighing, verbalizations) (Block, Kremer, & Gaylor, 1980; Lousberg, Schmidt, & Groenman, 1992; Turk, Kerns, & Rosenberg, 1992). Conversely, when a spouse negatively reacts, such as yelling or complaining to the injured partner, there is a higher frequency of partner emotional distress (Kerns, Haythornthwaite, Southwick, & Giller, 1990).

Reiss's (1989) family paradigms and cognitive schema suggest the importance of family appraisals, beliefs, and behaviors related to interactions with a family member with chronic pain. Very similar to how the individual with chronic pain perceives and reacts to his/her pain, family members' appraisals can dictate whether the entire family adapts well to the circumstances or becomes dysfunctional with life revolving around the injured loved one (Kerns & Payne, 1996). For families who reward an injured member's wellness behavior (e.g., when he or she exercises, watches weight, is productive) instead of reinforcing illness behaviors, this operant conditioning generally shows positive outcomes for decreasing pain behaviors (Fordyce, 1976; Sanders, 1996). Counselors can teach family members which behaviors to reinforce versus those that should be ignored. What unfortunately happens all too often is that family members sympathize with, and pay positive attention to, pain behaviors that have statistically been shown to increase with positive reinforcement (Kerns & Rosenberg, 1995; Lousberg et al., 1992; Otis et al., 2004; Turk et al., 1992).

Various studies have also suggested ethnic and racial differences in response to pain. In a study of 337 African Americans and Caucasians during an experimental pain threshold and tolerance comparison, African Americans reported less pain tolerance, higher levels of clinical pain, and greater perceived disability (Edwards, Doleys, Fillingim, & Lowery, 2001; Edwards & Fillingim, 1999). African Americans also perceive pain as more problematic than Caucasians in cases of glaucoma, jaw pain, migraine headaches, and myofascial pain (Faucett, Gordon, & Levine, 1994; Widmalm, Gunn, Christiansen, & Hawley, 1995).

Bates and Edwards (1992) studied Hispanic, Caucasians, Irish, Italians, French Canadians, and Polish pain clinic patients with regard to pain perceptions and behaviors. Although there were minor differences between these groups, the major finding was that Hispanic patients differed significantly from others in terms of more pain expressions, feeling less healthy, not working, frequency of pain complaints, and feeling resigned to their pain and the belief that an unhappy life was inevitable. Interestingly, persons of Hispanic backgrounds and other minorities generally receive poorer health care, and are prescribed less medication and less treatment than Caucasians (Chibnall & Tait, 2005; Todd, Samaroo, & Hoffman, 1993; Woodrow, Friedman, Siegelaub, & Collen, 1972).

Returning Injured Workers to Work

Worksite DM programs have empirically been shown to be effective in returning injured workers back to work (Shrey, 1995). The basic premise of DM programs is to have established in-house rehabilitation counselors or DM specialists working at the worksite with employees. Shrey (1995, p. 5) defines DM as "an active process of minimizing the impact of an impairment (resulting from illness, injury, or disease) on the individual's capacity to participate competitively in the environment". It is a proactive process that gives labor and management joint responsibility in designing and coordinating work-place interventions, such as disability prevention programs, wellness programs, and safe RTW programs, to control personal and economic costs of work injuries. DM specialists are trusted employees who work among the employees, and facilitate ongoing communication between management and the injured worker, giving both parties control over the RTW process, and conveying genuine concern in the worker's well-being. This communication and empathic concern minimizes lawsuit costs and workers generally RTW sooner (Cantlon, 1995; Conte & Van Antwerp, 1995; Shrey, 1995).

Boschen (1989) summarized early intervention with injured workers as having several positive psychosocial effects. Specifically, injured workers and their families are supported during the process before psychological problems develop, feelings of loneliness and abandonment are minimized, constant contact minimizes resentment and enhances trust, workers do not feel that they are getting the "runaround," secondary gains are minimized, and the injured worker is less likely to become comfortable in the sick role. Walker (1992) described how the long-wait periods, with little or no communication with injured workers in workers' compensation cases, often lead to experience helplessness and a sense of no control for the injured worker. Cost savings in workers' compensation claims where DM programs are available are well documented (Fruen, 1992; Habeck, 1991; Patenaude, 1989; Taulbee, 1991; Weinstein, 1993).

CONCLUSION

The psychological stress brought on to a chronically injured worker who in the end is unable to RTW is even more traumatic to the majority who suffer from chronic pain as well. A vicious behavioral cycle fueled by the fear of reinjury leads many injured workers to refrain from most physical activities that often facilitate an increase in deconditioning and weight gain. Without appropriate early intervention, many injured workers and their families soon experience financial difficulties, role changes, and communication problems. Psychologically, male injured workers frequently experience anxiety, depression, anger, and frustration worrying about the future and dealing with a confusing and often contradictory medical system. Vastly opposing medical opinions regarding ability to RTW and a seemingly uncaring employer often lead to distrust and eventually an embroiled litigation. Many injured workers socially withdraw, report a loss of self-esteem, and, in extreme cases, become addicted to prescription painkillers and/or alcohol.

Conversely, injured workers who cope better tend to be more optimistic and feel in control regarding their recovery; believe, trust, and participate in their physicians and the rehabilitation process; and have families who reinforce wellness behaviors as opposed to illness behaviors. Externally, these individuals are also more likely to have enjoyed their work and want to return, have a supportive employer, and are motivated to RTW. In addition, injured workers who are not involved in litigation or are not able to collect WCB statistically RTW sooner more often.

REFERENCES

Ahern, D., Adams, A., & Follick, M. (1985). Emotional and marital disturbance in spouses of chronic low back pain patients. *Clinical Journal of Pain, 1,* 69–64.

Antoniazzi, M., Celinski, M., & Alcock, J. (2002). Self-responsibility and coping with pain: Disparate attitudes toward psychosocial issues in recovery from work place injury. *Disability and Rehabilitation, 24*(18), 948–953.

Arnoff, G. M. (1998). *Evaluation and treatment of chronic pain.* Baltimore, MD: Williams & Wilkins.

Asmundson, G. J., & Norton, G. R. (1995). Anxiety sensitivity in patients with physically unexplained chronic back pain: A preliminary report. *Behavioral Resource Therapy, 33,* 771–777.

Atkinson, J. H., Slater, M. A., Patterson, T. L., Grant, I., & Garfin, S. R. (1991). Prevalence, onset, and risk of psychiatric disorders in men with chronic low back pain: A controlled study. *Pain, 45,* 111–121.

Banks, S. M., & Kerns, R. D. (1996). Explaining high rates of depression in chronic pain: A diathesis-stress framework. *Psychological Bulletin, 119,* 95–110.

Barnes, D., Smith, D., Gatchel, R. J., & Mayer, T. G. (1989). Psychosocioeconomic predictors of treatment success/failure in chronic low-back pain patients. *Spine, 14,* 427–430.

Bates, M. S., & Edwards, W. T. (1992). Ethnic variations in the chronic pain experience. *Ethnicity and Diseases, 2*(1), 63–83.

Beals, R. K. (1984). Compensation and recovery from injury. *Western Journal of Medicine, 40,* 276–283.

Beals, R. K., & Hickman, N. W. (1972). Industrial injuries of the back and extremities. *The Journal of Bone and Joint Surgery, 54*(8), 1593–1610.

Bevan, T. W. (1996). State workers' compensation programs. In S. L. Demeter & G. B. Andersson (Eds.), *Disability evaluation* (pp. 36–43). Chicago, IL: Mosby.

Biddle, J., Roberts, K., Rosenman, K. D., & Welch, E. M. (1998). What percentage of workers with work-related illnesses receive workers' compensation benefits? *Journal of Occupational and Environmental Medicine, 40,* 325–331.

Binder, L. (1992). Force choice testing provides evidence of malingering. *Archives of Physical Medicine and Rehabilitation, 73*(4), 377–380.

Blanchard, E. B. (1987). Long-term effects of behavioral treatment of chronic headache. *Behavior Therapy, 18,* 375–385.

Block, A., Kremer, E., & Gaylor, M. (1980). Behavioral treatment of chronic pain: The spouse as a discriminative cue for pain behavior. *Pain, 9,* 243–252.

Boschen, K. A. (1989). Early intervention in vocational rehabilitation. *Rehabilitation Counseling Bulletin, 32,* 34–45.

Brooker, A. S., Frank, J. W., & Tarasuk, V. S. (1997). Back pain claims rates and the business cycle. *Social Science and Medicine, 45,* 429–439.

Bureau of Labor Statistics. (1991). *Occupational injuries and illnesses in the United States by industry, 1989* (U.S. Department of Labor, Bulletin No. 2379). Washington, DC: U.S. Government Printing Office.

Burton, A. K., Tillotson, K. M., Main, C. J., & Hollis, S. (1995). Psychosocial predictors of outcome in acute and sub-chronic low back trouble. *Spine, 20,* 722–728.

Cantlon, S. (1995). Integrated disability management and claims management: An employer-centered alternative to costly litigation. In D. E. Shrey, & M. Lacerte (Eds.), *Principles and practices of disability management in industry* (pp. 451–463). Winter Park, FL: GR Press.

Chapman, C. R., & Okifuji, A. (2004). Pain: Basic mechanisms and conscious experience. In R. H. Dworkin, & W. S. Breitbart (Eds.), *Psychosocial aspects of pain: A handbook for health care providers* (pp. 3–27). Seattle, WA: IASP Press.

Chibnall, J. T., & Tait, R. C. (2005). Disparities in occupational low back injuries: Predicting pain-related disability from satisfaction with case management in African Americans and Caucasians, *Pain Medicine, 6*(1), 39–48.

Chubon, R. (1994). Work and rehabilitation: The value of work. In R. A. Cubon (Ed.), *Social and psychological foundations of rehabilitation* (pp. 189–199). Springfield, IL: Thomas.

Cole, D. C., Mondlock, M. V., & Hogg-Johnson, S. (2002). For the early claimant cohort prognostic: Modeling group. Listening to injured workers: How recovery expectations predict outcomes— A prospective study. *Canadian Medical Association Journal, 166,* 749–754.

Conte, L. E., & Van Antwerp, M. K. (1995). Legal perspectives on disability resolution and industrial rehabilitation. In D. E. Shrey, & M. Lacerte (Eds.), *Principles and practices of disability management in industry* (pp. 433–449). Winter Park, FL: GR Press.

Corbishley, M., Hendrickson, R., & Beutler, L. (1990). Behavior, affect, and cognition among psychogenic pain patients in group expressive psychotherapy. *Journal of Pain and Symptom Management, 5*, 241–248.

Crook, J., Milner, R., Schultz, I. Z., & Stringer, B. (2002). Determinants of occupational disability following a low back injury: A critical review of the literature. *Journal of Occupational Rehabilitation, 12*, 277–295.

Deyo, R. A. (1986). The early diagnostic evaluation of patients with low back pain. *Journal of General Internal Medicine, 1*, 328–338.

Deyo, R. A., & Tsui-Wi, Y. J. (1987). Descriptive epidemiology of low back pain and its related medical care in the United States. *Spine, 12*, 264–268.

Deyo, R. A., Walsh, N. E., & Martin, D. (1990). A controlled trial of transcutaneous electrical nerve stimulation (TENS) and exercise for chronic low back pain. *New England Journal of Medicine, 322*, 1627–1634.

Division of Workers' Compensation. (2007). Retrieved from http://www.dir.ca.gov/dwc/Return ToworkRates/ReturnToWorkRates.pdf

Dodier, N. (1985). Social uses of illness at the workplace: Sick leave and moral evaluation. *Social Science and Medicine, 20*(2), 123–125.

Drukteinis, A. M. (2004). Disability. In R. I. Simon, & L. H. Gold (Eds.), *The American psychiatric textbook of forensic psychiatry* (pp. 287–301). Washington, DC: American Psychiatric Press.

Dworkin, R. H., & Breitbart, W. S. (2004). *Psychosocial aspects of pain: A handbook for health care providers.* Seattle, WA: IASP Press

Dworkin, S. F., & Massoth, D. L. (1994). Temporomandibular disorders and chronic pain: Disease or illness? *Journal of Prosthetic Dentistry, 7*, 29–38.

Edwards, R. R., Doleys, D. M., Fillingim, R. B., & Lowery, D. (2001). Ethnic differences in pain tolerance: Clinical implications in a chronic pain population. *Psychosomatic Medicine, 63*, 316–323.

Edwards, R. R., & Fillingim, R. B. (1999). Ethnic differences in thermal pain processes. *Psychosomatic Medicine, 61*, 346–354.

Erickson, W., Lee, C., & Von Schrader, S. (2010, March). *Disability statistics from the 2008 American Community Survey.* Ithaca, NY: Cornell University Rehabilitation Research and Training Center on Disability Demographics and Statistics (StatsRRTC). Retrieved from www.disability statistics.org.

Faucett, J., Gordon, N., & Levine, J. (1994). Differences in postoperative pain severity among four ethnic groups. *Journal of Pain Symptom Management, 9*, 383–389.

Fallenbaum, R. (2003). The injured worker. *Studies in Gender and Sexuality, 4*(1), 72–92.

Fernandez, E., & Turk, D. C. (1995). The scope and significance of anger in the experience of chronic pain. *Pain, 16*(2), 165–175.

Feuerstein, M., Menz, L., Zastowny, T. R., & Barron, B. A. (1994). Chronic back pain and work disability: Vocational outcomes following multidisciplinary rehabilitation. *Journal of Occupational Rehabilitation, 4*, 229–251.

Flor, H., & Turk, D. C. (1989). Psychophysiology of chronic pain: Do chronic pain patients exhibit symptom-specific psychophysiological responses? *Psychological Bulletin, 105*, 215–259.

Fordyce, W. E. (1976). *Behavioral methods for chronic pain and illness.* St Louis, MO: C.V. Mosby.

Fordyce, W. E. (1995). *Back pain in the workplace.* Seattle, WA: IASP Press.

Fruen, M. (1992). Disability management focuses on prevention. *Business & Health, 10*(10), 27–29.

Gatchel, R. J. (1996). Psychological disorders and chronic pain: Cause and effect relationships. In R. J. Gatchel & D. C. Turk (Eds.), *Psychological approaches to pain management: A practitioner's handbook* (pp. 33–52). New York: Guilford Pess.

Gatchel, R. J., & Turk, D. C. (1996). *Psychological approaches to pain management: A practitioner's handbook.* New York, NY: Guilford Press.

Gilbride, D., Stensrud, R., Ehlers, C., Evans, E., & Peterson, C. (2000). Employer's attitudes towards hiring persons with disabilities and vocational rehabilitation services. *Journal of Rehabilitation, 66,* 17–25.

Greene, C. S., & Laskin, D. M. (1974). Long-term evaluation of conservative treatments for myofascial pain dysfunction syndrome. *Journal of the American Dental Association, 89,* 1365–1368.

Gribich, C., McGartland, M., & Polgar, S. (1998). Regulating workers compensation: The medico legal evaluation of injured workers in Victoria. *Australian Journal of Social Issues, 33*(3), 241–263.

Habeck, R. (1991). Managing disability in industry. *NARPPS Journal and News, 6*(3&4), 141–146.

Hadler, N. M., Carey, T. S., & Garrett, J. (1995). North Carolina back pain project: The influence of indemnification by workers' compensation insurance on recovery from acute backache. *Spine, 20,* 2710–2715.

Hadjistavropoulos, T. (1999). Chronic pain on trail: The influence of litigation and compensation on chronic pain syndromes. In A. R. Bolck, E. F. Kremer, & E. Fernandez (Eds.), *Handbook of pain syndromes* (pp. 59–76). Mahwah, NJ: Lawrence Erlbaum.

Hanson, R. W., & Gerber, K. E. (1990). *Coping with chronic pain: A guide to patient self-management.* New York, NY: Guilford Press.

Hashemi, L., Webster, B. S., Clancy, E. A., & Volinn, E. (1997). Length of disability and cost of workers' compensation low back pain claims. *Journal of Occupational Environmental Medicine, 39,* 937–945.

Hazard, R. G., Haugh, L., Green, P., & Jones, P. (1994). Chronic low back pain: The relationship between patient satisfaction and pain, impairment and disability outcomes. *Spine, 19,* 881–887.

International classification of disability-10-CM, (2010). Eden Praire, MN: Ingenix.

Jensen, M. P., Romano, J. M., Turner, J. A., Good, A. B., & Wald, L. H. (1999). Patient beliefs predict patient functioning: Further support for a cognitive-behavioral model of chronic pain. *Pain, 81,* 91–104.

Kerns, R. D., Haythornthwaite, J., Southwick, S., & Giller, E. L. (1990). The role of marital interaction in chronic pain and depressive symptom severity. *Journal of Psychosomatic Research, 34,* 401–408.

Kerns, R. D., & Payne, A. (1996). Treating families of chronic pain patients. In R. J. Gatchel & D. C. Turk (Eds.), *Psychological approaches to pain management: A practitioner's handbook* (pp. 283–304). New York, NY: Guilford Press.

Kerns, R. D., Rosenberg, R., & Jacob, M. C. (1994). Anger expression and chronic pain. *Journal of Behavioral Medicine, 17,* 57–68.

Krause, S. J., Wiener, R. L., & Tait, R.C. (1994). Depression and pain behavior in patients with chronic pain. *The Clinical Journal of Pain, 10,* 122–127.

Lewinsohn, P. M., Clarke, G. N., Hops, H., & Andrews, J. A. (1990). Cognitive-behavioral treatment for depressed adolescents. *Behavioral Therapy, 21,* 385–401.

Linton, S. J. (2000). A review of psychological risk factors in back and neck pain. *Spine, 25,* 1148–1156.

Lousberg, R., Schmidt, A. J., & Groenman, N. H. (1992). The relationship between spouse solicitousness and pain behavior: Searching for more experimental evidence. *Pain, 51,* 75–79.

Magni, G., Caldieron, C., Rigatti-Luchini, S., & Merskey, H. (1990). Chronic musculoskeletal pain and depressive symptoms in the general population: An analysis of the 1st National Health and Nutrition Examination survey. *Pain, 43,* 299–307.

Marini, I. (2003). What rehabilitation counselors should know in assisting SSDI/SSI beneficiaries in becoming employed. *Work, 18,* 37–43.

Marini, I., & Reid, C. R. (2001). A survey of rehabilitation professionals as alternative provider contractors with social security: Problems and solutions. *Journal of Rehabilitation, 67*(2), 36–41.

Matkin, R. E. (1995). Private sector rehabilitation. In S. E. Rubin & R. T. Roessler (Eds.), *Foundations of the vocational rehabilitation process* (pp. 375–398). Austin, TX: Pro-ed.

Maruta, T., Osborne, D., Swenson, D. W., & Holling, J. M. (1981). Chronic pain patients and spouses: Marital and sexual adjustment. *Mayo Clinic Proceedings, 56,* 307–310.

Melzack, R., & Wall, P. (1965). Pain mechanisms: A new theory. *Science, 50,* 971–979.

Newman, S. S., Perry, D. A., & Pan, E. L. (1985). Characteristics of the private rehabilitation client: Implications for the rehabilitation specialist. In L. J. Taylor, M. Gotter, G. Gotter, & T. E. Becker (Eds.), *Handbook of private sector rehabilitation* (pp. 115–137). New York, NY: Springer.

Otis, J. D., Cardella, L. A., & Kerns, R. D. (2004). The influence of family and culture on pain. In R. H. Dworkin & W. S. Breitbart (Eds.), *Psychosocial aspects of pain: A handbook for health care providers* (pp. 29–45). Seattle, WA: IASP Press.

Patenaude, S. (1989). Promoting functional ability in industry. *Industrial Rehabilitation Quarterly, 2*(1), 34, 40–41.

Pati, G. C. (1985). Economics of rehabilitation in the workplace. *Journal of Rehabilitation, 51*, 22–30.

Philips, H. C. (1987a). Avoidance behavior and its role in sustaining chronic-pain. *Behavior Research and Therapy, 25*, 273–279.

Picus, T., Burton, A. K., Vogel, S., & Field, A. P. (2002). A systematic review of psychological factors as predictors of chronicity/disability in prospective cohorts of low back pain. *Spine, 27*(5), E109–E120.

Polatin, P. B. (1996). Integration of pharmacotherapy with psychological treatment of chronic pain. In R. J. Gatchel, & D. C. Turk (Eds.), *Psychological approaches to pain management: A practitioner's handbook* (pp. 305–328). New York, NY: Guilford Press.

Polatin, P. B., & Mayer, T. G. (1992). Quantification of function in chronic low back pain. In D. G. Turk & R. Melzack (Eds.), *Handbook of pain assessment* (pp. 37–48). New York, NY: Guilford Press.

Portnoy, R. (1994). Opioid therapy for chronic nonmalignant pain: Current status. In H. Fields & J. Liebeskind (Eds.), *Progress in pain research and management* (pp. 247–287). Seattle, WA: International Association for the Study of Pain Press.

Reiss, D. (1989). Families and their paradigms: An ecologic approach to understanding the family and its social world. In C. N. Ramsey, Jr. (Ed.), *Family systems in medicine* (pp. 119–134). New York, NY: Guilford Press.

Robles, B. B., & Marini, I. (2005). Supplemental security income and social security disability insurance. In W. Crimando, & T. F. Riggar's , *Utilizing community resources: An overview of human services* (2nd ed.) (pp. 169–184). Prospect Heights, IL: Waveland Press.

Rogers, R., & Payne, J. W. (2006). Damages and rewards: Assessment of malingered disorders in compensation cases. *Behavioral Sciences and the Law, 24*, 645–658.

Rubin, L. B. (1979). *Worlds of pain: Life in the working class family.* New York, NY: Basic.

Rudy, T. E., Kerns, R. J., & Turk, D. C. (1988). Chronic pain and depression: Toward a cognitive-behavioral medication model. *Pain, 35*, 179–183.

Sachs, P. R., & Ellenberg, D. B. (1994). The family system and adaptation to an injured worker. *The American Journal of Family Therapy, 22*(3), 263–272.

Sager, L., & James, C. (2005). Injured workers' perspectives of their rehabilitation process under the New South Wales workers compensation system. *Australian Occupational Therapy Journal, 52*, 127–135.

Samra, J., & Koch, W. J. (2002). The monetary worth of psychological injury. In J. R. P. Ogloff (Ed.), *Taking psychology and law into the twenty-first century* (pp. 285–322). New York, NY: Kluwer-Plenum.

Sanders, S. H. (1996). Operant conditioning with chronic pain: Back to basics. In R. J. Gatchel & D. C. Turk (Eds.), *Psychological approaches to pain management: A practitioner's handbook* (pp. 112–130). New York, NY: Guilford Press.

Scheer, S. (1995). The role of the physician in disability management. In D. E. Shrey & M. Lacerte (Eds.), *Principles and practices of disability management in industry* (pp. 175–205). Winter Park, FL: GR Press.

Schoefferman, J. (1994). *The use of medications for pain of spinal cord origin.* Paper presented at "The Final Link to Therapeutic Success" course, Seton Medical Center, San Francisco, CA.

Schultz, I. Z., Crook, J., Meloche, G. R., Berkowitz, J., Milner, R., Zuberbier, O. A. et al. (2004). Psychosocial factors predictive of occupational low back disability: Towards development of a return-to-work model. *Pain, 107*, 77–85.

Sengupta, I., & Reno, V. (2007). Recent trends in workers' compensation. *Social Security Bulletin, 67*(1), 17–26.

Shrey, D. E. (1995). Worksite disability management and industrial rehabilitation: An overview. In D. E. Shrey & M. Lacerte (Eds.), *Principles and practices of disability management in industry* (pp. 3–53). Winter Park, FL: GR Press.

Sternbach, R. A. (1974). *Pain patients: Traits and treatment.* New York, NY: Academic Press.

Sternbach, R. A., Wolf, S. R., Murphy, R. W., & Akeson, W. H. (1973). Trait of pain patients: The low-back "loser." *Psychosomatics, 14*, 226–229.

Tait, R. C. (2004). Compensation claims for chronic pain: Effects on evaluation and treatment. In R. H. Dworkin, & W. S. Breitbart (Eds.), *Psychosocial aspects of pain: A handbook for health care providers* (pp. 547–569). Seattle, WA: IASP Press.

Tarasuk, V., & Eakin, J. M. (1995). The problem of legitimacy in the experience of work-related back injury. *Qualitative Health Research, 5*, 204–222.

Taulbee, P. (1991). Corralling runaway workers' comp costs. *Business & Health, 9*(4), 46–55.

Todd, K., Samaroo, N., & Hoffman, J. (1993). Ethnicity as a risk factor for inadequate emergency department analgesia. *JAMA, 269*, 1537–1539.

Turk, D. C. (1996). Biopsychosocial perspective in chronic pain. In R. H. Dworkin & W. S. Breitbart (Eds.), *Psychosocial aspects of pain: A handbook for health care providers* (pp. 3–32). Seattle, WA: IASP Press.

Turk, D. C. (2002). A diathesis-stress model of chronic pain and disability following traumatic injury. *Pain Research & Management, 7*, 9–19.

Turk, D. C. (2004). Fibromyalgia: A patient-oriented perspective. In R. H. Dworkin & W. S. Breitbart (Eds.), *Psychosocial aspects of pain: A handbook for health care providers* (pp. 309–338). Seattle, WA: IASP Press.

Turk, D. C., Kerns, R. D., & Rosenberg, R. (1992). Effects of marital interaction on chronic pain and disability: Examining the down side of social support. *Rehabilitation Psychology, 37*, 259–274.

Turk, D. C., Okifuji, A., & Scharff, L. (1995). Chronic pain and depression: Role of perceived impact and perceived control in different age cohorts. *Pain, 61*, 93–102.

Turpin, S. (2010). Fact facts & figures about social security, 2010. *Social Security Administration, Office of Retirement and Disability Policy, Office of Research Evaluation, and Statistics*, Washington, DC: SSA Publication, No. 13–11785.

Waddell, G. A., & Sawney, P. (2002). *Back pain, incapacity for work, and social security benefits: An international review and analysis*. London, UK: Royal Society of Medicine Press.

Walker, J. M. (1992). Injured worker helplessness: Critical relationships and systems level approach for intervention. *Journal of Occupational Rehabilitation, 2*(4), 201–209.

Webster, B. S., & Snook, S. H. (1989). The cost of 1989 workers' compensation low back pain claims. *Spine 1994, 19*, 1111–1116.

Weinstein, M. (1993). Proactive prevention. *Risk and Insurance, 4*(2), 1, 12–13.

Widmalm, S., Gunn, S., Christiansen, R., & Hawley, L. (1995). Association between CMD signs and symptoms, oral parafunctions, race, and sex, in 4–6 year-old African and white children. *Journal of Oral Rehabilitation, 22*, 95–100.

Wiesenfeld-Hallin, Z., & Hallin, R. G. (1984). The influence of the sympathetic system on mechanoreception and nociception: A review. *Human Neurobiology, 3*, 41–46.

Williams, A. C. (2004). Assessing chronic pain and its impact. In R. H. Dworkin & W. S. Breitbart (Eds.), *Psychosocial aspects of pain: A handbook for health care providers* (pp. 97–115). Seattle, WA: IASP Press.

Williams, D. A., & Keefe, F. J. (1991). Pain beliefs and the use of cognitive-behavioral coping strategies. *Pain, 46*, 185–190.

Willis, E. (1986). Commentary: RSI as a social process. *Community Health Studies X, 2*, 210–219.

Woodrow, K., Friedman, G., Siegelaub, A., & Collen, M. (1972). Pain tolerance: Differences according to age, sex, and race. *Psychosomatic Medicine, 34*, 548–556.

INSIDER PERSPECTIVE

The Story of Gino Sonego

The transition from an unemployed quadraplegic to the field of employment for me was fairly quick and only by chance. I had gone through my rehabilitation at Lyndhurst Hospital and had just newly arrived home. When I say home I mean, Thunder Bay, Ontario and not in my own home but in an accessible housing unit as my own home was not completed as yet. So I was released from Lyndhurst rehab in Toronto and returned to Thunder Bay and was living in an accessible housing unit while I started to put the pieces back together.

I applied for accessible housing with the HAGI (Handicap Action Group Incorporated), and a unit came up for my wife and me to move into. So we moved out of my in-laws' home in the country to an accessible apartment in town. Slowly, we adjusted to living on our own, together as a newly married couple and dealing with this thing called quadriplegia.

My wife Lori, who has stood by me from day one through thick and thin, and has always been there for me till date, would go to work during the day and I would be left in the apartment to . . . to what . . . . what do you do when your world has abruptly stopped and taken a turn down a path you have no idea about or where you are going? How will we pay the bills, how do we finish off our home, what am I going to do for employment, how am I going to get around, how will our friends react, how is our marriage going to work, what about kids . . . and on and on?

So the solitary quiet time in the apartment was both good because you started to think about what all your challenges were, but I also started to think about the possible solutions and small steps in putting the puzzle back together. A short time later, we were in the mall one day and I ran into a former classmate, Don Wing, whom I had gone to high school with but didn't know very well. It wasn't until college that I got to know Don better as we were enrolled in the same course, architectural design. As fate would have it, that is where I met my wife Lori and went on to marry her later on in life. So Don asked how I was doing and what my plans were. We talked for a little while and he mentioned that they may be looking for someone to fill a position in their office. A few days later, he called me up and asked if I was interested in coming in for an interview, and so I said sure.

I couldn't believe what was happening. Here I was an unemployed quadriplegic just returned from my rehabilitation, and I was being asked to come in for an interview to work in the office of a construction company. Now, while the opportunity was great and I didn't want to pass it up, I started to question myself. Would I be able to handle an office job; would I have the qualifications; could I do what was being asked of me; would I fit in, and so on? I wasn't sure whether I would be able to live up to the expectations of the job, but I surely did want to be able to get back to working again.

I need to regress some so that my story can be fully appreciated. Let me take you back to October 20, 1984; it was the day that I got married to my college sweetheart Lori. We went to Confederation College together in 1978 and after many years of me avoiding the question, I finally proposed and we were married. I had graduated in 1978 from Confederation College as an architectural technician and found employment for a short period of time but was not happy working in an office setting. So I decided to go out and get a trade and put my college experience to work with my hands. I tried to get into carpentry but could not find anyone willing to offer me an apprenticeship, and so I had some contacts in the masonry field and decided to follow my father's footsteps and take on a masonry apprenticeship. I started my apprenticeship with Gasporotto Masonry and completed it in 1984. I was 24 years old, married to my college sweetheart, had just finished my apprenticeship as a bricklayer, and building my own home that Lori and I had designed together. Life seemed pretty good and we had goals ahead of us.

I was working out of town on and off that summer and got an opportunity to come home for the week. I would get a chance to spend some time with Lori and get some additional work done on the house. We were working on the roof at the time (August 5, 1985), putting the final sheets of plywood on and getting the roof ready for shingles. I was coming down the ladder, and as it started to move I lost my balance and fell backward down to the ground. The fall itself was not that far and I had fallen many times farther than that, but I must have landed wrong, perhaps on my head and when I tried to get up I couldn't move. I knew something was wrong, but I didn't know what. I tried to get up but couldn't. Lori and my parents were there and went over to call an ambulance to take me to the hospital. I was taken to the hospital by an ambulance, where I was diagnosed by the doctor on call as having had a spinal cord injury, causing paralysis from the chest down, and that I would have no use of my hands. I had a fracture dislocation at C5 and they put me in traction for a few days trying to get the disc back in place on its own. They tried the maximum traction on my neck to try and get the disc back into place without having to operate, but unfortunately it did not work and they had to operate to remove the fractured disc and then did a fusion from C4–C6. I had a halo vest put on to stabilize my neck while it healed. The operation was a success according to the doctors, but I was still not walking and had little hand movement. The nursing staff at McKellar General Hospital did their best to try and keep everything positive and to keep my spirits up. There were lots of friends, family, and well-wishers who would come in and see me at the hospital. Over time, I did get some hand movement back and some finger movement, which seemed to be a positive sign to me at the time.

It had been approximately a month since my accident, I had been operated on and I had this halo contraption on my head. I was stable, and so it was time for me to start the next step in my recovery, my rehabilitation process (September 1985). In my mind, I was still thinking that I would get better and would beat the odds and start walking again. The nursing staff were careful as to not give me false hope but at the same time not to tell me that I would probably never walk again. Thinking back now, it's not walking that is the biggest issue. While that in itself is a major item, it's all of the other things that you don't even think about, like writing your name, scratching your nose, or feeding yourself; being able to pick up something that has fallen on the floor; sensation to hot and cold, being able to control your bowel and urine function; and numerous other things that most people take for granted everyday. I decided to go to Lyndhurst Hospital in Toronto for my rehabilitation, partly because I heard they had a good rehabilitation centre and partly because I had relatives in the Toronto area. I went down to Lyndhurst at the beginning of September 1985 and spent my 25th birthday there.

I don't know what I expected to happen when I was in Lyndhurst, but I guess I expected that they had special treatments in the big city and that I would be better in no time. Well, reality slowly stared to sink in, and I started to see that with the limited function I had, I would need to maximize my ability to function as independently as I could. I would go to all my OT and PT therapy sessions and work at all of the challenges that they would introduce, such as getting up in bed on my own, finding my balance point and how to work around that limitation (since I was a quadriplegic with no stomach muscles or back muscles, I really need to be careful with balance so that I don't fall sideways or forward out of the wheelchair), dressing myself independently, transferring in and out of the wheelchair, bowel and bladder routine, and many other tasks that most people take for granted as part of their daily activities.

My rehabilitation was going great according to the physiotherapist and the occupational therapists, but to me it wasn't working as I still wasn't walking. In my mind, I really expected that the rehabilitation would get me back up and walking. It was around the time, when they wanted me to order my wheelchair so I would have it for when I would be released, that I really started to realize I probably would never walk again and I would need a wheelchair for the rest of my life. That was a rough day, because up to that point I was holding on to the dream that I would beat the odds and walk again. It was tough to take the next step of moving on mentally. It's not that I gave up on the vision of getting better, but I needed to accept the fact that I would need the wheelchair for my daily activities.

I went home for Christmas, and then returned to Lyndhurst in the new year to complete my rehabilitation. When I returned to Lyndhurst, I focused on all the life skills that I was being taught and started to think about what I would do when I was released and how I would move on. I knew I would not be able to return to my trade as a bricklayer, and so I started to think about what was available to a quadriplegic and what skills I may have that may make me employable. I took some computer classes at Lyndhurst to introduce me to the computer, as I believed that some sort of office job would be where I may be able to find employment. My thinking was that with my education as an architectural technician and my trade as a bricklayer I should be able to find something in the construction field. I have always been interested in construction and working with my hands to make things, and so this was the area I was thinking I would focus on.

I was probably ready for release by February of 1986, but I was not released until April 19, as I didn't have any proper accommodation in Thunder Bay. So I returned home, rehabilitated but unemployed. What do I do now? When you are in a hospital setting, you are taken care of, and you are in safe environment. You are encouraged to become as independent as you can, so you can deal with your daily routine when you get home, but it is not an easy transition.

I'm not sure as to what motivates people to move forward, whether it is necessity to survive, whether it's a strong support network that they have around them, their upbringing, their own personal drive to succeed, financial needs, or a combination of all these and other reasons. But, I knew I had to get back on that horse and I wasn't going to stay down. I had a house that was 60% completed, and our only income was my disability check and my wife's income as a part-time store manager. While we had enough income to live on, it was not enough to get us out of our accumulated financial burden. We had accumulated bills while I was in hospital and in Lyndhurst, and so I felt I had a responsibility to provide for my family.

You see, my injury was due to a fall while building my own home, and so I did not have any workers' compensation and no insurance coverage for being the owner of the property. I did not have any financial safety net to help me get back on my feet, and so I had a strong desire to get back to work in whatever capacity I could. I know of many people who have not returned to employment because of the fact that they would lose their disability check or they have other income, such as insurance income. So they choose to stay on disability and never really try to get back into the world of employment. I have never regretted making the decision to go back to work, and I look forward to getting up in the morning and going to work.

So that brings me back to my employment opportunity and my life after my accident. I started working with Wing Construction in early summer of 1986, less than a year after having had my accident. I was starting a new job, with a new employer, in a new career while still trying to learn how to cope with being a quadriplegic. I was nervous about the whole thing and how it would work out, but everyone at Wing Construction was great and supportive of my situation. They had to make some modifications to the washroom and entry to their building for wheelchair access, but this was fairly minor. There was a boardroom on the second floor of the building, and once a month we would have an office meeting, and so they would carry me upstairs to the boardroom for our meetings. I felt bad, but they didn't seem to mind and perhaps it was a way of bringing everyone together for a common purpose.

I had to learn how to fit into the office routine, and I was being groomed as their contract administrator. Many of my responsibilities were new to me, but my college training was helping me to fit in quick and to take on the duties as required. I quickly learned how to do the work that was requested of me, and I was one of the first people in the office to learn how to use the computer for our office needs.

I worked at Wing Construction from 1986 to 1997 and the management and staff were always more than accommodating and helpful. They treated me as an equal employee, and I gave them 100% dedication and loyalty. In 1997, the staff were told that the company was going to get out of the construction business and that they would be closing the doors. This came as a shock to all the employees as we never anticipated that this could ever happen. The company had done many projects over the years and seemed financially sound. So what do I do now? Would I be able to find another employer willing to take a chance on me and hire a quadriplegic? We had just started our family by adopting a young boy from Russia, and so I couldn't afford to be unemployed. (The adoption of our son, and the emotional roller coaster before, during, and afterwards, is a story in itself, but it's probably one of the best things that has happened in our lives and the joy that he has brought and continues to bring into our lives is immeasurable; we love you Levan.)

They say that things happen for a reason, and as we were being told that we were being laid off, and opportunity became available for me and the office estimator, Peter McCart, to start our own construction company and take on building a condominium for a developer whom we had worked for over the years when we were employed at Wing Construction. So, do we invest in ourselves and get back in the game or do we sit by the sidelines and watch the game being played?

So we jumped in with both feet and started Aurora Construction, and we have never looked back. We took the skills that we had working with Wing Construction and applied them to our own company. This will be our 13th year in business and we are both enjoying the challenges and rewards that come with being the owner of your own destiny. I get to the jobsites as much as possible, but spend most of my time in the office dealing with the day-to-day needs of the projects. I can't say that I have encountered any owners, architects, consultants, or trades people who have not treated me with respect. Sometimes people are a little apprehensive because of my disability, but I think it is because they have not encountered very many people working in the construction field and they see the wheelchair first rather than the person. But this usually doesn't last long.

I am enjoying what I am doing and I am living my dream of being a contractor even though I am on a wheelchair. I must say that I have never really looked back to say "why me?" Would I have chosen this path if I had a choice? Probably not. Do I have any regrets? None. I am fortunate to have friends and family who are there for us when we need them and we have needed them over the years. I have a wife and son who believe in me and love me for who I am . . . Who can ask for anything else?

DISCUSSION QUESTIONS

1. Solicit student stories re: someone they know who sustained a work injury and overall experience in dealing with WCB. How did they feel going through the process?
2. Solicit student stories re: someone they know who applied for and was either denied or accepted for SSDI and/or SSI. What was their experience in applying for benefits? How did they feel going through the process?
3. Ask for any examples from students of people they know who collect disability benefits but still work and what the students think about such situations.
4. Discuss student opinions re: their beliefs as to whether less than 5% of all pain patients exaggerate their symptoms versus those who keep working and underreport or downplay their pain.

EXERCISES

A. Have students research what the WCB laws are in their state re: formula benefits, wage replacement percentage while off work, maximum number of weeks workers can receive benefits, and what the most common work injuries are in their state.
B. Have students research what the five levels of application and appeal process are for persons applying for SSDI and/or SSI.
C. Have students interview someone they know who collects either WCB or SSDI/SSI benefits re: what their experience was to have to stop work, apply for assistance, and any problems with the system they encountered, whether it was the medical system, WCB, SSA, or other entities?

PART THREE

Pertinent Topics Concerning Psychosocial Issues of Disability

NINE

Disability and Quality of Life Over the Life Span

Noreen M. Glover-Graf

OVERVIEW

Quality of life is considered to be a vague, subjective, multidimensional concept that incorporates all life dimensions and experiences. It is both difficult to observe and difficult to measure (Bowling, 2001). The Centers for Disease Control and Prevention (CDC) defines quality of life as "a person or group's perceived physical and mental health over time" (CDC, 2010; para 1). Quality of life is a difficult construct to measure because it includes both tangible, measurable variables, such as how much income one has, and subjective variables, such as the satisfaction with one's relationships and perceived meaningfulness of experiences. Also, because people vary in the value they place on these variables, a good life for one person could be considered distressing by another person's standards. Clearly then, aside from the basic and essential survival needs, human service professionals will need to have an understanding of what else people require to live fulfilling and meaningful lives. They will need to understand what individual clients value as important and additive to their quality of life. Over the course of one's life, needs and desires are likely to change. Things important for an individual as a child or adolescent will change entirely, or in part, as they age and take on different roles and responsibilities. This chapter will explore the concept of quality of life, the impact of disability at various life stages, and the impact of various types of disabilities on quality of life.

THE CONCEPT OF QUALITY OF LIFE

Quality of Life and Health

Revicki et al. (2000) define *quality of life* as primarily subjective: "a broad range of human experiences related to one's overall well-being. It implies value based on subjective functioning in comparison with personal expectations and is defined by subjective experiences, states, and perceptions. Quality of life, by its very nature, is idiosyncratic to the individual, but intuitively meaningful and understandable to most people" (Revicki et al., 2000, p. 888). Others have included both objective and subjective indicators in the determination of quality of life that seems to have at the core, trying to get at the elements of life that create a condition of happiness or contentment.

Quality of life can also be viewed primarily through the lens of good health. The medical profession frequently uses the term *Health-Related Quality of Life* (HRQOL) as a means of better understanding the effect of illness and disability on day-to-day life. In order to understand the impact of health differences in Americans who do and do not have disabilities, the CDC has identified typical American health responses as follows:

- Americans feel physically or mentally unhealthy approximately 6 days per month.
- Americans feel full of energy and healthy approximately about 19 days per month.
- About one-third of Americans report some mental or emotional problem each month.
- Americans 18–24 years old report the most mental health distress.
- Older adults report the most physical limitation and poorest physical health.
- Adults with the lowest education or income reported more unhealthy days than those with higher education or income.
- Persons with disabilities and chronic illness report high levels of unhealthy days.

In comparing adults with and without disabilities, health-related quality-of-life measures show substantial differences. Adults with arthritis reported almost five more unhealthy days than adults without arthritis; women with breast cancer report about two additional unhealthy days when compared with women without breast cancer; persons with cardiovascular conditions and persons with diabetes each reported about twice as many unhealthy days as persons without those conditions.

Additional Quality-of-Life Indicators

While it makes sense that persons with chronic illness and disabilities would experience less healthy days, a number of other life domains are presumed to influence a person's perception regarding their quality of life. Objective indicators, such as income, employment, and socioeconomic status and support systems, have traditionally been a focus (Bishop & Feist-Price, 2001) for researchers, but these measures alone seem to be poor predictors of individuals' subjective perceptions about life satisfaction, happiness, well-being, or quality of life (Michalos, 1991; Myers & Diener, 1995). Thus, in addition to objective indicators, a number of subjective factors have been determined to be important influences of quality of life. "Core Domains" of quality of life include psychological health and life satisfaction (psychological well-being), physical health, interpersonal and social well-being, financial well-being, productivity and/or employment, and functional capacity (Bishop & Allen, 2003; Felce & Perry, 1996; George & Bearon, 1980). In a review of the literature related to quality of life, Hughes, Hwang, Kim, Eisenmand, and Killian (1995) identified the following factors as influential to quality of life:

- Physical and material well-being
- Social interactions and relationships

- Psychological well-being and personal satisfaction
- Recreation and leisure time
- Employment
- Individual and demographic indicators
- Autonomy, self-determination, and personal choice
- Personal development and fulfilment
- Personal competence
- Community integration
- Community adjustment and independent living skills
- Residential environment
- Normalization and support services received
- Social acceptance, social status, and ecological fit
- Civic responsibility

The 49 million people, 15 years and older, in the United States with disabilities or chronic health conditions (U.S. Census Bureau, 2005) have a number of pervasive disadvantages over those without disabilities that affect quality-of-life domains. For example, only 35% of Americans with disabilities are employed, 26% live in poverty compared with 9% of Americans without disabilities, 21% do not hold an HS degree compared with 10% of Americans without disabilities, more report inadequate transportation (31% versus 13%) and health care (18% versus 7%), they socialize less, over half are worried that they will be a burden to their families and unable to support or care for themselves, and considerably less life satisfaction is expressed by people with disabilities (National Organization of Disability/Harris Survey of Americans with Disabilities, 2004).

Rehabilitation Counseling and Quality of Life

Quality of life has been an increasing focus for rehabilitation counsellors and is philosophically consistent with rehabilitation practice and outcome, despite problems with construct ambiguity and measurement (Bishop, Chapin, & Miller; 2008; Bishop & Feist-Price, 2001; Crewe, 1980; Fabian, 1991; Livneh, 2001; Wright, 1980). Specifically, Fabian (1991) noted that measures of quality of life for persons with disabilities differed in studies and were alternately either measures of life satisfaction, adaptive functioning, or social integration as determined by variables such as socioeconomic status and employment rates. Compounding this problem is the difficulty in measuring quality of life for persons with severe disabilities who can provide no response or limited response to researchers.

Smart (2001) defined quality of life for persons with disabilities as having basic needs met, including medical and psychological care, social and economic independence to the extent possible, social and familial support, and self-actualization. For persons with disabilities, prejudice, lack of accommodation and opportunities, and discrimination needlessly diminish the quality of life. Counselors working to increase quality of life work from a holistic and wellness perspective to address the life issues beyond vocational and independence goals, toward inclusion, personal growth and development, environmental accessibility, and ending job discrimination (Rosseler, 1990; Rosseler, Neath, & Rumrill, 2007). Chubon (1994) explained:

> Because of the quest for more fulfilling lives by persons with disabilities, the concept of rehabilitation is becoming inextricably bound to quality-of-life issues. Its mission has now become that of enhancing life quality so that it is worth living and preserving. In essence, the role of rehabilitation in increasingly being accepted as that of enhancing opportunity for persons with disabilities to participate in all walks of life to the greatest extent possible, thereby supporting at least an acceptable life quality. (Chubon, 1994, p. 49)

Because quality of life is also a matter of perception, counselors have been attentive to client feelings and beliefs related to losses experienced due to disability for decades. In particular, researchers have studied how changes in values assist in adapting to the consequences of disability. Beatrice Wright (1960) proposed that persons' values may be adjusted following disability onset in that the scope of values enlarges so that their values are no longer in conflict with their disabilities. For example, if disability results in limiting work capacity, time spent with family may become more important than work. Adjustment might also entail subordination of the physique as a symbol of self-worth, containment of the effects of disability, and ceasing to make comparisons with others who are not disabled. When looking at quality of life, it may be important that such cognitive restructuring occurs in persons with disabilities because satisfaction in the most highly valued areas has the greatest influence on quality of life, and satisfaction in the valued domains may even compensate for dissatisfaction in other life areas (Frisch, 1999; Gladis, Gosch, Dishuk, & Crits-Christoph, 1999).

In the study of quality of life, the adaptive shifting of value priorities is sometimes referred to as "preference drift," "domain compensation," or "response shift" and represents a person's change of internal measurement standards, a change in values, or a change in the personal definition of life quality following the acquisition of disability (Schwartz & Sprangers, 2000). Response shift is considered a promising avenue for exploration in quality of life among persons with chronic illness and disability because the recalibration, reprioritization, and reconceptualization that take place over time may allow for quality of life to be perceived differently. Recalibration involves a change in acceptable standards of level of engagement in some activity; reprioritization involves a shift in the importance of life domains, and reconceptualization involves a change in domains important to quality of life. In a study of persons with cardiac conditions, patients were asked to rate their quality of life over time and their perceptions of their functioning. Patients' perceptions regarding what *areas* of life affect quality of life did not change. Those who used active coping strategies (as opposed to denial, avoidance, or other strategies) experienced greater response shift due to recalibration, a change of internal measurement standards. (Dempster, Carney, & McClements, 2010). In other words, adding to Wright's (1960) model of cognitive restructuring of values, some persons may come to recalibrate, and a lower level of functioning may become more acceptable than it was prior to the onset of the health condition.

According to Falvo (2009), what individuals believe about their quality of life is a main determining factor in services requested, treatment compliance, and satisfaction. Individuals' perception of how their disabilities affect their quality of life "is determined by the degree to which they feel they have control over their life circumstances or destiny" (Falvo, 2009, p. 26). Knowledge and involvement in decision making related to management and treatment of their disabilities can lead to enhanced quality of life regarding their needs, goals, and life circumstances.

LIFE STAGES AND QUALITY OF LIFE

From a developmental perspective, the work of Erikson (1963) has suggested that each life stage brings about challenges that will ultimately enhance or distract one from leading a fulfilled life. During each life stage a psychosocial crisis will likely occur based on having reached a particular level of psychological, social, and physical development, creating a need to develop new life skills, attitudes, outlooks, and/or emotional growth. The natural order of psychosocial crises is defined by Erikson (1963) as occurring in the life stages of infancy, toddler and early childhood, school-age child, adolescence, young adulthood, middle-age adulthood, and older adulthood. However, crises can occur or reoccur at any point in a person's lifetime, creating new opportunity for psychological and emotional growth (Sneed, Whitbourne, & Culang, 2006).

For persons with disabilities, the natural order of psychosocial development may be delayed due to a number of environmental, social, and medical factors. According to Falvo (2009), the reaction to disability and chronic illness are influenced by the developmental stage of an individual. Life skills, independence, and self-control are affected according to the needs, roles and responsibilities, and resources of individuals, which are dictated in part by their developmental stage.

Infancy

During this time, physical life tasks focus on the maturation of sensory, perceptual, and motor functions termed as *sensorimotor intelligence*. Early casual schemes are also being developed, leading the infant to understand the nature of cause and effect (if the child cries, someone will come to aid them). Emotional functions center around emotional attachment and the development of trust, in particular of one's caregiver. If the children appropriately bond and develop trust, they will acquire the virtues of hope and drive, and if not, they risk social withdrawal (Erikson, 1959). According to Erikson (1950), when the caregiver responds consistently to the needs of a child, the child will come to expect being comforted and gain a sense of predictability and inner security (Graves & Larkin, 2006). In the case of children with disabilities when they are unable to develop trust in the caregiver due to numerous hospitalizations, medical regimes, and other restrictions, they are at an increased risk for developing behavioral and emotional problems (Geldhill, Rangel, & Garralda, 2000).

Toddlerhood

During toddlerhood, language continues to develop, and children engage in fantasy play and begin to develop self-control over their bodies. They begin to explore their environment, briefly letting go and then returning to the trusted caretaker. According to Erikson (1950) the psychological task is to explore the world and gain an understanding of the self as autonomous from others. Emotionally, a child will gain a sense of mastery and autonomy or will develop shame and self-doubt. Successful accomplishment of tasks will lead to self-control and will power. Failure will result in impulsive and compulsive behavior patterns.

The caretakers have an important function in healthy psychosocial development at this stage in that they must allow the children to explore so as not to restrict their development. They must encourage exploration and curiosity, but they must also maintain sufficient contact so that the children do not feel unsupported or neglected, and apply sufficient discipline to protect the children. Setting boundaries for the children is particularly important to avoid the children developing a preoccupation with testing the limits of their power and control. According to Erikson (1950), too much shame or self-doubt in a child may lead to defiance and attempts to gain a sense of mastery and autonomy through getting away with undesirable actions (Graves & Larkin, 2006). Erikson wrote about this stage stating, "From a sense of self-control without loss of self-esteem comes a lasting sense of good will and pride; from sense of loss of self-control and of foreign over-control comes a lasting propensity for doubt and shame" (Erikson, 1950, p. 254).

The impact of disability at this stage may place physical limitations on exploration, hospitalizations can interrupt nurturing, caregivers can overprotect the child by restricting activities or interactions with others, or may fail to apply necessary behavior corrections due to sympathy for the child's condition (Falvo, 2005). Due to the recognition of the importance of the parent–child relationship at this developmental stage, a relationship-based approach with emphasis on the mother–child interaction is considered important to early intervention. Studies have demonstrated that the key to improved developmental outcomes in children with disabilities is maternal presence (or primary caregiver) and responsiveness. Professionals must work with families of infants and young children, understanding that "Family and cultural expectations and goals and improved parent–child relationships, rather than normative developmental milestones, are the targets of assessment and intervention. The cognitive domain no longer dominates. Affect is gaining recognition as the organizer of development, and increased emphasis is placed on emotional development of the child" (Atkins-Burnett & Allen-Meares, 2000, para. 9).

Preschool- and School-Age Children

Preschool-age children have primary relationships with their families. They learn to cooperate with others and begin to understand gender identification. They will engage in play for discovery and will need to learn to initiate actions and to make choices to avoid a sense of guilt over a lack of accomplishment. Successful development will result in a sense of purpose and direction, whereas deficits in abilities may lead to feelings of inferiority and incompetence and can result in ruthlessness and inhibition (Erikson, 1959).

During early school age, children leave their home environment and learn to interact with peers in a social environment and develop social relationships and friendships. Intellectually they will develop concrete operations, learn new skills, and begin to self-evaluate by comparing themselves with others (Falvo, 2005). Their developmental tasks will lead them to a feeling of achievement and a sense of accomplishment. Failure to progress may result in inertia (Erikson, 1959).

Disability during school-age childhood years may lead to disruption of school attendance and peer play and can interfere with the child's academic performance, peer acceptance, self-confidence, and psychological well-being. Family attempts to shelter the child from painful emotions may lead to increased social isolation and reduced self-confidence. The child will not be given the opportunity to assess his or her potential or to develop important social skills. Early school-age children with disabilities need encouragement to participate in social activities rather than protection from possible peer rejection (Falvo, 2005).

Adolescents

During this life stage, children transition to adulthood. Their bodies become physically mature, and they begin to explore their sexuality and sexual feelings and behaviors. Peer relationships, physical appearance, and attractiveness to others are of primary concern, and adolescents have a need to explore values and beliefs separate from the beliefs of their families, sometimes leading to rebellious behaviors and attitudes. Developmentally, adolescents strive to gain a sense of individuality and independence defined by Erikson (1959) as a stage of identity versus role diffusion in which role models and peers are used to experiment with various roles and identities. Successful psychological development leads to virtues of devotion and fidelity, whereas failure at this time leads to repudiation and feelings of separation from others.

While adolescents with physical disabilities strive to be like their peers, the literature reports a number of social and health differences from teens without disabilities, including less alcohol and illicit drug use, less healthy diets, less physical activity, fewer social activities, and greater difficulty making friends (Antle, Mills, Kalnins, & Rossen, 2007). The impact of disability during this time may cause problems with body image, self-concept, and sexual expression. Disability at this time can be disruptive to peer relationships and emotional development. Parents of adolescents with disabilities may become overly protective, creating a desire on the part of the adolescent to rebel against necessary treatment or medical regimens to fit in with peers or feel independent. Denial of the impact of disability or of imposed restrictions may also be a mechanism used to feel more connected to their peers, but this can lead to noncompliance and have detrimental effects on health (Falvo, 2005).

Parental support during this time is essential, and a number of studies have also shown that adolescents view their parental relationships as supportive and facilitative of their successes (Antle, 2004; Scal, 2002). In a study to examine parents' functioning to promote the health of adolescents with disabilities, Antle et al. (2007) discovered three main parental functions, including (1) promoting healthy behaviors and nutrition; (2) trying to foster opportunities for friendships, a more active social life, and a productive future; and (3) balancing independence with safety and attending to energy conservation so that the adolescents with physical disabilities would have sufficient time and energy for school and social life.

In reviewing the needs of adolescents with disabilities as they transition into adulthood, Schultz and Liptak (1998) identified helpful transition factors as having a high self-esteem and a positive social orientation, living in a warm and cohesive family with supportive but not overly protective parents, having adequate social supports, including friends with and without disabilities, being a contributing family member with chores and responsibilities, and having previously coped successfully with stressful experiences.

Early Adulthood

During early adulthood, individuals emphasize becoming productive members of society through vocation, intimate relationships, and social responsibilities. The psychological task of young adults is to establish intimacy and affection and focus on beginning a family, work, and lifestyle goals. Success in this area leads to feelings of love and affiliation but failure to do so leads to role confusion and a sense of isolation and not fitting in (Erikson, 1959).

Onset of disability at this time can influence vocation in that the limitations imposed by the condition may determine vocational training and selection rather than the interests or even abilities of the individual. Persons with disabilities at this age may also be delayed in gaining independence from their family of origin and experience restrictions from families that are more appropriate for young persons and may interfere with gaining autonomy, setting life goals, and finding a sense of purpose in life. The impact of disability during this time may lead to delays in dating and intimate relationships, delays in starting families because procreation may be difficult, and substantial issues related to the ability to provide adequate childcare and parenting (Falvo, 2005).

Middle Adulthood

During this life stage, adults are involved with managing a career and nurturing an intimate relationship. There may be a shift in caring relationships in that they will experience their own children leaving, but they may also become grandparents or caretakers for their own parents. It is also a time of life reexamination that may result in "mid-life crisis." Emotionally, persons are dealing with measuring the value of their accomplishments in comparison with earlier life goals and dreams, and reviewing perceived failures. It can be a time of passing knowledge and skill to younger generations and shifting from a self-focus to one of concern for children and grandchildren, and mentoring others. Ideally this stage results in a feeling of being needed and valued. Erikson (1959) saw this as a time of gaining a sense of generativity or stagnation. Generativity would be accomplished if the adult felt a sense of guiding and helping create the next generation; stagnation results from dissatisfaction with what had been accomplished and with the current life state (Graves & Larkin, 2006).

Generativity would result in feelings of care and productivity, whereas stagnation would lead to rejectivity (Erikson, 1959).

The impact of disability at this time causes interference with further career development and may lead to early retirement or may otherwise lead to financial difficulties. Because the person's partner is also likely to be experiencing a reexamination of life goals and desires, there is potential for disability to play a role in recommitment to the relationship, but there is also the possibility that the nondisabled partner may choose to leave. The ability to financially or emotionally support aging parents, grown children, and grandchildren may also diminish depending on the extent of the disability. Failure to meet these perceived obligations may result in problems with self-identity and self-esteem (Falvo, 2005).

Later Adulthood

According to Erikson (1959), later adulthood is a time of life review and more global concerns, and resolution about the meaning of life, leading to wisdom or feelings of disdain. Most of the research related to quality of life and life stage occurs with the later adulthood population. The elderly population is growing rapidly, which will lead to substantial increases in numbers of persons with disabilities in the United States. It is estimated that by 2050, over 21% of the total U.S. population will be 65 years or older (Smith, Rayer, & Smith, 2008). This life stage is a time of developing a psychohistorical perspective, a point of view about death, and learning to cope with the physical changes of aging. It is a time of accepting the life lived thus far, of work accomplished, and acceptance that death is imminent. According to Erikson (1959), persons will gain either a sense of integrity or feelings of despair, based on their conclusions about the kind of person they have been. A sense of integrity will result from a determination that their accomplishments and endeavors were worthwhile and meaningful. Persons who are dissatisfied with the life lived so far will feel unhappy and dissatisfied and live with feelings of despair and a fear of death (Graves & Larkin, 2006).

Physical and cognitive limitations and decreasing strength and stamina are expected in older-age persons as well as increasing impairment of hearing and vision. Impact of disability may lead to the surrender of their lifestyles and autonomy. They may need to seek assistance from extended family members since their spouse is likely to be at a similar life stage and at some point no longer able to provide assistance. The older adult may need to move into an assisted care facility when home supports are not sufficient, experiencing a loss of familiar surroundings that may be decades old. Financial issues related to health care may also emerge or increase because many older persons live on a fixed income and many have little in the way of health care benefits (Falvo, 2005).

Quality of life at this stage has been associated with standard of living and stability of finances; physical and mental health; activity involvement; accessible homes and communities; relationships with others that provide feelings of friendship, companionship, love; independence and making one's own choices; having a life purpose or role; and a sense of safety and security (Bowling, 2005; Farquhar, 1995; Grewal et al., 2006).

In a qualitative study of quality of life for older adults, Murphy, Cooney, Shea, and Casey (2008) examined 122 older persons with disabilities that included stroke, depression, arthritis, learning disability, dementia, and hearing and visual impairments. Although their participants placed value on their health and physical functioning as important to their quality of life, when they experienced a decline in physical functioning, they adjusted their definitions of being healthy by noting what they were still able to do such things as wash or dress themselves, and by comparing themselves to others who had less physical capacity. Thus, rather than devaluing health as an important factor of their quality of health, health remained important but was recalibrated in terms of how much was required.

This study also defined social connectedness as important to older persons' quality of life with family as a central component that provided for feeling loved and having companionship and necessary help. For persons who were not connected to a family, friends provided support and companionship but disability limited opportunities for interaction with friends. Older persons with dementia reported difficulty recognizing known persons, a reduction in social interactions, and they lamented the changes imposed when neighbors and friends moved or died, creating feelings of unfamiliarity and a lack of connectedness and belonging with the people in their communities.

Continuing in familiar roles and maintaining familiar activities was also noted as important to older persons' quality of life. Individuals expressed pride in their previous work roles and accomplishments but were generally successful in transition to retirement by directing their interests and skills to new activities. Persons forced to retire due to disability had greater difficulty in their transitions, experiencing a loss of self-confidence and grief over the loss of physical capacities and their work roles. Disability also impacted the ability to participate in desired activities due to physical and cognitive restraints, motivational difficulties, and transportation and accessibility problems.

Perhaps due to the challenges of living with a disability and aging, elderly persons with physical disabilities show higher rates of both depression and anxiety than do persons with disabilities who are not elderly (Brenes et al., 2008). For the elderly, social connectedness and social participation are vital parts of quality of life because "Social participation creates relationships and social networks that build a system of social support that contribute to health and well-being states, including life satisfaction and quality of life" (Stevens-Ratchford, 2008, p. 2).

QUALITY OF LIFE AND DISABILITY TYPE

There is no doubt that there are differences in quality of life based on the type of disability, although much of these differences may be attributable to social responses to different types of disabilities and available resources. Other factors, such as whether a disability is stable or progressive in nature, stigmatized or not, predictable or unpredictable in course, and how much it interferes with daily functioning, will also play a role in attainable quality of life. Falvo (2009) discussed the impact of body image on self-concept. Disability can create a change in body image based on visible changes, the significance of the body alteration on function, how rapidly the body was changed, the perceived importance of the limitations, and the reactions of other people.

Stigma also has an impact on how people feel about themselves and their lives and is sufficiently powerful to keep people from attaining their full potential. Individuals with stigmatized conditions will attempt to hide their conditions from others, which can interfere with treatment and adjustment to disability (Saylor, Yoder, & Mann, 2002). Invisible disabilities can have a similar effect in that others do not recognize that a person has a condition that may need accommodation or have unreasonable expectations for a person based on a lack of visible indication that the person is disabled. The unapparent condition may also create a lack of treatment compliance and movement toward adjustment. Finally, uncertainty in the prognosis or course of a disability makes planning and feeling in control difficult. Persons may hesitate to engage in activities or travel away from home due to fear of deterioration in their conditions. Family members may also overprotect their loved one in an attempt to keep the individual from future loss of functioning (Falvo, 2009).

Psychiatric Disability

In a study to examine differences in quality of life between persons with and without severe mental illness using the World Health Organization Quality of life (WHOQOL) measure (The WHOQOL Group, 1998), Murphy and Murphy noted that "the negative repercussions of mental illness encompassed almost all aspect of quality of life that individuals had ascertained to be important for satisfaction and wellbeing in everyday life" (Murphy & Murphy, 2006, p. 289). Specifically, quality-of-life assessments were found to be lower in the *physical domain* (needed more and less sleep than nondisabled persons), *psychological domain* (more negative feelings, less positive feelings, lower cognitive skills, and lower self-esteem), *independence domain* (more dependence on medication and treatment, less mobility, more difficulty with activities of daily living [ADL], and lower work capacity), *social relationships domain* (lower levels of personal relationships, social support, and sexual activity), and the *environment domain* (lower level of transportation and opportunity for information and skill acquisition). Only the *spirituality* domain showed no significant differences between the populations.

Developmental and Cognitive Disability

In a study to measure quality of life for persons with multiple profound impairments, including profound intellectual impairment, Petry, Maes, and Viakamp (2005) interviewed 76 caregivers, including parents and support staff. Quality of life was identified as comprising five domains of physical well-being, material well-being, social well-being, development and activities, and emotional well-being. *Physical well-being* was seen by caregivers as a need to attend to the lack of physical mobility that interfered with participation in activities; health issues such as nourishment, sleeping problems, neurological problems, and so on; hygiene issues such as changing and washing to avoid bedsores and discomfort; nourishment that frequently involved dealing with digestive problems and also paying attention to food preferences; and providing sufficient rest opportunities during the day and evening. *Material well-being* was seen as a function of a safe, comfortable, and accessible living environment with attention to room temperature, ventilation, and a pleasant atmosphere that included attention to lighting, furnishings, and music. Technical aids that assisted with comfort and posture and assisted with activity participation and transportation for excursions were also noted as important to material well-being. *Social well-being* involved attending to communication needs and expressions that were "often small and hard to notice behavioral signals" (Petry et al., 2005, p. 41); basic security, family bonds, which were primarily with parents who were most aware of their child's needs; social relationships that involved the presence of other persons, including others with profound multiple disabilities; individual attention; and social participation that utilized public services. The fourth *personal* domain of well-being included development and a broad range of activities. Attending to signals that indicate what persons want and do not want to do, and developing potential and increasing skills were seen as important to this domain. The final domain of *emotional well-being* included having a positive affect around clients, recognition of client individuality, a respectful approach, and providing an atmosphere that is nonstressful and pleasant. While the domains of quality of life for persons with profound impairments are similar to persons without disabilities, persons with profound impairments are very dependent on others for their quality of life, and many of them are unable to communicate through language their needs and desires. Additionally, support staff and members of society may find their appearances frightening, but quality of life is based on meeting many of the common human needs. Their situations require attention to those shared and distinctive elements that can contribute to an increase in quality of life.

In a review of studies from 1990 to 2004 aimed at increasing levels of happiness for persons with severe or profound learning disabilities, Lancioni, Singh, O'Reilly, Oliva, and Basili (2005) concluded that numerous activities and stimulations would increase the level of expressed pleasure. Despite being unable to communicate, consumers could express happiness by smiling, laughing, and excited movements. Participants could be given favorite items or positively stimulated through talking, tickling, or rubbing the arms. Microswitch-based stimulation has also been shown to increase pleasure responses in persons with brain injury and intellectual and multiple disabilities by providing a switch to the consumer for operation of electronic equipment to provide music, video clips, and massage devices upon activation (Lancioni et al., 2006, 2010).

Historically, deinstitutionalization has been recognized as contributing to the increase in quality of life for persons with learning impairments because it is assumed that integration into the social mainstream will lead to a more satisfying life (Barlow & Kirby, 1991; Emerson, 1985; Sullivan, Vitello, & Foster, 1988). In a study of older men who had severe learning impairments and who had moved from institutionalized living to sharing a three-bedroom home with direct care services provided by a nonprofit agency, participants indicated overall life satisfaction. However, a number of deficit areas were noted that negatively impacted their quality of life, including a lack of opportunity to make choices about daily routines, personal finances, housemates, and house selection. The authors conclude that merely moving individuals to preferred locations is insufficient if not accompanied by opportunities for meaningful choice-making because it is contrary to the concept of normalization (Wolfensburger, 1972) and denies consumers the right to achieve optimal autonomy, noting, "Respecting the values held by adults with severe learning difficulties, fostering choice-making opportunities, and honouring preferences, are imperative to supporting these adults in enhancing the quality of their lives" (Treece, Gregory, Ayers, & Mendis, 1999, p. 801). Higher functioning persons with learning disabilities also experience challenges to quality of life. Houghton found that persons with attention deficit hyperactivity disorder (ADHD) continued to have problems interacting with others throughout their lifetime, stating, "The research evidence seems to suggest that mentors across all periods of development across the lifespan can be beneficial to those with ADHD . . ." (Houghton, 2006, p. 270). In part, some of the behavior problems that exist in persons with learning disabilities and pervasive developmental disorders (PDDs) may be due to a lack of sufficient education and intervention programs in their early childhood, particularly for those with PDDs, resulting in substantial behavior problems, including self-aggression and aggression toward others, social withdrawal, and lethargy. Because many persons with PDDs are not able to verbally communicate, quality of life is viewed by a reduction in negative behaviors most frequently accomplished through behavioral techniques, including positive reinforcement for desired behaviors and negative reinforcement to extinguish aberrant behaviors (Gerber, Baud, Giroud, & Carminati, 2008).

There are distinct differences in quality of life for persons with traumatic brain injury (TBI) that are based on the experience of losing abilities that the person with a TBI once had. Barriers to higher quality of life have been noted as personal losses, social reactions of others, and loss of control (Kincaid, 1998). In a study of quality of life for persons with acquired head injuries, Degeneffe and Lee (2010) surveyed 279 siblings of persons with TBI. The majority of siblings viewed the injured person as having a negative quality of life primarily due to functional losses in the areas of self-care, physical health, employment, financial self-sufficiency, relationships, and active lifestyle. The siblings also noted that negative quality of life due to psychological factors included difficulties with adjustment, adaptation, and acceptance of their injuries. They discussed sadness, a lack of hope and ambition, and a loss of self-identity. Further, negative quality of life was attributed to a lack of sufficient professional care and family support. Contrarily, participants who believed that their family member had a more positive quality of life attributed it to positive family support and professional care. These families were seen as providing emotional support, encouragement, and financial support and professionals were viewed as acting in a caring and supportive manner. The authors point specifically to the negative impact of role limitations due to emotional and physical deficits of TBI that interfere with relationships, employment, and education as being detrimental to a good quality of life. Interestingly, Kreuter, Sullivan, Dahllof, and Siosteen (1998) found that marital status and educational attainment were not correlated to quality of life for persons with TBI but that lack work or student engagement, depression, low social and physical functioning, and greater severity of the injury were negatively correlated to quality of life.

Physical Disability

The attitudinal and behavioral shift toward attending to quality of life for persons with physical disability has occurred in part because of advances in medical care that have substantially extended the life span expectations for many persons with chronic illness and physical disabilities. A number of studies have examined quality of life in persons with stable injuries and illnesses and in persons with illnesses with an unpredictable or progressively declining course. The predictability or unpredictability of illness and resulting complications can affect the way persons live their day-to-day lives, their satisfaction with their lives, and their perceptions of quality of life.

In a study to compare the quality of life of persons with spinal cord injury (SCI) to persons without a disability, Barker et al. (2009) determined that quality of life was substantially lower for persons with SCI than for persons without disability. The level of quality of life among persons with SCI was not associated with the level of injury, the age of the person, or the time since the injury. Rather, two factors were determined to influence having a lower quality of life: a secondary impairment and the level of social participation. The presence of a secondary condition, such as urinary tract infections and neuropathic pain, was the most significant predictor of quality of life. Second, quality of life could be predicted by the level of community integration that included perceptions, beliefs, and attitudes about their connections to their communities. The more integrated and positively connected the persons with SCI perceived themselves to be, the higher they rated their quality of life.

Duggan and Dijkers (2001) conducted interviews with 40 persons with SCI and found that high levels of quality of life were prevalent among persons having a greater length of time since injury, material assets, financial security, and valuable social roles. Low levels of quality of life were associated with financial instability, few material resources, and reports of lower emotional and spiritual assets. Other variables that impact quality of life for persons with SCI were identified by Boswell, Dawson, and Heininger (1998) in a qualitative study that interviewed 12 participants with SCI. The domains identified as most important were life attitude, opportunity for work, and level of resources. These domains interacted with each other because resources, including basic needs such as housing, transportation, and food, were identified as necessary for positive attitude. Similarly, work opportunities strongly influenced life attitude.

In a study to assess the lives and emotions of 160 persons with amputations, Williamson, Schulz, Bridges, and Behan (1994) noted that less satisfactory social relationships and more restriction of activity increased emotional distress. Those who used their prostheses less had greater activity restriction and more depressive symptomatology. Underscoring the importance of family and social interaction, an investigation of quality of life between persons with tetraplegia and dependent on ventilators, and persons who had tetraplegia but were not ventilator assisted, determined that only 23.8% of those with ventilators expressed dissatisfaction with their lives and only 35.6% of those without ventilators expressed dissatisfaction. Life satisfaction, well-being, and quality of life were all generally positive and correlated with social and family interaction (Bach & Tilton, 1994).

Kreuter et al. (1998) specifically looked at the role of partner relationships in quality of life for persons with SCI. About half of the participants reported that they separated from their partners after their injuries. Marital status correlated with quality of life, although sexual functioning did not. Other factors that predicted a higher quality of life were being younger and being injured at a younger age. Vocational involvement also positively affected quality of life, although the level of education did not. Pain that interfered with functioning, depression, lower levels of social and physical functioning, and the feeling of loss of independence also negatively impacted quality of life.

Chronic Health Conditions

Similar to persons with SCI, pain also impacts quality of life in persons with multiple sclerosis (MS). Pain is frequently accompanied by fatigue, difficulty in sleeping, and depression pointing to a necessity of effective pain management in quality of life (Newland, Naismith, & Ullione, 2009). Overall, quality of life has been shown to be significantly lower for persons with chronic health conditions than for persons without disabilities. Quality of life of people with MS is impacted by the extent of medical condition, health care needs being met, help with ADL, and employment (Wu, Minden, Hoaglin, Hadden, & Frankel, 2007). Emotionally, patients report fear, anger, and sadness. They are emotionally overwhelmed by the diagnosis and have concerns about the course of the disease (White, White, & Russell, 2007). In a study of life satisfaction among persons with MS and progressive muscular dystrophy, Chen and Crewe (2009) determined that the best predictor of life satisfaction were the acceptance of disability and hope that was defined as the expectation of reaching one's goals. Other factors that influenced satisfaction with life included spiritual well-being and a number of demographic variables. For example, women and married persons with MS were more satisfied.

Like MS, diabetes is a degenerative disease associated with a declining quality of life (Brown et al., 2004). Diabetes requires numerous lifestyle changes, and adjustment is often difficult requiring continued dietary and medical compliance and self-motivation. Ayalon et al. (2008) found a number of factors predictive of quality of life. A higher quality of life could be predicted by higher educational attainment, less difficulty in meeting basic needs, no medical complications, lack of emotional distress, and physical activity. However, the authors also found that strict medical and dietary adherence could lower, rather than raise, the subjective quality of life, perhaps suggesting that people have a limit to the amount of regulation and restriction they are willing to accept. For this reason, some individuals may take health risks to increase quality of life.

For an increasing number of persons, cancer has become a curable disease. However, it may also have an unpredictable course. Frequently, those who recover from cancer live with fear of its recurrence. Issues of importance to cancer survivors related to quality of life determined by Avis et al. (2005) include personal growth and a number of concerns about physical appearance, financial problems, distress over a possible recurrence of cancer, and distress within the family. Additional factors that could negatively affect quality of life were identified by Luoma and Hakamies-Blomqvist (2004) as increased dependence on others and isolation that resulted from alterations in physical appearance.

Sensory Disability

Sensory disabilities have great potential to delay development and isolate individuals with these disabilities that may significantly impact their quality of life even at a very young age. Overall life satisfaction for youth who are deaf or hard of hearing has been shown to be significantly lower than for hearing youth (Gilman, Easterbrooks, & Frey, 2004). Persons who are deaf frequently have problems communicating with hearing people and may be socially isolated as a result of their disabilities. As students, in addition to typical academic and social demands, they may need supplemental services and education for communication and social skills, independent living skills, and career exploration. Learning is generally delayed in persons born deaf or who acquire hearing loss at an early age, owing to less exposure to language, and many are functionally illiterate as a result of communication and education barriers that greatly impact employment opportunities later in life (Hardwell Byrd, 2004; Ries, 1994).

While some persons in the deaf community frown on cochlear implants as a means of restoring hearing capacity, in a recent study of 88 families of deaf children, Roland and Tobey (2010) found that profoundly deaf children who received cochlear implants had a quality of life equal to hearing children on the dimensions of physical health, mental and emotional health, academic performance, self-esteem, and relationships with friends and family.

In a study of the psychological well-being of 343 adults with acquired hearing loss, Helvik, Jacobsen, and Hallberg (2006) determined that well-being was influenced by greater social participation, more activity, and greater sense of humor. Females in the study reported lower levels of positive well-being, self-control, general health, and vitality, and higher levels of anxiety and depression. Interestingly, the level of hearing impairment was not a factor associated with overall well-being. Interestingly, the type of communication strategy (CS) used was also not associated with well-being. CS for persons with hearing impairment included maladaptive strategies, such as avoiding communicating with others or pretending to understand others; verbal strategies, such as acknowledging hearing problems; and nonverbal strategies, such as watching the speaker closely. Despite the CS used, well-being was not shown to be impacted.

There is a paucity of literature related to quality of life for persons with visual impairment, although considerable work has been done in the area of adjustment to vision loss, suggesting that depression is a likely reaction to vision loss and that adaptation is facilitated by higher intellect, educational attainment, and self-efficacy (Livneh & Antonak, 1997). For persons who become visually impaired, a loss of the driving ability is associated with feelings of a loss of freedom because a lack of mobility can lead to job loss and restrictions in socialization and recreation (Montarzino et al., 2007). Several studies have demonstrated that as visual acquity decreases, so does quality of life (Broman et al., 2002; Globe, Wu, Azen, & Varma, 2004).

A few studies have looked at age-related sensory impairment and quality of life. Adolescents with visual impairment report a lower overall quality of life, lower psychosocial functioning, and lower school functioning than adolescents with normal vision (Wong, Machin, Tan, Wong, & Saw, 2009). In older adults, age-related sensory impairment is not uncommon; over 18% of adults older than 70 are visually impaired, over 33% are hearing impaired, and over 8% have both types of impairment. Older adults with visual and hearing impairments are likely to experience a functional decrease and are at increased risk of hip fracture and depression. They will also need to rely more on family or on caregivers for their ADL and transportation (Campbell et al., 1999) that may greatly affect quality of life.

CURRENT QUALITY-OF-LIFE TOPICS

End of Life and Quality of Life

End of life is also a time to be considerate of maintaining quality of life to the extent possible and is an important new aspect of rehabilitation counseling demonstrated by the addition of a new standard to the rehabilitation code of ethics that addresses end-of-life issues for terminally ill persons, including counselor competence and quality of care (CRCC, 2010). While physicians may be reluctant to have end-of-life discussions with their patients who are nearing death, studies have shown that such discussions are helpful to the client in understanding choices related to prolonging life and frequently result in do-not-resuscitate orders and can decrease stress, depression, and anxiety in family members. In addition, more aggressive medical treatment has been associated with a lower quality of life in patients and increased depression in family members (Wright et al., 2008).

Davison (2002) argues that prolonging life for terminal patients may cause them to suffer needlessly. In her discussion on quality of life and end-stage renal disease (ESRD), she notes that patients are not assessed for quality of life and frequently die isolated from the community and family because the focus of physicians is on dialysis schedules to prolong life. A lack of communication with the patient creates false hope, and patients do not accept that they are dying and they are not given opportunity to focus on decisions related to pain management, symptom control, psychological supports, and communication that might afford them a higher quality of life. A lack of quality-of-life assessment may in part be based on why patients wait until very late in the disease to withdraw from dialysis with little time or energy remaining to communicate preferences, values, and goals or to work toward a meaningful death. With this in mind, Davison (2002) outlines end-of-life discussion content as needing to include:

- Realistic information with respect to prognosis and expectations on dialysis.
- An exploration of patients' values, expectations, goals, beliefs, and fears.
- Questions that need to be asked of patients include:

  What is important in life to you?
  How does your illness/dialysis make you feel?
  How has your illness affected your ability to do the things you enjoy/your day-to-day life?
  What is your understanding of your prognosis?
  What do you want out of your treatment?

What do you want to achieve?
What frightens you about death?
What limitations, if any, would make you want to stop dialysis (treatment)?
(Davison, 2002, p. 43)

Interviews based on understanding clients' wishes and concerns could result in assisting persons in constructing a plan regarding their end-of-life care that includes their values, goals, and ideas about what makes for a meaningful end of life. While aggressive medical treatment is not advocated as necessarily conducive to quality of life, aggressive pain management and management of depression are considered to be essential components to quality of life at the end of life.

Spirituality, Religiosity, and Quality of Life

There is a growing body of literature on the impact of religion and spirituality on numerous disabilities, including heart disease, cancer, arthritis, chronic pain, SCI, and other conditions (Abraido-Lanza, Vasquez, & Echeverria, 2004; Graf, Marini, Baker, & Buck, 2007; Kozak, 2001; Levin, 2001; Marini & Graf, 2010; Rippentrop, 2005; Warfield & Goldstein, 1996). Although religiosity and spirituality are excluded from a number of quality-of-life measures, researchers from a variety of disciplines have begun to examine the impact of these factors on quality of life. In a study of nearly 500 persons with cancer diagnoses, spiritual well-being was noted to be a significant contributor to quality of life and found to be positively associated with a fighting spirit and negatively associated with a sense of hopelessness and helplessness (Whitford, Olver, & Peterson, 2008). Similarly, Brillhart (2005) explored spirituality and SCI in relation to quality of life and life satisfaction with 230 participants with SCI and found a moderate positive correlation ($r = 0.65$) between the psychological/spiritual subscale and quality of life.

Religiosity has also been found to have an impact on quality of life at the end of life. In a study of 499 elderly persons who were 12 months or less from death, more religious persons were healthier and they found life more exciting. Overall, quality of life over the last year of life was found to be positively associated with religious involvement (Idler, McLaughlin, & Kasl, 2009).

CONCLUSION

Quality of life is a difficult construct to measure because it is impacted by numerous objective and subjective variables and individual preferences. For people with disabilities, additional factors related to their health conditions may challenge attaining optimum quality of life. In addition, developmental progression may both have an effect on, and be affected by, disability because roles, responsibilities, goals, and outlooks are affected by life stage. Quality of life will also be influenced by the type of disability and the factors associated with it, including associated stigma, whether a disability is stable or progressive in nature, whether it has a predictable or unpredictable course, and how much it interferes with daily functioning.

REFERENCES

Abraido-Lanza, A. F., Vasquez, E., & Echeverria, S. E. (2004). En las manos de dios (In God's hands): Religious and other forms of coping among Latinos with arthritis. *Journal of Consulting and Clinical Psychology, 72*, 91–102.

Antle, B. J. (2004). Seeking strengths in young people with physical disabilities examining factors associated with self-worth. *Health and Social Work, 29*, 167–175.

Antle, B. J., Mills, W., Steele, C., Kalnins, I., & Rossen, B. (2007). An exploratory study of parents' approaches to health promotion in families of adolescents with physical disabilities. *Child Care, Health and Development, 34*, 185–193.

Atkins-Burnett, S., & Allen-Meares, P. (2000). Infants and toddlers with disabilities: Relationship-based approaches. *Social Work, 45*(4), 371–379. Retrieved on May 16, 2011 from EBSCO*host*.

Avis, N. E., Smith, K. W., McGraw, S., Smith, R. G., Petronis, V. M., & Carver, C. S. (2005). Assessing quality of life in adult cancer survivors (QLACS). *Quality of life Research, 14*, 1007–1023.

Ayalon, L., Gross, R., Tabenkin, H., Porath, A., Heymann, A., & Porter, B. (2008). Determinants of quality of life in primary care patients with diabetes: Implications for social workers. *Health and Social Work, 33*, 229–236.

Bach, J. R., & Tilton, M. C. (1994). Life satisfaction and well-being measures in ventilator assisted individuals with traumatic tetraplegia. *Archives of Physical Medicine and Rehabilitation, 75*, 626–632.

Barker, R. N., Kendall, M. D., Amsters, D. I., Pershouse, K. J., Haines, T. P., & Kuipers, P. (2009). The relationship between quality of life and disability across the lifespan for people with spinal cord injury. *Spinal Cord, 47*, 149–155.

Barlow, J., & Kirby, N. (1991). Residential satisfaction of persons with an intellectual disability living in an institution or in the community, *Australia and New Zealand Journal of Developmental Disabilities, 17*, 7–23.

Bishop, M., & Allen, C. A. (2003). Epilepsy's impact on quality of life: A qualitative analysis. *Epilepsy & Behavior, 4*, 226–233.

Bishop, M., & Feist-Price, S. (2001). Quality of life in rehabilitation counseling: Making the philosophical practical. *Rehabilitation Education, 15*, 201–212.

Bishop, M., Chapin, M., & Miller, S. (2008). Quality of life assessment in the measurement of rehabilitation outcomes. *Journal of Rehabilitation: Special Issue on Rehabilitation Outcomes, 74*(2), 45–55.

Boswell, B. B., Dawson, M., & Heininger, E. (1998). Quality of life as defined by adults with spinal cord injuries. *Journal of Rehabilitation, 64*, 27–32.

Bowling, A. (2001). *Measuring disease: A review of disease specific quality of life measurement scales* (2nd ed.). Buckingham, UK: Open University Press.

Bowling, A. (2005). *Aging well: Quality of life in old age*. Berkshire, UK: Open University Press.

Brenes, G. A., Penninx, B. W. J. H., Judd, P. H., Rockwell, E., Sewell, D. D., & Wetherell, J. L. (2008). Anxiety, depression and disability across the lifespan. *Aging & Mental Health, 12*, 158–163.

Brillhart, B. (2005). A study of spirituality and life satisfaction among persons with spinal cord injury. *Rehabilitation Nursing, 19*, 191–197.

Broman, A. T., Munoz, B., Rodriguez, J., Sanchez, R., Quigley, II. A., Klein, R. et al. (2002). The impact of visual impairment and eye disease on vision-related quality of life in a Mexican-American population: Proyecto VER. *Investigative Ophthalmology & Visual Science, 43*, 3393–3398.

Brown, D. W., Balluz, L. S., Giles, W. H., Beckles, G. L., Moriarty, D. G., Ford, E. S. et al. (2004). Diabetes mellitusand health-related quality of life among older adults. Findings from the behavioral risk factor surveillance system (BRFSS). *Diabetes Research and Clinical Practice, 65*, 105–115.

Campbell, V. A., Crews, J. E., Moriarty, D. G., Zack, M. M., & Blackman, D. K. (1999). Surveillance for sensory impairment, activity limitation, and health-related quality of life among older adults—United States, 1993–1997. *Centers for Disease Control and Prevention*. Retrieved from http://www.cdc.gov/mmwr/preview/mmwrhtml/ss4808a6.htm

Centers for Disease Control and Prevention. (2010). *Health related quality of life*. Retrieved from http://www.cdc.gov/hrquality of life/index.htm

Chen, R. K., & Crewe, N. M. (2009). Life satisfaction among people with progressive disabilities. *The Journal of Rehabilitation, 75*(2), 50–58.

Chubon, R. A. (1994). *Social and psychological foundations of rehabilitation.* Springfield, IL: Charles C. Thomas Publisher.

CRCC (2010). *New Code of Professional Ethics for Rehabilitation Counselors Effective January 1, 2010: Top 10 changes.* Retrieved January 17, 2011, from http://www.crccertification.com/filebin/pdf/CRCC_COE_Top10Changes.pdf

Crewe, N. M. (1980). Quality of life: The ultimate goal in rehabilitation. *Minnesota Medicine, 63,* 586–589.

Davison, S. (2002). Quality end-of-life care in dialysis units. *Seminars in Dialysis, 15,* 41–44.

Degeneffe, C. E., & Lee, G. K. (2010). Quality of life after traumatic brain injury: Perspectives of adult siblings. *Journal of Rehabilitation, 76*(4), 27–36.

Dempster, M., Carney, R., & McClements, R. (2010). Response shift in the assessment of quality of life among people attending cardiac rehabilitation. *British Journal of Health Psychology, 15,* 307–319.

Duggan, C. H., & Dijkers, M. (2001). Quality of life after spinal cord injury: A qualitative study. *Rehabilitation Psychology, 46,* 3–27.

Emerson, E. B. (1985). Evaluating the impact of deinstitutionalization on the lives of mentally retarded people. *American Journal of Mental Deficiency, 90,* 277–288.

Erikson, E. H. (1950). *Childhood and society.* New York, NY: W. W. Norton & Company.

Erikson, E. H. (1959). *Identity and the life cycle; selected papers.* New York, NY: International Universities Press.

Erikson, E. H. (1963). *Childhood and society* (2nd ed.) (Rev. & Enl.). New York, NY: Norton.

Fabian, E. S. (1991). Using quality of life indicators in rehabilitation program evaluation. *Rehabilitation Counseling Bulletin, 34,* 344–356.

Falvo, D. (2005). *Medical and psychosocial aspects of chronic illness and disability.* Sudbury, MA: Jones and Barlett Inc.

Falvo, D. R. (2009). *Medical and psychosocial aspects of chronic illness and disability.* Sudbury, MA: Jones and Barlett Inc.

Farquhar, M. (1995). Elderly people's definitions of quality of life. *Social Science Medicine, 41,* 1439–1446.

Felce, D., & Perry, J. (1996). Exploring current conceptions of quality of life: A model for people with and without disabilities. In R. Renwick, I. Brown, & M. Nagler (Eds.), *Quality of life in health promotion and rehabilitation: Conceptual approaches, issues, and applications* (pp. 52–62). Thousand Oaks, CA: Sage.

Frisch, M. B. (1999). Quality of life assessment/intervention and the Quality of Life Inventory (QOLI®). In M. R. Maruish (Ed.), *The use of psychological testing for treatment planning and outcome assessment* (pp. 1227–1331). Hillsdale, NJ: Lawrence-Erlbaum.

George, L., & Bearon, L. (1980). *Quality of life in older persons.* New York, NY: Human Sciences Press.

Gerber, F., Baud, M. A., Giroud, M., & Galli-Carminatim, G. (2008). Quality of life of adults with pervasive developmental disorders and intellectual disabilities. *Journal of Autism and Developmental Disorders, 38,* 1654–1665.

Gilman, R., Easterbrooks, S., & Frey, M. (2004). A preliminary study of multidimensional life satisfaction among deaf/hard of hearing youth across environmental settings. *Social Indicators' Research, 66,* 143–166.

Gladis, M. M., Gosch, E. A., Dishuk, N. M., & Crits-Christoph, P. (1999). Quality of life: Expanding the scope of clinical significance. *Journal of Consulting and Clinical Psychology, 67,* 320–331.

Gledhill, J., Rangel, L., & Garralda, M. E. (2000). Surviving chronic physical illness: Psychosocial outcome in adult life. *Archives of Disease in Childhood, 83,* 104–110.

Globe, D. R., Wu, J., Azen, S. P., & Varma, R. (2004). The impact of visual impairment on self-reported visual functioning in Latinos: The Los Angeles Latino Eye Study. *Ophthalmology, 111,* 1141–1149.

Graf, N. M., Marini, I., Baker, J., & Buck, T. (2007). The perceived impact of religious and spiritual beliefs for persons with chronic pain. *Rehabilitation Counseling Bulletin, 51*(1), 21–33.

Graves, S. B., & Larkin, E. (2006). Lessons from Erikson: A look at autonomy across the lifespan. *Journal of Intergenerational Relationships, 4,* 61–71.

Grewal, I., Lewis, J., Flynn, T., Brown, J., Gond, J., & Coast, J. (2006). Developing attributes for a generic quality of life measure for older people: Preferences or capabilities? *Social Science and Medicine, 62,* 1891–1901.

Hardwell Byrd, S. (2004, December 12). Deaf students seek help to master English texts. *Los Angeles Times,* p. A36.

Helvik, A. S., Jacobsen, G., & Hallberg, L. (2006). Psychological well-being of adults with acquired hearing impairment. *Disability and Rehabilitation, 28,* 535–545.

Houghton, S. (2006). Advances in ADHD research through the lifespan: Common themes and implications. *International Journal of Disability, Development and Education, 53,* 263–272.

Hughes, C., Hwang, B., Kim, J., Eisenman, L., & Killian, D. (1995). Quality of life in applied research: A review and analysis of empirical measures. *American Journal on Mental Retardation, 99,* 623–641.

Idler, E. L., McLaughlin, J., & Kasl, S. (2009). Religion and the quality of life in the last year of life. *Journals of Gerontology Series B: Psychological Sciences & Social Sciences, 64B,* 528–537.

Kincaid, C. A. (1998). Quality of life and secondary disabling conditions among individuals with traumatic brain injury. *Dissertation Abstracts International, 59*(01), 93.

Kozak, D. (2001). Faith eases chronic pain. *Prevention, 53,* 50.

Kreuter, M., Sullivan, M., Dahllof, A. G., & Siosteen, A. (1998). Partner relationships, functioning, mood and global quality of life in persons with spinal cord injury and traumatic brain injury. *Spinal Cord, 36,* 252–261.

Lancioni, G. E., Singh, N. N., O'Reilly, M. F., Oliva, D., & Basili, G. (2005). An overview of research on increasing indices of happiness of people with severe/profound intellectual and multiple disabilities. *Disability and Rehabilitation, 27,* 83–93.

Lancioni, G. E., Singh, N. N., O'Reilly, M. F., Oliva, D., Smaldone, A., Tota, A., et al. (2006). Assessing the effects of stimulation versus microswitch-based programmes on indices of happiness of students with multiple disabilities. *Journal of Intellectual Disability Research, 50,* 739–747.

Lancioni, G. E., Singh, N. N., O'Reilly, M. F., Sigafoos, J., Buonocunto, F., Sacco, V. et al. (2010). Persons with acquired brain injury and multiple disabilities access stimulation independently through microswitch-based technology. *Perceptual and Motor Skills, 111,* 485–495.

Levin, J. (2001). *God, faith, and health: Exploring the spirituality healing connection.* Hoboken, NJ: Wiley & Sons.

Livneh, H. (2001). Psychosocial adaptation to chronic illness and disability: A conceptual framework. *Rehabilitation Counseling Bulletin, 44,* 151–160.

Livneh, H., & Antonak, R. F. (1997). *Psychosocial adaptation to chronic illness and disability.* Gaithersburg, MD: Aspen.

Luoma, M., & Hakamies-Blomqvist, L. (2004). The meaning of quality of life in patients being treated for advanced breast cancer: A qualitative study. *Psychooncology, 13,* 729–739.

Marini, I., & Graf, N. M. , (2010). Spirituality among persons with spinal cord injury: Attitudes, beliefs and practices. *Rehabilitation Counseling Bulletin, 54,* 82–92.

Michalos, A. C. (1991). *Global report on student well-being: Volume I: Life satisfaction and happiness.* New York, NY: Springer-Verlag.

Montarzino, A., Robertson, B., Aspinall, P., Ambrecht, A., Findlay, C., Hine, et al. (2007). *Visual Impairment Research, 9,* 67–82.

Murphy, K., Cooney, A., Shea, E. O., & Casey, D. (2008). Determinants of quality of life for older people living with a disability in the community. *Journal of Advanced Nursing, 65,* 606–615.

Murphy, H., & Murphy, E. K. (2006). Comparing quality of life using the World Health Organization Quality of life measure (WHOQUALITY OF LIFE-100) in a clinical and non-clinical sample: Exploring the role of self-esteem, self-efficacy and social functioning. *Journal of Mental Health, 15,* 289–300.

Myers, D. G., & Diener, E. (1995). Who is happy? *Psychological Science, 6,* 10–19.

National Organization on Disability/Harris Survey of Americans with Disabilities. (2004, June 24). Landmark survey finds pervasive disadvantages. *Internet TV for Assistive Technology.* Retrieved from http://www.at508.com/040624_national_press_club.cfm

Newland, P. K., Naismith, R. T., & Ullione, M. (2009). The impact of pain and other symptoms on quality of life in women with relapsing-remitting multiple sclerosis. *Journal of Neuroscience Nursing, 41*, 322–328.

Petry, K., Maes, B., & Viaskamp, C. (2005). Domains of quality of life of people with profound multiple disabilities: The perspective of parents and direct support staff. *Journal of Applied Research in Intellectual Disabilities, 18*, 35–46.

Revicki, D. A., Osoba, D., Fairclough, D., Barofsky, I., Berzon, R., Leidy, N. K., et al. (2000). Recommendations on health-related quality of life research to support labeling and promotional claims in the United States. *Quality of Life Research, 9*, 887–900.

Ries, P. W. (1994). *Prevalence and characteristics of persons with hearing trouble: United States, 1990–91* (Vital and Health Statistics, Series 10, No. 188; DHHS Publication No. PHS 94-1516). Hyattsville, MD: National Center for Health Statistics.

Rippentrop, E. A. (2005). A review of the role of religion and spirituality in chronic pain populations. *Rehabilitation Psychology, 50*, 278–284.

Roland, P., & Tobey, E. (2010, February 25). Deaf children with cochlear implants report similar quality of life to that of normal-hearing kids, UT Southwestern survey finds. *Southwestern Medical Center.* Retrieved from http://www.utsouthwestern.edu/utsw/cda/dept353744/files/577530.html

Rosseler, R. T. (1990) A quality of life perspective on rehabilitation counseling. *Rehabilitation Counseling Bulletin, 34*(2), 82–90.

Rosseler, R. T., Neath, J., McMahon, B. T., & Rumrill, P. D. (2007). Workplace discrimination outcomes and their predictive factors for adults with multiple sclerosis. *Rehabilitation Counseling Bulletin, 50*(3), 139–152.

Saylor, C., Yoder, M., & Mann, R. J. (2002). Stigma. In I. M. Lubkin & P. D. Larsons (Eds.), *Chronic illness: Impact and interventions* (pp. 53–76). Sudbury, MA: Jones & Bartlett.

Scal, P. (2002). Transition for youth with chronic conditions: Primary care physicians' approaches. *Pediatrics, 110*, 1315–1321.

Schultz, A. W., & Liptak, G. S. (1998). Helping adolescents who have disabilities negotiate transitions to adulthood. *Issues in Contemporary Nursing, 21*, 187–201.

Schwartz, C. E., & Sprangers, M. A. G. (2000). *Adaptation to changing health: Response shift in quality of life research.* Washington, DC: American Psychological Association.

Smart, J. (2001). *Disability, society, and the individual.* Gaithersburg, MD: Aspen.

Smith, S. K., Rayer, S., & Smith, E. A. (2008). Aging and disability: Implications for the housing industry and housing policy in the United States. *Journal of the American Planning Association, 74*, 289–306.

Sneed, J. R., Whitbourne, S. K., & Culang, M. E. (2006). Trust, identity, and ego integrity: Modeling Erikson's core stages over 34 years. *Journal of Adult Development, 13*, 148–157.

Stevens-Ratchford, R. G. (2008). Aging well through long-standing social occupation: A closer look at social participation and quality of life in a sample of community-dwelling older adults. *Forum on Public Policy Online*, Spring 2008 edn. Retrieved from http://www.forumonpublicpolicy.com/archivespring08/stevens-Ratchford.pdf

Sullivan, C. A. C., Vitello, S. J., & Foster, W. (1988). Adaptive behaviour of adults with mental retardation in a group home: A case study. *Education and Training in Mental Retardation, 23*, 76–81.

Treece, A., Gregory, S., Ayers, B., & Mendis, K. (1999). 'I always do what they tell me to do': Choice-making opportunities in the lives of two older persons with severe learning difficulties living in a community setting. *Disability & Society, 14*, 791–804.

U.S. Census Bureau. (2005). *Americans with disabilities, 2005.* Retrieved from http://www.census.gov/hhes/www/disability/sipp/disab05/d05tb1.pdf

Warfield, R. D., & Goldstein, M. B. (1996). Spirituality: The key to recovery from alcoholism. *Counseling and Values, 40*, 196–205.

White, M., White, C. P., & Russell, C. S. (2007). Multiple sclerosis patients talking with healthcare providers about emotions. *Journal of Neuroscience Nursing, 39*, 89–101.

Whitford, H. S., Olver, I. N., & Peterson, M. J. (2008). Spirituality as a core domain in the assessment of quality of life in oncology. *Psycho-Oncology, 17*, 1121–1128.

The WHOQOL Group (1998). The World Health Organization Quality of life Assessment (WHOQOL): Development and general psychometric properties. *Social Science & Medicine, 46,* 1569–1585.

Williamson, G. M., Schulz, R., Bridges, M. W., & Behan, A. M. , (1994). Social and psychological factors in adjustment to limb amputation. *Journal of Social Behavior and Personality, 9,* 249–268.

Wolfensburger, W. (1972). *The principle of normalization in human services.* Toronto: National Institute on Mental Retardation.

Wong, H. B., Machin, D., Tan, S. B., Wong, T. Y., & Saw, S. M. (2009). Visual impairment and its impact on health-related quality of life in adolescents. *American Journal of Ophthalmology, 147,* 505–511.

Wright, B. A. (1960). *Physical disability: A psychological approach.* New York, NY: Harper & Row.

Wright, G. (1980). *Total rehabilitation.* Boston, MA: Little, Brown & Co.

Wright, A., Zhang, B., Ray, A., Mack, J. W., Trice, E., Balboni, T. et al. (2008). Associations between end-of-life discussions, patient mental health, medical care near death, and caregiver bereavement adjustment. *Journal of the American Medical Association, 300,* 1665–1673.

Wu, N., Minden, S. L., Hoaglin, D. C., Hadden, I., & Frankel, D. (2007). Quality of life in people with multiple sclerosis: Data from the Sonya Slifka Longitudinal Multiple Sclerosis Study. *Journal of Health and Human Services Administration, 30,* 233–267.

INSIDER PERSPECTIVE
The Story of Richard Daggett

The first indication that something was wrong was on Friday morning, July 17, 1953, waking up with a stiff neck and back. My parents took me to our family physician, and he suggested that I should be taken to the Los Angeles County General Hospital. I was a month past my 13th birthday. That night my legs began to ache, and shortly after midnight I started to have trouble sitting up. I don't remember anyone using the word polio or telling me what it was that they suspected I had, but by now I knew that whatever it was, I had it for sure. The next morning they performed a tracheotomy. The operation was done with a local anesthetic and I could watch the doctors bending over me as they worked.

Until this time I had moments of apprehension, but I was never really frightened. Some of the tests hurt, and I wondered what was happening, but everybody acted as though things were going fine. Then the doctor doing the tracheotomy made one final cut and air started being sucked in and out of the hole he made in my throat. I thought he must have done something wrong. I tried to ask him what had happened, but every time I tried to talk more air bubbled up out of the hole. I was really frightened. When tracheotomy was done I was put in a tank respirator, more commonly known as an iron lung. I started to vomit blood.

My mother drove to the hospital to visit me almost every afternoon, and both my parents came in the evenings. I'm sure that it was a difficult time for them. It was probably more difficult for them than for me. Everyone had to wear gowns and masks when they were on the patient units. Men, who I assumed were doctors, would often stop by my respirator. They would talk *about* me, but never *to* me. This heightened my sense of apprehension. Were they preparing to do some different tests? Would they be painful?

I was very naive and no one told me what was going on. I really had no conception of how serious my condition was. Oh, I knew that I was completely paralyzed, but the long-term impact did not sink in. My greatest concern was that I might miss the first day of school. After 3 weeks, I was moved to Rancho Los Amigos and was treated by a physiotherapist. She began to stretch the muscles that had tightened on disuse. My therapist had a habit of bringing student PTs with her so that they could observe the therapy sessions. She was followed by four to six students, asked if I were dressed, and proceeded with her demonstration. If I said that I was not dressed she would pull the curtain. Sometimes, but not always, she would leave the sheet over my body. These were the only concessions to privacy. The students were usually females and, more often than not, very attractive. For a young teenage boy it was quite unsettling.

Like most of the other patients in a tank respirator, I had several personal items hanging near my head. I had a photo of my brother in his army uniform, and a photo of me throwing a football. It was the last picture taken before I was hospitalized. Looking back, I think having it on my respirator might have been my way of saying, "This is the *real* me. Not the weak, emaciated kid you see with his head sticking out of this tank respirator." I slowly regained breathing tolerance: 10 minutes, three times a day, 15 minutes, then 20, and so on. When I could breathe about 1 hour on my own I was moved from the tank respirator to a bed. After a year tracheostomy was stopped.

Since nobody was sick, in the usual sense of the word, it was different from what a person might think of as being in a hospital. The main complaint we all had, usually unspoken, was the lack of privacy. Even at night there were several low-level, indirect lights on. We had no way of knowing when a member of the staff would be walking by our beds. As teenagers, we were probably more concerned about this than most of the other patients. I remember: once an older teenage couple went out on one of the balconies of the administration building. Someone found them in an amorous embrace. It was something most high-school students would find quite ordinary, but some of the hospital staff had a fit.

That sort of thing didn't happen very often, but there was one nurse who behaved like a warden. She seemed to have two rules. Rule number one was, "Patients should do exactly as told." Rule number two was, "Everything else is forbidden." It helped to pass the time if you had a good imagination. The ceilings on the wards had random patterns built into them, and I would conjure up images of things I pretended to build; a go-cart, a rocket ship, a house, and so on. Sometimes I would conjure up images of female body parts.

I was "horny" much of the time. I'm sure most teenage boys of my age were the same. The main difference was that I lived in a hospital. Most boys could arrange their own privacy. They could lock the bathroom door, or at least expect to be left alone when they were in their beds at night. They wouldn't usually have any trouble finding a place or time to masturbate. My problem was that I would wake up in the night on the verge of a wet dream. I had three choices. I could suppress it and be miserable in the morning; I could try to go back to sleep and hope I would pick up the dream where I left off, which seldom worked; or, I could try to masturbate without being caught. This was difficult with limited strength in my upper extremities.

I spent most of my free time in the solarium looking at medical textbooks. I probably learned more about anatomy and physiology than most boys of my age. We also had wheelchair races in the halls. Another of our favorite projects was seeing how much free literature we could get. We sent for information on all sorts of subjects and from all sorts of places. We requested pamphlets and brochures from such diverse sources as the American Petroleum Institute, the U.S. Printing Office, and Planned Parenthood. The Planned Parenthood packet brought some raised eyebrows from the hospital staff. The package of information on sex and birth control had obviously been opened by someone before I got it. We always used my address: Richard Daggett, 502D, Rancho Los Amigos.

I had several appointments at the Scoliosis Clinic over the following two years. Usually the chief of the Orthopedic Department would have doctors look on as he described the patient's history. Then he would ask for recommendations. It seemed that in my case they always said "operate!" It was ordered that I have a complete set of X-rays: front, back, side, standing, and lying down. I also had a series of photographs taken. A girl on our ward had pictures taken at the same time. To say it was embarrassing for both of us would be an understatement. I was just a month past my 15th birthday, and the girl was about 6 months younger to me. We were together in this small room, wearing nothing but very loose G strings. The girl also had what appeared to be a small piece of ace bandage that was supposed to cover her breasts. It didn't do a very good job and she knew it. I could tell by her expression that it bothered her a lot. I must admit that I peeked a little while she was having her pictures taken. I don't know why they didn't take our photographs separately. I guess it was an example of institutional insensitivity. The photographer told us that he would put black spots over our faces and, anyway, nobody but the doctors would see the photographs. Our friends on the ward teased us for weeks about the "nude" photographs.

I hadn't really had an opportunity to see my whole body since contracting polio, and it was pretty discouraging to see these photographs. I guess I was about 9 or 10 years old when I first became aware of my physical appearance. I could never seem to develop a tan, and I thought I looked rather soft and "puny." Then, just before my polio onset at the age of 13, I could look into the mirror and see the development of muscles and the beginnings of a potential adult. Now, here I was, 15 years old and, almost literally, nothing but skin and bones. It was a real blow to my ego. It was obvious that I had matured physically. I had the usual secondary sex characteristics, but I looked like a corpse. I happened to see these photographs again, many years later. I looked like the people in the concentration camps during World War II. I'm still thin, and in some ways more visibly disabled than I was then, but I hope I've filled out a little bit.

Another embarrassing thing happened about the same time period. It seems funny, looking back, but it wasn't then. I had to fill out a psychological questionnaire when I was immobilized with casts. One of the teen volunteers, or candy stripers as they were, offered to help. She would ask the questions and fill in my answers. Most of the questions were rather mundane, such as, "What is your favorite color?" or "What animal would you like to be if you weren't human?" It worked fine until she came to a series of very personal questions about my sexual experiences and fantasies. I remember thinking, "I'm 15 years old, and I live in a hospital. What kind of sexual experiences do they think I've had?" Even if I'd had any real sexual experiences it would have been too embarrassing to tell them to the attractive young girl sitting by my bed. After several awkward moments, we made it to the end. It would have made a great comedy sketch.

I was discharged from the hospital in 1956. Although I was still visibly disabled, I had regained a high level of function. I continued school with a home teacher because in those days, students with a disability were not encouraged to attend regular classes. There were some differences in the courses offered to me too, although it might have been just a peculiarity of my teachers. Course requirements included "Senior Problems"; a mixture of things that included a mild sort of sex education called "Family Life." My teacher said of Family Life, "We can skip this if you want. I'm sure you know it anyway, and you'll probably never need it." I was too polite to tell him that he was showing his ignorance about people with disabilities. He probably thought like many people do, that if a person is disabled they lose interest in sexual matters. Another course requirement was driving education. Although it was very unlikely that I would ever have the physical strength to drive, he still made me take the textbook part of the course. He probably felt more comfortable teaching me how to drive than he did talking about sex.

I think I benefited from having a home teacher academically. Having a teacher on a one-to-one basis meant that I couldn't fake it. If I was having a problem with a certain subject, the teacher knew it immediately. Overall, it was probably good for me. But I missed taking science lab courses and mixing with the other students. I lacked a social life. My neighborhood friends thankfully would still come over, and I was invited to a few parties, but not very often. This was compounded by the social "rituals" of the time. It was usually the male's responsibility to provide transportation and to pay for meals and entertainment. I didn't drive and I had very little income of my own.

I probably had a pretty low physical self-image, too. I was well liked, and felt at ease with individuals or in small groups, but I was uncomfortable in many situations. This was especially true when I was around girls I had known before I contracted polio. The stereotype is of a teenager looking into a mirror and saying, "I can't go out tonight. I've got this great big zit on my nose." They think that everyone is going to be staring at their pimple. It's much worse if you walk with braces and have limited use of your upper extremities. I often thought that everyone in the room was watching me. I've worked hard to overcome this, but I still struggle with it occasionally.

In 1980, I was elected president of the Polio Survivors Association, a nonprofit corporation. I served as an advocate for those with severe physical disabilities, and I write articles on disability and home-based long-term care. I have never had the stamina to hold down a full-time job. Instead, I have become a full-time volunteer, serving on several boards and commissions. In the early 1980s, I was interviewed by a psychologist who appeared regularly on local television. He asked about my relations with other people, if I had considered marriage, and if not, why not. I explained some of the disincentives built into our "system" that people with severe disabilities must think about before getting married. A person will almost always lose eligibility for income maintenance programs, and will often lose their medical coverage. I explained that in my case, I could live with a person, and as long as I called that person my provider of personal assistance services or attendant, we could have an adequate income. But, if I married that same person, our income would be cut almost in half. This applies to employment too. A person would need a well-paying job or be independently wealthy to compensate for this loss. I told him about people I know who have tried both options; marriage and/or employment. A few are successful. Some barely struggle by. Many end up divorced and/or quit their job in frustration. The "system" often punishes those who try the hardest. My portion of the interview never made it on the air. He appeared to be more interested in the physical relationships of disabled people.

Because of the late effects of polio, my physical condition has deteriorated. This was anticipated but is still frustrating. I walked unaided for more than 30 years, but now I use a power wheelchair. I have had to modify my home to make it accessible. Unfortunately, this also means that I can't get into my friends' houses. I've had to turn down many social invitations. My pulmonary capacity has diminished, too. Through the 1960s and 1970s I breathed without the aid of a respirator, but now I use one most of the time.

Almost every time a reporter interviews me, he/she says something about how "brave" I am. I tell them, as politely as possible, that bravery has nothing to do with it. Bravery is when a person consciously puts their own life in danger to save or protect someone else. A person who happens to have a disability has not made a conscious effort to be disabled. It just happened. They still have the desire to live as full a life as possible just like everybody else. You don't have to be brave to do this.

I was asked once by a television reporter what I thought my life would have been like had I not contracted polio. I replied that people can't, or at least shouldn't, dwell on things that might have been, because no one knows "what might have been." You just do the best you can. You make decisions based on the information and circumstances at the time. There are things that I haven't done that I would have liked to do, but I've had an interesting and enjoyable life. I've traveled extensively, met many political leaders and celebrities, and appeared on local and national television several times. I've been blessed with a supportive family and by the encouragement of friends.

Over the past several years I've received a few letters from polio survivors who are angry. They feel that they were encouraged, even pushed, to go out and make an active life. They feel that this is why they are having trouble now. While I certainly sympathize with them, I don't agree with this outlook. I'm not sure I would have done things much differently even if I'd known about post-polio's late onset effects. I'm a richer person for the people I've met and the things I've done.

DISCUSSION QUESTIONS

1. Have students make a list of their top five personal values and then discuss the impact of personal values on quality of life.
2. Discuss anyone's experience with a family member they believe has a poor quality of life. What are the reasons for this life quality being evaluated as poor?

3. Ask students to identify differences in persons who use religious/spiritual and non-religious/spiritual coping. What kind of differences do they perceive, if any, in terms of quality of life?

4. Discuss the case of a person who chooses to use aggressive life sustaining measures to prolong life. What are the positive and negative consequences of this choice?

5. Solicit student stories about experiences with end of life and give reactions to the process of dying and quality of life at the end of life.

EXERCISES

A. For a class activity, have students create a timeline of the important events in their lives and how each impacted their quality of life.

B. For a class group activity, form groups and give each group a list of the same questions (e.g., What are you most worried about?), and have them answer the questions as if they were in different psychosocial life stages. Have groups share their answers.

C. For a homework assignment, have students interview a person with a disability using and online support group about what is important to their quality of life.

TEN

Implications of Social Support and Caregiving for Loved Ones With a Disability

Irmo Marini

OVERVIEW

Caregiving in America is perhaps one of the most misperceived, underappreciated, sometimes stressful, and otherwise rewarding acts of unconditional love. Yet, depending on which study or author you are reading, caregiving is often described at one of two contradictory ends of the spectrum; "a curse or opportunity" (Hulnick & Hulnick, 1981). Olkin (1999) and Wright (1988) are critical of some researchers' bias in presuming certain research conclusions before conducting a study, or alternatively, twisting the findings toward their research hypothesis. Olkin (1999) in particular outlines a number of research studies in which the title is formulated prior to conducting the study, where researchers use all too common identifiers, such as "burden, caregiver burnout, and caregiver stress," regarding caring for a family member (pp. 47–48). She cites numerous studies with the concept of burden and negative implications of caring for a disabled family member as a foregone conclusion. Yuker (1994) attempted to declare a moratorium on research focusing on the horrific negative affects of caring for a child with a disability.

Wright (1988) discusses the insider versus outsider perspective, in that when speaking to family members of a loved one with a disability (insider perspective) versus someone who has never experienced the situation (outsider perspective), generally two different perceptions of what it must be like (outsider) versus what it is actually like (insider) to care for a disabled child begin to emerge. Overall, these studies point to insider perspectives that often translate into the benefits and rewards of caregiving, whereas many outsider perspectives continue to be saddled by the belief that caregiving drains the emotional, physical, and financial reserves from the caregiver(s) (Argyle, 2001; Bogdan & Taylor, 1989; Heller & Factor, 1993; Hulnick & Hulnick, 1981; Quittner, Opipari, Regoli, Jacobsen, & Eigen, 1992; Tangri & Verma, 1992; Wickham-Searl, 1992; Wright, 1988). In this chapter, we review all aspects of this phenomenon, as well as delve into caregiving for loved ones with a specific type of disability, including Alzheimer's disease, neuromuscular disorders, traumatic brain injury, psychiatric disabilities, spinal cord injury, and congenital disabilities, such as muscular dystrophy and cerebral palsy. Ellenbogen, Meade, Jackson, and Barrett (2006) indicate there are significant group differences in caregiving responsibilities and demands between disability types. Aside from the psychological impact of caregiving, we also explore the dynamics of caregiver abuse, and the often painful decision to place a loved one in a long-term care facility. First, we explore the significance of having social support in caring for a loved one with a disability at home.

THE SIGNIFICANCE OF SOCIAL SUPPORT

Related to caregiving, there is a plethora of literature regarding social support and disability, and its significance is critical to the well-being of loved ones. Numerous theories and construct definitions exist. Cohen and Wills (1985) differentiate between structural and functional components of social support. *Structural* support defined as the quantity and frequency of persons in the network, noting the type (partner, spouse, coworkers) and frequency in engaging with one's social network and social activities. *Functional* support is broken down into instrumental, informational, and emotional support (Chak, 1996; Cohen, 1988). Instrumental support refers to providing personal assistance with activities of daily living, finances, and other tangible types of assistance. Informational support refers to providing information and education to assist individuals' through difficult times. Emotional support pertains to listening, being empathetic, and offering counsel to individuals experiencing difficulties (Cohen, 1988). Chronister (2009) outlines empirical findings for structural and functional support, noting several interesting overall results. Concerning structural support, several studies suggest higher mortality for persons with fewer social supports as well as lower rates of chronic illness and disability (Berkman, 1995; Cohen, Doyle, Skoner, Rabin, & Gwaltney, 1997; Schwarzer & Leppin, 1991). Functional support studies show some fairly consistent findings with regard to physical and psychological well-being, as it appears to act as a buffer against stress and stress-related illness (Cohen & Wills, 1985; Pearlin, Lieberman, Menaghan, & Mullan, 1981; Wills & Filer, 2000).

Chronister, Chou, Frain, and Cardoso (2008) conducted a meta-analysis regarding perceived social support for various rehabilitation populations. They found small effect sizes related to perceived support and physical health; medium effect sizes for psychological health, quality of life, and employment; and, large effect size for adjustment to disability. This latter finding is supported by other studies as well, noting specifically that with strong family support, family members with disabilities generally adapt and accept their disabilities better (Li & Moore, 1998; Varni, Rubenfeld, Talbot, & Setoguchi, 1989).

Although social support is generally found to have a positive influence on recipients with disabilities, there are studies that indicate there can indeed be negative consequences with dysfunctional social supports (Abbey, Abramis, & Kaplan, 1985). Persons with substance abuse problems returning to an environment where friends and family also abuse substances is an example of this occurrence. Related instances where people with disabilities are in an abusive relationship and unable to defend themselves likely creates greater vulnerability to psychological well-being (McFarlane et al., 2001; Nosek, Foley, Hughes, & Howland, 2001). In dysfunctional or abusive relationships, caregiving and/or social support may lead to depression, increased negative affect, social withdrawal, and deleterious physical well-being (Abbey et al., 1985; Nosek et al., 2001; Evans, Palasano, LePore, & Martin, 1989). Overall, for better or worse, functional and structural social support following a disability may be the most significant indicator of an individual's ability to adapt to his or her disability.

PREVALENCE AND DYNAMICS OF CAREGIVING

It is estimated that approximately 120 million adult Americans or 57% have in the past provided or currently provide caregiving services to a family member or friend (National Alliance for Care-giving and American Association of Retired Persons, 2004). About 80% of all family caregiving services in the United States are unpaid, and for the approximate 57% of caregivers who are also employed, they report having to leave work early, take sick and vacation leave, or go to work late on numerous occasions. The average caregiver is a mid-40s female in 50%–66% of cases, most often caring for an ageing parent or loved one over 50 (National Alliance for Caregiving and American Association of Retired Persons, 2004). Approximately, 14% of family caregivers care for their disabled child in 55% of cases, estimated to be approximately 17 million people in the United States. It is estimated that unpaid family caregiving would cost over $300 billion per year, twice the amount spent on nursing homes and home health care services combined (Peter Arno, personal communication, January 2006).

Caregiving can perhaps best be summarized on a continuum of care, for young and old alike who have physical and/or cognitive limitations that require assistance performing *activities of daily living* and *instrumental activities of daily living.* Activities of daily living (ADL) include providing assistance with personal hygiene and grooming, dressing and undressing, feeding, transferring (in/out of bed, car), bowel and/or bladder management, and ambulation. Assistance with instrumental activities of daily living (IADL) includes providing assistance with housekeeping, paying bills, managing money, meal preparation, grocery or related shopping, and medications. In many instances, caregiving may also include caring for a pet, caring for a patient's child, transportation to/from appointments, health maintenance, and being a companion. Some individuals require less than 1 hour a day of assistance, whereas others with more severe disabilities may require 24/7 care, 365 days per year.

NEGATIVE HEALTH IMPLICATIONS OF CAREGIVING

There are numerous studies examining the physical and psychological health implications of perceived caregiving stress and burden (Brehaut et al., 2009; Drentea & Goldner, 2006; Haley et al., 1995; Roth, Perkins, Wadley, Temple, & Haley, 2009;

Schwarz & Roberts, 2000; Talley & Crews, 2007). Although Olkin (1999) objects to some researchers' stereotypical assumptions regarding caregiver stress, there is an abundance of evidence of the negative health implications for caregivers who perceive themselves to be in high-strain roles, particularly those caregivers who clock more hours per day with more severely disabled loved ones (Byrne, Hurly, Daly, & Cunningham, 2010; Roth et al., 2009). Byrne et al. (2010) found female caregivers of children with cerebral palsy reported poorer physical and mental health than noncaregivers, particularly those mothers who spent more time caregiving.

Brehaut et al. (2009) analyzed population-based data regarding caregiver health of 3,633 healthy children versus 2,485 children with health problems in Canada. Caregivers of the children with health problems reported more chronic health conditions, activity limitations, poorer health, and higher depressive symptoms. Over 88% of the sample was the biological mother, and over 65% had beyond a high-school education with an average household income of over $49,000. With Canada having universal health care, one would think that education and income would be positive factors in shielding some of the caregiver health problems, but this did not appear to be the case in this study. Other studies, however, have shown lower income and education to be contributing factors to poor physical and/or mental health of caregivers (Canning, Harris, & Kelleher, 1996; Imran et al., 2010; Manuel, 2001; Saunders, 2009). In further exploring physical health problems only, studies supporting specific health problems are vague other than low-back pain and headaches (Brehaut et al., 2009; Grosse, Flores, Ouyang, Robbins, & Tilford, 2009; Murphy, Christian, Caplin, & Young, 2006; Tong et al., 2003).

Studies regarding the psychological impact of caregiving are much more common and delineate more specifically the type of problems, most commonly depression and anxiety (Canning et al., 1996; Grosse et al., 2009; Imran et al., 2010; Mulvihill et al. 2005; Murphy et al., 2006; Roth et al., 2009). Imran and associates, for example, examined anxiety, depression, and family burden of 100 Pakistani primary caregivers caring for a family member with a psychiatric illness. Results indicated a high rate of depression and anxiety among male and female caregivers (86% and 85% respectively) who expressed concerns regarding the future, fear of being alone, and having the sole responsibility for the family member, coping with family member behavioral problems, social isolation, and the stigma associated with mental illness. MacDonald and Callery (2007) reported the projected complexity of caring for a family member without adequate respite. Some of the time-related difficulties for caregivers include isolation and fatigue, recognition of lost dreams, and lost identity.

POSITIVE ASPECTS OF CAREGIVING

Although there are far more studies addressing caregiver stress and subsequent physical and mental health problems, there are fewer, yet significant studies supporting the positive aspects of caregiving for loved ones with a disability (Bogdan & Taylor, 1989; Buchanan, Radin, Chakravorty, & Tyry, 2009; Janoff-Bulman, 2004; Krause, Coker, Charlifue, & Whiteneck, 1999; Matheis et al., 2006). Buchanan et al. (2009) surveyed

530 caregivers (78% were spouses, 54% male) of a loved one with multiple sclerosis, almost half of which provided 20 or more hours of caregiving per week. Approximately 25% of caregivers reported they could benefit from counseling, over half indicated that although caregiving was demanding, time consuming, or a challenge, 90% reported being happy that they could help. In addition, approximately 65% indicated caregiving was rewarding, and over 80% expressed they were proud of the care they provided.

In studies related to "social exchange reciprocity" (see Call, Finch, Huck, & Kane, 1999; Dwyer & Miller, 1990), in instances where a loved one with a disability is perceived as being able to reciprocate love, communicate, and provide companionship, caregivers generally report mutual benefits, reciprocity, and reduced perceived burden. Reid, Moss, and Hyman (2005) assessed 56 caregivers with a burden inventory, self-esteem inventory, and caregiver reciprocity scale. Results indicated that increased reciprocity, such as warmth and balance, was inversely related to physical, social, emotional, and developmental burden. In addition, contrary to expectations, expressed disabled family member love was related to decreased emotional burden of caregivers, but intrinsic motivation to provide care was more highly related when reciprocal love was perceived. In other words, intrinsic motivation did not come from within the caregiver, but was more driven by extrinsic reasons (reciprocal love). Bogdan and Taylor (1989) also described a "sociology of acceptance" perceived reciprocation, even with caregivers whose child was profoundly developmentally disabled and unable to verbally communicate.

Lindblad, Holritz-Rasmussen, and Sandman (2007) reported similar findings in a group of 13 parents caring for a child with a disability in Sweden. In-depth narrative interviews were conducted, resulting in three overlapping themes: "being gratified by experiences of the child as having a natural place in relation with others, being provided a room for sorrow and joy, and being enabled to live an eased and spontaneous life" (p. 238). As with Bogdan and Taylor (1989), parents had a defined social place for their child in the family. The child was equally valued and appreciated. Parents also acknowledged the family openness and support to discuss their sadness and worries, and conversely to experience joyous occasions intermixed. Finally, the ability to live an eased and spontaneous life was described as the family social support network of grandparents and friends who would spontaneously assist with the family needs. This interdependency was appreciated and "life enriching" for all caregivers concerned (p. 244).

CAREGIVING STUDIES WITH SPECIFIC POPULATIONS

It is always less time consuming to talk or write about people with disabilities as one homogeneous group; however, there are vast intergroup differences. The lived experience of individuals born with severe developmental disabilities is essentially entirely different from that of individuals who sustain a spinal cord injury later in life. The caregiving experience of caregivers who work with loved ones with various disabilities may also experience varying levels of reciprocity, stress, fulfillment and, or burden. We now briefly explore the inside perspective of some of these caregivers.

Spinal cord injury: The demographics of spinal cord injury (SCI) in the United States indicate 80% of all injuries occur to males for mainly risky behaviors (e.g., car accidents, sports, falls, violence), and generally between the ages of 15 and 24 (Livneh & Antonak, 1997). About half of these injuries involve impairment of all four limbs (tetraplegia), while the other half involves some level of lower-extremity paralysis (paraplegia). Unless the SCI additionally involves a traumatic brain injury (TBI), the primary functional limitations of this population is mobility, and the ability to physically carry out their instrumental and other activities of daily living (ADL) (Britell & Hammond, 1994). In most instances of low-level paraplegia, little or no caregiving is necessary, as many of these individuals live virtually totally independent. For those with higher-level tetraplegia; however, many will be partially or totally dependent on a caregiver for dressing, grooming, bowel and bladder evacuation, feeding, cleaning, and transportation.

Caregiver research has been conducted with family and spousal caregivers (Blanes, Carmagnani, & Ferreira, 2007; Elliott & Berry, 2009; Elliott, Brossart, Berry, & Fine, 2008; Elliott, Shewchuk, & Richards, 2001; Post, Bloemen, & de Witte, 2005). Post et al. (2005) studied partner burden of 265 couples. Results showed high perceived burden in approximately 25% of the sample for partners with more severe SCI, and about 4% for those with minor ADL needs. Significant predictors in order of importance included amount of care provided, partner with SCI psychological problems (defined as being dependent and asking for help, accepting the SCI, and sexual problems), partner age and gender (most were female with a mean age of 49), and time since injury. Essentially, the more severe the disability requiring more personal care, the greater the likelihood of perceived caregiver burden.

Blanes et al. (2007) completed a cross-sectional descriptive study with 60 primary caregivers of persons with high- and low-level paraplegia regarding health-related quality-of-life in São Paulo, Brazil. Eighty one percent of participants were female with a mean age of 35, many who reported spending an average 11 hours per day caregiving. Approximately 25% each were wives or sisters, with the remaining being relatives. Results indicated about 38% of caregivers reported their own chronic diseases, such as pain, and the authors note in previous studies where caregiver physical complaints frequently have psychosomatic origins (Karlin & Retzlaff, 1995). The primary quality-of-life complaint for caregivers was an inaccessible environment regarding transportation and access to medical services. Environmental access barriers have also been frequently reported as a source of frustration and anger for Americans with SCI despite 20-year-old legislation (Graf, Marini, & Blankenship, 2009; Li & Moore, 1998; Marini, Bhakta, & Graf, 2009).

Elliott and Berry (2009) explored problem-solving training with 30 caregivers of a loved one with SCI versus a control group of 30 other caregivers and followed them for 1 year posttraining. They found that although those caregivers who had the problem-solving training showed no difference in depression level 1 year later, they did show a decrease in dysfunctional problem-solving styles (careless decision making) over time, as well as increased social functioning that had a palliative effect on their physical functioning. The authors conclude that caregiving issues have long since been ignored by professionals who tend to focus more on the individual with a disability; however, recommend that any type of training is better than none at all, and ultimately leads to better caregiving and indirectly better health for all parties concerned.

Traumatic brain injury: Head injuries (TBI) in the United States mimic some of the same demographics as etiology for SCI, including twice as many males than females, most common age group is 15 to 24, and similar causation with motor vehicle accidents, falls, occupational accidents, sports, and child abuse (National Institutes of Health (NIH), 1999). Unlike SCI, which has an incidence rate of 10,000 to 12,000 new injuries per year, NIH estimates indicate 1.5 million to 2 million new head injuries per year, with 70,000 to 90,000 individuals experiencing long-term functional impairments. Although approximately 75% of all head injuries are diagnosed as mild in nature with few subsequent symptoms, those with more severe injuries can experience symptoms such as short- and/or long-term memory problems, headaches, fatigue, disinhibition, inappropriate social and sexual functioning, low stress tolerance, substance abuse, impulsiveness/hostility, depression, and physical limitations in more serious cases (Degeneffe, 2001).

Family members or others who take on the caregiving role are typically faced with a number of challenges, not so much with physical direct care ADLs (except for more severe or profound cases), but more so supervisory, as many caregivers indicate they are essentially looking after a child (Blake, 2008). Kreutzer, Gervasio, and Camplair (1994) noted unhealthy family functioning similar to families who care for a member with a psychiatric illness, and that caregiver depression, anxiety, stress, and burden may not dissipate over time (Brooks, 1991; Douglas & Spellacy, 2000; Lefebvre, Cloutier, & Levert, 2008; Oddy, 1995). A common observation by nondisabled spouses is that the spouse with a head injury is not the same person they married, possessing a different personality. Spouses report decreased leisure time, social isolation, loneliness, and a greater domestic workload caring for children, needing to become the breadwinner, and dealing with dwindling finances (Brooks & McKinley, 1983; Kreutzer et al., 1994; Lezak, 1988). Lefebvre et al. (2008) surveyed 21 family caregivers of a loved one with a moderate or severe TBI, finding after 10 years that caregivers continue to report physical and emotional exhaustion, family disruption, daily stress, ongoing supervision to complete ADLs, learn memory games, and so on.

Similar to Elliott and Berry's (2009) study, caregivers who are provided education, problem-solving training, respite can positively cognitively reframe their situations, and given resources, generally fare better regarding psychosocial well-being than caregivers who do not receive such assistance (Campbell, 1988; Chan, 2007; Douglas & Spellacy, 2000; Tyerman & Booth, 2001). And as with related studies, there appears to be a silver lining for some caregivers working with family members with TBI. Again, the selfless act of helping a loved one, periodic reciprocal love, have a sense of meaning and purpose, better communication, a closer family bond, and holding traditional *caregiver ideology* (defined as natural, caring, sense of duty, and virtuous) lead to caregiver satisfaction (Elliott & Kurylo, 2000; Lawrence, Murray, Samsi, & Banerjee, 2008; Lefebvre et al., 2008; Wells, Dywan, & Dumas, 2005).

In two related caregiver coping studies, Hanks, Rapport, and Vangel (2007) explored functional status, coping style, social support, and caregiver appraisal of 60 primary caregivers. Results revealed that appraisals of caregiver burden, mastery, and relationship satisfaction moderately to strongly relate to perceived social support and family functioning. Where social support is perceived to be good, this minimizes stressful feelings and provide some sense of control over the circumstances. In addition, 70% of caregivers in this study were African American and reported high levels of traditional caregiver ideology, as did 32 minority caregivers in the Lawrence et al. (2008) findings. A related caregiver coping study was by Sander et al. (2007) of 195 caregivers, of whom 75% were White and 25% Black/Hispanic. The authors found that minority participants reported lower levels of education and income, and were more likely to be caring for an extended family member. Race/ethnicity significantly predicted caregiver's use of coping strategies of distancing and accepting responsibility. The fact that most minority respondents held to the traditional caregiver ideology was also associated with increased distress. Minority caregivers, especially Blacks, use more prayer, faith, and religion as a coping strategy, and tend to report lesser perceived burden than Whites (Macera et al., 1992; Wood & Parham, 1990; Wykle & Segall, 1991).

Psychiatric disabilities. In discussions about psychiatric disabilities, the primary ones that dominate U.S. research include schizophrenia, bipolar mood disorders, and personality disorders (Cook, Cohler, Pickett, & Beeler, 1997). The alarming steady rise of persons with psychiatric disabilities, and more recently children diagnosed with a disorder, have called greater attention to this illness (Marini, 2001a; Marini & Reid, 2001). Marini (2001a) cited Social Security Administration (SSA) statistics indicating that persons with mental illness represent the largest segment of SSA beneficiaries (approximately 27%), with 76% of this population being under age 39. There is also an alarming dual-diagnosis comorbidity of substance abuse and mental illness estimated between 41% to 65% lifetime occurrence (Kessler et al., 1996; Mueser, Bennett, & Kushner, 1995; Regier et al., 1990). Biegel, Ishler, Katz, and Johnson (2007) note how the literature often separates substance abuse and mental illness pertaining to caregiving. Specifically, they indicate virtually no literature regarding caregiver burden in the substance abuse field, but a plethora of such studies concerning psychiatric disabilities.

The types of behaviors typically diagnosed concerning people with psychiatric disabilities varies depending on the diagnosis. It is beyond the scope of this chapter to list out all the possible symptoms; however, the reader is encouraged to consult with the *Diagnostic and Statistical Manual of Mental Disorders* (4th ed, text revision; *DSM-IV-TR*, 2000). Briefly, according to the *DSM-IV-TR* (2000), persons diagnosed with types of schizophrenia may include symptoms of psychosis (hallucinations and delusions), disorganized speech, flat affect, low energy, low goal-directed behavior, confusion of thought and understanding, and social and occupational dysfunction. Bipolar mood disorders comprise four types; mania, depression, hypomania, and mixed disorders. Most persons diagnosed experience depression more so than mania, and these symptoms typically include shifts in mood, energy, judgment, anxiety, sleep, sex drive, concentration, and delusions/hallucinations in severe cases.

Caregiver studies show similar findings to other disability studies (Biegel et al., 2007; Greenberg, Greenley, & Brown 1997a; Greenberg, Kim & Greenley, 1997b; Kravetz, Faust, & Dasberg, 2002; Lefley, 1996; Provencher, Perreault, St-Onge, & Rousseau, 2003). Provencher et al. (2003) surveyed 154 family caregivers regarding predictors of psychological distress using hierarchical regression analysis. Results showed that younger, female, less than full-time employed caregivers reported higher levels of psychological distress. Disabled family member problematic behaviors (hallucinations, delusions, violent behavior and para-suicide) were the second primary stressor causing psychological distress for the caregiver. Subjective burden (perceived loss, worry, and feelings of distress) and objective secondary burden (physical complaints, financial problems, and diminished social life) also contributed to caregiver distress. Interestingly, support from friends actually increased psychological distress in this study, as did frequent contact with the primary health care provider. Caregivers who held full-time jobs reported less distress, likely indicating that work and time away from caregiving acted as a buffer. The authors noted that most critical to caregivers, was effectively dealing with their caregiving duties, family routine disruptions, restrictions in social activities, personal reaction to the family member's personality, and worries about the future of their relatives. The authors recommended improving problem-solving skills and communication with family members, respite for caregivers for social and leisure time, and establishing a support network.

Cook et al. (1997) described the complex implications of deinstitutionalization, where formally state-funded institutions were the home of many persons with chronic psychiatric illnesses. Harding, Zubin, and Strauss (1987), however, note that although the deinstitutionalization ideology was good, communities were not prepared or funded for the release of thousands of these individuals. The authors indicate that many persons with psychiatric disabilities lifestyles are as disabling as their mental illness, compromised by poverty level Supplemental Security Income, residing in unsafe and/or unwelcoming neighborhoods, homelessness, housed in prison for abnormal behavior in public, and the stress experienced by family members (Cook, Hoffschmidt, Cohler, & Pickett, 1992). Persons with psychiatric disabilities often go through life experiencing cyclical periods of decompensation, hospitalization, stabilization, and reentry into the community. Although the negative side effects of medications in and of themselves are debilitating, individuals are generally able to function better with, than without, psychopharmacology.

Finally, dual-diagnosis studies of substance abuse and mental illness are few, despite approximately 50% of cases that are so diagnosed (Kessler et al., 1996). Biegel et al. (2007) examined 82 family caregivers and 87 females dually diagnosed and family members regarding predictors of family caregiver burden. Results showed that family caregivers reported moderate levels of subjective burden (worry and displeasure) and lower levels of stigma. Family caregivers were also negatively affected by member behavioral problems. In addition, although social support in general was not predictive of reduced caregiver burden, specific support for the care recipient did minimize caregiver burden. The authors recommend that substance abuse agencies involve family members in treatment, which can have a positive impact on substance abstinence. Caregiver needs must also be treated regarding depressive symptoms, family education, social support, and strategies to address behavior problems and the myriad of potential worries.

Neuromuscular diseases: This family of diseases includes many diagnoses, including spina bifida, cerebral palsy (CP), multiple sclerosis (MS), muscular dystrophy (MD), amyotrophic lateral sclerosis (ALS), Parkinson's disease, Huntington's disease, myasthenia gravis, and a host of related diseases. Some of these disabilities may or may not involve mental retardation or cognitive impairment, but all do involve gradual or immediate and relatively stable loss of muscle functioning from birth or later in life (Corcoran, 1981). Many of these disabilities will either immediately or gradually involve increased caregiver assistance in ADLs and IADLs as their loved ones' physical impairments become more severe. There is inconsistent evidence, however, suggesting that caregivers who have high caregiving demands perceive any more or less burden then caregivers with lesser demands (Lo Coco et al., 2005; Mah, Thannhauser, McNeil, & Dewey, 2008).

There have been numerous studies regarding caregiver perceptions and coping abilities with these different groups (Schrag, Hovris, Morley, Quinn, & Jahanshahi, 2006). Khan, Pallant, and Brand (2007) interviewed and assessed 62 caregivers regarding perceived strain, quality of life, and caregiver self-efficacy. Forty two percent reported strain in having to emotionally adjust to their partners with MS, endure sleep disruptions, time demands, and lifestyle changes. Perceived burden was higher for those caregivers whose partner with MS was more depressed and anxious. Caregiver perceived quality of life also correlated with caregiver strain. No correlation was found between caregiver strain and self-efficacy scores. Recommendations for caregivers were to access community respite services.

Spina bifida and CP are congenital disabilities typically originating at birth.

Grosse et al. (2009), for example, noted their sample of 49 parents of children with spina bifida compared with a control group, reported lower quality of life, few social activities, loss of sleep, and often feeling blue or unhappy. The authors note that little research has examined the long-term implications of caring for a child with a disability into adulthood. As children with neuromuscular diseases such as spina bifida and CP age, they become heavier, can experience developmental growth problems, such as osteoporosis, require adaptive equipment for transferring in/out of the wheelchair as well as adapted van with a lift, and may place caregivers at increased risk for low-back injuries (Yilmaz, Aki, Duger, Kayihan, & Karaduman, 2004), and the disabled loved one is at increased risk for secondary complications, such as pressure sores, urinary tract infections, and respiratory problems (Easton & Halpern, 1981).

Dagenais et al. (2006) assessed caregiver satisfaction with regard to having received appropriate education and disclosure by health care professionals regarding their child's diagnosis and how to manage it. Much like Elliott and Berry's (2009) recommendations regarding educating and training caregivers, Dagenais and associates reported 62% of caregivers were satisfied with the information disclosure process, 69% were hopeful, and 92% appreciated the candor or honesty from the professional. Further, it appears this disclosure moderated scores of perceived stress for caregivers, as the information removed many of the worrisome uncertainties for them in raising a child with CP.

Finally, severe neuromuscular diseases requiring ventilator support might otherwise seem to be a daunting and very demanding condition for caregivers, especially in the case of children. Past caregiver studies regarding caregiving for such children indeed show some parents become depressed, anxious, worried, and experience intense isolation over their situations (Carnevale, Alexander, Daoud, Dooley, & Gordon, 2004; Davis, Rennick, & Troini, 2006; Nereo, Fee, & Hinton, 2003). Mah et al. (2008) conducted semistructured interviews with 19 parents of children with spinal muscular atrophy, muscular dystrophy, and unspecified myopathy who were ventilator dependent regarding their experiences. All parents were concerned about providing their child with the best quality of life possible. Parents also reported that although the initial adjustment was stressful, once the routine became "normal," stress was reduced (p. 985). Parents also expressed guilt over not being able to give equal attention to their other children. Many of the mothers restricted their social outings because they required too much effort to coordinate and did not want to risk their child's health with exposure to other sick individuals. The mothers also chose to avoid negative reactions of strangers. As a result, many felt lonely and isolated. This feeling was often mediated by family support providing respite breaks. Living with loss and uncertainty was also a common theme, but many parents discussed changing their perspectives (reframing) and focusing on the positives in their lives. This study once again demonstrates both the rewards and stresses placed on caregivers.

Alzheimer's disease: Alzheimer's disease and dementia are estimated to affect over 24 million people worldwide, with over 4 million reported cases in the United States and expectations to quadruple by 2043 (Ferri et al., 2005; Karlawish et al., 2003). Persons diagnosed with Alzheimer's generally experience a progressive loss of cognitive abilities and ability to perform instrumental activities of the living, while concomitantly developing behavioral and psychiatric symptoms (Chen, Borson, & Scanlan, 2000). Rabins, Mace, and Lucas (1982) indicate that for caregivers, the behavioral and psychiatric symptoms often cause them more distress than a loved one's memory loss. Often, as a loved one with Alzheimer's disease deteriorates physically and mentally, caregivers experience greater levels of physical and psychological health problems themselves (Eisdorfer & Cohen, 1981). Mannion (2008) noted that a loved one's unpredictable behavior, wandering off, and requiring constant supervision, are commonly reported as chronically stressful worries for caregivers.

Pang et al. (2002) investigated caregiver distress between 31 Chinese, 89 Taiwanese, and 169 American caregivers. American caregivers expressed a significantly higher rate of caregiver depression then Taipei or Hong Kong caregivers, and also expressed more apathy than caregivers in Taipei or Hong Kong. All three groups, however, reported similar distress caused by their loved ones' delusions, hallucinations, agitation, disinhibition, and aberrant motor behavior. Similar distress signs were evident regardless of whether the caregiver was a spouse. The authors suggest that perhaps Asian culture deference to their elders and harmonious interpersonal relationships may have accounted for traditional caregiver ideology and the expectation to care for loved ones.

Vellone, Piras, Talucci, and Cohen (2007) interviewed 32 Italian caregivers regarding quality of life in caring for a family member with Alzheimer's disease.

Caregivers associated a good quality of life with psychological well-being, freedom, financial status, tranquility and good health, and poor quality of life with worrying about their loved ones' disease progression and the stress of caregiving. Takano and Arai (2005) found that females in their caregivers' study of 24 family members with early onset Alzheimer's disease, reported a higher correlation of caregiver burden (personal and role strain) for female caregivers when the loved one was a younger age. This group also expressed financial worries because there was not enough financial support to meet the extra costs of medical care. Unlike other studies, in which caregivers report distress over common behavioral problems (incontinence, irritability, agitation, aggression, wandering), no significant correlations were found. The authors cite other studies in which female caregivers report a higher level of caregiver burden and depression, noting that the difference may be in perceived nurturing roles. Males may view caregiving as a new job, whereas females may be more emotionally attached (Stevenson, 1990; Zarit, Todd, & Zarit, 1986).

ABUSE BY CAREGIVERS

One of the hypothesized consequences of caregiver stress and burden is that some caregivers will strike back at the individuals they are caring for physically or verbally (Anetzberger, 1987; Fulmer, 1990). Payne (2005) estimates prevalence rates between 500,000 to two million cases of elder abuse or neglect annually, not including child abuse. One theory of why abuse occurs is due to individual or family stress defined as sociological theory (Parke & Collmer, 1975). Another theory is the psychiatric model based on some flawed characteristic of the caregiving abuser, such as abusing substances or psychiatric illness (Miller, 1959). Violence is most prevalent on elderly women in 70% of cases of women 65 years or older (Nadien, 1995). Paveza et al. (1992) found that persons with Alzheimer's disease were 2.25 times more likely to be abused than other elder persons. Coyne, Reichman, and Berbig (1993) surveyed 342 caregivers of cognitively impaired adults and found those caregivers who were more likely to abuse typically worked longer hours, had been the caregiver for many years, worked with persons requiring a higher level of care, and, were more likely to be depressed. In addition, caregiver abusers reported being more likely to have been physically assaulted by their care recipients.

Nadien (1996) describes various types of abuse, including physical, psychological, and material. *Physical abuse* involves "physical assault, sexual abuse, slapping, grabbing, pushing, or restraining... physical neglect pertaining to denial of food, medicine, shelter, and physical assistance." (p. 159). *Psychological abuse* involves coercion, ridicule, verbal aggression, confinement, abandonment, and threats of aggression, including sexual or nonsexual. *Material abuse* generally involves legal or financial abuse, such as theft, exploitation, or other personal property matter, and material neglect is defined as withholding legal help and information (Johnson, 1991; Nadien, 1996, 2006). Caregiver abuse may be inferred from many signs, including fractures, sprains, bruises, cigarette burns, abrasions, and overmedication. Other forms may include eating disturbances, sleeping disorders, untreated pressure sores, malnutrition or dehydration, lack of clean clothes, and denial of hearing aids, visual aids, or ambulation devices (Nadien, 2006).

Some of the general characteristics of persons with disabilities who are more statistically vulnerable to various forms of abuse include those who are more dependent for activities of daily living, have fewer support resources, and have less power. Older women more so than men, and in one study of caregiver abuse regarding younger persons with developmental disabilities, it appears that those with more mild, moderate, or severe mental retardation who can interact have a higher frequency of abuse than those with profound mental retardation. Specifically, those individuals who interact but whose interactions involved maladaptive behavior (e.g., rebellious, hyperactive, violent, or disruptive) are more susceptible to caregiver abuse (Friedrich & Boriskin, 1976; Martin, 1982; Zirpoli, Snell, & Loyd, 2001). Zirpoli et al. (2001) assessed teacher ratings of residential caregiver abuse for 91 abused persons with mental retardation, noting a statistically significant relationship between abuse status and the level of functioning (mild to profound mental retardation) and frequency of maladaptive behaviors. Nadien (2006) concurs regarding interaction type and dependency, and cites differences with caregivers who find caregiving fulfilling versus those who are resentful and/or are paid poorly.

Gainey and Payne (2006) studied the role of caregiver burden in 751 suspected elder abuse cases of persons with Alzheimer's disease and compared this with other non-Alzheimer's-type disabilities. They found that the impact of burden and abuse was no different between Alzheimer's and other types of disabilities, calling into question the stress or burden causation theory as to why caregivers abuse their recipients. O'Brien et al. (1994) and Korbin, Antzberger, & Eckert (1990) have indicated that perhaps the overstressed explanation is oversimplified, noting that only some caregivers abuse, while most do not under similar circumstances. The authors suggest that interventions should focus not only on the caregiver in better dealing with their anger/frustration but also on care recipients in minimizing conflicts with their caregivers.

THE DECISION TO MOVE A LOVED ONE INTO A NURSING HOME

What may be one of the most difficult and psychologically painful tasks for any family member is having to make the decision to place a loved one into a long-term care facility (Reuss, Dupuis, & Whitfield, 2005). This section addresses the dynamics, circumstances, and reasons behind making such difficult decisions. The Agency for Health Care Policy and Research (1998) indicate that four out of 10 Americans in the United States will spend some time in a nursing home in their lives. The decision to place a loved one into a nursing home is generally a difficult one in most instances; however, numerous studies cite the psychological and financial stresses caregivers report regarding the toll of caring for a loved one at home (Dupuis, Epp, & Smale, 2004; Grosse et al., 2009). The perceived stress of the caregiver, perceived and actual support or lack of it, financial constraints, severity of care recipient disability (e.g., ventilator and/or feeding tube), and age of the caregiver are all significant factors in making such a decision (Dellasega & Mastrian, 1995; Fisher & Lieberman, 1999;

Reinhardy, 1993, Wackerbarth, 1999). It is not uncommon for caregivers to experience simultaneous feelings of loneliness, guilt, resentment, sense of failure, sadness, anger, loss of control, rushed decision making, and peace of mind with the process (Dellasega & Mastrian, 1995; Dellasega & Nolan, 1997; Nolan & Dellasega, 2000).

Reuss et al. (2005) surveyed family members in southern Ontario, Canada regarding what factors were most influential in facilitating a positive transition for their loved ones into long-term care institutions. Results indicated several key factors, including the experience during the waiting process, preparation for the move, ease of the actual move, control over decisions, communication throughout the process, support from others, and family and resident perceptions and attitudes toward the move." (p. 17). Nolan et al. (1996) specified that when significant family members and the care recipient (a) are able to plan and rationally prepare for the move, (b) are equal participants in actually choosing a setting, (c) have time to express reactions and sentiments about the choices, and (d) are provided information to make informed decisions about the alternatives, then final decisions and a positive transition are more likely (pp. 269–271).

Grasel (2002) was interested in studying caregiver physical and mental health after having placed a loved one in a long-term care facility. He interviewed 720 German primary caregivers of dementia patients prior to placing their loved ones, and followed up with 681 1 year later after the loved one was in long-term care. Two groups were distinguished: active caregivers still caring for their loved one at home after 12 months, and caregivers who were at least 6 months postplacing their loved one in long-term care. Grasel's results showed several interesting changes between groups. The active caregiving group showed no major health changes after 1 year, but the frequency of illnesses was up moderately with a mild increase of medication. This continuing active caregiving group did not have an increase in somatic complaints or physician visits. For the group who was no longer providing care, their average physician visits almost doubled. Grasel attributed this occurrence to the caregivers now having time to visit their physicians. And despite their dramatic increase in physician visits, the former caregivers subjectively perceived themselves to be feeling much better, and their medications had not increased. In contrast to the sense of feeling better with the perceived burden or stress of caregiving in Grasel's study, there are studies where caregivers become worse health-wise. It is not uncommon for women caregivers, in particular, to become lonely, express guilt, become depressed, and potentially physically ill postplacement (Baumgarten, Hanley, Infante-Rivard, et al., 1994; Collins, Stommel, Wang, et al., 1994; Gaugler, Leitsch, Zarit, et al., 2000). Overall, numerous factors go into making a long-term care placement decision, and Gaugler, Roth, Haley, and Mittelman (2008) advise counseling and support to reduce caregiver negative feelings in making such decisions.

CONCLUSION

From the hundreds of studies regarding caregiver physical and mental health in general as well as the health of caregivers who work with loved ones with specific disabilities, several important overall conclusions can be summarized. First, there appears to be some consistent (but not exclusive) literature that supports the more hours of direct care and related severity of the disability (especially when behavioral problems exist), the greater the level of reported caregiver physical and mental health problems (Canning et al., 1996; Grosse et al., 2009; Imran et al., 2010; Mulvihill et al., 2005; Roth et al., 2009).

Second, although a number of studies show a reported decline in caregiver physical health, it remains unclear, in many studies, as to exactly how physical health is negatively impacted, and whether perceived poorer caregiver health translates into actual physical health problems (Grosse et al., 2009; Murphy et al., 2006). Low-back pain appears to be the most common symptom reported (Tong et al., 2003). Several studies noted here show that caregivers report declining physical health and not having the time to attend to their own health concerns; however, the nature of the physical health problems other than low-back pain and perhaps headache remains unknown in many studies.

Third, mental health has been studied more extensively, showing caregivers are most often at greater risk for depression and anxiety. Presumably, loss of sleep, fear of their loved one's uncertain health status, reduction in social support, leisure and pleasure deriving activities facilitates these emotions (Grosse et al., 2009; Hanson, 1995; Murphy et al., 2006). Restricted lifestyle and lack of pleasurable engagement has been a lifelong study of Peter Lewinsohn (1974). Lewinsohn's major premise here is that when individuals are unable or unwilling to engage in what otherwise for them were once pleasurable activities (socializing, dining out, attending events, etc.) they can become more susceptible to depression. As such, when caregivers either perceive or actually have no choice but to socially withdraw from doing once pleasurable activities in order to care for a loved one, depression or dysthymia may result. Joiner, Lewinsohn, and Seeley's (2002) study of loneliness and pleasurable engagement among over 1,500 adolescents found small effect sizes supporting that lack of pleasurable engagement is directly related to loneliness and subsequently related to depression. Caregivers often report this sense of isolation (Borg & Hallberg, 2006; Brehaut et al., 2009; Roth et al., 2009).

Fourth, it would appear that it is not the family member's disability and actual caregiving involved that directly causes stress and stress related illness for caregivers, but rather it is their "perception" of the situation as being burdensome, and their perceived lack of control to change the situation and feeling trapped that may facilitate illness (Grant et al., 2007; Miller, 1979; Thompson, 1985). When under duress, our immune system becomes compromised, making it more difficult to fight off flu, colds, pain, negative affect, and other stress-related illnesses (Cohen & Lazarus, 1983; Rosenhan & Seligman, 1984; Selye, 1956, 1985). Basically, if we perceive our situation to be hopeless and uncontrollable, the greater is the likelihood for physical and mental health problems to occur (Rosenhan & Seligman, 1984).

Fifth, perceptions and reactions to caregiving are, as noted earlier, on a continuum: neither good nor bad, stressful or nonstressful. It is more often ultimately a combination of both, comprising rewards and sacrifices. The rewards are documented as giving the caregiver meaning and purpose, the reciprocation of love, companionship, sense of virtue, and the joy of giving (Bogdan & Taylor, 1989; Buchanan et al., 2009; Janoff-Bulman, 2004; Reid et al., 2005). Conversely, reported sacrifices can include depression, anxiety, reduced pleasurable activities, social isolation, disrupted sleep, and physical health problems, including chronic low-back pain (Grosse et al.,

2009; Joiner et al., 2002; Murphy et al., 2006; Shewchuk, Richards, & Elliott, 1998; Yilmaz et al., 2004).

Six, families who are taught or otherwise use problem-solving skills to manage caregiving responsibilities, implement rules, and delegate equally to other members, positively reinforce one another, and view caregiving as a virtuous and critical family obligation, generally adapt better to their circumstances (Elliott & Berry, 2009; Knestrict & Kuchey, 2009; Park & Folkman, 1997; Wagnild & Young, 1990; Williams, Wiebe, & Smith, 1992). Evidence also suggests that spiritual faith and prayer is practiced more by minorities and appears to be a good coping strategy in reducing perceived burden (Macera et al., 1992; Sander et al., 2007). Somewhat paradoxical is the traditional caregiver ideology practiced mainly by persons of ethnic minority. Although this ideological belief generally provides a sense of purpose, virtue, and reward for the caregiver, these selfless acts of kindness tend to be associated with increased distress as well for those caregivers who take on most, if not all, caregiving responsibilities.

Seven, it appears in instances where (a) caregivers are caring for a loved one who is highly dependent on them physically and mentally; (b) the care recipient can interact and displays rebellious, hyperactive, violent, or antagonizing behavior toward the caregiver; (c) the care recipient is female and older; and (d) the caregiver feels overworked and under financial restraints, that these circumstances sometimes facilitate caregiver physical, verbal, and/or material abuse toward the care recipient (Friedrich & Boriskin, 1976; Martin, 1982; Zirpoli et al., 2001). In instances where caregivers are not abusive, but nevertheless experience the above stressors, the painful decision to place a loved one into a long-term care institution or nursing home threatens their own perceived well-being. In these situations, careful planning and psychological readiness become critical for a positive transition into long-term care and out of the home (Reuss et al., 2005).

Finally, it appears in many instances that once caregivers become accustomed to their routine over time, they are able to delegate responsibilities equally, and can support and communicate to each other positively; these are all strong predictors of family adjustment and accommodation to a family member with a disability (see Penner, 2004). In addition, personal characteristics discussed in the positive psychology chapter, including resilience, hardiness, a sense of becoming stronger through adversity, internal locus of control, and posttraumatic growth, all contribute to positive well-being (Janoff-Bulman, 2004; Schafer, 1996). Nonetheless, when the onus of caregiving falls to one person (typically the mother or daughter) with little or no support, the mental and physical care demands of the loved one are high with no respite available; caregiver mental and physical health problems are likely a foregone conclusion of deteriorating health problems for the caregiver (Grosse et al., 2009).

REFERENCES

Abbey, A., Abramis, D. J., & Caplan, R. D. (1985). Effects of different sources of social support and social conflict on emotional well-being. *Basic and Applied Psychology, 6*, 111–129.

Agency for Health Care Policy and Research. (1998). *Research on long-term care.* Washington, DC: AHCPR.

American Psychiatric Association. (2000). *Diagnostic and statistical manual of mental disorders* (4th ed., text rev.). Washington, DC: Author.

Anetzberger, G. (1987). *The etiology of elder abuse by adult offspring.* Springfield, IL: Charles C. Thomas.

Argyle, E. (2001). Poverty, disability and the role of older carers. *Disability & Society, 16*(4), 585–595.

Baumgarten, T., Hanley, J. A., Infante-Rivard, C., et al. (1994). Health of family members caring for elderly persons with dementia: A longitudinal study. *Annals of Internal Medicine, 120,* 126–132.

Berkman, L. F. (1995). The role of social relations in health promotion. *Psychosomatic Medicine, 57,* 245–254.

Biegel, D. E., Ishler, K. J., Katz, S., & Johnson, P. (2007). Predictors of burden of family care-givers of women with substance use disorders or co–occurring substance and mental disorders. *Journal of Social Work Practice in the Addictions, 7*(12), 25–49.

Blake, H. (2001). Care-giver stress in traumatic brain injury. *International Journal of Therapy and Rehabilitation, 15*(6), 263–271.

Blanes, L., Carmagnani, M. I., & Ferreira, L. M. (2007). Health-related quality of life of primary care-givers of persons with paraplegia. *Spinal Cord, 45,* 399–403.

Bogdan, R., & Taylor, S. (1989). Relationships with severely disabled people: The social construction of humanness. *Social Problems, 36,* 135–148.

Borg, C., & Hallberg, I. R. (2006). Life satisfaction among informal care-givers in comparison with non-care-givers. *Scandinavian Journal of Caring Sciences, 20,* 427–438.

Brooks, D. N. (1991). Presidential address, Innsbruck: The head-injured family. *Journal of Clinical and Experimental Neuropsychology, 13,* 155–188.

Brooks, N., & McKinlay, W. (1983). Personality and behavioural change after severe blunt head injury- A relative's view. *Journal of Neurology, Neurosurgery, and Psychiatry, 46,* 336–344.

Brehaut, J. C., Kohen, D. E., Garner, R. E., Miller, A. R., Lach, L. M., Klassen, A. F. et al. (2009). Health among care-givers of children with health problems: Findings from a Canadian population-based study. *American Journal of Pubic Health, 99*(7), 1254–1262.

Britell, C. W., & Hammond, M. C. (1994). Spinal cord injury. In R. M. Hays, G. H. Kraft, & W. C. Stolov (Eds.), *Chronic disease and disability: A contemporary rehabilitation approach to medical practice* (pp. 142–160). New York, NY: Demos.

Buchanan, R. J., Radin, D., Chakravorty, B. J., & Tyry, T (2009). Informal care-giving to more disabled people with multiple sclerosis. *Disability and Rehabilitation, 31*(15), 1244–1256.

Byrne, M. B., Hurley, D. A., Daly, L., & Cunningham, C. G. (2010). Health status of care-givers of children with cerebral palsy. *Child: Care, Health & Development, 36*(5), 696–702.

Call, K. T., Finch, M. D., Huck, M. A., & Kane, S. M. (1999). Caregiver burden from a social exchange perspective: Caring for older people following hospital discharge. *Journal of Marriage and the Family, 61,* 688–699.

Campbell, C. (1988). Needs of relatives and helpfulness of support groups in severe head injury. *Rehabilitation Nursing, 13,* 320–325.

Canning, R. D., Harris, E. S., & Kelleher, K. J (1996). Factors predicting distress among care-givers to children with chronic medical conditions. *Journal of Pediatric Psychology, 21,* 735–749.

Carnevale, F. A., Alexander, E., Davis, M., Rennick, J., & Troini, R. (2006). Daily living with distress and enrichment: The moral experience of families with ventilator-assisted children at home. *Pediatrics, 117,* 48–60.

Chak, A. (1996). Conceptualizing social support: A micro or macro perspective? *Psychologia, 39,* 74–83.

Chan, J. (2007). Carers' perspective on respite for persons with acquired brain injury. *International Journal of Rehabilitation Research, 30*(2), 137–146.

Chen, J. C., Borson, S., & Scanlan, J. M. (2000). Stage-specific prevalence of behavioral symptoms in Alzheimer's disease in a multi-ethnic community sample. *American Journal of Geriatric Psychiatry, 8*(2), 123–133.

Chronister, J. (2009). Social support and rehabilitation: Theory, research and measurement. In F. Chan, E. Da Silva Cardoso, & J. A. Chronister (Eds.), *Understanding psychosocial adjustment to chronic illness and disability: A handbook for evidence-based practitioners in rehabilitation* (p. 149–183). New York, NY: Springer.

Chronister, J., Chou, C. C., Frain, M., & Cardoso, E. (2008). The relationship between social support and rehabilitation related outcomes: A meta-analysis. *Journal of Rehabilitation, 74,* 16–32.

Cohen, F., & Lazarus, R. S. (1983). Coping and adaptation in health and illness. In D. Mechanic (Ed.), *Handbook of health, health care, and the health professions.* New York, NY: Free Press.

Cohen, S. (1988). Psychosocial models of social support in the etiology of physical disease. *Health Psychology, 7,* 269–297.

Cohen, S., Doyle, W. J., Skoner, D. P., Rabin, B. S., & Gwaltney, J. M. (1997). Social ties and susceptibility to common cold. *Journal of the American Medical Association, 277,* 1940–1944.

Cohen, S., & Wills, T. A. (1985). Social support, stress and the buffering hypothesis. *Psychological Bulletin, 98,* 310–357.

Collins, C., Stommel, M., Wang, S. et al. (1994). Care-giving transitions: Changes in depression among family care-givers of relatives with dementia. *Nursing Research, 43,* 220–225.

Cook, J. A., Hoffschmidt, S., Cohler, B. J., & Pickett, S. A. (1992). Predicting marital satisfaction among parents of off-spring with severe mental illness living in the community. *American Journal of Orthropsychiatry, 62*(4), 552–563.

Cook, J. A., Cohler, B. J., Pickett, S. A., & Beeler, J. A. (1997). Life-course and severe mental illness: Implications for care-giving within the family of later life. *Family Relations, 46,* 427–436.

Corcoran, P. J. (1981). Neuromuscular disease. In W. C. Stolov & M. R. Clowers (Eds.), *Handbook of severe disability* (pp. 83–100). Washington, DC: U.S. Department of Education Rehabilitation Services Administration.

Coyne, A. C., Reichman, W. E., & Berbig, L. J. (1993). The relationship between dementia and elder abuse. *American Journal of Psychiatry, 150,* 643–646.

Dagenais, L., Hall, N., Majnemer, A., Birnbaum, R., Dumas, F., Gosselin, J. et al. (2006). Communicating a diagnosis of cerebral palsy: Care-giver satisfaction and stress. *Pediatric Neurology, 35*(6), 408–414.

Daoud, A., Dooley, J. M., & Gordon, K. E. (2004). Depression in parents of children with duchenne muscular dystrophy. *Pediatric Neurology, 31,* 16–19.

Degeneffe, C. E. (2001). Family care-giving and traumatic brain injury. *Health & Social Work, 26*(4), 257–268.

Dellasega, C., & Mastrian, K. (1995). The process and consequences of institutionalizing an elder. *Western Journal of Nursing Research, 17*(2), 123–140.

Dellasega, C., & Nolan, M. (1997). Admission to care: Facilitating role transition amongst family carers. *Journal of Clinical Nursing, 6,* 443–451.

Douglas, J., & Spellacy, F. (2000). Correlates of depression in adults with severe traumatic brain injury and their carers. *Brain Injury, 14*(1), 71–88.

Drentea, P., & Goldner, M. A. (2006). Care-giving outside of the home: The effects of race on depression. *Ethnicity & Health, 11,* 41–57.

Dupuis, S. L., Epp, T., & Smale, B. J. (2004). *Care-givers of persons with dementia: Roles, experiences, supports and coping.* Waterloo, ON: Murray Alzheimer's Research and Education Program.

Dwyer, F. W., & Miller, M. K. (1990). Differences in care-giving network by area of residence: Implications for primary care-giver stress and burden. *Family Relations, 39,* 27–37.

Easton, J. K., & Halpern, D. (1981). Cerebral palsy. In W. C. Stolov & M. R. Clowers (Eds.), *Handbook of severe disability* (pp. 137–154). Washington, DC: U.S. Department of Education Rehabilitation Services Administration.

Eisdorfer, C., & Cohen, D. (1981). Management of the patient and family coping with dementing illness. *Journal of Family Practice, 12*(5), 831–837.

Ellenbogen, P. S., Meade, M. A., Jackson, M. N., & Barrett, K. (2006). The impact of spinal cord injury on the employment of family caregivers. *Journal of Vocational Rehabilitation, 25,* 35–44.

Elliott, T., & Kurylo, M. (2000). Hope over disability: Lessons from one young woman's triumph. In C. R. Snyder (Ed.), *The handbook of hope: Theory, measures, and applications* (pp. 373–386). New York, NY: Academic Press.

Elliott, T., Shewchuk, R., & Richards, J. S. (2001). Family care-givers social problem-solving abilities and adjustment during the initial year of the care-giving role. *Journal of Counseling Psychology, 48,* 223–232.

Elliott, T. R., Brossart, D., Berry, J. W., & Fine, P. R. (2008). Problem-solving training via videoconferencing for family care-givers of persons with spinal cord injuries; A randomized controlled trail. *Behavior Research and Therapy, 46,* 1220–1229.

Elliott, T. R., & Berry, J. W. (2009). Brief problem-solving training for family care-givers of persons with recent-onset spinal cord injuries: A randomized controlled trial. *Journal of Clinical Psychology, 65*(4), 406–422.

Evans, G. W., Palasano, M. N., LePore, S. J., & Martin, J. (1989). Residential density and psychological health: The mediating effects of social support. *Journal of Personality and Social Psychology, 57*, 994–999.

Ferri, C. P., Prince, M., Brayne, C., Brodaty, H., Fratiglioni, L., Ganguli, M. et al. (2005). Global prevalence of dementia: A Delphi consensus study. *The Lancet, 366*(9503), 2112–2117.

Fisher, L., & Lieberman, M. A. (1999). A longitudinal study of predictors of nursing home placement for patients with dementia: The contribution of family characteristics. *The Gerontologist, 39*(6), 677–686.

Friedrich, W. N., & Boriskin, J. A. (1976). Primary prevention of child abuse: Focus on the special child. *Hospital and Community Psychiatry, 29*, 248–251.

Fulmer, T. (1990). "The debate over dependency as a relevant predisposing factor in elder abuse and neglect" *Journal of Elder Abuse & Neglect, 2*(1/2), 51–57.

Gainey, R., & Payne, B. K. (2006). Care-giver burden, elder abuse and Alzheimer's disease: Testing the relationship, *Journal of Health and Human Services Administration, 29*(2), 245–259.

Gaugler, J. E., Leitsch, S. A., Zarit, S. H. et al. (2000). Care-giver involvement following institutionalization: Effects of pre-placement stress. *Research on Aging, 22*, 337–359.

Gaugler, J. E., Roth, D. L., Haley, W. E., & Mittelman, M. S. (2008). Can counseling and support reduce burden and depressive symptoms in care-givers of people with Alzheimer's disease during the transition to institutionalization? Results from the New York University care-giver intervention study. *Journal of the American Geriatrics Society, 56*, 421–428.

Graf, N. M., Marini, I., & Blankenship, C. (2009). 100 Words about disability. *Journal of Rehabilitation, 75*(2), 25–34.

Grant, G., Ramcharan, P., & Flynn, M. (2007). Resilience in families with children and adult members with intellectual disabilities: Tracing elements of a psychosocial model. *Journal of Applied Research in Intellectual Abilities, 20*, 563–575.

Grasel, E. (2002). When home care ends- Changes in the physical health of informal care-givers caring for dementia patients: A longitudinal study. *Journal of the American Geriatrics Society, 50*, 843–849.

Greenberg, J. S., Greenley, J. R., & Brown, R. (1997a). Do mental health services reduce distress of families of people with serious mental illness? *Psychiatric Rehabilitation Journal, 21*, 40–50.

Greenberg, J. S., Kim, H. W., & Greenley, J. R. (1997b). Factors associated with subjective burden in siblings of adults with severe mental illness. *American Journal of Orthopsychiatry, 67*, 231–241.

Grosse, S. D., Flores, A. L., Ouyang, L., Robbins, J. M., & Tilford, J. M. (2009). Impact of spina bifida on parental care-givers: Findings from a survey of Arkansas families. *Journal of Child Family Studies, 18*, 574–581.

Haley, W. E., West, C. A., Wadley, V. G., Ford, G. R., White, F. A., Barrett, J. J., et al. (1995). Psychological, social, and health impact of care-giving: A comparison of black and white dementia family care-givers and non-care-givers. *Psychology and Aging, 10*, 540–552.

Hanks, R. A., Rapport, L. J., & Vangel, S. (2007). Care-giving appraisal after traumatic brain injury: The effects of functional status, coping style, social support and family functioning. *NeuroRehabilitation, 22*, 43–52.

Hanson, J. G. (1995). Families' perceptions of psychiatric hospitalization of relatives with a severe mental illness. *Administration and Policy in Mental Health, 22*(5), 531–541.

Harding, C., Zubin, J., & Strauss, J. (1987). Chronicity in schizophrenia: Fact, partial fact, or artifact? *Hospital and Community Psychiatry, 38*, 477–486.

Heller, T., & Factor, A. (1993). Aging family caregivers: Support resources and changes in burden and placement desire. *American Journal of Mental Retardation, 98*, 417–426.

Hulnick, M. R., & Hulnick, H. R. (1981). Life's challenges: Curse or Opportunity? Counseling families of persons with disabilities. In R. P. Marinelli, & A. E. Dell Orto (3rd eds.), *The psychological & social impact of disability* (pp. 258–268). New York, NY: Springer.

Imran, N., Bhatti, R., Haider, I. I., Azhar, L., Omar, A., & Sattar, A. (2010). Caring for the care-givers: Mental health, family burden and quality of life of care-givers of patients with mental illness. *Journal of Pakistan Psychiatric Society, 7*(1), 23–28.

Janoff-Bulman, R. (2004). Posttraumatic growth: Three explanatory models. *Psychological Inquiry, 15*(1), 30–34.

Johnson, T. F. (1991). *Elder mistreatment: Deciding who is at risk.* Westport, CT: Greenwood Press.

Joiner, T. E., Lewinsohn, P. M., & Seeley, J. R. (2002). The core of loneliness: Lack of pleasurable engagement –More so than painful disconnection-Predicts social impairment, depression onset, and recovery from depressive disorders among adolescents. *Journal of Personality Assessment, 79*(3), 472–491.

Karlawish, J. H., Casarett, D. J., James, B. D., Tenhave, T., Clark, C. M., & Asch, D. A. (2003). Why would care-givers not want to treat their relative's Alzheimer's disease? *Journal of the American Geriatrics Society, 51*, 1391–1397.

Karlin, N. J., & Retzlaff, P. D. (1995). Psychopathology in care-givers of the chronically ill: Personality and clinical syndromes. *Hospital Journal, 10*, 55–61.

Kessler, R. C., Nelson, C. B., McGonagle, K. A., Edlund, M. J., Frank, R. G., & Leaf, P. J. (1996). The epidemiology of co-occurring addictive and mental disorders: Implications for prevention and service utilization. *American Journal of Orthopsychiatry, 66*, 17–31.

Khan, F., Pallant, J., & Brand, C. (2007). Caregiver strain and factors associated with care-giver self-efficacy and quality of life in a community cohort with multiple sclerosis. *Disability and Rehabilitation, 29*(16), 1241–1250.

Knestrict, T., & Kuchey, D. (2009). Welcome to Holland: Characteristics of resilient families raising children with severe disabilities. *Journal of Family Studies, 15*, 227–244.

Korbin, J. E., Anetzberger, G. J., & Eckert, J. K. (1990). "Elder abuse and child abuse: A consideration of similarities and differences in intergenerational family violence" *Journal of Elder Abuse & Neglect, 1*(4), 1–14.

Krause, J. S., Coker, J., Charlifue, S., & Whiteneck, G. G. (1999). Depression and subjective well-being among 97 American Indians with spinal cord injury: A descriptive study. *Rehabilitation Psychology, 44*, 354–372.

Kravetz, S., Faust, M., & Dasberg, I. (2002). A comparison of care consumer and care provider perspectives on the quality of life of persons with persistent and severe psychiatric disabilities. *Psychiatric Rehabilitation Journal, 25*(4), 388–397.

Kreutzer, J. S., Gervasio, A. H., & Camplair, P. S. (1994). Patient correlates of care-givers' distress and family functioning after traumatic brain injury. *Brain Injury, 8*, 211–230.

Lawrence, V., Murray, J., Samsi, K., & Banerjee, S. (2008). Attitudes and support needs of black Caribbean, south Asian and white British carers of people with dementia in the UK. *The British Journal of Psychiatry, 193*, 240–246.

Lefebvre, H., Cloutier, G., & Levert, M. J. (2008). Perspectives of survivors of traumatic brain injury and their care-givers on long-term social integration. *Brain Injury, 22*(7–8), 535–543.

Lefley, H. P. (1996). *Family care-giving in mental illness.* Thousand Oaks, CA: Sage.

Lewinsohn, P. M. (1974). A behavioral approach to depression. In R. J. Friedman & M. M. Katz (Eds.), *The psychology of depression: Contemporary theory and research* (pp. 264–279). Washington, DC: Winston-Wiley.

Lezak, M. (1988). Brain damage is a family affair. *Journal of Clinical and Experimental Neuropsychology, 10*, 111–123.

Lindblad, B., Holritz, B., & Sandman, P. (2007). A life enriching togetherness-meanings of informal support when being a parent of a child with disability. *Scandinavian Journal of Caring Sciences, 21*, 238–246.

Li, L., & Moore, D. , 1998. Acceptance of disability and its correlates. *Journal of Social Psychology, 138*(1), 13–25.

Livneh, H., & Antonak, R. F. (1997). *Psychosocial adaptation to chronic illness and disability.* Gaithersburg, MD: Aspen.

Lo Coco, G., Lo Coco, D., Cicero, V., Oliveri, A., Lo Verso, G., Piccoli, F. et al. (2005). Individual and health-related quality of life assessment in amyotrophic lateral sclerosis patients and their care-givers. *Journal of the Neurological Sciences, 238*, 11–17.

MacDonald, H., & Callery, P. (2007). Parenting children requiring complex care: A journey through time. *Child: Care, Health and Development, 34*(2), 207–213.

Macera, C. A., Eaker, E. D., Goslar, P. W., Deandrade, S. J., Williamson, J. S., Cornman, C., et al. (1992). Ethnic differences in the burden of care-giving. *American Journal of Alzheimers Disease & Other Dementias, 7*(5), 4–7.

Manuel, J. C. (2001). Risk and resistance factors in the adaptation of the mothers of children with juvenile rheumatoid arthritis. *Journal of Pediatric Psychology, 26,* 237–246.

Marini, I. (2001a). Characteristics of SSDI/SSI beneficiaries as rehabilitation clients. *The Rehabilitation Professional, 9*(3), 40–42.

Marini, I., & Reid, C. R. (2001). A survey of rehabilitation professionals as alternative provider contractors with social security: Problems and solutions. *Journal of Rehabilitation, 67*(2), 36–41.

Marini, I., Bhakta, M. V., & Graf, N. (2009). A content analysis of common concerns of persons with physical disabilities. *Journal of Applied Rehabilitation Counseling, 40*(1), 44–49.

Martin, H. (1982). The clinical relevance of prediction and prevention. In H. R. H. Starr, Jr. (Ed.), *Child abuse prediction: Policy implications* (pp. 175–190). Cambridge, MA: Ballinger.

Matheis, E. N., Tulsky, D. S., & Matheis, R. J. (2006). The relation between spirituality and quality of life among individuals with spinal cord injury. *Rehabilitation Psychology, 51,* 265–271.

Mah, J. K., Thannhauser, J. E., McNeil, D. A., & Dewey, D. (2008). Being the lifeline: The parent experience of caring for a child with neuromuscular disease on home mechanical ventilation. *Neuromuscular Disorders, 18,* 983–988.

Mannion, E. (2008). Alzheimer's disease: The psychological and physical effects of the care-giver's role. Part 1. *Nursing Older People, 20*(4), 27–32.

McFarlane, J., Hughes, R. B., Nosek, M. A., Groff, J. Y., Swedlund, N., & Mullen, P. D. (2001). Abuse assessment screen-disability (AAS-D): Measuring frequency, type, and perpetrator of abuse toward women with physical disabilities. *Journal of Women's Health and Gender-Based Medicine, 10,* 861–866.

Miller, D. S. (1959). Fractures among children. *Minnesota Medicine, 42,* 1209–1213.

Miller, S. M. (1979). Controllability and human stress: Method, evidence and theory. *Behaviour Research and Therapy, 17,* 287–304.

Mueser, K. T., Bennett, M., & Kushner, M. G. G. (1995). Epidemiology of substance use disorders among persons with chronic illness. In A. F. Lehman & L. B. Dixion (Eds.), *Double jeopardy: Chronic mental illness and substance use disorders* (pp. 9–25). Chur, Switzerland: Harwood Academic Publishers.

Mulvihill, B. A., Wingate, M. S., Altarac, M., Mulvihill, F. X., Redden, D. T., Telfair, J., et al. (2005). The association of child condition severity with family functioning and relationship with health care providers among children and youth with special health care needs in Alabama. *Maternal and Child Health Journal, 9,* S87–S97.

Murphy, N. A., Christian, B., Caplin, D. A., & Young, P. C. (2006). The health of care-givers for children with disabilities: Care-givers perspectives. *Child: Care, Health and Development, 33*(2), 180–187.

Nadien, M. B. (1995). Elder violence (maltreatment) in domestic settings. In L. L. Adler & F. L. Denmark (Eds.), *Violence and the prevention of violence* (pp. 177–190). Westport, CT: Praeger.

Nadien, M. B. (1996). Aging women: Issues of mental health and maltreatment. *Annals of the New York Academy of Sciences* (pp. 129–145). New York, NY: New York Academy of Sciences.

Nadien, M. B. (2006). Factors that influence abusive interactions between aging women and their caregivers. *Annals of the NewYork Acadamy of Sciences, 1087,* 158–169.

National Alliance for Care-giving, the American Association of Retired Persons (2004). *Care-giving in the US.* Washington, DC: NAC and AARP.

National Institutes of Health (1999). *Report of the NIH consensus development conference on the rehabilitation of persons with traumatic brain injury.* Bethesda, MD: U.S. Department of Health and Human Services.

Nereo, N. E., Fee, R. J., & Hinton, V. J. (2003). Parental stress in mothers of boys with duchenne muscular dystrophy. *Journal of Pediatric Psychology, 28,* 473–484.

Nolan, M., & Dellasega, C. (2000). I really feel I've let him down: Supporting family carers during long-term care placement for elders. *Journal of Advanced Nursing, 31,* 759–767.

Nolan, M., Walker, G., Nolan, J., Williams, S., Poland, F., Curran, M., et al. (1996). Entry to care: Positive choice or fait accompli? Developing a more proactive nursing response to the needs of elder people and their carers. *Journal of Advanced Nursing, 24,* 265–274.

Nosek, M. A., Foley, C. C., Hughes, R. B., & Howland, C. A. (2001). Vulnerabilities for abuse among women with disabilities. *Sexuality and Disability, 19,* 177–189.

O'Brien, M. E. (1994). "Elder abuse: How to spot it-How to help" *North Carolina Medical Journal, 55*(9), 409–411.

Oddy, M. (1995). He's no longer the same person: How families adjust to personality change after head injury. In M. Chamberlain, V. Neumann, & V. Tennant (Eds.), *Traumatic brain injury rehabilitation: Services, treatment and outcomes* (pp. 167–179). London: Chapman and Hall Medical.

Olkin, R. (1999). *What psychotherapists should know about disability.* New York, NY: The Guilford Press.

Pang, F. C., Chow, T. W., Cummings, J. L., Leung, V. P., Chiu, H. F., Lam, C. W., et al. (2002). Effects of neuropsychiatric symptoms of Alzheimer's disease of Chinese and American care-givers. *International Journal of Geriatric Psychiatry, 17,* 29–34.

Parke, R. D., & Collmer, C. W. (1975). Child abuse: An interdisciplinary analysis. In E. M. Hetherington (Ed.), *Review of child development research* (pp. 509–590). Chicago, IL: University of Chicago Press.

Park, C. L., & Folkman, S. L. (1997). Meaning in the context of stress and coping. *Review of General Psychology, 1,* 115–144.

Paveza, G. J., Cohen, D., Eisdorfer, C., Freels, S., Semla, T., Ashford, J. W. et al. (1992). "Severe family violence and Alzheimer's disease" *The Gerontologist, 12,* 493–497.

Payne, B. K. (2005). *Crime and elder abuse: An integrated perspective.* Springfield, IL: Charles C. Thomas.

Pearlin, L. T., Lieberman, M. A., Menaghan, E. G., & Mullan, J. T. (1981). The stress process. *Journal of Health and Social Behavior, 22,* 337–356.

Penner, L. A. (2004). Volunteerism and social problem: Making things better or worse? *Journal of Social Issues, 60*(3), 645–666.

Post, M. W., Bloemen, J., & de Witte, L. P. (2005). Burden of support for partners of persons with spinal cord injuries. *Spinal Cord, 43,* 311–319.

Provencher, H. L., Perreault, M., St. Onge, M., & Rousseau, M. (2003). Predictors of psychological distress in family care-givers of persons with psychiatric disabilities. *Journal of Psychiatric and Mental Nursing, 10,* 592–607.

Rabins, P. V., Mace, N. L., & Lucas, M. J. (1982). The impact of dementia on the family. *Journal of the American Medical Association, 248*(3), 333–335.

Regier, D. A., Farmer, M. E., Rae, M. E., Locke, B. Z., Judd, L. L., & Goodwin, F. K. (1990). Comorbidity of mental disorders with alcohol and other drug abuse. *Journal of the American Medical Association, 264,* 2511–2518.

Reid, C. E., Moss, S., & Hyman, G. (2005). Care-givers reciprocity: The effect of reciprocity, carer self-esteem and motivation on the experience of care-giver burden. *Australian Journal of Psychology, 57*(3), 186–196.

Reinhardy, J. R. (1993). Decisional control in moving to a nursing home: Post admission adjustment and well-being. *The Gerontologist, 32*(1), 96–103.

Reuss, G. F., Dupuis, S. L., & Whitfield, K. (2005). Understanding the experience of moving a loved one to a long-term care facility: Family members' perspectives. *Journal of Gerontological Social Work, 46*(1), 17–46.

Rosenhan, D. L., & Seligman, M. E. (1984). *Abnormal psychology.* New York, NY: Norton.

Roth, D. L., Perkins, M., Wadley, V. G., & Temple, E. M. (2009). Family caregiving and emotional strain: Associations with quality of life in a large national sample of middle-aged and older adults. *Quality of Life Research, 18,* 679–688.

Sanders, A. M., Davis, L. C., Struchen, M. A., Atchison, T., Sherer, M., Malec, J. F. et al. (2007). Relationship of race/ethnicity to care-givers' coping, appraisals, and distress after traumatic brain injury. *Neurological Rehabilitation, 22,* 9–17.

Schafer, W. (1996). *Stress management for wellness.* Orlando, FL: Harcourt Brace.

Schrag, A., Hovris, A., Morley, D., Quinn, N., & Jajanshahi, M. (2006). Care-giver-burden in Parkinson's disease is closely associated with psychiatric symptoms, falls, and disability. *Parkinsonism and Related Disorder, 12*, 35–41.

Schwarz, K., & Roberts, B. (2000). Social support and strain of family care-givers of older adults. *Holistic Nursing Practice, 14*, 77–90.

Schwarzer, R., & Leppin, A. (1991). Social support and health: A theoretical and empirical overview. *Journal of Social and Personal Relationships, 8*, 99–127.

Selye, H. (1956). *The stress of life.* New York, NY: McGraw-Hill.

Selye, H. (1985). History and present status of the stress concept. In A. Monat & R. S. Lazarus (Eds.), *Stress and coping* (2nd ed.). New York, NY: Columbia University Press.

Shewchuk, R., Richards, J. S., & Elliott, T. (1998). Dynamic processes in health outcomes among care-givers of patients with spinal cord injuries. *Health Psychology, 17*, 125–129.

Stevenson, J. (1990). Family stress related to home care of Alzheimer's disease patients and implications for support. *Journal of Neuroscience Nursing, 22*, 179–188.

Takano, M., & Arai, H. (2005). Gender difference and care-givers' burden in early-onset Alzheimer's disease. *Psychogeriatics, 5*, 73–77.

Talley, R. C., & Crews, J. E. (2007). Framing the public health of care-giving. *American Journal of Public Health, 97*, 224–228.

Tangri, P., & Verma, P. (1992). A study of social burden felt by mothers of handicapped children. *Journal of Personality and Clinical Studies, 8*, 117–120.

Thompson, S. C. (1985). Finding positive meaning in a stressful event and coping. *Basic and Applied Social Psychology, 6*(4), 279–295.

Tong, H. C., Haig, A. J., Nelson, V. S., Yamakawa, K. S., Kandala, G., & Shin, K. Y. (2003). Low back pain in adult female care-givers of children with physical disabilities. *Archives of Pediatrics and Adolescent Medicine, 157*, 1128–1133.

Tyerman, A., & Booth, J. (2001). Family intervention after traumatic brain injury: A service example. *Neurological Rehabilitation, 16*(1), 59–66.

Quittner, A., Opipari, L., Regoli, M. J., Jacobsen, J., & Eigen, H. (1992). The impact of care-giving and role strain on family life: Comparisons between mothers of children with cystic fibrosis and matched controls. *Rehabilitation Psychology, 37*, 275–290.

Varni, J. W., Rubenfeld, L. A., Talbot, D., & Setoguchi, Y. (1989). Family functioning, temperament, and psychologic adaptation in children with congenital or acquired limb deficiencies. *Pediatrics, 84*(2), 323–330.

Vellone, E., Piras, G., Talucci, C., & Cohen, M. (2007). Quality of life for care-givers of people with Alzheimer's disease. *Journal of Advance Nursing, 5*, 222–231.

Wackerbarth, S. (1999). What decisions aremade by family care-givers? *American Journal of Alzheimers Disease, 14*(2), 111–119.

Wagnild, G., & Young, H. M. (1990). Resilience among older women. *IMAGE: Journal of Nursing Scholarship, 22*, 252–255.

Wells, R., Dywan, J., & Dumas, J. (2005). Life satisfaction and distress in family care-givers as related to specific behavioral changes after traumatic brain injury. *Brain Injury, 19*(3), 1105–1115.

Wickham-Searl, P. (1992). Mothers with a mission. In P. M. Ferguson, D. L. Ferguson, & S. J. Taylor (Eds.), *Interpreting disability.* New York, NY: Teachers College Press.

Williams, P. G., Wiebe, D. J., & Smith, T. W. (1992). Coping processes as mediators of the relationship between hardiness and health. *Journal of Behavioral Medicine, 15*, 237–255.

Wills, T. A., & Filer, M. (2000). Social networks and social support. In A. Baum & T. Revenson (Eds.), *Handbook of health psychology* (pp. 209–234). Mahwah, NJ: Erlbaum.

Woods, J. B., & Parham, I. A. (1990). Coping with perceived burden: Ethnic and cultural issues in Alzheimer's family care-giving. *Journal of Applied Gerontology, 9*, 325–339.

Wright, B. A. (1988). Attitudes and the fundamental negative bias: Conditions and corrections. In H. E. Yuker (Ed.), *Attitudes toward persons with disabilities* (pp. 3–21). New York, NY: Springer.

Wykle, M., & Segall, M. A comparison of black and white family care-givers experience with dementia. *Journal of the National Black Nurses Association, 5*, 29–41.

Yilmaz, O., Aki, E., Duger, T., Kayihan, H., & Karaduman, A. (2004). Susceptibility of mothers of children with muscular dystrophy to chronic back pain. *Journal of Back and Musculoskeletal Rehabilitation, 17*, 51–55.

Yuker, H. E. (1994). Variables that influence attitudes toward persons with disabilities: Conclusion from that data. *Psychosocial Perspectives on Disability: A Special Issue of the Journal of Social Behavior and Personality, 9*, 3–22.

Zarit, S., Todd, O., & Zarit, J. (1986). Subjective burden of husbands and wives as care-givers: A longitudinal study. *Gerontologist, 26*, 260–266.

Zirpoli, T. J., Snell, M. E., & Loyd, B. H. (2001). Characteristics of persons with mental retardation who have abused by care-givers. *The Journal of Special Education, 21*(2), 37–40.

INSIDER PERSPECTIVE

The Story of Verne Sanford

I would like to begin with brief descriptions of my "disability," education, career, wife and family, and retirement activities. Then, in a chronological manner, discuss how I lived and coped with my physical problems. Finally, I'll presume to give a few recommendations to rehabilitation counselors.

I've been legally blind for approximately 60 years, due to macular degeneration in both eyes. My present ophthalmologist attributes my loss of central vision to an eye infection, possibly linked to a childhood disease. Furthermore, my left eye has had glaucoma and surgeries for detached retina and cataract, and is of little use to me.

My formal education includes two degrees in the field of mathematics from the University of North Dakota: Bachelor of Philosophy and Master of Science. Also, I hold two degrees from the University of Michigan: Master of Public Health and Doctor of Philosophy, both in biostatistics. During my years of study, various vocational rehabilitation services provided books and supplies, a human reader, and eyeglasses with strong magnification.

For 27 years, I taught college mathematics at Valparaiso University, Valparaiso, IN, retiring in 1993. Here again, vocational rehabilitation assisted with specialized lighting, closed-circuit television enlarger, white cane, sunglasses, talking calculator, and computer monitor, and so on.

Marie and I have been together since our marriage in 1958. We have two sons, three daughters, and 12 grandchildren. For many years Marie augmented the family income by working part-time as a registered nurse. Also, for 11 summers our family operated a camp store in a nearby state park.

Retirement time has literally been overflowing with a wide variety of activities. Woodworking is a favorite hobby. I make children's toys (wooden cars, trucks, puzzles, games, toy boxes, small beds, bookcases, tables, step stools, etc.). One day each week I make hospital calls for my church. I have dabbled in writing most of my life. Now I write poems and short stories with determined attempts to publish. So far I have published one poem and one short story. Needless to say, I have a plump file of rejection letters! Did I mention our 12 grandchildren? Much retirement time is gladly spent enjoying them. We travel now and then, usually by train. Elderhostels have proven to be both educational and a lot of fun. Retirement has been a busy and happy time. But then, so were my career years. In general, my life has been pleasant, prosperous, and gratifying. I work hard at making everyday a good day.

Now then, this story actually begins with my birth on September 4, 1935, in Waukegan, IL. It was the middle of the Great Depression, and that fact certainly affected the way we lived our daily lives. My father always had work, so we never went to bed hungry. I do remember what seemed like an endless diet of oatmeal; somehow I still like it to this day!

I was a middle child with two sisters, one older and one younger. In Waukegan, my father installed large appliances for the local gas company. Later, in North Dakota, he was a brakeman and conductor for the Great Northern Railway. My mother was a housewife. As my story continues, it will become apparent just how important it was that Mom was always at home.

My mother noticed nothing wrong with my eyes when I was an infant. Later the problem became obvious. The earliest recollection I have of my poor vision is one traumatic day in the second grade. I wasn't able to read what the teacher had written on the blackboard, and so she made me leave my desk and stand close to the board. I was totally embarrassed, standing there squinting at the words, still unable to read them. From then on the teacher gave me large-print copies of blackboard assignments or read them to me. In an attempt to help, an eye doctor prescribed magnifying eyeglasses that were, in my opinion, quite useless. The low magnification they provided was not nearly enough for me to read print or see the blackboard. I was ashamed to wear glasses and wore them only when forced to do so. In those days no one called my eye condition macular degeneration, nor did they suggest coping strategies.

Of necessity, I became a good listener at a very early age, an attribute that has served me well throughout my life, especially in my teaching career. I found grade school to be easy because teachers usually spoke what they were writing on the board. My mother, God bless her, with only an eighth-grade education, read my assignments to me, and I listened. Did I ever listen! High school was more difficult, with longer assignments and much more reading. Mom kept reading and I kept listening! I was able to graduate with my class; an exciting day for me.

My father told me over and over again to get a good education because many jobs would be closed to me. Dad had graduated from high school and attended a small community college for only 6 weeks before he had to withdraw and find a paying job. I took my father's advice and completed the academic degrees mentioned earlier. I never learned Braille because large print worked for me. Writing was never my problem. Instead, it was the persistent frustration of trying to read what was written. At first I used grocers' grease pencils and crayons to write letters and words large enough to read. The invention of the felt marker was a dream-come-true. Suddenly I could write clearly *and* read my own writing!

Most of the time, coping with my legal blindness on a daily basis seemed rather natural. I've been able to do just about everything I've wanted to do, but everyday was and still is a challenging process of adaptations. I was forever inventing special ways to do what might have been routine for someone with normal vision. For many activities my fingers see as well as my eyes, and my hearing is acute. I touch the heads of screws to locate their slots or the Velcro covers on the f-key and j-key in order to properly position my fingers on the keyboard. Walking lightly in stocking feet helps find dropped objects. I often orient myself by counting stairs, rows of chairs, houses along city streets, and so on. Watching and listening to moving traffic reveals the color of a traffic signal. From early on I listened to radio broadcasts. To this day, I often carry a battery-operated radio. In lieu of reading newspapers or magazines, I listen intently to radio and television. For years I rode a bicycle on familiar streets, and I now use a computer with accessible software (scanner/reader and synthesized-speech screen reader) and a closed-circuit television enlarger. Recognizing people is difficult, but their voices, sizes, shapes, and the way they move all provide good clues. I do wish I could train all people to identify themselves as they approach me.

I rarely have a bad day, but I can think of two things that continue to sadden me. The fact that people "have no faces," and not being able to read books to my grand-children. Somehow a positive attitude and lots of good humor have helped me through everyday. I recall the time I reached down and picked up our dog's white tail, thinking it was a piece of paper. As one might have expected, the poor dog flew out from under the chair like a rocket being launched! Humor I learned from my mother. She came from independent, homesteading German parents, whose days were filled with hard work and practical jokes. From my father I learned assertiveness, without which I could never have come this far. I suppose it was I who taught myself adaptation. These three, "humor," "assertiveness," and "adaptation," have made me independent and successful. I have always worked hard and had a lot of fun while doing it. Such a lifestyle just can't be beat. I must add that I have received unlimited positive support from my family, friends, and colleagues. Everyday I needed and received assistance from someone. Thank goodness my assertiveness made me bold enough to ask for that help. I sometimes wonder where I would be if no one had read to me or if my college classmates had been unwilling to share carbon copies of their class notes. And, I may have faltered in my teaching if my students hadn't helped me find those equations I'd "lost" on the blackboard. Then there's my wife, Marie. She's also of German descent and strongly independent, but willing to help me whenever needed. On the other hand, her independence has probably made *me* much more independent, also.

Of course I cannot drive a car, but I surely would like to do so. Modern automobiles are really cool! What I truly desire is to own a pickup truck. Now and then it does frustrate me that I can't drive, but only now and then. Driving must produce a strong feeling of independence and I could always use a little more of that.

Allow me a moment to discuss how a person with macular degeneration is able to use only peripheral vision to walk and run and ride a bicycle, and see so many objects. Hopefully, this information will help a counselor understand how it is possible for a person to see without central vision. Macular degeneration (MD) limits or com-pletely obliterates acute detailed vision by "degenerating" or destroying the macula (a 5% center portion of the retina) in one or both eyes. MD seldom affects periph-eral vision (vision from the remaining 95% of the retina). Peripheral vision does not see fine detail, but it is good vision that is extremely useful in everyday-life activities.

In order to use peripheral vision effectively, it is necessary to drastically change the way the eye "looks" at things. The MD eye sees a blind spot (sees nothing at all) when the eye looks directly at an object. Therefore, in order to see an object clearly, but with much less detail than with a normal eye, the MD eye must look to one side or above or below the object. At the same time the brain must concentrate on the object, not on the blind spot. This process of seeing by looking elsewhere may seem, at first, very clumsy for anyone who has had normal vision, but it can be done, and with great success.

When walking or shopping or moving about at home, the "seeing" trick is to keep the eyes moving continuously, so as to avoid letting the blind spot block out any one object. By training the eyes and the brain to "look" at one thing and "see" another, peripheral vision can help greatly to overcome MD.

Before I close this chapter, I would like to suggest some things rehabilitation counselors might do to better serve disabled persons. A disabled person is a complete person, with ambitions, feelings, abilities, talents, etc., but who may have difficulty walking, seeing small objects, or using accepted table manners. Although I wish no disability on anyone, it may enhance a counselor's perspective to "walk" in the shoes of disabled persons. That is, counselors or trainees should spend time in a wheelchair with legs bound together, or don a blindfold and operate a computer with nothing but keystrokes, no mouse, no point, no click. I believe that counselors are fine, dedicated individuals, but counselors with clear understandings of disabilities are even better. Disabled persons have specialized lifestyles, whether or not their disabilities are chronic. Counselors could gain firsthand knowledge by temporarily adopting these same lifestyles.

Counselors must not be good listeners, they must be *great* listeners! They must never assume remedies for the disabled without first listening carefully to their needs and paying even closer attention to their feelings. Only then should they suggest appropriate assistance. Each person, especially each disabled person, has a unique way of solving life's daily problems. I can't emphasize this enough—assistance *must* be based on daily struggles of each disabled person, not on what "seems appropriate" to a counselor or on what some textbook might mandate.

One more comment seems appropriate. In my experience, there are few things slower than rehabilitation offices. In all fairness, their caseloads are surely heavy and their time severely limited. Since it is inevitable that there will be lengthy time delays, it would be thoughtful and very helpful to the disabled if someone would occasionally contact them with a progress report. Waiting with no information is frustrating.

Finally, I consider rehabilitation counseling to be one of the noblest of professions, and I am proud of anyone who accepts such a demanding challenge. We who receive your help are grateful; please know that you are appreciated.

DISCUSSION QUESTIONS

1. Discuss what would be the perceived costs and benefits of being a primary caregiver to a loved one with a disability.
2. How is caregiving performing ADLs the same and different for an older person with a disability as opposed to a newborn child for his or her first 2 years of life?

3. How true is the concept that it is not the actual act of caregiving itself that many caregivers find burdensome and stressful, but rather their perception of caregiving as being stressful?
4. How difficult and under what circumstances would it take to place a loved one into a nursing home?

EXERCISES

A. As a class assignment, have students set up appointments to go visit, tour, and interview the director to learn more about an assisted living residence, a nursing home, and a residential care home. Write and turn in a three-page report for grade.
B. Seek out and interview a primary caregiver of a child or adult with a disability, asking what they do for their loved one on a typical day, and what the caregiver perceives to be the costs and rewards of caregiving?

ELEVEN

Thriving Versus Succumbing to Disability: Psychosocial Factors and Positive Psychology

Irmo Marini

OVERVIEW

Perhaps the most crucial and significant question rehabilitation researchers have sought to answer since the past several decades is: *How is it that some persons with disabilities appear to excel and succeed in life beyond all expectations, whereas others seemingly succumb or yield to the limits imposed by their disabilities and society?* This chapter explores the multiple factors that contribute to this dichotomy. It is an extension beyond what is discussed in Chapter 5 regarding the various theories of adjustment to disability, and focuses on disability from a salutogenic orientation (focusing on the traits of healthy and successful persons) as opposed to the traditional pathological approach (focusing on the reasons and treatment of those beleaguered with ongoing mental and physical health problems) (Antonovsky, 1987). In the January 2000 issue of *American Psychologist*, Seligman and Csikszentmihalyi (2000) called for a new era of concentrated empirical study devoted to positive psychology, noting that the vast majority of past research was pathological in nature. By focusing study toward a salutogenic orientation, researchers are encouraged to explore factors related to wellness and what makes and keeps us happy, healthy, and satisfied in life. This orientation considers such factors as quality of life, resiliency, hope, optimism, spirituality, subjective well-being, hardiness, flow, self-efficacy, motivation, self-determination, and posttraumatic growth. As such, we explore not only the literature behind positive psychology but also the environmental and social barriers that obstruct wellness, as well as the U.S. demographic statistics surrounding substance abuse, depression, and suicide. Although wellness and positive psychology requires much from the individual in terms of attitude and perseverance, this alone cannot lead to transcendence from one's disability or posttraumatic growth without an amenable environment.

A SYNOPSIS OF SOCIETAL EXPECTATIONS TOWARD DISABILITY

This topic was thoroughly covered in earlier chapters; however, a brief overview of generalized societal attitudes and expectations toward those with disabilities provides a reminder of some of the stereotypical perceptions about this population. Historically, many persons with disabilities were persecuted and shunned in various regions across the globe predating the fourth century for economic reasons or a punishment by God (Gallagher, 1995; Sigerist, 1951). Leading up to the 20th century, persons with disabilities were warehoused in asylums away from the public, tortured, killed in the name of humanity, and sometimes burned for being witches (Chubon, 1994; Deutsch, 1949; Kramer & Sprenger, 1971). Charles Darwin and his followers in the late 1800s pursued the concept of natural selection and survival of the fittest, espousing that the weaker of the species should not be allowed to propagate their kind lest we dilute and eventually cause extinction of the human race. This led the United States, beginning in 1907, to sterilize some individuals diagnosed with mental illness, mental retardation, and epilepsy. This practice continued in Germany in the 1930s, culminating in the eventual T4 murder program of over an estimated 300,000 Germans with disabilities from 1939 to 1941 (Gallagher, 1995).

In the United States, the latter half of the 20th century and the 21st century has seen much more humane treatment of persons with disabilities. Sentiment seemingly began to change after the World Wars, with returning veterans with disabilities who had served their country. The federal government stepped in with legislation to assist disabled veterans, and eventually U.S. citizens with disabilities, in pursuing employment, education, and independence (Rubin & Roessler, 2008). Many Americans polled feel either pity or admiration for persons with certain disabilities, much of it fueled by sensationalized media coverage of charity telethons and superhuman stories of people with disabilities excelling in their lives (Lou Harris & Associates, 1991). Attitude research also suggests, however, that persons with disabilities are often viewed as sick, helpless, and incapable (DeJong, 1979a; English, 1971). This perception has likely contributed to the high unemployment rate of persons with disabilities. Franklin Delano Roosevelt tried to hide from all media the fact that he had polio, so as to not be perceived as weak or incapable of leading (Gallagher, 1994; Honey, Meager, & Williams, 1998). Even many parents are wooed into the belief that their disabled child will never be able to work. Statistics show an over 70% unemployment rate among persons with disabilities, underemployment for many who do work, and the highest poverty rates among any other group, especially for minority women with disabilities (Szymanski, Ryan, Merz, Trevino, & Johnston-Rodriguez, 1996).

It is important to note that these are not exclusive attitudes expressed by all non-disabled Americans, and that many Americans possess positive attitudes or at least ambivalent attitudes (Makas, 1988). Societal attitudes and expectations toward persons with disabilities are important since person-environment interactions appear to influence one's ability to adjust or adapt to disability (DiTomasso & Spinner, 1997; Li & Moore, 1998; Olkin, 1999; Trieschmann, 1988; Vash & Crewe, 2004; Wright, 1983).

With this in mind, we next explore some of the statistical realities facing people with disabilities from the traditional pathological side of study.

CORRELATES OF SUCCUMBING TO DISABILITY

There are hundreds of different types of diagnosable disabilities, many of which are vastly different physiologically and with regard to functional abilities. We often lump persons with disabilities into one homogeneous category for simplicity of discussion; however, their overall functional differences are often great. The groupings are sometimes broken down into physical disabilities (e.g., spinal cord injury, muscular dystrophy, arthritis), sensory disabilities (vision and hearing loss), cognitive disabilities (e.g., traumatic brain injury, mental retardation), and emotional disabilities (e.g., psychiatric conditions such as schizophrenia, bipolar disorder, anxiety, and personality disorders). However, there are also often vast differences within these groups. For example, despite the fact that persons with spinal cord injuries and muscular dystrophy most often use wheelchairs, persons with SCI typically sustain those injuries later in life, whereas persons with MD are born with their condition. Similarly, being blind versus being deaf, share few, if any, similarities. As such, in exploring the demographic statistics and incidence of substance abuse, depression, and suicide in relation to race and ethnic differences, these differences become more apparent.

Substance Use Disorder

Heinemann (1993) cites substance use in approximately 68% of traumatic disabling injuries, noting it to be a sign of poor psychosocial adjustment for some persons with physical disabilities. Similarly, the incidence of comorbid alcohol dependence and depression is approximately 50%, and anxiety disorders concomitant with drug dependency is approximately 43% (Grant et al., 2004). For those with schizophrenia, comorbid occurrences of substance use disorders (SUDs) across various studies of individuals in treatment settings range from 20% to 65%, essentially six times more than the general population (Bennett, 2009; Kessler et al., 1994; Mueser, Bennett, & Kushner, 1995). Bennett and Gjonbalaj (2007) describe the serious consequences in functioning for persons with dual diagnoses of schizophrenia and SUD, including poorer compliance with treatment, poorer outcomes, greater risk of violence and homelessness, poor life functioning, and greater risk of physical illness. Women are more likely than men to experience mental illness and SUD later in life, but tend to experience more severe problems over a briefer period of time (Daughters, Bornovalova, Correia, & Lejuez, 2007).

Substance use disorder is also common for persons with traumatic brain injuries (TBI). Graham and Cardon (2008) outline the fact that the dual diagnosis of TBI and SUDs predicts increased disability, delayed recovery, and poorer prognosis. With an estimated 1.5–2 million new cases of TBI a year, approximately 85% of which are diagnosed as mild cases, Walker, Cole, and Logan (2007) note how the symptoms of TBI (e.g., depression, cognitive deficits, irritability, headaches, fatigue) lead many individuals to seek drugs that provide them with an emotionally numbing experience.

Again, as with other disabilities, the incidence of moderate-to-heavy alcohol use disorder and TBI is estimated to be approximately 66% (Kreutzer et al., 1991). Two larger studies found similar high rates of dual diagnosis of moderate to heavy drinking and TBI among individuals 81% of whom had a previous arrest history and 47% of whom did not (Kreutzer, Marwitz, & Witol, 1995; Kreutzer, Witol, & Marwitz, 1996). In their review of 346 mental-health retrospective screenings of returning Iraqi and Afghanistan veterans, Graham and Cardon (2008) found the incidence of posttraumatic stress disorder and TBI carried past and current alcohol use ranging between 65.9% and 53.7%, respectively. Of these individuals, over 75% were also diagnosed with a depressive disorder and 22% with a panic disorder.

Substance use disorder is not limited to comorbidity of disability and SUD. Specifically, SUD involving two or more types of substances is prevalent as well. Stinson et al. (2005) found 12-month prevalence rates of over 55% for individuals with an alcohol disorder and drug use disorder. Clinical sample studies further suggest that the comorbid incidence of cocaine dependence and alcohol use disorder ranges from 62% to 68% (Carroll, Rounsaville, & Bryant, 1993; Tsuang, Shapiro, Smith, & Schuckit, 1994). Rounsaville, Petry, and Carroll (2003) have advocated for moving away from research involving a single drug, and instead assessing individuals for a wide range of drug use with the intent of determining a principal substance of abuse, and working to treat this problem for effectiveness. Griffin, Kolodziej, and Weiss (2009) have outlined problems with this approach, primarily with the fact that there is no empirically supported research as to how best to identify what the principal substance of abuse may be.

Li and Moore (2001) have identified some contributing factors and explanations regarding why there may be such a high incidence of disability and SUD. The authors define the concept of *secondary deviance* from Labeling Theory as a potential explanation for the phenomenon. Specifically, persons with various disabilities (the primary deviance regarding labeling stigma) (Goffman, 1963) are already societally stigmatized, and therefore may develop an entitlement attitude toward substance use and abuse. The authors suggest that perceived discrimination is associated with the acceptance of disability, and those who perceive themselves discriminated against may turn to illicit drug use (secondary deviance) as a form of escapism or to become emotionally numb as described earlier (Walker et al., 2007). Li and Moore (2001) indicate that many persons with disabilities buy into societal value systems of beauty and health as being desirable, and can succumb to the notion that they are not "normal." For those who do, they may use substances as a defense mechanism (Lemert, 1967). Scheff (1966) suggests that stigma and discrimination may cause individuals to feel damaged, which, in turn, can lead them on a continued secondary deviance path of illicit drug behavior. In Li and Moore's (2001) Medication and Other Drug Use Survey of 1,876 individuals with various disabilities, 304 responded to having used illicit drugs following their injuries. Their findings suggest that reactions to social discrimination and self-acceptance of disability were indirectly related with whether these individuals engaged in using illicit drugs. In addition, individuals of low socioeconomic status and education were more likely to perceive social discrimination and more likely to have favorable attitudes toward entitlement to use substances.

Depression

Depression for persons with and without disabilities is one of the most insidious and commonly recognized disabling conditions in America today. The National Institute of Mental Health (NIMH) indicates that approximately 21 million Americans or 9.5% of the population is affected by a depressive disorder each year (Kessler, Chiu, Demler, & Walters, 2005a). Major depressive disorder is the leading cause of disability for ages 15–44 and is more prevalent in women than men, with a median onset of age 32 (Kessler et al., 2005a; Kessler, Berglund, Demler, & Walters, 2005b). Depression is also the second most common cause of lost work productivity, costing an estimated $31 billion per year.

When depression is not the sole, primary disabling condition, but rather secondary in relation to a co-occurring chronic illness or disability, the prevalence rates are higher. Cuijpers, de Graff, and van Dorsselaer (2004) found in their Dutch study of 7,076 persons interviewed at 1- and 3-year time intervals for minor depression that 8% of those with a functional disability reported more pronounced symptoms of major depression after 2 years. Turner and McLean (1989) reported that persons with physical disabilities were 3–4 times more likely to be diagnosed with depression than the general population. In relation to this, Wilz (2007) found that of 104 persons who sustained a stroke, those perceiving themselves as more impaired functionally reported greater depression, consistent with previous studies indicating about a 24% incidence at 3 months postinjury (Burvill et al., 1995; Turner-Stokes & Hassan, 2002). Wilz (2007) found a diagnosed depression for those who had a stroke correlated with a decrease in socializing and greater isolation. He noted that even though depression had lessened for many at 12 months postinjury, it continued to be a long-term problem for those who remained more functionally impaired and had fewer opportunities for socialization.

Chronic pain, most commonly low-back pain, is statistically the most common and prevalent type of disabling pain condition, costing an estimated $125 billion annually for treatment and lost productivity in the United States (Aronoff, 2003). Persons with chronic pain report co-occurring depression rates of 30% to 54% (Banks & Kerns, 1996). An increasing incidence of depression and anxiety with persistent or chronic low-back pain is well documented, with poorer recovery rates for those with a co-occurring psychiatric condition (Bener et al., 2006; Louch, 2009; Von Korff & Simon, 1996). Dickens (2001) notes, however, that not everyone with pain reports symptoms of depression.

It is important to reiterate that not all individuals who sustain a disability become clinically depressed (Dickens, 2001; Olkin, 1999; Silver, 1982). As with Wilz's (2007) findings, many persons with disabilities adapt to their situations over time. Silver (1982) found that his participants with spinal cord injuries reportedly returned to a preinjury emotional baseline adaptation level somewhere around 2 months postinjury. Koch, Uyttenboogaart, Harten, Heerings, and Keyser (2008) similarly found in their 10-year longitudinal study of persons with multiple sclerosis that roughly the same 38% of patients who reported fatigue and depression at the initial onset persisted with these symptoms at the 10-year follow-up. However, those who did not report fatigue or depression at the onset continued to report no symptoms even 10 years later.

Overall, it appears that the incidence of depression as a reaction to a chronic illness or disability is higher for persons with various disabilities compared with the general population. It also appears evident that in many instances, depressive symptoms subside over time as individuals adapt to their situations. Depending on the disability and individual personal attributes, some persons will become depressed and may remain so years later. Others, however, may not become depressed following their disabilities, or develop depressive symptoms later in life. For the percentage of persons who do become depressed, counselors must pay close attention to those who express suicidal thoughts.

Suicide

Concomitantly linked to depression is the incidence of suicide. In 2006, approximately 33,300 persons died by suicide in the United States (Centers for Disease Control and Prevention [CDC], 2010). Of this group, more than 90% had a diagnosable mental disorder, most commonly a depressive disorder and/or SUD (Conwell & Brent, 1995). Although the highest suicide rates are among White males over age 85, women attempt suicide 2–3 times more often than men, but males are four times more likely to die by suicide (Kochanek, Murphy, Anderson, & Scott, 2004). Adolescence between ages 15 and 24 has seen the greatest increase in suicide over the past decade (CDC, 2010). Depression and subsequent suicide frequently co-occurs with some other medical illness, such as heart disease, cancer, and chronic pain, as well as overall poor health conditions (Lee, Chan, Chronister, Chan, & Romero, 2009).

Epidemiologically, suicide rates are highest among Caucasians, with males aged 64 and older leading the way, 10 times higher than that of Black females. These rates are particularly high among Caucasians whose country of origin is Hungary, Austria, Germany, Lithuania, or one of the Scandinavian countries. Suicide rates are higher for lower socioeconomic groups except when divorce is considered. Those who are socially isolated, such as the divorced, widowers, and those living alone or with a few family or social supports, commit suicide more often. When considering a disabling condition, major depression combined with substance abuse is one of the strongest predictors of suicide at 7–10 times that of the general population (Maris, Berman & Silverman, 2000). Lester (2000) notes that as many as 18% of alcoholics eventually commit suicide, and that evidence of alcohol or drug consumption is often found at the scene.

After considering major depression and substance abuse, statistics regarding suicide in relation to other disabilities is complex and generally contingent on other factors (Goldblatt, 2000). Goldblatt notes that persons undergoing kidney dialysis are 14.5% more likely to commit suicide, persons with malignant neoplasms of the head or neck 11.4% more likely, and persons with HIV/AIDS 6.6% more likely. DeVivo and Stover (1995) found that persons with spinal cord injuries were 4.8 times more likely to commit suicide than the general population. Goldblatt's (2000) extensive literature review of physical illness and suicide further suggests that persons with multiple sclerosis, cancer, epilepsy, lupus, and Huntington's disease are at increased risk for suicide or suicidal behavior.

Again, it is important to note overall, and Goldblatt (2000) affirms this, that most persons with acute or chronic disabilities *do not* commit or even attempt suicide simply because they have a disability. In relation to this, not everyone who has a disability becomes depressed. In both instances, there are always other complex factors, such as comorbid conditions, including preexisting psychopathology, personality traits, ethnicity, age, ability to manage stress, social support, and other considerations that must be factored on a case-by-case basis. Rehabilitation researchers have been exploring pathology and its treatment for decades, but many contemporary researchers have begun to focus their sights on individuals who thrive despite adversity with the exploration of positive psychology and posttraumatic growth.

INDIVIDUAL TRAITS RELATED TO THRIVING WITH A DISABILITY

Until this point in the chapter, we have been exploring what social scientists and researchers have been discussing for decades: the pathological exploration, assessment, and potential treatment for mental illness and other chronic illness and disabilities. The remainder of this chapter takes a 180-degree turn away from studying pathology, and is instead devoted to the salutogenic exploration of factors related to health and wellness (Marini & Chacon, 2007; Seligman & Csikszentmihalyi, 2000). Specifically, what factors, conditions, and personal traits make up those individuals who, despite having a disability, are otherwise mentally and physically healthy, successful in their careers and socially, and report a high quality of life and life satisfaction? And just as we have noted that not all persons with disabilities become depressed, abuse substances, or commit suicide, likewise, not all persons with a chronic illness or disability are able to excel, transcend, and thrive following adversity.

Positive Psychology

The empirical support for positive psychology continues to grow over the past decade (Peterson & Park, 2009). Strength-based or asset-focused rehabilitation according to Wright (1983) must consider how environmental or external conditions may be facilitating a handicap, the personal assets and traits persons with disabilities possess to affectively deal with adversity, and how such individuals perceive themselves in relation to how they perceive others view them. Wright's coping versus succumbing framework of adjusting to disability explores these value-laden beliefs, noting that persons who have experienced a traumatic disability will likely initially mourn their losses before they begin the road to recovery (Wright, 1983, p. 194). But, positive psychology goes beyond simply adjusting, adapting, or responding to a disability as discussed in Chapter 5, and explores those personal strengths, virtues, and environmental conditions that enable the well-being experienced by persons with and without disabilities to excel and optimally perform exceptionally in life across all domains.

Seligman and Csikszentmihalyi (2000) noted that a major premise of positive psychology is to understand what makes life worth living, how to flourish, and be well both mentally and physically, and in addition, what makes us not only care for ourselves but also care for others in the larger community as well. The authors believe that humans have within them the desire to do well and improve themselves, consistent with humanistic theorists such as Abraham Maslow and Carl Rogers regarding striving for self-actualization. Seligman and Csikszentmihalyi describe three levels of analysis for positive psychology: the subjective level, the individual level, and the group level. The subjective level includes understanding an individual's subjective experiences, such as perceived happiness, subjective well-being, self-determination, hope, optimism, flow, and satisfaction. The individual level includes traits such as perseverance, resilience, spirituality, forgiveness, interpersonal skills, future-mindedness, capacity to love, bravery, and hardiness. Finally, the group level involves outward focused caring, including civic virtues, altruism, work ethic, citizenship, responsibility, and essentially giving back to the community (Marini & Chacon, 2007; Peterson & Park, 2009; Seligman & Csikszentmihalyi, 2000). We next briefly describe some of these common factors that continue to build empirical support.

Subjective-level indicators

Happiness: Perhaps one of the most fascinating research areas over the past decade relates to what makes us happy (Ben-Shahar, 2007; Diener, Lucas, & Scollon, 2006; Diener & Seligman, 2002; Lucas, 2007; Marinic & Brkljacic, 2008; Myers, 2000; Ryan & Deci, 2000, 2001; Seligman, 2002). Quite literally, the pursuit of happiness is so popular that Ben-Shahar, a Harvard psychologist, indicates that it is the most popular and sought-after course on campus. There are several theories of happiness: *hedonic happiness* (Ryan & Deci, 2001; Lucas, 2007), *eudiamonic happiness* (Ryan & Deci, 2000), and *authentic happiness* (Seligman, 2002). Hedonic happiness occurs when we seek out and experience activities (e.g., purchasing material goods, engaging in sex, socializing) that bring us pleasure and gratify us. Unfortunately, as Lucas (2007) and others have found, we generally adapt or return to a "set point" after a short period of time (Frederick & Loewenstein, 1999). They described this as the hedonic treadmill, whereby we continually pursue pleasure, shortly become accustomed or adapted to it, then seek out something new (e.g., buying new clothes or electronics). Marketing agencies seem to be particularly tuned in to this American mindset of bigger and better. Eudiamonic happiness has a different focus; not by pursuing pleasurable material things, activities, and so on, but rather engaging in self-development and self-growth, such as obtaining an advanced degree and, in essence, delaying immediate gratification for some longer-term sense of mastery. Finally, Seligman's (2002) book on *Authentic Happiness* combines both hedonic and eudiamonic happiness in search of a good and meaningful life that integrates hedonic and eudiamonic happiness. In essence, it is the balanced combination of temporary strings of fleeting happy moment pleasures, along with pursuing long-term delayed gratification goals that brings a sustained lasting happiness.

Empirical research supporting the concept of happiness is growing. Martin Seligman has, at the University of Pittsburgh, developed a Web site devoted to the topic, including self-assessment, literature, and Web lectures. Marinic and Brkjacic (2008) conducted a correlational study between happiness and life satisfaction between persons with and without a physical disability. Although both groups expressed positive levels of happiness and life satisfaction over many domains, those without disabilities scored higher overall. Specifically, less than 15% of persons with disabilities reported being extremely happy compared with 40% of the nondisabled group. The nondisabled group was significantly happier with their health, family, friends, feelings of physical safety, and community acceptance. Those with disabilities were significantly less satisfied with family, friend relationships, and community acceptance. The authors cite barriers and stigmatization as likely having a factor in their findings, and the resulting negative impact on personal adjustment has been documented elsewhere (DiTomasso & Spinner, 1997; Graf, Marini, & Blankenship, 2009; Li & Moore, 1998).

Other research on happiness suggests that individuals have happy personality traits when possessing traits such as extroversion, optimism, internal locus of control, and self-confidence (Diener & Lucas, 1999). Lykken's (1999) study of twins found that 50% of the variance was explained by momentary feelings of happiness attributed to genetics. He also found that 80%–98% of persons who were happy described returning to a "set point" of happiness similar to a body weight set point. Other variables dealing with a set point of happiness suggest that married persons are happier than unmarried ones (Myers, 2000), having close family and friendships contribute to feelings of happiness (Argyle, 2001; Diener & Seligman, 2002), and being employed, well educated, job satisfied, and feeling successful all correlate with happiness (Argyle, 2001; Diener & Lucas, 1999). For persons with disabilities, these latter objective quality-of-life factors (employment, job satisfaction, education) may not be attainable; however, such individuals still generally indicate a positive subjective quality of life due to appreciating family and friends more, a spirituality/religious connection, and greater appreciation of life in general (Bishop, 2005; Myers, 2000). Finally, once people report their basic needs having been met (e.g., food, shelter, safety), those who earn a modest income versus those who are excessively wealthy show very minute differences in reported increased happiness (Kaliterna-Lipovcan & Prismic-Larson, 2006; Seligman, 2002).

Subjective well-being: Subjective well-being (SWB) is described as a person's "cognitive and affective evaluations of his or her life" (Diener, Lucas, & Oishi, 2005, p. 53). Central to this concept is the fact that it pertains exclusively to an individual's subjective appraisal or perceptions regarding satisfaction in life, and not the events themselves, but rather our interpretation of those events (Diener, 2000; Diener et al., 2005). Diener (2000) describes three central components of SWB: adaptation, goals, and temperament. Adaptation refers to the hedonic treadmill concept discussed earlier where we are temporarily happy, habituate or get used to the new activity/person/event, and over time return to a relatively established emotional set point. Striving for realistic goals and obtaining them provides for longer-term happiness by building competence, self-efficacy, and self-esteem (Bandura, 1997; Diener, 2000). As Bandura (1997) noted with self-efficacy theory, however, if a desired goal is perceived as too much work, or the costs outweigh the gains, we will likely not be motivated to continue or pursue such goals. As Marini and Stebnicki (1999) found in working with Social Security beneficiaries, the costs of losing medical and wage replacement benefits outweighed the benefits of applying/obtaining a job. It comes as no surprise then that less than 1% of all Social Security beneficiaries ever return to gainful employment. Finally, temperament refers to traits associated with well-being, including tolerance for stress and emotional stability, trust in others, having a sense of humor, self-actualization, and hardiness or a strong sense of commitment and control.

Self- determination theory. This concept refers to human motivation and personality traits (Ryan & Deci, 2000). The authors describe three psychological needs related to self-determination theory (SDT): autonomy, competence, and relatedness. Autonomy refers to an individual's perceptions of mastery over their environment and the perception of being in control of situations. Achieving this has been found to be difficult for many persons with disabilities, as evidenced in study findings pertaining to environmental and societal barriers, including negative employer attitudes in hiring and lack of physical access to jobs and socialization experiences (Graf et al., 2009; Li & Moore, 1998; Marini, Bhakta, & Graf, 2009). Such environmental barriers, real or perceived, often block individuals' perception of mastery or control over their circumstances. Ryan and Deci (2000) describe cognitive evaluation theory (CET) as a subcomponent of SDT, noting how social and environmental factors may impede individuals' intrinsic motivation to accomplish their goals. The authors state that people are often driven by extrinsic punitive motivating factors, such as coercion, threats, deadlines, and other externally imposed goals. Competence refers to the sense of pride people feel from working hard to develop skills to perform some task(s) competently, and being recognized for those skills. This psychological need can often be met through athletics, work, or volunteer efforts (Harter, 1978). As such, persons with disabilities who are unable to work may still obtain feelings of competence through Special Olympics, volunteer activities, or other hobbies.

Hope. The construct of hope and Hope Theory (Snyder, 2000) assumes that human behavior is goal directed, and for persons with high hope who become successful in accomplishing their goals, they tend to experience greater and lasting happiness. Conversely, those with low hope tend to have problems overcoming barriers to goal attainment, and as a result experience more negative emotions (Lopez, Snyder, & Teramoto-Pedrotti, 2003). Snyder (1994) describes hope as a cognitive process whereby individuals set goals, develop strategies to achieve them (pathways thinking), and develop and sustain the motivation to accomplish one's goals (agency thinking). Snyder (2002) hypothesized that goals and their attainment bring about positive emotions, and that goal failure brings about negative emotions. Snyder and Lopez (2002) indicate that more attention needs to be devoted to overlapping constructs, such as hope and optimism. In addition, as Bandura (1997) describes with self-efficacy theory, we are only motivated to pursue goals we perceive are worth the effort and subsequent rewards. Snyder, Rand, and Sigmon (2002) indicate that goals, pathway thinking, and agency thinking all reciprocally influence each other and increase motivation whenever benchmarks are achieved. In considering persons with disabilities once again, environmental and societal barriers may block goal attainment to where the individual either gives up or devises strategies to circumvent any real or perceived barriers.

Snyder (2002) further asserted that hope involves an overlapping understanding of attitude formation, processes of change, potentially distorted or false cognitive thinking, spirituality and life meaning, and maintaining self-concept. As such, it can include learned helplessness (Seligman, 1998), internal versus external locus of control (Rotter, 1966), self-efficacy (Bandura, 1997), and self-defeating thoughts (Seligman, 1998). Regarding disability, a key counseling trait is to empower clients and instill hope in what may be perceived as a hopeless or helpless situation. Learned helplessness and hopelessness generally result when individuals perceive that their situations are uncontrollable, thus succumbing or giving up their dreams (Peterson, Maier, & Seligman, 1995). Depression and pessimism can result, but some individuals become even more resilient and work to disprove self or others' low expectations (Dyer & McGuinness, 1996). Several studies involving persons with the unpredictable progression of multiple sclerosis scored higher on levels of helplessness, depression, and low self-efficacy than did persons with a severe, but stable, prognosis of spinal cord injury (Shnek, Foley, LaRocca, Smith, & Halper, 1995; Shnek et al., 1997).

Research findings point to persons with hope having an internal locus of control, higher self-efficacy, optimism, good coping skills, and the spiritual belief that they will be okay (Moore & Stambrook, 1995; Puchalski, 1999; Shnek et al., 1997; Stanton, Danoff-Burg, & Huggins, 2002). Stotland (1969) noted that hope and anxiety can be influenced by the attitudes of others, thus stressing the need to instill hope in others. This concept has previously been confirmed in the perceptions of those with disabilities when experiencing perceived discrimination and the resulting negative impact (DiTomasso & Spinner, 1997; Graf et al., 2009; Li & Moore, 1998). Finally, Rosenbaum and Rosenbaum (1999) indicate that for persons who have sustained a trauma or loss, developing a positive attitude and conveying to others the ability to successfully adapt, there is a reciprocal effect on how others react (Snyder, 1998).

Optimism: Closely related to hope is the concept of optimism (Snyder & Lopez, 2002; Seligman, 1998). Peterson (2000) indicated that optimism is correlated with effective problem solving, occupational and academic success, positive affect, better health, and lower mortality, whereas pessimism is correlated with depression, anxiety, perceived failure, poorer health, and higher mortality. Seligman (1998) describes findings suggesting that optimists who tend to attribute success to internal qualities, however, attribute failure to external causes or influences. Pessimists on the other hand attribute failure internally as a perceived personal flaw, and attribute success to luck or some external cause. Seligman believes that optimism can be learned just as becoming a pessimist can be unlearned.

Taylor and Brown (1988) conclude that humans have three positive illusions. The first is that we have the ability to improve ourselves or self-enhance. Second is unrealistic optimism, the belief that we are generally invincible health-wise and that our lives will be gratifying. Finally, we often have an exaggerated perception of personal control over circumstances. Positive and overly optimistic beliefs of health recovery have been associated with a stronger immune system and quicker recovery times for persons with cancer, bypass surgery, and other illnesses (Stone, Cox, Valdimarsdottir, Jandorf, & Neale, 1987; Taylor, 1983). Oettingen (1996), however, observes that unrealistic or naïve optimism may have deleterious effects on health if we ignore disease onset symptoms in the belief that we are invincible. Although this is a logical assertion, Lazarus (1983) acknowledged that positive denial may be an asset for a stronger immune system when individuals do not become stressed.

Flow: Csikszentmihalyi (1975, 1978, 1999) describes the concept of *flow* as an experience of optimal involvement in an activity we find challenging but sufficiently matching one's skills, involving deep concentration performing the activity, and is of great intrinsic interest to the individual. Although Csikszentmihalyi asserts that individuals involved in flow experiences do not necessarily derive a sense of happiness from being in the moment during the optimal experience, they do ultimately enjoy longer-term fulfillment, competence, and satisfaction from having mastered their art or skill. Csikszentmihalyi describes the opposite of flow as being that of entropy, being unchallenged and bored when we are involved in repetitive or underwhelming experiences, such as watching television. Optimal growth experiences are individually defined but can include one's job, sports, reading, and social interactions (Csikszentmihalyi, 1999).

Research suggests that persons with disabilities can experience flow. Delle Fave (1996) and Delle Fave and Maletto (1992) found that persons who were blind or sustained a spinal cord injury experienced transformational flow, whereby they were able to engage in previous or new optimal experiences that they found to be challenging and satisfying. For the majority of individuals with chronic illness and disability, who do not or are unable to work, flow may be derived from involvement in volunteering, sports, hobbies, and social relationships (Csikszentmihalyi, 1999). Csikszentmihalyi additionally pointed out that what might be considered mundane for some, may be optimal experiences for others. For example, although some individuals may perceive golfing or hiking as boring activities, those persons who are intrinsically interested find these activities challenging and become competent performing them and derive deep satisfaction from these experiences.

Life satisfaction: The final subjective concept discussed is that of life satisfaction. Perceived life dissatisfaction and quality of life (QOL) are viewed as highly correlating concepts (Bishop, 2005a; Dijkers, 1997; Huebner, 2004), and Dijkers distinguishes between objective and subjective quality of life. Persons with disabilities often report a lower objective quality of life described earlier concerning functional limitations and poor vocational opportunities, but generally report relatively high subjective QOL and life satisfaction when considering material status (Huebner, 2004; Marinic & Brkljacic, 2008; Seligman, 2002). Hope and optimism have also been found to contribute to adolescent life satisfaction, as has locus of control (Ash & Huebner, 2001; Edwards, 2004; Huebner, 1991).

Individual-level indicators

Resilience: Resilience theory relates to an individual's ability to positively adapt in response to some significant trauma or adversity (Dyer & McGuinness, 1996). Resilient people are those who not only simply adapt to their situations but also thrive from the experience and adjust much better than expected (Dykens, 2005; Luthar, Cicchetti, & Becker, 2000). Kumpfer (1999) notes that resilience is multifaceted, resulting from factors related to the individual, his or her unique situation, and interaction with the environment. Individual factors will, for example, include problem-solving skills, attitude, self-efficacy, and self-esteem (Thompson, 2002). Situational factors in considering disability might include type of injury and time of onset, functional limitations, and how the value of any functional losses is perceived by the individual. Environmental factors can either exacerbate or minimize the psychosocial impact of disability, and may include finances, family support, social networks, and available community resources (Arman, 2002; Grant, Ramcharan & Flynn, 2007; Kumpfer, 1999; Vash & Crewe, 2004; Walsh, 2003; Werner & Smith, 1982). Aldwin (1994) describes resilient coping mechanisms as a form of an "inoculation effect" whereby the individual effectively deals with adverse situations by expanding their coping repertoires, improved mastery of adverse situations, and subsequently increases self-confidence, sense of control, inner-strength, and self-esteem.

Wagnild and Young (1990) found that older women who had adjusted to a significant-other loss cited five qualities in relation to resilience, including a balanced perspective or outlook of life circumstances, self-belief, perseverance despite adversity, ability to make sense of life's purpose, and the acknowledgment that certain experiences must be faced alone. In Grant et al.'s (2007) literature review of factors related to family caregiving resilience, the authors found several consistent themes that included rationalizing normative conflicts, whereby family members' were able to move on regarding existential questions concerning "why" the disability happened, or why they had to raise a child with a disability. Cognitive coping concerned reframing the circumstances to lessen the impact of stress. The third theme was acknowledging the coexistence of caregiving as providing both rewards and stresses, but otherwise reinforcing the importance of the role. The embrace of paradox described conflicting personal goals versus the need to care for a disabled loved one. The fifth theme dealt with the concept of reciprocity, whereby even nonverbal loved ones were seen as contributing back in terms of love, communication, and gratitude. Other themes included perceiving a sense of control, contingency planning, and regulation of internal and external support.

Related, Knestrict, and Kuchey (2009) interviewed 20 pairs of parents regarding their caregiving for a child with a severe disability. They found that the more resilient families possessed a higher income. Resilient families also displayed the ability to reflect and reconfigure family responsibilities, and establish a rhythm described as establishing consistent rules, rituals, and routines regarding expectations. This sense of rhythm has previously been acknowledged by McCubbin and McCubbin (1988), and essentially addresses the temporal importance of becoming accustomed to one's situation and positively responding to the needed changes. As previously addressed in the chapter on adjustment to disability, once an individual and/or the family have dealt with the initial shock, anxiety, mourning, and chaos of the situation, a gradual transition and emotional stabilization often occurs along with subsequent cognitive reframing, sense of control, and enhanced problem-solving abilities (Kendall & Buys, 1998; Livneh, 1991).

Spirituality: The role of religion and spirituality in counseling has received considerable attention in the past 10 to 15 years (Graf, Marini, Baker, & Buck, 2007; Levin, 2001; Vash & Crewe, 2004). Its place in positive psychology and coping lies in the notion that individuals who believe in God or a spiritual power (G/SP) ultimately take comfort in the belief that some higher entity is looking out for them (Levin, 2001). Numerous correlational studies suggest that involvement in religious activities, such as praying, churchgoing, religious fellowship, and faith, statistically lead to lower rates of divorce, depression, suicide, substance abuse, risky behavior, loneliness, and mortality (Batson, Schoenrade, & Ventis, 1993; Levin, 2001; Seligman, 1988). Myers (2000) also states that persons who report being close to God are generally happier than nonbelievers.

There appears to be consistent evidence suggesting that belief in G/SP is indeed a positive coping mechanism for dealing with stress and maintaining mental health (Abraido-Lanza, Vasquez, & Echeverria, 2004; Graf et al., 2007; Johnstone, Glass, & Oliver, 2007; Marini & Glover-Graf, 2011; Matheis, Tulsky, & Matheis, 2006). Graf et al. (2007) found that persons with chronic pain relied on their faith to help them cope, gave them a purpose and meaning in life, and was a source of happiness for them. Similarly, Marini and Glover-Graf's (2011) survey of 157 persons with spinal cord injury found that 72% of participants believed that G/SP gave them a purpose in life, 62% expressed a closer connection to others as a result of their injuries, and 48% believed that their injuries was to serve a higher purpose. The theme of making meaning of adversity was also evident in a study of 79 veterans with spinal cord injuries (deRoon-Cassini, de St. Aubin, Valvano, Hastings, & Horn, 2009). The authors found that veterans who reported a higher level of psychological well-being perceived their functional losses to be less severe. In addition, positive well-being was significantly related to those who perceived that they lead meaningful and purposeful lives.

It also appears that families who believe in G/SP may benefit mental health-wise as a buffer against stress and effective coping mechanism. Jonker and Greeff (2009) interviewed 34 South African family members about caring for a member diagnosed with mental illness, and grouped the data in three categories involving internal resources within the home, external resources in the community, and factors related to treatment. Overall, religion and spirituality played the key role in family adaptation through their faith in God. Kloosterhouse and Ames (2002) similarly found that parents' spiritual beliefs helped them cope during times when their child was hospitalized, regardless of whether the parents had a religious affiliation. The presence of others, prayer, and acts of kindness have also been identified in reducing stress and psychological coping for Southern Baptist families (Stone, Cross, Purvis, & Young, 2004).

Spirituality or a religious affiliation, however, does not always correlate with positive well-being. A minority of people with disabilities perceive their impairments to be a punishment from God, report being angry with God, and/or are resentful for having their disability (Graf et al., 2007; Marini & Glover-Graf, 2011; Selway & Ashman, 1998). In addition, there is no empirical evidence so far to suggest that belief and practice of religion or spirituality can cure or otherwise have any direct impact on minimizing the physiology of a disability, despite anecdotal or sensationalized unexplained inferences of miracle recoveries (Park, 2007).

Hardiness: The concept of hardiness was originally developed by Kobasa (1979), and refers to a personality trait comprising three related tendencies: challenge, commitment, and control. Kobasa defined challenge as one's outlook on life in considering adversity or need for change more as an opportunity for growth as opposed to a threat or something to be feared. *Change* is perceived as a natural part of life, rather than being stable or content. *Commitment* refers to one's perceived value and belief in pursuing goals, and ultimately provides the individual with a sense of purpose and meaning. The term *control* pertains to a belief that we have control over our life events, within reason, and this sense of mastery over our environment provides a feeling of competence, confidence, and self-esteem. Conversely, those who do not have a hardy personality are described as fearful of making changes, lacking a sense of control or the confidence to do so, and ultimately bored and powerless to change their lives or situational circumstances (Kobasa, Maddi, & Kahn, 1982a).

Previous studies hypothesized that hardiness improves health by buffering against stress (Kobasa et al., 1982a; Rhodewalt & Zone, 1989); however, other researches suggest that hardiness may have a more direct effect on health by minimizing stress-related illnesses (Banks & Gannon, 1988; Kobasa & Puccetti, 1983; Kobasa, Maddi, Puccetti, & Zola, 1985; Pollock, 1986). Hardiness is viewed as an approach-oriented coping strategy, behaviors associated with better health, and problem-solving coping (Williams, Wiebe, & Smith, 1992). Again, the sense of meaning and purpose emanates with this theory, and in deRoon-Cassini et al.'s (2009) study of veterans with spinal cord injury, the authors describe global "meaning-making appraisals" as having clear aims in life, feeling as though life goals are being achieved, and sensing that daily activities are worthwhile (Park & Folkman, 1997). In addition, veterans reframed their perceived loss of physical ability as an opportunity to generate new meaning and purpose in life (Janoff-Bulman, 1992).

Group-level indicators

Civic virtue, altruism, and caring: These concepts overlap in definition and, therefore, are discussed together. All three represent an outward focus of the individual toward helping others, some in dire situations. Volunteering and charitable donations all interrelate with this category. The concept of downward comparison is well documented, whereby persons who view the plight of others as more debilitating than their own often derive a positive affect that their own circumstances are not worse (Klein, 1997; Wills, 1991). As discussed earlier, even though employment is viewed by many as an objective good quality-of-life (QOL) indicator, many persons with disabilities who are unable to work report high subjective QOL due to the satisfaction obtained from volunteer and other perceived helping activities (Bach & Tilton, 1994; Krause, Coker, Charlifue, & Whiteneck, 1999; Matheis et al., 2006). Altruism and volunteerism have been extensively studied, indicating that these traits are related to subjective well-being, empathy, self-efficacy, and a psychological sense of community (see Penner, 2004; Piliavin & Charng, 1990; Wilson, 2000).

Bruhin and Winkelmann (2009) examined altruism, subjective well-being, and happiness between parents and their adult children. The authors extracted annual German Socio-Economic Panel data from 2,577 surveyed parents in Germany and noted that the interdependent parental and children's life satisfaction, and children's subjective well-being through parental altruistic behavior toward them was significant for approximately 25% of the group. Seligman and Csikszentmihalyi (2000) cite one's capacity to love, civility, citizenship, and altruism as important variables for positive well-being.

POSTTRAUMATIC GROWTH

Posttraumatic growth (PG) is a relatively new concept, although Vash (1981) described a similar concept (transcendence) 30 years ago. Vash and Crewe (2004) noted that "before disability can be transcended, it must first be acknowledged at the three designated levels: recognition of the facts, acceptance of the implications, and embracing the experience" (Vash & Crewe, 2004, p. 154). Transcendence is described as rising above imposed physical limitations by escaping the physical body and exploring one's spiritual growth or higher level of consciousness. The authors offer anecdotal personal stories connoting transcendence, however, no empirical evidence. The concept of PG conceptualized by Tedeschi and Calhoun (1988, 1995, 1996) explores the ability for certain individuals with disabilities being able to eventually thrive, reporting the paradox that their disabilities brought both suffering and positive changes to their lives. Five main areas of positive change include a greater sense of personal strength, a greater overall appreciation of life, closer relationships with others, spiritual change, and new opportunities and possibilities (Tedeschi & Calhoun, 1996). Calhoun and Tedeschi (2004) describe other foundations for posttraumatic growth to occur, and one major factor is a strong and supporting social network. Another key foundation is the cognitive reframing or development of new cognitive schema postinjury that needs to occur in establishing a new philosophy and in pursuing new opportunities (Janoff-Bulman, 1992; Kendall & Buys, 1998; Kobasa et al., 1982a). Janoff-Bulman (2004) cites our cultural popular lore from Nietzsche that whatever does not kill us makes us stronger. Some trauma survivors are able to rise up by discovering new-found strength and new coping skills. Also, consistent with related research, PG addresses spiritual connectedness, making meaning of one's situation, and feeling better prepared/stronger to deal with future crises (Graf et al., 2007; Kendall & Buys, 1998; Matheis et al., 2006).

Empirical support for PG is growing, despite its fairly recent advent (see Linley & Joseph, 2000). Tedeschi and Calhoun's (1996) Post Traumatic Growth Inventory (PTGI) has been used in a number of studies concerning persons with various disabling conditions (Morrill et al., 2008; Pollard & Kennedy, 2007; Powell, Ekin-Wood, & Collin, 2007; Steel, Gamblin, & Carr, 2008). Powell et al. (2007), for example, investigated PG for 48 persons with head injuries at two time intervals 1–3 years postinjury ($n = 23$), and 9–12 years postinjury ($n = 25$). Results indicated the most important factor for survivors was social support from family, friends, and significant others. The second most important factor was individual personal skills, determination, and belief in oneself. The only statistically significant difference between groups was that the older injury group reported their lives to have been made richer and fuller since the injury.

Morrill et al. (2008) interviewed 161 women previously treated for early-stage breast cancer. The women were assessed using the PTGI, a QOL scale, a depression scale, and a posttraumatic stress symptoms scale. Results indicated that women reporting PG reported less depression, less posttraumatic stress, and a better quality of life. These results are similar to other cancer studies investigating PG (Cordova & Andry-kowski, 2003; Stanton, Bower, & Low, 2006). In addition, Steel et al. (2008) tested 120 persons diagnosed with hepatobiliary cancer using the PTGI, a depression scale, functional assessment of cancer therapy scale, and also administered the PTGI to family members. Results suggested that PG occurred early in the process of diagnosis and treatment for the cancer, and at the time of testing, patients were actually receiving a second opinion and had been aware of their diagnoses between 1 and 8 weeks prior. The authors note that only 50% of their sample reported positive growth, whereas the others reported no change or negative changes since diagnosis. Their findings were consistent with previous studies indicating 60%–90% of patients reporting positive changes to a cancer diagnosis (Fromm, Andrykowski, & Hunt, 1996; Petrie, Buick, Weinman, & Booth, 1999).

Pollard and Kennedy (2007) tested 87 persons with SCI at 12 weeks postinjury and were able to follow up 10 years later with 37 participants. Several measures were used, including the PTGI, coping strategies inventory, a depression scale, an anxiety inventory, social support scale, and functional independence measure. Results indicated that for individuals who reported rates of depression and anxiety at 12 weeks, they continued to do so at 10 years postinjury. The authors also found a strong positive relationship between psychological distress and posttraumatic growth. This supports Tedeschi and Calhoun's (1995) assertion that individuals can experience both distress and growth simultaneously, essentially a paradoxical effect. Elfstrom, Kreuter, Ryden, Persson, and Sullivan (2002) found similar results, with participants reporting feelings of helplessness and intrusion. Znoj (1999) perhaps best explains this phenomenon in that although individuals can experience adversity and negative affect, the personal growth from such experiences appears to be a survival mechanism that serves to minimize the effects of trauma.

CONCLUSION

Pollard and Kennedy (2007) concluded their study with an interesting observation worthy of future research. They noted that Seligman and Csikszentmihalyi's (2000) promotion of studying the qualities of people who seem to perpetually maintain mental and physical well-being may be missing an important component. Specific to persons with disabilities, can some people possess many of these positive psychology traits, be generally happy and satisfied in their lives, perceive themselves as stronger and having personally grown as a result of a traumatic injury, yet simultaneously at times experience a negative affect? It appears this may well be the case, and healthy versus unhealthy is not an either/or situation. Personal observations of celebrities, who appear to be the happiest, healthiest, and most successful individuals by most standards, reveal that they are not immune to suicide, depression, and substance abuse problems.

In addition, the person-environment interaction once again appears to be an important element of positive psychology and well-being. A strong support network of family and friends has consistently shown to be perhaps the most important factor to well-being and self-esteem. No matter how mentally strong an individual may be, if there is no support network or the available support is dysfunctional at best, it would likely be more difficult for an individual to thrive in such surroundings. Group-level indicators, such as capacity to love, care, and give to others would appear to be diminished. Also, when people with disabilities are cut off from others and their communities, and are otherwise unable to enjoy pleasurable activities (restaurants, movies, events, etc.) due to transportation, physical access barriers, or lack of attendant care, the isolation is also sure to thwart well-being (DiTomasso & Spinner, 1997; Graf et al., 2009; Li & Moore, 1998). As such, researchers and counselors must remain cognizant of the reality that facilitating the well-being of clients must also include acknowledging environmental barriers, and advocating with, and on behalf of clients to remove them.

REFERENCES

Abraido-Lanza, A. F., Vasquez, E., & Echeverria, S. E. (2004). En las manos de dios (In God's hands): Religious and other forms of coping among Latinos with arthritis. *Journal of Counseling and Clinical Psychology, 72*, 91–102.

Aldwin, C. M. (1994). *Stress, coping and development: An integrative perspective.* New York, NY: The Guilford Press.

Antonovsky, A. (1987). *Unraveling the mystery of health: How people manage stress and stay well.* San Francisco, CA: Jossey-Bass.

Argyle, M. (2001). *The psychology of happiness* (2nd ed.). London, UK: Routledge.

Arman, J. F. (2002). A brief group counseling model to increase resiliency of students with mild disabilities. *Journal of Humanistic Counseling, Education and Development, 41*, 120–128.

Aronoff, G. M. (2003). Evaluating and rating impairment caused by pain. In S. L. Demeter & G. B. Anderson (Eds.), *Disability evaluation* (pp. 552–566). St Louis, MO: Mosby.

Ash, C., & Huebner, E. (2001). Environmental events and life satisfaction reports of adolescents: A test of cognitive mediation. *School Psychology International, 22*, 320–336.

Bach, J. R., & Tilton, M. C. (1994). Life satisfaction and well-being measures in ventilator assisted individuals with traumatic tetraplegia. *Archives of Physical Medicine Rehabilitation, 75*, 626–632.

Bandura, A. (1997). *Self-efficacy. The exercise of control.* New York, NY: Freeman.

Banks, J. K., & Gannon, L. R. (1988). The influence of hardiness on the relationship between stressors and psychosomatic symptomatology. *American Journal of Communication Psychology, 16*, 25–37.

Banks, S. M., & Kerns, R. D. (1996). Explaining high rates of depression in chronic pain: A diathesis-stress frame-work. *Psychological Bulletin, 119*, 95–110.

Batson, C. D., Schoenrade, P. A., & Ventis, W. L. (1993). *Religion and the individual: A social psychological perspective.* New York, NY: Oxford University Press.

Ben-Shahar, T. (2007). *Happier.* New York, NY: McGraw-Hill.

Bener, A., El-Rufair, O. F., Kamran, S., Georgievski, A. B., Farooq, A., & Rysavy, M. (2006). Disability, depression and somatization in a low back pain population. *Asia Pacific League of Associations Journal of Rheumatology, 9*, 257–263.

Bennett, M. E. (2009). Assessment of substance use and substance use disorders in schizophrenia. *Clinical Schizophrenia & Related Psychoses, 3*(1), 50–63.

Bennett, M. E., & Gjonbalaj, S. (2007). The problem of dual diagnosis. In M. Turner & D. Beidel (Eds.), *Adult psychopathology and diagnosis.* New York, NY: John Wiley & Sons.

Bishop, M. (2005a). Quality of life and psychosocial adaptation to chronic illness and acquired disability: A conceptual and theoretical synthesis. *Journal of Rehabilitation, 71*(2), 5–13.

Bruhin, A., & Winkelmann, R. (2009). Happiness functions with preference interdependence and heterogeneity: The case of altruism within the family. *Journal of Population Economist, 22*, 1063–1080.

Burvill, P. W., Johnson, G. A., Jamrozik, K. D., Anderson, C. S., Stewart-Wayne, E. G., & Chakera, T. M. (1995). Prevalence of depression after stroke: The Perth Community Stroke Study. *British Journal of Psychiatry, 166*, 320–327.

Calhoun, L. G., & Tedeschi, R. G. (2004). The foundations of posttraumatic growth: New considerations. *Psychological Inquiry, 15*(1), 93–102.

Carroll, K. M., Rounsaville, B. J., & Bryant, K. J. (1993). Alcoholism in treatment-seeking cocaine abusers: Clinical and prognostic significance. *Journal of Studies on Alcohol, 54*, 199–208.

Centers for Disease Control and Prevention, National Center for Injury Prevention and Control. (2010, April). *Web-based Injury Statistics Query and Reporting System (WISQARS)*. Retrieved on October 23, 2010, from www.cdc.gov/ncipc/wisqars.

Chubon, R. A. (1994). *Social and psychological foundations of rehabilitation*. Springfield, IL: Charles C. Thomas.

Cordova, M. J., & Andrykowski, M. A. (2003). Responses to cancer diagnosis and treatment: Post-traumatic stress and post-traumatic growth. *Seminar Clinical Neuropsychiatry, 8*, 286–296.

Conwell, Y., & Brent, D. (1995). Suicide and aging: Patterns of psychiatric diagnosis. *International Psychogeriatrics, 7*(2), 149–164.

Csikszentmihalyi, M. (1975). *Beyond boredom and anxiety*. San Francisco, CA: Jossey-Bass.

Csikszentmihalyi, M. (1978). Attention and the holistic approach to behavior. In K. S. Pope & J. L. Singer (Eds.). *The stream of consciousness* (pp. 335–358). New York, NY: Plenum.

Csikszentmihalyi, M. (1999). If we are so rich, why aren't we happy? *American Psychologist, 54*, 821–827.

Cuijpers, P., de Graaf, R., & van Dorsselaer, S. (2004). Minor depression: Risk profiles, functional disability, healthcare use and risk of developing major depression. *Journal of Affective Disorders, 79*(1-3), 71–80.

Daughters, S. B., Bornovalova, M. A., Correia, C., & Lejuez, C. W. (2007). Psychoactive substance use disorders: Drugs. In M. Hersen, S. M. Turner, & D. C. Beidel (Eds.), *Adults psychopathology and diagnosis*. Hoboken, NJ: John Wiley & Sons.

DeJong, G. (1979a). Independent living: From social movement to analytic paradigm. *Archives of Physical Medicine and Rehabilitation, 60*, 435–446.

Delle Fave, A. (1996). The process of flow transformation in a sample of subjects with spinal cord injuries. In F. Massimmi, P. Inghilleri, & A. Delle Fave (Eds.), *La selezione psicologica umana* (pp. 615–634). Milan: Cooperativa Libraria IULM.

Delle Fave, A., & Maletto, C. (1992). Attention processes and the quality of subjective experience. In D. Galati (Ed.), *La psicologia dei non vedenti* (pp. 321–353). Milan: Franco Angeli.

deRoon-Cassini, T. A., de St. Aubin, E., Valvano, A., Hastings, J., & Horn, P. (2009). Psychological well-being after spinal cord injury: Perception of loss and meaning making. *Rehabilitation Psychology, 54*(3), 306–314.

Deutsch, A. (1949). *The mentally ill in America* (2nd ed.). New York, NY: Columbia University Press.

DeVivo, M. J., & Stover, S. L. (1995). Long-term survival and causes of death. In S. L. Stover, J. L. DeLisa, & G. G. Whiteneck (Eds.), *Spinal cord injury: Clinical outcomes from the model systems* (pp. 289–316). Gaithersburg, MD: Aspen.

Dickens, C. (2001). The burden of depression in patients with rheumatoid arthritis. *Rheumatology, 40*(12), 1327–1330.

Diener, E. (2000). Subject well-being: The science of happiness and a proposal for a national index. *The American Psychologist, 55*, 34–43.

Diener, E., & Lucas, S. (1999). Personality and subjective well-being. In E. Diener & N. Schwartz (Eds.), *Well being: The foundations of hedonic psychology* (pp. 213–229). New York, NY: Russell Sage Foundation.

Diener, E., & Seligman, M. (2002). Very happy people. *Psychological Science, 13*, 81–84.

Diener, E., Lucas, R. E., & Oishi, S. (2005). Subjective well-being: The science of happiness and life satisfaction. In C. R. Snyder & S. J. Lopez (Eds.), *Handbook of positive psychology* (pp. 63–73). New York, NY: Oxford University Press, Inc.

Diener, E., Lucas, R. E., & Scollon, C. (2006). Beyond the hedonic treadmill: Revising the adaptation theory of well-being. *American Psychologist, 61*, 305–314.

Dijkers, M. (1997). Measuring quality of life. In M. J. Fuhrer (Ed.), *Assessing medical rehabilitation practices: The promise of outcome research* (pp. 153–180). Baltimore, MD: Paul H. Brooks.

DiTomasso, E., & Spinner, B. (1997). Social and emotional loneliness: A re-examination of Weiss' typology of loneliness. *Personality and Individual Differences, 22,* 417–427.

Dyer, J. G., & McGuinness, T. M. (1996). Resilience: Analysis of the concept. *Archives of Psychiatric Nursing, 10,* 276–282.

Dykens, E. (2005). Happiness, well-being and character strengths: Outcomes for families and siblings of persons with mental retardation. *Mental Retardation, 43,* 360–364.

Edwards, L. M. (2004). *Factors contributing to subjective well-being in Mexican-American adolescents.* Unpublished doctoral dissertation. Lawrence, KS: University of Kansas.

Elfstrom, M. L., Kreuter, M., Ryden, A., Persson, L. O., & Sullivan, M. (2002). Effects of coping on psychological outcome when controlling for background variables: A study of traumatically spinal cord lesioned persons. *Spinal Cord, 40,* 408–415.

English, R. W. (1971). Correlates of stigma toward physically disabled persons. In R. P. Marinelli & A. E. Dell Orto (Eds.), *The psychological & social impact of physical disability* (pp. 162–182). New York, NY: Springer.

Frederick, S., & Loewenstein, G. (1999). Hedonic adaptation. In D. Kahneman, E. Diener, & N. Schwarz (Eds.), *Well-being: The foundations of hedonic psychology* (pp. 302–329). New York, NY: Sage.

Fromm, K., Andrykowski, M. A., & Hunt, J. (1996). Positive and negative psychosocial sequelae of bone marrow transplant: Implications for quality of life assessment. *Journal of Behavioral Medicine, 19,* 221–240.

Gallagher, H. G. (1994). *FDR's splendid deception.* Arlington, VA: Vandarmere.

Gallagher, H. G. (1995). *By trust betrayed: Patients, physicians, and the license to kill in the third Reich* (Rev. ed.). Arlington, VA: Vandamere.

Goffman, E. (1963). *Stigma.* Englewood Cliffs, NJ: Prentice-Hall.

Goldblatt, M. J. (2000). Physical illness and suicide. In R. W. Maris, A. L. Berman, & M. M. Silverman (Eds.), *Comprehensive textbook of suicidology* (pp. 342–356). New York, NY: Guilford Press.

Graf, N. M., Marini, I., Baker, J., & Buck, T. (2007). The perceived impact of religious and spiritual beliefs for persons with chronic pain. *Rehabilitation Counseling Bulletin, 51*(1), 21–33.

Graf, N. M., Marini, I., & Blankenship, C. (2009). 100 Words about disability. *Journal of Rehabilitation, 75*(2), 25–34.

Graham, D. P., & Cardon, A. L. (2008). An update on substance use and treatment following traumatic brain injury. *New York Academy of Sciences, 1141,* 148–162.

Grant, G., Ramcharan, P., & Flynn, M. (2007). Resilience in families with children and adult members with intellectual disabilities: Tracing elements of a psycho-social model. *Journal of Applied Research in Intellectual Disabilities, 20,* 563–575.

Grant, B. F., Stinson, F. S., Dawson, D. A., Chou, S. P., Dufour, M. C., Compton, W. et al. (2004). Prevalence and co-occurrence of substance use disorders and independent mood and anxiety disorders: Results from the National Epidemiologic Survey on Alcohol and Related Conditions. *Archives of General Psychiatry, 61*(8), 807–816.

Griffin, M. L., Kolodziej, M. E., & Weiss, R. D. (2009). Measuring principal substance of abuse in comorbid patients for clinical research. *Addictive Behaviors, 34,* 826–829.

Harter, S. (1978). Effectance motivation reconsidered: Toward a developmental model. *Human Development, 1,* 661–669.

Heinemann, A. W. (1993). *Substance abuse & physical disability.* New York, NY: Haworth Press.

Honey, S., Meager, N., & Williams, M. (1998). *Employers' attitudes towards people with disabilities.* Grantham, England: Institute for Employment Studies.

Huebner, E. S. (1991). Correlates of life satisfaction in children. *School Psychology Quarterly, 6,* 103–111.

Huebner, E. S. (2004). Research on assessment of life satisfaction of children and adolescents. *Social Indicators, 66,* 3–33.

Janoff-Bulman, R. (2004). Posttraumatic growth: Three explanatory models. *Psychological Inquiry, 15*(1), 30–34.

Janoff-Bulman, R. (1992). *Shattered assumptions: Towards a new psychology of trauma.* New York, NY: Free Press.

Johnstone, B., Glass, B. A., & Oliver, R. E. (2007). Religion and disability: Clinical, research and training considerations for rehabilitation professionals. *Disability and Rehabilitation, 29,* 1153–1163.

Jonker, L., & Greeff, A. P. (2009). Resilience factors in families living with people with mental illness. *Journal of Community Psychology, 37*(7), 859–873.

Kaliterna-Lipovcan, L., & Prizmic-Larsen, Z. (2006). What makes Croats happy? Predictors of happiness in representative sample. In A. D. Fave (Ed.), *Dimensions of well-being. Research and intervention* (pp. 53–59). Milano, Italy: Franco Angeli.

Kendall, E., & Buys, N. (1998). An integrated model of psychosocial adjustment following acquired disability. *Journal of Rehabilitation, 64*(3), 16–20.

Kessler, R. C., McGonagle, K. A., Zhao, S., Nelson, C. B., Hughes, M., Eshleman, S., et al. (1994). Lifetime and 12-month prevalence of DSM-III-R psychiatric disorders in the United States. Results from the National Comorbidity Survey. *Archives of General Psychiatry, 51*(1), 8–19.

Kessler, R. C., Chiu, W. T., Demler, O., & Walters, E. E. (2005a). Prevalence, severity, and comorbidity of twelve-month DSM-IV disorders in the National Comorbidity Survey Replication (NCS-R). *Archives of General Psychiatry, 62*(6), 617–627.

Kessler, R. C., Berglund, P. A., Demler, O., & Walters, E. E. (2005b). Lifetime prevalence and age-of-onset distributions of DSM-IV disorders in the National Comorbidity Survey Replication (NCS-R). *Archives of General Psychiatry, 62*(6), 593–602.

Klein, W. M. (1997). Objective standards are not enough: Affective, self-evaluative, and behavioral responses to social comparison information. *Journal of Personality and Social Psychology, 72,* 763–774.

Kloosterhouse, V., & Ames, B. D. (2002). Families' use of religion/spirituality as a psychosocial resource. *Holistic Nursing Practice, 17*(1), 61–76.

Knestrict, T., & Kuchey, D. (2009). Welcome to Holland: Characteristics of resilient families raising children with severe disabilities. *Journal of Family Studies, 15,* 227–244.

Kobasa, S. C. (1979). Stressful life events, personality, and health: An inquiry into hardiness. *Journal of Personality and Social Psychology, 37,* 1–11.

Kobasa, S. C., Maddi, S. R., & Kahn, S. (1982a). Hardiness and health: A prospective study. *Journal of Personality and Social Psychology, 42,* 168–177.

Kobasa, S. C., & Puccetti, M. C. (1983). Personality and social resources in stress resistance. *Journal of Personality and Social Psychology, 45,* 839–850.

Kobasa, S. C., Maddi, S. R., Puccetti, M. C., & Zola, M. A. (1985). Effectiveness of hardiness, exercise, and social support as resources against illness. *Journal of Psychosomatic Research, 29,* 525–533.

Koch, M., Uyttenboogaart, M., Harten, A. V., Heerings, M., & Keyser, J. D. (2008). Fatigue, depression and progression in multiple sclerosis. *Multiple Sclerosis, 14,* 815–822.

Kochanek, K. D., Murphy, S. L., Anderson, R. N., & Scott, C. (2004). Deaths final data for 2003. *National Vital Statistics Reports, 53*(5), 1–115.

Kramer, H., & Sprenger, J. (1971). *The Malleus Maleficarum of Heinrich Kramer and James Sprenger.* Dover, DE: Dover Publications.

Krause, J. S., Coker, J., Charlifue, S., & Whiteneck, G. G. (1999). Depression and subjective well-being among 97 American Indians with spinal cord injury: A descriptive study. *Rehabilitation Psychology, 44,* 354–372.

Kreutzer, J. S., Wehman, P. H., Harris, J. A., Burns, C. T., & Young, H. F. (1991). Substance abuse and crime patterns among persons with traumatic brain injury referred for supported employment. *Brain Injury, 5,* 177–187.

Kreutzer, J. S., Marwitz, J. H., & Witol, A. D. (1995). Interrelationships between crime, substance abuse, and aggressive behaviors among persons with traumatic brain injury. *Brain Injury, 9,* 757–768.

Kreutzer, J. S., Witol, A. D., & Marwitz, J. H. (1996). Alcohol and drug use among young persons with traumatic brain injury. *Journal of Learning Disability, 29,* 643–651.

Kumpfer, K. (1999). Factors and processes contributing to resilience: The resilience framework. In M. D. Glantz & J. L. Johnson (Eds.), *Resilience and development: Positive life adaptations* (pp. 179–224). New York, NY: Kluwer Academic/Plenum Publishers.

Lazarus, R. S. (1983). The costs and benefits of denial. In S. Benitz (Ed.), *Denial of stress* (pp. 1–30). New York, NY: International Universities Press.

Lee, E. J., Chan, F., Chronister, J., Chan, J. Y., & Romero, M. (2009). Models, research, and coexisting depression for people with chronic illness and disability. In F. Chan, E. D. S. Cardoso, & J. Chronister (Eds.), *Understanding psychosocial adjustment to chronic illness and disability: A handbook for evidence-based practitioners in rehabilitation* (pp. 75–107). New York, NY: Springer.

Lemert, E. M. (1967). *Human deviance, social problems, and social control.* Englewood Cliffs, NJ: Prentice-Hall.

Lester, D. (2000). Alcoholism, substance abuse, and suicide. In R. W. Maris, A. L. Berman, & M. M. Silverman (Eds.), *Comprehensive textbook of suicidology* (pp. 357–375). New York, NY: Guilford Press.

Levin, J. (2001). *God, faith, and health: Exploring the spirituality healing connection.* Hoboken, NJ: Wiley & Sons.

Li, L., & Moore, D. (1998). Acceptance of disability and its correlates. *Journal of Social Psychology, 138*(1), 13–25.

Li, L., & Moore, D. (2001). Disability illicit drug use: An application of labeling theory. *Deviant Behavior, 22*(1), 1–21.

Linley, P. A., & Joseph, S. (2000). Positive change following trauma and adversity: A review. *Journal of Traumatic Stress, 17*(1), 11–21.

Livneh, H. (1991). On the origins of negative attitudes toward people with disabilities. In R. P. Marinelli, & A. E. Dell Orto (Eds.), *The Psychological & Social Impact of Disability* (pp. 111–138). New York, NY: Springer.

Lopez, S. J., Snyder, C. R., & Teramoto-Pedrotti, J. (2003). Hope: Many definitions, many measures. In S. J. Lopez, & C. R. Synder (Eds.), *Positive psychological assessment: A handbook of models and measures* (pp. 91–107). Washington, DC: American Psychological Association.

Lou Harris and Associates. (1991). *Public attitudes toward persons with disabilities.* New York, NY: International Center for the Disabled.

Louch, P. (2009). Understanding the impact of depression. *Practice Nurse, 37*(9), 43–48.

Lucas, R. E. (2007). Adaptation and the set-point model of subjective well-being: Does happiness change after major life events? *Current Directions in Psychological Science, 16*, 75–79.

Luthar, S. S., Cicchetti, D., & Becker, B. (2000). The construct of resilience: A critical evaluation and guidelines for future work. *Child Development, 71*, 543–562.

Lykken, D. (1999). *Happiness: The nature and nature of joy and contentment.* New York, NY: St. Martin's Press.

Makas, E. (1988). Positive attitudes toward disabled people: Disabled and nondisabled persons' perspectives. *Journal of Social Issues, 44*(1), 49–61.

Marini, I., Bhakta, M. V., & Graf, N. (2009). A content analysis of common concerns of persons with physical disabilities. *Journal of Applied Rehabilitation Counseling, 40*(1), 44–49.

Marini, I., & Chacon, M. (2007). The implications of positive psychology and wellness for rehabilitation counselor education. In R. P. Marinelli, & A. E. Dell Orto (Eds.), *The psychological & social impact of physical disability* (pp. 551–581). New York, NY: Springer.

Marini, I., & Glover-Graf, N. M. (2011). Religiosity and spirituality among persons with spinal cord injury: Attitudes, beliefs, and practices. *Rehabilitation Counseling Bulletin, 54*(2), 82–92.

Marini, I., & Stebnicki, M. (1999). Social security's alternative provider program: What can rehabilitation administrators expect. *Journal of Rehabilitation Administration, 23*(1), 31–41.

Marinic, M., & Brkljacic, T. (2008). Love over gold-the correlation of happiness level with some life satisfaction factors between persons with and without physical disability. *Journal of Development and Physical Disability, 20*, 527–540.

Maris, R. W., Berman, A. L., & Silverman, M. M. (2000). *Comprehensive textbook of suicidology.* New York, NY: Guilford Press.

Matheis, E. N., Tulsky, D. S., & Matheis, R. J. (2006). The relation between spirituality and quality of life among individuals with spinal cord injury. *Rehabilitation Psychology, 51*, 265–271.

McCubbin, H., & McCubbin, M. (1988). Typologies of resilient families: Emerging roles of social class and ethnicity. *Family Relations, 37*, 247–254.

Moore, A. D., & Stambrook, M. (1995). Cognitive moderators of outcome following a traumatic brain injury: A conceptual model and implications for rehabilitation. *Brain Injury, 9*(2), 109–130.

Morrill, E. F., Brewer, N. T., O'Neill, S. C., Lillie, S. E., Dees, E. L., Carey, L. A. et al. (2008). The inter-action of post-traumatic growth and post-traumatic stress symptoms in predicting depressive symptoms and quality of life. *Psycho-Oncology, 17,* 948–953.

Mueser, K. T., Bennett, M. E., & Kushner, M. G. (1995). Epidemiology of substance abuse among persons with chronic mental disorders. In A. Lehman & L. Dixon (Eds.), *Substance abuse disorders among persons with chronic mental illness.* New York, NY: Harwood Academic Publishers.

Myers, D. (2000). The funds, friends and faith of happy people. *The American Psychologist, 55,* 56–67.

Oettingen, G. (1996). Positive fantasy and motivation. In P. M. Gollwitzer & J. Bargh (Eds.), *The psychology of action: Linking cognitive and motivation to behavior* (pp. 236–259). New York, NY: Guilford Press.

Olkin, R. (1999). *What psychotherapists should know about disability.* New York, NY: The Guilford Press.

Park, C. (2007). Religiousness/spirituality and health: A meaning systems perspective. *Journal of Behavioral Medicine, 30,* 319–328.

Park, C. L., & Folkman, S. L. (1997). Meaning in the context of stress and coping. *Review of General Psychology, 1,* 115–144.

Penner, L. A. (2004). Volunteerism and social problems: Making things better or worse? *Journal of Social Issues, 60*(3), 645–666.

Peterson, C., Maier, S. F., & Seligman, M. E. (1995). *Learned helplessness: A theory for the age of personal control.* Oxford, UK: Oxford University Press.

Peterson, C. (2000). The future of optimism. *American Psychologist, 55,* 44–55.

Peterson, C., & Park, N. (2009). Positive psychology. In I. Marini & M. Stebnicki (Eds.), *The professional counselor's desk reference* (pp. 791–799). New York, NY: Springer.

Petrie, K. J., Buick, D. L., Weinman, J., & Booth, R. J. (1999). Positive effects of illness reported by myo-cardial infarction and breast cancer patients. *Journal of Psychosomatic Research, 47*(6), 537–543.

Piliavin, J. A., & Charng, H. W. (1990). Altruism: A review of recent theory and research. *Annual Review of Sociology, 16,* 27–65.

Pollard, C., & Kennedy, P. (2007). A longitudinal analysis of emotional impact, coping strategies and post-traumatic psychological growth following spinal cord injury: A 10-year review. *British Journal of Health Psychology, 12,* 347–362.

Pollock, S. E. (1986). Human responses to chronic illness: Physiological and psychosocial adaptation. *Nurses Resources, 35,* 90–95.

Powell, T., Ekin-Wood, A., & Collin, C. (2007). Post-traumatic growth after head injury: A long-term follow-up. *Brain Injury, 21*(1), 31–38.

Puchalski, C. M. (1999). *Touching the spirit: The essence of healing. Spiritual life.* Washington, DC: Discalced Carmelite Friars of the Washington Province.

Rhodewalt, F., & Zone, J. B. (1989). Appraisal of life change, depression, and illness in hardy and non-hardy women. *Journal of Personality Social Psychology, 56,* 81–88.

Rosenbaum, E. H., & Rosenbaum, I. R. (1999). *Inner-fire: Your will to live: Stories of courage, hope and deter-mination.* Austin, TX: Plexus.

Rounsaville, B. J., Petry, N. M., & Carroll, K. M. (2003). Single versus multiple drug focus in substance abuse clinical trails research. *Drug and Alcohol Dependence, 70,* 117–125.

Rotter, J. B. (1966). Generalized expectancies for internal versus external control of reinforcement. *Psychological Monographs, 80,* 244–248.

Rubin, S. E., & Roessler, R. T. (2008). *Foundations of the vocational rehabilitation process* (6th ed.). Austin, TX: Pro-Ed.

Ryan, R. M., & Deci, E. L. (2000). Self-determination theory and the facilitation of intrinsic motivation, social development and well-being. *American Psychologist, 55,* 68–78.

Ryan, R. M., & Deci, E. L. (2001). On happiness and human potentials: A review of research on hedonic and eudaimonic well-being. *Annual Review of Psychology, 52,* 141–166.

Scheff, T. (1966). *Being mentally ill.* Chicago, IL: Aldine.

Seligman, M. E. (1998). Building human strength: Psychology's forgotten mission. *APA Monitor, 29,* 2.

Seligman, M. E. P., & Csikszentmihalyi, M. (2000). Positive psychology: An introduction. *American Psychologist, 55,* 5–14.

Seligman, M. (2002). *Authentic happiness: Using the new positive psychology to realize your potential for lasting fulfillment*. New York, NY: Free Press.

Selway, D., & Ashman, A. F. (1998). Disability, religion and health: A literature review in search of the spiritual dimensions of disability. *Disability & Society, 13*(3), 429–439.

Shnek, Z. M., Foley, F. W., LaRocca, N. G., Smith, C. R., & Halper, J. (1995). Psychological predictors of depression in multiple sclerosis. *Journal of Neurologic Rehabilitation, 9*(1), 15–23.

Shnek, Z. M., Foley, F. W., LaRocca, N. G., Gordon, W. A., DeLuca, J., Schwartzman, H. G., et al. (1997). Helplessness, self-efficacy, cognitive distortions, and depression in multiple sclerosis and spinal cord injury. *Annals of Behavioral Medicine, 19*(3), 287–294.

Sigerist, H. E. (1951). *A history of medicine*. New York, NY: Oxford University Press.

Silver, R. L. (1982). *Coping with an undesirable life event: A study of early reactions to physical disability*. Unpublished doctoral dissertation. Evanston, IL; Northwestern University.

Snyder, C. R. (1994). *The psychology of hope*. New York, NY: The Free Press.

Snyder, C. R. (1998). A case for hope in pain, loss, and suffering. In J. H. Harvey, J. Omarzy, & E. Miller (Eds.), *Perspectives on loss: A sourcebook*. Washington, DC: Taylor & Francis.

Snyder, C. R. (Ed.) (2000). *Handbook of hope: Theory, measures, and applications*. San Diego, CA: Academic Press.

Snyder, C. R. (2002). Hope theory: Rainbows in the mind. *Psychological Inquiry, 13*, 249–275.

Snyder, C. R., & Lopez, S. J. (2002). The future of positive psychology: A declaration of independence. In C. R. Snyder & S. J. Lopez (Eds.), *Handbook of positive psychology* (pp. 751–767). London, UK: Oxford University Press.

Snyder, C. R., Rand, K. L., & Sigmon, D. R. (2002). Hope theory: A member of the positive psychology family. In C. R. Snyder & S. J. Lopez (Eds.), *Handbook of positive psychology* (pp. 257–276). London, UK: Oxford University Press.

Stanton, A. L., Bower, J. E., & Low, C. A. (2006). Post-traumatic growth after cancer. In L. G. Calhoun & R. G. Tedeschi (Eds.), *Handbook of post-traumatic growth* (pp. 138–175). Mahwah, NJ: Lawrence Erlbaum Associates, Inc.

Stanton, A. L., Danoff-Burg, S., & Huggins, M. E. (2002). The first year after breast cancer, diagnosis: Hope and coping strategies as predictors of adjustment. *Psycho-Oncology, 11*, 93–102.

Steel, J. L., Gamblin, T. C., & Carr, B. I. (2008). Measuring post-traumatic growth in people diagnosed with hepatobiliary cancer: Directions for future research. *Oncology Nursing Forum, 35*(4), 643–650.

Stinson, F. S., Grant, B. F., Dawson, D. A., Ruan, W. J., Huang, B., & Saha, T. (2005). Comorbidity between DSM-IV alcohol and specific drug use disorders in the United States: Results from the National Epidemiologic Survey on alcohol and related conditions. *Drug and Alcohol Dependence, 80*, 105–116.

Stone, A. A., Cox, D. X., Valdimarsdottir, H., Jandorf, L., & Neale, J. M. (1987). Evidence that secretory IgA antibody is associated with daily mood. *Journal of Peronality and Social Psychology, 52*, 988–993.

Stone, H., Cross, D. R., Purvis, K., & Young, M. J. (2004). A study of church members during times of crisis. *Pastoral Psychology, 52*(5), 405–421.

Stotland, E. (1969). *The psychology of hope*. San Francisco, CA: Jossey-Bass.

Szymanski, C. R., Ryan, C., Merz, M. A., Trevino, B., & Johnson-Rodriguez, S. (1996). Psychosocial and economic aspects of work: Implications for people with disabilities. In E. M. Szymanski & R. M. Parker (Eds.), *Work and disability: Issues and strategies in career development and job placement* (pp. 9–38). Austin, TX: Pro-ed.

Taylor, S. E. (1983). Adjustment to threatening events: A theory of cognitive adaptation. *American Psychologist, 38*, 1196–1173.

Taylor, S. E., & Brown, J. D. (1998). Illusion and well-being: A social psychological perspective on mental health. *Psychological Bulletin, 110*, 193–210.

Tedeschi, R. G., & Calhoun, L. G. (1988). *Perceived benefits in coping with physical handicaps*. Paper presented at the meeting of the American Psychological Association, Atlanta, GA.

Tedeschi, R. G., & Calhoun, L. G. (1995). *Trauma and transformation: Growing in the aftermath of suffering*. Thousand Oaks, CA: Sage.

Tedeschi, R. G., & Calhoun, L. G. (1996). The posttraumatic growth inventory: Measuring the positive legacy of trauma. *Journal of Traumatic Stress, 9,* 455–471.

Thompson, N. (2002). *Building the future: Social work with children, young people and their families.* Lyme Regis, UK: Russell House Publishing.

Trieschmann, R. (1988). *Spinal cord injuries: Psychological, social, and vocational rehabilitation* (2nd ed.). New York, NY: Demos.

Tsuang, J. W., Shapiro, E., Smith, T. L., & Schuckit, M. A. (1994). Drug use among primary alcoholic veterans. *American Journal of Drug and Alcohol Abuse, 20,* 483–493.

Turner, R. J., & McLean, P. D. (1989). Physical disability and psychological distress. *Rehabilitation Psychology, 34,* 225–242.

Turner-Stokes, L., & Hassan, N. (2002). Depression after stroke: A review of the evidence base to inform the development of an integrated care pathway. Part 1: Diagnosis, frequency and impact. *Clinical Rehabilitation, 16,* 231–247.

Vash, C. L. (1981). *The psychology of disability.* New York, NY: Springer.

Vash, C. L., & Crewe, N. M. (2004). *Psychology of disability* (pp. 288–299). New York, NY: Springer.

Von Korff, M., & Simon, G. (1996). The relationship between pain and depression. *British Journal of Psychiatry, 30,* 101–108.

Wagnild, G., & Young, H. M. (1990). Resilience among older women. *IMAGE: Journal of Nursing Scholarship, 22,* 252–255.

Walker, R., Cole, J. E., Logan, T. K., & Corrigan, J. D. (2007). Screening substance abuse treatment clients for traumatic brain injury: Prevalence and characteristics. *Journal Head Trauma Injury Rehabilitation, 22,* 360–367.

Walsh, F. (2003). Family resilience: Strengths forged through adversity. In F. Walsh (Ed.), *Normal family processes* (3rd ed., pp. 399–423). New York, NY: Guilford Press.

Werner, E. E., & Smith, R. S. (1982). *Vulnerable but invincible: A longitudinal study of resilient children and youth.* New York, NY: McGraw-Hill.

Williams, P. G., Wiebe, D. J., & Smith, T. W. (1992). Coping processes as mediators of the relationship between hardiness and health. *Journal of Behavioral Medicine, 15,* 237–255.

Wills, T. A. (1991). Similarity and self-esteem in downward social comparison. In J. M. Suls & T. A. Wills (Eds.), *Social comparison* (pp. 51–78). Hillsdale, NJ: Erlbaum.

Wilson, J. (2000). Volunteering. *Annual Review of Sociology, 26,* 215–240.

Wilz, G. (2007). Predictors of subjective impairment after stroke: Influence of depression, gender and severity of stroke. *Brain Injury, 21*(1), 39–45.

Wright, B. (1983). *Physical disability: A psychosocial approach* (2nd ed.). New York, NY: Harper & Row.

Znoj, H. J. (1999). *European and American perspectives on post-traumatic growth: A model of personal growth: Life challenges and transformation following loss and physical handicap.* Talk given at the APA conference 1999, Boston.

INSIDER PERSPECTIVE

The Story of Dave Shannon

Carpe diem might perhaps best describe the philosophy of how I have lived my life so far as I approach age 50. I'm not exactly sure as to how my life would have turned out if not for my injury, but it certainly has been a life lived to this point. I'm reminded of the classic line Tim Robbins' character says to fellow inmate Morgan Freeman in Shawshank prison the day Robbins breaks out after 20 years of wrongful imprisonment: "Get busy living, or get busy dying."

It's 1981, I am 18 years of age, and I'm an invincible rugby player just having returned from Thunder Bay representing Nova Scotia in the Canada Summer

Games. And I'm excited because now my sights are set on the University of Waterloo in Ontario as a member of its varsity rugby team. During practice the week before school starts in September, I find myself trapped at the bottom of a scrum with players from both teams piling on top of me until I hear this excruciating crunching noise in my neck and my body immediately goes limp. Although it's medically termed a C4 spinal cord injury or tetraplegia, in lay person's language I had just broken my neck. Strangely, the pain was not severe. I felt an electrical current start from my neck then radiate downward and out my feet. Then, total immobility, confusion, fear, and desperation.

Arriving in hospital, the severity began to take on a greater degree of clarity. No physicians needed to tell me that this was serious when I lay on an x-ray bed paralyzed, my breathing becoming shallow, and the attending staff staying so silent that the sound of the scissors cutting my rugby jersey imploded on my ear drum in a crunching soprano shrill that signified the severance of my sweater and spinal cord.

I then lay in bed for almost the entirety of the next 14 weeks. True friendships were tested as it appeared that I may need new supports, but the response from so many was overwhelming. My parents and extended family came immediately. Several friends flew more than 2 hours from Halifax to Waterloo to be at my bedside. They left school for 2 weeks to raise my spirits to assure me that things would be O.K., and perhaps find a way to cope with their own shock at the awareness we are vulnerable. These were not just medically critical times, but my emotional stability was also equally at risk. Emerging from those early visits, although much remained in a cognitive haze, I gained the germination of a certainty that relationships would remain as dear and profound as they were before my injury. A change in physicality could not alter our humanity and internal fire of aspiration to be our best.

I also started to develop ways of filling the gaps of activity that immobility can create. After the first few weeks of surgery, a severe bladder infection and a halo vest that did not fasten correctly (meaning it was screwed back into my skull before the anesthetic took hold) meant a long stay in hospital. I learned to find patience through meditation. Although quite young and unexposed to mindful introspective retreats, the situation forced me to learn these techniques. It helped me to suspend my intellectual and spiritual self above the physical boundaries holding me down. It also allowed my dreams to continue to take flight, setting the stage for new goals and a feeling of success with each minor and major achievement.

Having left the acute care, I went to Lyndhurst Hospital in Toronto for rehabilitation for what were to be several months of rigorous physical and occupational therapy. It was the first time that I met other guys just like me from all walks of life and all ages with similar or different spinal cord injuries like mine. Their stories are all surreal and fascinating, and, much like me, their lives had changed in the blink of an eye. A couple of guys were injured playing hockey (Irmo Marini is one). One elderly Portuguese guy falls off a street corner curb the wrong way and breaks his neck. Another guy collides on his motocross bike with another bike on a hill. And some guy falls out of the tree doing housework at home. We learn that not everybody survives a spinal cord injury, and at this point still grieving our loss of former lifestyle and function, we are not sure whether that is a blessing or a curse. Some of us aren't sure whether we can do this, but my carpe diem philosophy doesn't allow me to think about giving up or letting this get the best of me. After all, I wasn't dead yet.

And so after periodic insight into the value of human relationships tempered with less frequent moments of despair, sorrow, and immense sadness, I slowly began the mental journey back among the living and getting on with my life, albeit now in a power wheelchair. First stop, back to Thunder Bay to begin an English degree and political science minor at Lakehead University.

I had been born in Thunder Bay and still had some extended family there. More importantly, this city was ahead of its time in the provision of independent living services. Attendant care was available in my own apartment, a parallel transit service was well established and there was a strong advocacy group that had a good relationship with the City Council and the Mayor. This seemed at first to be a perfect place to live in while I transitioned out of rehab and gained an undergraduate degree. This was true to some extent, but the experience was for the most part dichotomous.

The wonderful friends I mentioned earlier were now 3,000 miles away. My parents were almost as far. The climate was harsh. This became a lonely time. My basic service or physical needs were being met, but little was being done for my emotional well-being.

By year two and three of undergraduate studies things began to pick up. I was exposed to the world of great thinkers, poets, and social visionaries. A budding interest in social change and human rights was taking off, and the campus had what every heterosexual 20-year-old wants, that is, several thousand women in one location.

After completing my bachelors degree in 1986, I moved back home to Nova Scotia and attended Dalhousie University, taking a full-time load of courses at the Honours English level. I had always been intrigued by law and started thinking about what kind of jobs a guy in a wheelchair might get hired to do, knowing that nobody might hire me at all, and in thinking about starting my own practice, I knew I could hire myself. By 1990, after four more grueling years of academia, I graduated with my Bachelors of Law degree.

Most importantly, I was back home to those dear friends who had supported me from day one. A full student and campus life was ahead of me with parties, dates and heartaches, and many new friends, but it was with a core support system that I was able to grow to levels that I knew would be impossible for other quadriplegics who did not have the people around them who fortunately were there for me. So during that period I not only attended law school but also became Student Union President, took on leadership positions with Disabled Persons Organizations whose mission supported an independent living philosophy, and started to scratch some of my wanderlust with trips to Nicaragua, Europe, and Africa.

In 1990, equipped with several degrees in an otherwise ready for the world of work, I decided to move to Los Angeles and try my hand at acting since I had a drama background. This proved to be an interesting 2 years for me living on Sunset Boulevard with my attendant, who ultimately turned out to be both gay and a thief impersonating me with my credit card when he went out, but that's another story. I auditioned for a number of parts while there, and of course much like today, people with disabilities are barely on the radar in Hollywood for being seriously considered for acting parts. Nevertheless, I was of course rejected on countless occasions. Perhaps the most rewarding rejection came when I read for a pineapple company commercial. Standing in line with hundreds of beautiful girls wearing bathing suits waiting to audition wasn't the worst experience I've had. Serendipitously, I did get a couple parts playing a lawyer in the People's Court-type half-hour show, signaling to me that since being a lawyer requires being a part entertainer, I might not be so bad at it. At any rate, after a number of interesting experiences, I decided to come back to reality and returned to Canada briefly, next having made the decision to go to the London School of Economics in England for a Masters of Law degree.

My graduate experience in England was in many respects an intellectual haven. Students engaged in vigorous debates on interesting topics of the law, fascinating lectures, amidst the eclectic buzz of London. While there, I needed a capstone experience in England to quench my eccentric side, and this involved literally being roped up with mountain climbing gear to my manual wheelchair like a calf for branding and being thrown off a crane plunging to my death until of course the bungee cord holding me yanked back my fall.

I could have stayed forever, and truly wanted to launch into a career in international human rights in London or elsewhere in Europe. This however, was not to be. I brought two attendants with me to bolster my support systems and avoid burning them out. Shortly after arriving, one became homesick and crashed into a serious depression. The other drank so heavily that he eventually put my safety and security at risk. As a result, I had to return to leave school early and return to Thunder Bay.

My mother was living in Thunder Bay by that time. So there I was, a promising career in international law crashed, high student debt, 30 years old, and living at my mothers house. The core supports whom I had trusted just ruthlessly turned on me, and I had no job.

It was now time to apply the skills that I had learned since my injury. I had to trust in myself, knowing that this was a low point, but I had been lower. And if I wasn't defeated before, then the traits and skills I used in the hospital would help me succeed again. It was important to reach out to those who truly cared for me, believe in my instincts, and set short- and long-term goals for my future. I had the added advantage of having acquired many academic and professional skills since my accident. Therefore, I reached out to a budding network of colleagues and set my sights first on work that comported with my interests and passions. The combination of this experience had to bear fruit and turn things around.

I began my clerkship articling in a poverty law clinic before becoming a member of the Ontario Law Bar in 1996. This was also the year that I met my first wife Alison who I dated until 2002, got married, then divorced in 2007. Like any couple who ends up divorcing, our marriage was filled with high and low points best kept private.

Professionally, in looking back, I observed once again that I was all educated up and technically ready to begin working, but still had a passionate itch to scratch. One of the research passions I pursued obtaining my law degrees was Civil Rights legislation for persons with disabilities nationally and internationally. I didn't like how I was occasionally ignored, condescended, and paternalized by ignorant able-bodied persons, and I wanted to heighten the public's awareness of just what people with disabilities were capable of doing.

So, instead of beginning a law practice, in 1997 after much planning, marketing and corporate sponsorship, I decided to trek cross Canada in my power wheelchair to raise spinal cord injury cure research money and awareness about the abilities of people with SCI.

This physical journey tested me and my crew both physically and mentally from beginning to end. The journey began in April on the east coast in an intense winter storm, passing through the intense heat of the prairies during harvest time, and crossing the Rocky Mountains just before winter set in again. I rolled my chair into a ditch and broke three ribs along the way, but our focus was on finishing the journey.

The rationale for this major event was to produce an opportunity for highly targeted mass communications that portrayed the potential of persons with a disability. One needed to look no further than Darth Vader or the Jerry Lewis telethon to know that there was a barrage of messages in popular culture and in the mainstream media that showed negative stereotypes of persons with a disability. We wanted to play our part in contributing to turning the tide of this discrimination. It was a monumental task, and deep prejudices persist against the disabled within Canadian and American society, and so we did not build Rome with one wheel across Canada, but I like to think that the perspective of many was challenged, refreshed, and maybe changed.

After some rest but relatively still sore from the country tour, I settled in to begin practicing law in Thunder Bay in 1998. The Northern Ontario winters are unimaginably frigid for anyone who has never lived in such conditions. Average daily highs in January and February are often $-30°$ below zero without a wind chill, nights even colder. The sun rises after 8:30 a.m. and sets around 4:30 p.m., and so for several months people come and go to work in the dark. Being in a wheelchair makes living in such conditions even more challenging. I often would bundle up with only the slits of my eyes showing and trek down the street or sidewalk (whichever was cleared of snow) in my power wheelchair. I'm sure that people thought I was nuts, and I wasn't sure whether I could rationally convince them otherwise on the coldest days. But, I needed to make a living, and the para-transit van wasn't always reliable.

And so I began practicing my passion: helping those with disabilities pursue their civil rights. I have done this in a variety of ways over the years, but the themes have been two pronged. I continue to take on major public awareness projects and advocate for the substantive equal rights of persons with a disability before Administrative Tribunals and the Courts. After all, I want to work hard as well as play hard.

My law practice from the start set out to provide excellence in advocacy for all individuals, with a particular emphasis on persons with a disability. I will often appear before mental health review boards or what is termed in Ontario as The Consent and Capacity Board. This body hears matters related to persons detained involuntarily in a psychiatric hospital or found incapable of consenting to treatment. Also, I have been able to represent individuals with a physical disability in human rights matters before Appellate Courts, and work for policy and legislative changes. This has meant a period as the founding Chair of the Accessibility Advisory

Council under the former Ontarians with Disabilities Act. I also represented Independent Living Canada in New York during deliberations to draft the United Nations Convention on the Rights of Persons with Disabilities.

The law and policy work was fun and I felt it was also rather important, but I couldn't exclusively push a pen (or in my case type with a pen in my mouth). The itch for adventure returned. As if Thunder Bay was not cold enough, I had to go further. In April 2009, I planted a wheelchair accessible parking sign on the North Pole. This has for centuries been symbolic of barriers that humanity faced and felt compelled to overcome, and I believe that the 650 million persons across the world, who live with a disability, face such challenges more profoundly than anyone else on Earth on a daily basis. I wanted to lead a team that turned this barrier on its head, and so almost exactly one century to the day after the first successful expedition to the North Pole, Chris Watkins and I arrived for the first time in history on behalf of all persons with a disability to at least symbolically make it wheelchair accessible.

We had not had enough that year. In December, Chris and I did a sky dive near New Orleans with me setting a world record for a wheelchair user at an altitude of approximately 28,500 feet. This was very close to the able-bodied civilian record. I paid a price by breaking my left femur, and now carrying a prosthetic hip, but I am now recovered and found joy in participating in such a positive demonstration of embracing the boundless.

My view is that advocacy must be broad and holistic to have effect. Therefore, changes in public portrayal, the law, policy, community supports, personal empowerment, and litigation must combine to move the yardstick of human rights and civil liberties for the 50 million persons living with a disability in the United States and Canada. This was the model for change proposed in my first book, *The Six Degrees of Dignity: Disability in an Age of Freedom*. Although I am currently on the adjudicative side of this coin because I am a part-time member of the Human Rights Tribunal of Ontario and must pull back somewhat from direct advocacy, I believe that this remains a sound approach to creating an inclusive community and enhancing the self-esteem and self-worth of persons with disabilities. It is a theme that I intend to investigate further as I study how equality is enforced by the judiciary in the United States, Canada, and the United Kingdom while continuing my PhD in the Faculty of Law at the University of Leeds over the next few years.

My advice to students in training and veteran counselors is simple and straightforward. Too many in society sell us (the disabled) short in so many ways. Don't prejudge or underestimate our abilities physically or mentally. History shows that many of us have done and continue to do exemplary things far exceeding most able-bodied persons (e.g., FDR, Stephen Hawking, Stevie Wonder, Beethoven, Wilma Rudolph, etc.). We need a chance and we need you to give your very best to us. We need your understanding, empathy (not sympathy or pity), and support. We have career aspirations, sexual needs, social support needs, and to live life equally among those who take these things for granted. And we need you to treat us with the same dignity and respect that you would want for yourself or your loved ones.

As for me, my journey continues. I'm not a psychologist and so I don't really know how to explain my psychological makeup. All I do know is that what hasn't killed me (literally) so far has only made me stronger. Professionals and doctors telling me I couldn't do something only made me more resilient. Enduring the most sad and painful of times only makes me appreciate even more the simple joys of watching a sunset with my girlfriend Darlene. I did not choose to break my neck, but I have chosen and taken control of my life since then. I got busy living.

DISCUSSION QUESTIONS

1. Name and discuss people with disabilities who appear to have thrived and succeeded despite their circumstances. List any qualities or traits learned in positive psychology they appear to have mastered.
2. Name and discuss people who are not disabled who appear to have thrived and succeeded. List any qualities or traits learned in positive psychology they appear to have mastered.
3. What is success and how would you measure it?
4. What are the similarities and differences between what society believes/tells us through the media and mass marketing is a successful and happy person versus what positive psychology research shows?

EXERCISES

A. Have students write a paper re: what, if any, changes they need to make in their lives to thrive and experience well-being and sustained happiness.
B. Have students interview and write a reaction paper on someone they know with or without a disability who they believe best exemplifies the traits and qualities described in positive psychology. Interview questions should include how the interviewees perceives themselves, their environment, and what they think, do, and feel about how they conduct their affairs. In other words, what is their worldview and how do they fit into the larger picture.

PART FOUR

Counseling Strategies and Insights for Working With Persons With Disabilities

Which Counseling Theories and Techniques Work Best With Different Disability Populations and Why

Michael Jay Millington

OVERVIEW

The identity of rehabilitation counseling is rooted in the constructs of counseling psychology and is expressed through current best practice. To ask which theories and techniques work best and why is to ask, "Who are we?" or more specifically, "Who are we becoming?" Rehabilitation adopted counseling's lineage, history, and culture early on and has been pursuing its unique identity within the counseling community ever since. If an evidence base is the measure, we are only beginning to define ourselves. We can see the form of our discipline emerging from the field. The fundamental mission of full community inclusion drives the process and discerns what is of value in each theory and each technique. We pursue a pragmatic eclecticism that chooses the "best fit" for our clients and ourselves—not atheoretical, but pan-theoretical. Through our choices, we build a unified approach to serve a diverse population.

In this chapter, we will trace the emerging threads of rehabilitation counseling through the generic counseling theories and techniques. We will not attempt to catalog and differentiate the evidence base, which is beyond the scope of this text (see Chan, Cardoso, & Chronister, 2009; Stout & Hayes, 2005). In order to address the existential questions, what works and why, we will instead focus on the relevance of theory to the community of rehabilitation counseling and an accounting of successful applications of theory to practice. We will start at the roots of counseling and move outward—from common factors to schools of thought—and attempt to show how counseling fits into our community-based world. From the broader view that best embraces evidence-based and emerging practice as signs of our struggle for identity, we hope to better address the teleological question of our becoming.

COMMON FACTORS OF COUNSELING AND BASIC TECHNIQUES

Perhaps 70% of the therapeutic effect of counseling is attributable to conditions that are common to all forms (Wampold, 2000). A great deal of research has been carried out for identifying and validating these common factors, and they are at the core of any claims to evidence. What is striking about these conditions is how fundamentally common they are. The core conditions are a therapeutic interpretation of the golden rule. The therapeutic alliance is an ethos of communion. The basic techniques are the engine of collaborative work in any context. The foundation of counseling is community.

Empathy, Congruence, and Unconditional Positive Regard (Agape)

Empathy, congruence, and unconditional positive regard are the core conditions of a therapeutic counseling relationship. Empathy is a threefold way of subjectively, objectively, and interpersonally knowing the client's experience (Clark, 2010). Subjective empathy arises out of the internal resonance one feels in experiencing the narrative of the other. The subjective response is visceral, affective, and experienced through identification, intuition, and imagination. Objective empathy arises out of data elicited from the client's frame of reference (Clark, 2007). Self-report inventories and other evaluation tools provide the raw materials on which the counselor acts in building a client schema. Objective empathy is a concrete and critical appraisal of the knowledge at hand. The most Rogerian way of knowing a client's experience is through interpersonal empathy. Interpersonal empathy transpires in a here-and-now relationship between counselor and client. It is a way of knowing through communication. It is not enough to passively listen to the client's story; the counselor must actively engage in understanding the story through questions and encouragement. In this active engagement, the counselor communicates empathy back to the client. It is not enough for the counselor to feel empathy for it to be interpersonal; the client must experience the counselor's empathy as well. Through interpersonal empathy, the counselor (a) comes as close as possible to the phenomenological source experience, (b) reflects what is experienced, and (c) explores for deeper comprehension.

Clark (2010) calls for an integration and synthesis of all forms of empathic knowledge. Regardless of the counseling strategy, the counselor builds a clear and detailed phenomenological understanding of the client that will inform future interventions. Of the core conditions, empathy is the fundamental one. Congruence and unconditional positive regard are arguably instrumental aspects of empathy. Congruence is the quality of genuineness or authenticity that the counselor brings to the relationship. It is also the absence of counselor baggage; a counseling-specific mindfulness, focused completely on the subject at hand. Unconditional positive regard reflects a genuine valuing of the other-in-themselves. Unconditional positive regard is love, in the sense of *agape*, an unconditional and voluntary love of humankind.

Working Alliance

The therapeutic (or working) alliance refers to the qualities of the client/counselor relationship that arise out of the implementation of the core conditions. The working alliance builds on four client/counselor themes: (a) collaboration; (b) emotional bonding; (c) correspondence on goals, process, and tasks (Horvath & Symonds, 1991); and (d) motivation to work toward those goals (Wampold, 2001). There is strong evidence, supported by comprehensive meta-analysis, that the working alliance has a direct and moderate therapeutic effect (Martin, Garske, & Davis, 2000) across counseling strategies.

Microskills (communication and verbal skills)

The particulars of intervention, the individual tactics that make up the work of the working alliance, are known as microskills (Daniels & Ivey, 2007). They are the vocabulary of the working alliance. The basic microskills (Kuntze, van der Molen, & Born, 2009) set the stage for further development:

- *encouraging communication*, brief verbal indications that the client is being heard;
- *asking questions*, facilitating the client's attempts to put thoughts into words;
- *paraphrasing content*, rephrasing and returning the client's message in a common language that communicates understanding;
- *reflecting feelings*, mirroring back the emotions expressed in the client narrative;
- *concreteness*, facilitate client precision in describing their issues and situations;
- *summarizing*, structuring the story by putting order to the main points of the narrative; and
- *clarifying*, identifying ambiguities or misunderstandings in the counseling process.

Advanced microskills are differentiated by their goal of facilitating client insight (Kuntze et al., 2009):

- *advanced accurate empathy*, a counselor-generated interpretation of the client's narrative that sharpens the view for both;
- *confrontation*, a form of advanced accurate empathy that generates a distinctly different and yet cogent interpretation of the narrative for client exploration of discrepancies in cognition, affect, or behavior (Strong & Zeman, 2010);
- *positive relabeling*, a constructive and positive reframing of formerly negative aspects of the presenting problem to alter negative self-images;
- *counselor disclosure*, a sharing of personal experience to clarify points and demonstrate empathy; and
- *directedness*, a dedication to frank, open discussion about the here-and-now.

Microskills are the means by which theory is translated into practice. They are used in different combinations for different results, but the assembly serves as the foundation for the myriad of theories and models.

Applied Basic Techniques

The working alliance sets the stage upon which fundamental techniques can be used. The intentional meeting of counselors and clients implies that clients have something they wish to accomplish or change, a problem they want to resolve, or a plan they wish to put into action. The counselor uses basic verbal and nonverbal skills through the process of an interview to surface the issues, learn about the client, set the goals, develop a plan, implement the plan, and deal with various issues in the world and in the client (e.g., conflict, resistance to change along the way). This is the basic logic model that is interpreted and reinterpreted in every counseling method (see Koch, McReynolds, & Rumrill, 2004).

Application is universal and the evidence is overwhelming. Counseling is fundamentally human and accessible. The most powerful mechanism of psychotherapy is not some obscure and dangerous intervention; it is applied humanity. Counseling provides a discipline for skill refinement, but the basic skill set is universal, communal, and accessible to any person who cares enough to listen.

PSYCHODYNAMIC ROOTS: ADLERIAN PSYCHOTHERAPY

The roots of counseling inevitably lead to the psychodynamic origins of psychotherapy. More for philosophy than science, the psychodynamic perspective will be discussed here, providing rehabilitation counseling with insight into deeper psychological conflicts, but not much in the way of quantifiable outcomes. We will focus on Adlerian psychotherapy (Mosak & Maniacci, 2010) as the most philosophically attuned to community.

Adlerian Concepts

Adler perceived humans as social entities that cannot be studied or treated in isolation (Mosak & Maniacci, 2010). Our social identities are constantly emerging and dynamic. We express ourselves through ongoing active relationships. Our identities are bound up in this active sense, in what Adler referred to as a lifestyle. His individual psychology held that all behavior is goal directed (Rule, 2004) and that these goals are pursued through an endless progression of choices based on an established set of cognitive convictions—the lived lifestyle. People pursue perfection, mastery, self-realization, power, and other individual growth needs in a social world through the guidance of their convictions.

Healthy social interaction is preferred. We desire to see and be seen with positive regard. Normality is finding your identity in being part of the group. Neurosis is the block, the "yes-but" that stops the individual from engaging in a healthy relationship with the community. Neurosis, one could say, is a self-imposed form of community exclusion. The contexts where lifestyle is expressed and choices are made are the tasks of life: engaging in society, work, sex, spiritual life, and coping with ourselves. Psychological health is measured by success and failure in these tasks.

Adler valued family constellations as the fundamental social context and the origin of healthy or neurotic lifestyles. Birth order is highly influential in Adler's thinking. The early socialization of the child sets the convictions on which the lifestyle will be built. Children develop convictions about themselves early on, often based on faulty information and limited cognitive ability. However contrived, they move in the world "as-if" these convictions were true. Where dysfunctional convictions take root, conflicts arise between "who I am" and "who I should be," between right and wrong, and between self and the nature of the world.

Inferiority emerges out of discrepancy between the real and ideal self. Compensation is the primary defense mechanism that comes into play to protect the psyche from these feelings of inferiority. Lifestyle creates the perspective of daily reality. It colors what is seen, how it is seen, what is ignored, and leads one to both successes and failures (Rule, 2004). A lifestyle built on unworkable convictions, inferiority, and compensatory response leads to challenges in the tasks of life.

Adlerian Practice

Adlerian counseling is positive, collaborative, and social. Clients in the Adlerian parlance are discouraged (rather than dysfunctional) and the direct therapeutic response is encouragement. The counseling process is a cooperative education—a mutually engaged venture to reorient the lifestyle, uncover and change faulty convictions, develop a healthy social interest, decrease feelings of inferiority, seek out and replace faulty motivation, develop an appreciation for others as valuable members of the community, and becoming a contributing member of the community.

The counselor is a role model, but very human. The counselor is encouraged to be seen as fallible and humorous. Adlerian techniques include imagery and imagination as a means of making alternate lifestyles more real and approachable. For instance, when the client says "If only I could. . .," the counselor engages the client in practicing living in the desired state that follows, and making decisions "as if" that desired state were true. The experience provides fodder for counseling exploration.

The push-button technique is used to demonstrate the link between cognitions and affect, and how the client can control emotions by changing thought processes. In the push-button technique, the client is asked to imagine a past positive event and to reexperience the corresponding affect. The activity is then repeated with a negatively charged experience, and then again repeated with a positive recollection.

Catching oneself is a technique in which the client becomes sensitized to and mindful of situations where old, dysfunctional thoughts arise, and learns to stop "going there." Analysis covers the life tasks, and work is done in all areas. Goals and tasks are developed collaboratively and adjusted to the level of competence and motivation of the client. Since all action is intentional and all movement is toward a positive end, the client in Adlerian counseling is working toward a moment of insight, an "aha" moment, where one sees the choices they make from a new more healthy perspective.

Application in Rehabilitation

As is the case with other psychodynamic psychotherapies, there is more theoretical application than proof. Adlerian techniques have been used successfully in group couples therapy to facilitate marital adjustment to mental illness (Croake & Kelly,

2002). Adlerian techniques have been developed for use as an adjunct to the following: cognitive therapy (CT) in the prevention of depressive relapses (Waller, Carlson, & Englar-Carlson, 2006), guided visual imagery for stress and coping (Kaufman, 2007), lifestyle analysis for treating anxiety (Hjertaas, 2009), childhood adjustment to deafness (Farrugia, 1986), and adjustment to orthopedic disabilities (Sigmon, 1986). However, little empirical research has been forthcoming to support these potential applications.

The Adlerian approach is presently most useful to rehabilitation as a philosophy and for the case it makes for community inclusion. There is substantial research into the impact of unfulfilled need to belong, a concept central to the substance of mental health in Adlerian psychotherapy (Shifron, 2010), on cognitive, affective, and behavioral outcomes (Gere & MacDonald, 2010), and with this a growing interest in applications for social justice, specifically through the mechanism of community inclusion (see Todman & Mansager, 2009). Adlerian approaches have been used organizationally and may be an intervention that serves the purpose of creating a more receptive and inclusive environment.

HUMANISTIC THEORIES AND TECHNIQUES

The humanistic theories resonate with the practice of rehabilitation counseling, and for good reason. Both celebrate the basic goodness and constructive nature of human beings. Roger's person-centered approach focuses on the dyad, the creation of a communicative space where insight happens. Frankl's logo therapy (1986) focuses on the search for, and centrality of, meaning in our lives. Both see people as strengths and potential.

Person-Centered Counseling

Carl Rogers posited that people were fundamentally good, could direct their own affairs, and would do so in positive ways ... with the appropriate encouragement. His approach was less theory and strategy and more of an expression of values through action. Person-centered counseling creates a space for personal exploration and the contemplation of change. Empathy, positive regard, and genuineness are behaviorally expressed values that focus therapy and not on technique *per se*, but on the relationship between counselor and client, and they are the necessary and sufficient conditions for therapy (Rogers, 1957).

Concepts

Person-centered counseling grounds self-actualization in instinct. Self-actualization is akin to a primal drive. Issues come from bad experiences that become part of the self-concept. Self-concept is learned behavior; it flourishes in the presence of unconditional love and positive regard. When love becomes conditional, self-concept is thwarted by these interjected values, and the resultant personality becomes its own obstacle to self-actualization. The disconnection between the natural proclivity for self-actualization and the shell of defense mechanisms that builds up around a frustrated personality is the source of conflict and anxiety. Therapy becomes the weakening of defense mechanisms to allow the healthy and natural self to emerge. Relationships are the target and context of therapy (See & Kamnetz, 2004). Appropriate counseling relationships are defined by 6 conditions.

1. The client and the counselor are in psychological contact.
2. The client is in a state of "incongruence" or internal conflict.
3. The counselor is congruent (genuine) in the relationship.
4. The counselor communicates unconditional positive regard for the client.
5. The counselor communicates an empathic understanding of the client's point of view by relating what is perceived.
6. Empathy and positive regard are communicated to the client.

Roger's focused on demonstrating genuineness, empathy, and positive regard results in an honest exploration of the client issues. The approach is nondirective, trusting that clients will address what they need to address.

Application in rehabilitation

Over 50 years of research supports the basic tenets of person-centered therapy inasmuch as they reflect most clearly the "common factors" that undergird all counseling models (Greenberg, Elliot & Lietaer, 1994; Lambert & Bergin, 1994; Wampold, 2000). These factors, particularly as interpreted by Rogers, have become accepted canon in the rehabilitation counseling literature over the years (see Rubin & Roessler, 2001; See, 1986; Thomas, Thoreson, Parker, & Butler, 1998). Outcome studies specific to the field suggest evidence supporting its utility in improving vocational outcomes in terms of employment, income, psychological well-being, and job satisfaction (Bozarth & Rubin, 1978).

Person-centered counseling is a foundational tool with generally positive effects across populations and contexts. These positive effects are necessary, but not sufficient, for the efficacious delivery of rehabilitation services, facilitating, and yet requiring technical proficiency (Kanfer & Goldstein, 1991) in specific interventions. Techniques include attending, reflecting, and confrontation.

See and Kamnetz (2004) outline how a person-centered approach can be integrated into the continuum of rehabilitation service by stages. In the first stage the counselor-client relationship is being established as they work through the evaluation process. Rapport is established through the facilitative conditions, and the client explores early feelings and moves toward a determination that positive change is both possible and desirable. In the planning and implementation stages, person-centered counseling is supporting rather than driving the processes; available for dealing with inner conflicts that arise as plans and strategies are made.

CONSIDERATIONS. Real-life experience (See & Kamnetz, 2004) is a necessary foundation for person-centered counseling. To the degree that life experiences have been impoverished, isolated, passive, there is less experience to draw upon. The client's worldview must accept introspection as a means to change, posing a cross-cultural challenge (Freeman, 1993). Person-centered counseling leans heavily on the framework of communication and tends to be a highly verbal exchange. Relationships are built on language: the less verbal the client, the harder it will be to establish the facilitative conditions and engage inner conflicts.

The nondirective nature of person-centered counseling does not lend itself to the directed and time-limited work of rehabilitation counseling. It works best as a foundational tool and a means to sharpen focus on the working alliance.

Logotherapy

Victor Frankl's Logotherapy (1988) is in the framework of rehabilitation philosophy. It emerges out of the depth psychology of psychodynamic approaches (Mendelowitz & Schneider, 2008), but from the ontological perspective as opposed to the biological. Spirituality played an important role in Frankl's construct. His particular brand of existentialism was firmly rooted in the exchange between the self and the world, how identity is created as a commitment to action. Healing is an expression of personal meaning through action in the world. Logotherapy is not about primal drives; it is a search for meaning in existence. This is philosophy applied to the personal; what does it mean to be me, a person with a disability? It is for the counselor to assist in the search for answers (Ososkie & Holzbauer, 2004).

Life has meaning across the space and span of life (see Super, 1990). People are moved by force of will toward a search for meaning and all meaning is related to life. (Why do I want this sandwich? Because I am hungry. Why am I hungry? Because I need to eat. Why do I need to eat? So that I can live. Why do I need to live?). We are free to pursue a will to meaning. The dimensions of the self, engaged in this pursuit of meaning are mind (psyche), body (soma), and spirit (noetic). Spirit is the uniquely human aspect of life and the primary guide to action beyond the drives of biology and psychology. After spirituality, freedom is the next defining characteristic of human experience. We are free to choose how we view our experience, how we think about it, and how we will respond within it. The third defining characteristic of the human experience is responsibility, which ties the person to the community. In our freedom to respond, we find freedom to act on behalf of and in communion with someone or something beyond ourselves. Responsibility sets the field that completes identity; human identity is not simply the satisfaction of animal drives, but what we freely choose to do on behalf of others.

Meaning is revealed through the exercise of values. Frankl (1984) defines three:

- Creative values arising out of work and its consequences
- Experiential values arising out of aesthetic experience
- Attitudinal values arising out of the events and suffering of their lives

Dysfunction arises out of disengagement from life (that which brings meaning to the world). The isolated client views the world in a chronic apperception of meaninglessness. Frankl believed that meaninglessness was also found in the direct pursuit of pleasure and happiness for their own sake. True happiness, according to Frankl, was to be found in the pursuit of meaning, never fully realized. Suffering and struggle are the means of meaning-making. True happiness is the fruit of existential struggle.

Techniques

The prime intervention of Logotherapy is meaning analysis, a psychodynamic principle brought down into common philosophy and the core of treatment. In the course of the counseling dialog, microskill techniques are applied to open communication. Dereflection involves shifting the client's focus away from obsessive dwelling upon the negative aspects of physical, psychological, or sociological problems. In this initial stage, the focus shifts to (a) identifying what is under the client's control, (b) releasing that which is not, and (c) building on the positive aspects of lived experience. The client learns to detach from the conflicts of their lives, contemplate objectively, plan strategically, and take control of their situational attitudes. Openness to change occurs when thinking is no longer monopolized by attending to symptoms or the cognitions and affect that habitually coincide with them. At this point, the client is prepared to search for new meaning, to move beyond self-absorption to an interpretation of self as engaged in the world.

Application in rehabilitation counseling

Frankl's existential philosophy is a spiritual fit with the origins of rehabilitation theory as laid out in Wright's (1983) Somatopsychological model. The study of self-transcendence in the context of life-threatening illness (e.g., cancer, HIV, AIDS) demonstrates the connection (Lukas & Hirsch, 2002). The psychology of transcending and succumbing are covered in detail in an accompanying chapter, but here they are played out in existential terms. The profession of rehabilitation counseling exists to address community exclusion of people with disabilities. Isolation from life and the challenge of dealing with loss, chronic symptomology, progressive illness, and impending death have biological, psychological, sociological, and spiritual ramifications that are fully illustrated in logotherapy (Gould, 1993). While logotherapy research has been limited, the possibilities are open. It is a promising venue for integrating the spirituality of religious clients. In the meanwhile it has value simply for its foundational contribution to behavioral, cognitive, and affective approaches.

BEHAVIORAL, COGNITIVE, AND AFFECTIVE APPROACHES

From behavioral, to cognitive-behavioral, to rational-emotive behavior we find variations on a theme of A-B-C. An event (A), usually negative, engages irrational beliefs (B) (Nieuwenhuijsen, Verbeek, de Boer, Blonk, & van Dijk, 2010). Irrational beliefs lead to dysfunctional consequences (C), that is, thoughts, emotions, and behaviors. Each theoretical approach stakes out a different perspective of this communication dynamic. The counseling distinction between them is a matter of degree (Beck & Weishaar, 2010) and style. In all facets, counselors began to engage the client in the here-and-now, with regard to immediately changeable behaviors within the client's control.

Behavioral Therapy

Human social behavior, functional or otherwise, is learned behavior. Maladaptive behaviors are those that served some specific purpose in the past that now ultimately work against the client's best interests. The behavior continues, despite growing dysfunction because it has become habituated, and new learning is needed to undo the current behavior and replace it with a more constructive behavior, such as coping skills, communication skills, and responses to emotional conflicts (Wilson, 2000).

Techniques

There are two basic approaches to behavior therapy. Classical conditioning is learning via the classic Pavlovian response where a conditioned stimulus (CS) is paired with an unconditioned stimulus (US), resulting in the development of a conditioned response (CR). When a CR has been established, the client may generalize this learning to a set of cues (e. g., fear of dogs) or discriminate to the specific cue under any context (e. g., fear of *that* dog). Factors that influence classical conditioning are (a) the order (CS proceeds US), (b) time (delay between CS and US), (c) repetition (number of trials), and (d) characteristics of the CS and US. Techniques based on classical conditioning are generally about "unlearning" maladaptive CRs through such techniques as systematic desensitization (stepwise introduction of anxiety-provoking stimulus paired with a relaxation to remove the CR), flooding (exposing clients to anxiety-provoking stimuli with opportunity to escape), implosive therapy (imaging a flooding experience), and aversive therapy (replacing the CR with an unpleasant CR).

Operant conditioning is interactive learning based on the idea that people will pursue and learn behaviors that are reinforced and avoid behaviors that are punished. Positive reinforcement occurs when you get something you want. Negative reinforcement occurs when you get less of something that you do not want. Positive punishment is an increase in unwanted consequences. Negative punishment is a decrease in desirable consequences. Schedules of reinforcement shape and maintain behavior through the strategic manipulation of these four possible consequences. Operant conditioning extinguishes maladaptive behaviors, but unlike classical conditioning, it is equally effective in building new behaviors. Factors that influence the efficacy of operant conditioning are:

- the contingent relationship between the target behavior and the reinforcer;
- immediacy, strength, schedule, and prompts of reinforcement; and
- generalizability of the learned behavior.

Techniques include behavioral contracts (Kazdin, 2000), token economies, and social skills training. Behavioral contracts are generated through the working relationship between the client and the counselor. It specifies target behaviors, reinforcers, conditions by which the contract can be modified to fit the needs of the client progress, alternate reinforcers, and a feedback process that provides frequent updates on client progress. Token economies reinforce desirable behavior with tokens that can be traded for other desirable reinforcers. They have well-defined target behaviors, contingent reinforcement with tokens, a consistent monitoring and evaluation system, and a plan to transition the client behavior from a token economy to a real one (James & Gilliland, 2003). Social skill training is not strictly a behavioral approach, but it depends heavily on the reinforcement of classical and operant conditioning. Techniques often employed include rehearsal of behaviors, modeling, coaching, feedback, and homework.

Rehabilitation counseling applications

Research has been pursued in a variety of disability contexts, including substance abuse, (Rotgers, 1996), traumatic brain injury (Giles, Ridley, Dill, & Frye, 1997), developmental disabilities (Griffiths, Feldman, & Tough, 1997), psychiatric disabilities (Corrigan & Liberman, 1994), and chronic pain (McCracken, 1997). Substance abuse was one of the early adopters of behavioral techniques (Stoll, 2004). Covert sensitization (conditioning an aversive CR to imagined alcohol consuming situations) has been used to mixed results. Manipulating reinforcers in the community (creating alternative activities that are more attractive than substance abuse) has demonstrated positive effect on sobriety, employment, and family involvement (Hunt & Azrin, 1973). Psychological modeling has been shown to be an effective and fast approach, particularly when abstinence is the goal (Rotgers, 1996).

Traumatic brain injury applications have been studied and found effective in ameliorating behavioral loss, mediating behavior excess, and replacing maladaptive behaviors with constructive alternatives (Giles et al., 1997). The timing of reinforcement for clients with TBI is crucial and immediate. Counseling is approached as a psychoeducational intervention. The client is fully informed of the goals and processes of intervention, as well as what will and will not be reinforced. Goal behaviors are chosen and analyzed, and training for the behavior is broken down into steps sufficiently small enough to be accomplished. A variety of reinforcers are employed judiciously to shape and maintain behavior. Treatment schedules are long term and continuous. Fading does not occur until the behavior is well established (Lewis & Bitter, 1991). Timeout has been used in training people with TBI, although memory loss limits efficacy (Marr, 1982). Overcorrection involves the repeated practice of an appropriate behavior that is not compatible with the maladaptive behavior. It is particularly effective with people who have memory loss and or reduced executive function, such as planning, because it simultaneously practices and rewards the desired behavior, while interfering with opportunities for expression and practice of the maladaptive behavior.

Clients with developmental disabilities have been the primary candidates for behavioral programs. Early application focused on ADLs such as toileting and household chores (Madle & Neisworth, 1990) and job training employment (Systematic instruction). Shaping, prompting, reinforcing, and chaining are essential steps in the process. Other applications are used for removing maladaptive behaviors, such as pica (eating nonfood items, such as hair, dirt, etc.), self-injurious stimulation (head banging, slapping, biting), and impulsivity (Dixon et al., 1998).

Cognitive and Cognitive-Behavioral Therapy

For the sake of space, we will combine cognitive and cognitive-behavioral space into a single unit, with the recognition that there are differences. CT is founded on the centrality of information processing in individual survival. Perception and cognition are the primary modes of analysis and intervention. Affect and behavior are treated as consequences of cognition. Thinking is organized in schemas; faulty schemas cause faulty emotions and behaviors.

Cognitive-behavioral therapy (CBT) embraces the same cognition-affect-behavior cycle with a similar focus on cognition. However, the concept of experience is promoted to the instrumental mode; cognitions and behaviors reinforce each other and cognitions can be changed through learning new behaviors. The distinction between the two is largely a matter of degree on a spectrum of possible approaches (Beck & Weishaar, 2010).

CT and CBT assume that the maladaptive behavior and affect of psychological disorders are learned maladaptive ways of dealing with the world and maladaptive ways of thinking about oneself in the context of the world. By intervening at the level of cognition, CT and CBT identify these maladaptive and destructive ways of thinking in an effort to change the pattern: learning to think differently to evaluate the world differently, thereby respond to the world differently, and thereby change the affective response. The CT information-processing perspective focuses on the development of recurrent and identifiable schema that reflect and respond to psychological problems. For instance, a person with high trait anxiety tends to process information with a bias toward perceiving danger, and it follows that the perception of danger leads to high-state anxiety. Personality is built on a foundation of such schema, creating cognitive vulnerabilities (Beck & Weishaar, 2010) that lead to problems in the here-and-now. The CT focuses on information processing. CBT focuses on experience. The shared objective is to modify cognitions, teach new behaviors, reduce the cognitive vulnerabilities, and engage in the community.

Concepts

What is known about a given situation is drawn from direct, past experience. Experience in the present is interpreted through the schema of expectations, beliefs, attitudes, and prejudices that have developed over time. We respond both affectively and behaviorally to the cognitive appraisals we make. Cognitions create reality. Cognition distortions create dysfunctional realities, through faulty reasoning processes, such as (Beck & Weishaar, 2010):

- *arbitrary inference*, drawing conclusions without evidence or in the face of contradicting evidence;
- *selective abstraction*, magnifying certain details, while minimizing others to fit preexisting bias;
- *overgeneralization*, magnifying or minimizing and event beyond the rational in context;
- *personalization*, attributing self-responsibility for external events without supporting evidence; and
- *dichotomous thinking*, either total success or total failure . . . no in between.

Cognitively distorted thinking leads to, and is maintained by, three dystopian schemas: negative views of self, the world, and the future. Depression is the low concordance of the three. Mania would be the inverse. When cognitions lead to the apperception of constant danger, phobias and panic result. Anxiety disorder is the hyperfunctioning of the survival mechanism and regression to primal thinking. Obsession and compulsion is disrupted schema, stuck on uncertainty. Suicide is the consequence of perceived hopelessness and a decrease in cognitive problem-solving ability brought on by depression (see James, Reichelt, Carlsonn, & McAnaney, 2008).

Technique

The client is trained to the model, engaged as an active participant, and "colleague" (collaborative empiricism; Beck & Weishaar, 2010) in the treatment process. Therapy takes place in dialog as they determine goals; elicit and provide feedback; develop and test hypotheses, discerning the underlying logic of one's thinking through Socratic questioning; and use facts and logic to explore current thinking and try new thinking. The counselor and the client develop an understanding of the mechanics of the psychological issues at hand, seek early identification and treatment for that which is dysfunctional, gain control over cognitive and behavioral symptoms, and minimize the negative impact of stress (Basco & Rush, 1996).

The client and counselor explore how the client evaluates life events. They approach this evaluation through collaborative empiricism and guided discovery. The client is treated as a thinking and rational persons who can objectively collect and analyze the experiences of their lives and respond in a rational way. Looking at problem situations, the client describes personal responses in thinking, feeling, and acting; observes the consequences; identifies similar patterns in other aspects of life; suggests alternative ways of thinking and tries them out; and evaluates the differential effect. Behavioral and educational programs are used to disrupt the negative cognitions and actions and to facilitate learning of new strategies (James et al., 2008).

Cognitive techniques

Cognitive techniques intervene in negative thoughts (James & Gilliland, 2003) through a pragmatic scientific approach. Facilitated by the counselor, the client (1) identifies maladaptive thoughts and causally links them to the negative feelings and behaviors that follow; (2) monitors internal dialog, the "self-talk" that precipitates these events; (3) investigates the reciprocal relationship between cognitions, affect, and behavior; (4) identifies more functional and constructive thinking patterns; and (5) tests the efficacy of new hypotheses. A variety of counseling techniques are used to encourage, direct, and shape the process.

- *Distancing*: to remove oneself subjectively from the experience. By analyzing events objectively, it is possible to consider other frames of reference coolly and without preconditions. By stepping out of the learned and customary (subjective role) role and by separating thought from affect, the technique demonstrates that change is possible.
- *Redefining*: to bring situations that are perceived to be out of the client's control into the realm of control. For example, "Nobody wants to know me" becomes "I need to get out and meet people."
- *Decentering*: to realign the client's place in the world, not as the center of all things, but one in a community. Used to deal with situational anxiety, where clients believe that they are the center of public scrutiny and judgment. Schema-based hypotheses

are developed in the process of Socratic dialog and tested *in situ* (Beck & Weishaar, 2010).

- *Reattribution*: to reassign different, more positive interpretations of events. This is used particularly well with issues of personalization. It encourages the client to test the assumption of responsibility through a thorough analysis of the situation (Beck & Weishaar, 2010).
- *Decatastrophizing*: to reduce the affective response to a negative event by putting the scale of the issue in proper perspective. Often a "what if" technique is used to confront the inflated nature of catastrophic thinking (Beck & Emery, 1985).
- *Thought stopping*: to identify negative self-talk, interrupt with a sudden physical or cognitive stimulus, and redirect attention and thinking to a more positive line of thinking.
- *Relaxation and meditation*: to calm emotions, focus attention, clear thinking, and relax the body through meditation and relaxation exercises. Meditation is focusing attention singularly on an imagined or real "object" such that it is not possible to simultaneously maintain focus and ruminate on negative thoughts. Relaxation is similar to meditation, focusing on the body. By alternately tensing and relaxing various muscle groups, attention is brought into and focused on the body and wellness, displacing negativity.
- *Systematic desensitization*: to confront anxiety-producing situations and reduce their ability to affect your independent emotional state through guided experience. Techniques include mental imagery, cognitive modeling, cognitive restructuring, reframing, and stress innoculation. Many of these are techniques that are taught to the client and practiced in session. Systematic desensitization is quite behavioral in its application. In it, clients master basic relaxation techniques, and then employ them as they are exposed to imagined situations that illicit problematic levels of anxiety. This process desensitizes stepwise through a series of graduated (anxiety-causing scenarios x relaxation) techniques. Mental imagery directs the client through an imagined scenario that captures the essence of the counseling problem and challenges the client to imagine new, more efficacious ways of coping. Cognitive modeling pairs learning new, positive self-talk with actual performance of constructive behaviors. Cognitive restructuring and stress inoculation involve learning ways to cope by replacing negative self-talk with positive self-talk and acting on it. This involves developing a vocabulary of positive self-talk, practice, and homework and usually includes many of the techniques described herein.

These techniques are often provided through psychoeducational programs in conjunction with counselor guidance or "self-help" programs for self-maintenance (Cuipers, 1997).

Cognitive–behavioral techniques (CBT)

CBT posits that cognitions (thoughts, beliefs, expectations, etc.) are very powerful determinants of behavior and emotions. Behavioral techniques are used to challenge assumptions, interrupt automatic thoughts, and provide an opportunity to practice new cognitions. These concepts overlap, differing in part by emphasis.

- *Homework*: Focus on self-observation and monitoring (Beck & Weishaar, 2010; Kazantzis, 2000). If stress is a problem, client and counselor engage it, assess it, identify cognitions, and practice new cognitions.
- *Hypothesis testing*: Formulating tests of expectations; testing and trying on new hypotheses.
- *Exposure therapy*: Visiting situations that are assumed to create stress. Dealing with the experience and often finding that the fears (cognitions) were unfounded.
- *Role-play*: Practicing behavior *in situ* or in an educational environment.
- *Activity scheduling*: Tracking mood fluctuations during the day, rating them, observing the changes. Often challenging assumptions (e.g., one is never happy, or always stressed . . .) that prevent or hinder improvement.
- *Graded-task Assignment*: Moving from within a comfort zone to increasingly difficult or graduated levels of difficulty. As with phobias, practice helps to dispel automatic thoughts and cognitive distortions and replace them with more stable thoughts.

Rehabilitation application

CBT was designed specifically to deal with issues of anxiety and depression (Beck, 2008). There is considerable evidence of its applicability in these situations (see Bruce, Spiegel, & Hegel, 1999; Gloaguen, Cottraux, Cucherat, & Blackburn, 1998; Heimberg et al., 1998; Hofmann & Spiegel, 1999; Hollon, Stewart, & Strunk, 2006), including the elderly (Laidlaw, Thompson, Dick-Siskin, & Gallagher-Thompson, 2003).

Applications in dealing with chronic pain grew out of CBT success in depression and anxiety. Maladaptive cognitions put clients at risk for developing chronic pain following injury, and reduce the efficacy of rehabilitation from chronic pain that develops. A meta-analysis shows that CBT has a role in alleviating pain complaints in integrative treatment regimes (Borkum, 2010; Morley, Eccleston, & Williams, 1999) where CBT strategies are used to encourage the most adaptive beliefs, appraisals, and expectations about pain (cognitions) (Johnson & Kazantzis, 2004; Robertson, Smith, Ray, & Jones, 2009). Pain complaints are also magnified by depression, and so CBT also works to reduce pain complaints by reducing depression (see Robinson & Riley, 1999). CBT has been effective in treating bulimia nervosa (Agras, Walsh, Fairburn, Wilson, & Kraemer, 2000) and dually diagnosed SUD and bulimia (Sysko & Hildebrandt, 2009). CBT appears helpful in Bipolar disorder control of symptoms and medical compliance (Basco & Rush, 1996). With chronic fatigue syndrome, CBT shows promise in stress management in group format with significant reduction in stress compared with relaxation alone (Deale, Chalder, Marks, & Wessely, 1997). CBT techniques have been successfully used to identify self-defeating behaviors and create problem-solving interventions in psychoeducational formats for career development for persons with disabilities (Farley, 1987). Emerging application with cancer survivor supports dealing with the issues of anxiety, depression, and fatigue associated with cancer treatment and survival using CBT models (e.g., "guided self-help" homework assignments) to facilitate function, decision-making, and treatment compliance decisions (Ferguson, Cassel, & Dawson, 2010) while coping with pain, nausea, and psychological stress.

CT has demonstrated utility with meta-analyses (Butler, Chapman, Forman, & Beck, 2006), finding large effect size for depression, generalized anxiety, social phobia (Eng, Roth, & Heimberg, 2001); moderate effect size, with anger (see Beck, 1999) and chronic pain; and small effect size for eating disorders (Bowers, 2001; Pike, Walsh, Vitousek, Wilson, & Bauer, 2003) and schizophrenia. CT has demonstrated utility for panic disorder (Clark, 1996), substance abuse (Carroll & Onken, 2005), and posttraumatic stress disorder (Gillespie, Duffy, Hackmann, & Clark, 2002).

Stress innoculation training (Meichenbaum, 1985), an application of CBT, has been developed for use with people with traumatic brain injury to deal with impulsive behaviors that often emerge, including physical aggression, socially inappropriate sexuality, and stealing. Aeschleman and Imes (1999) report overall decrease in observed impulsivity measures but wide variability in a small clinical sample. It is possible that memory impairment makes the application of new skills (stopping impulse behaviors through cognitions) difficult.

Rational-Emotive Behavior Therapy (REBT)

CT and CBT therapies build on the assumed importance and centrality of schemas in underlying pathology. Rational-emotive behavior therapy (REBT) does not make such distinctions (Beck & Weishaar, 2010). REBT is arguably a variant on CBT and part of a cognitive-affective-behavioral spectrum. It can be differentiated from CT by its aggressively persuasive approach and use of psychoeducational and "emotive-vocative" (Ellis, 2008, p. 210) methods, but otherwise the differences are largely a matter of emphasis and degree (Dryden & David, 2008). Regardless, REBT stands on its own in the literature and earns a separate appraisal.

REBT was created by Albert Ellis in the 1950s as an early form of cognitive-affective-behavioral therapy (Ellis, 1962). Among the cognitive-behavior therapies it is deeply anchored in a philosophy, an ethos of right thinking about oneself in the world and the treatment of others (Ellis, 2004).

Concepts

REBT follows an augmented ABC model: negative event (A) engages irrational belief (B), leading to dysfunctional consequence (C), which becomes an activating event (D), engaging second-order irrational beliefs (E), and resulting in metaconsequences compounding the dysfunction (F). Ellis stresses that it is the belief, not the activating event, that causes the negative consequences, and thus the key to treatment is the identification and restructuring of these irrational beliefs.

REBT has evolved over time and yet remains true to its basic concepts (Ellis, 2008). People are both rational and irrational creatures, as likely to fall into superstition as think critically, and capable of sliding from one to the other. They grow into rationality, being more susceptible to irrational thought while young, but these ways of thinking become habits that get carried forward and become problematic. Thoughts, emotions, and behaviors are instantaneous, or nearly so, and charge the events of our lives. Behavior is thoughtful. Thoughts are charged with emotion. Because these three constructs are so inextricably intermingled, interventions are drawn from every possible behavioral, affective, or cognitive angle. Active-directive, interventions are more effective. The underlying goals are unconditional self-acceptance (no contingencies, value for simply existing, and value in the presence of fallibility and shortcomings) and a similar appraisal of others and life in general. Neurotic problems can be minimized by confronting the distorted thinking that causes them with "logic-empirical and pragmatic thinking" (Ellis, 2008, p. 198). Rigid beliefs are at the crux of psychological problems in REBT. Rigid beliefs lead to a variety of unnecessarily negative framing of the world. Awful beliefs, low frustration tolerance beliefs, and self-deprecating beliefs undermine the person's efficacy. There are healthy negative emotions, such as properly felt remorse, but negative framing results in dysfunctional emotions, such as guilt. REBT focuses on the metaemotional, how we respond to our situation. Seeking to dispute irrational beliefs and to reinforce stronger rational beliefs, REBT sees moderation and flexibility as healthy psychological goals.

Process

Counselors eschew extended client history, moving instead to a quick identification of basic dysfunctional beliefs and engaging the client in a challenge to these beliefs. Focus is directed not at the feelings that are presented, but at the thoughts behind the feelings. The counselor will point out inconsistencies in logic, expound upon the philosophy of REBT in session, explaining and pointing out that "shoulds" and "musts" lead to logically indefensible conclusions, and encourage the client to see these things in themselves. Working alliance is there, but there is a cool, analytical distance between the counselor and client. Counselors talk much and are much more directive, taking a teaching role much of the time (Ellis, 2008).

The topics of conversation revolve around irrational and rational beliefs. Irrational beliefs can be reduced to three fundamental areas of concern (Garske & Bishop, 2004; Livneh & Wright, 1995).

- *Beliefs about the self.* Unreasonable demands of self-perfection, righteousness, mastery, prowess, and any other self-attribute on which one hangs one's identity and self-esteem, creates stress inasmuch as they can be sustained, anxiety in the apperception of threats to self-image, self-esteem, and shame, guilt, and depression (Ashby, Rice, & Martin, 2006) in ones inevitable failures. Avoidance and withdrawal lead to conflicted self-loathing.
- *Beliefs about other people.* Unreasonable demands made upon social relationship in terms of complete and unwavering respect, deference, consideration, admiration, love ... whatever drives the relationship, sets up an unavoidable conflict when the other does not conform to rigid expectations. Judgment is extreme; punishment is exacted, either from the unworthy self or the unworthy other. Unresolved anger, rage, and resentment leads to isolation, escalating conflict, and violence.
- *Beliefs about the world.* Unreasonable sense of entitlement and rigid expectations of comfort, safety, excitement, pleasure ... whatever defines the good life, creates a lived experience of growing dissatisfaction. When "wants" become "needs" the

world is unworthy even in affluence, and in times of struggle it becomes a terrible, unjust, hell-on-earth. Self-pity, frustration, and resentment lead to withdrawal and depression.

Cognitive techniques
Disputing of irrational beliefs is central to REBT. Four identified strategies have been described (Beal, Kopec, & DiGiuseppe, 1996): (a) point out flaws in logic, (b) challenge the client to produce evidence to back up irrational belief; (c) reveal the unnecessary price paid for irrational belief (e. g., how's that working for you?); and (d) restructure a more logical, more effective, and more provable belief. There are techniques to support the strategy.

- *Semantic precision* cleans up language and clarifies thoughts where self-defeating beliefs hide.
- *Reframing* confronts the negative conceptualizations in a more realistic way.
- *Referenting* examines both sides of a topic, searches out both the positive and the negative, and uses humor to reveal the illogical or to lighten the mood.
- *Rational coping* encourages the development of new rational beliefs by practicing self-statements at critical junctures (Garske & Bishop, 2004).

Behavioral techniques
Psychoeducational approaches are very behavioral. REBT makes strong use of homework, including studying REBT, working through self-help exercises, and practicing behaviors. Often a system of rewards and punishment is set up with the clients to encourage participation in activities they will initially find uncomfortable. Social skills training, systematic desensitization, and the use of imagery are techniques used to practice new behaviors that emerge from taking on new beliefs.

Emotive techniques
Even though REBT sees cognitions, affect, and behaviors as simultaneous phenomena, emotions are not the emphasis for change. It is simply easier to dispute cognitions than it is to dispute emotions. What is done is to explore how emotions play into the process. For instance, rational-emotive imagery provides exercises where the client imagines the problem situation, perhaps in a worst-case scenario, and begins to understand that even in this situation the event would not be as catastrophic as imagined. Clients can then imagine how they would respond to a restructured belief. Similarly, emotions can be explored in role-playing. Shame-attacking is a more empirical way of actually experiencing the emotion by engaging in the behaviors they fear the most (e. g., talking to strangers, public speaking, etc.).

Application
It is a brief, directed approach that lends itself to the structure of rehabilitation counseling (Garske & Bishop, 2004), particularly with its central intrinsic valuing of the individual and intrinsic emphasis on adjustment (Balter & Unger, 1997). Ellis (1997)

emphasized the role of REBT in helping persons with disabilities address and developing high frustration tolerance to facilitate good mental health in dealing with the daily challenges of navigating a less-than-accommodating world.

The pragmatic utility of the tools are evident in more tactical, situational applications. It has direct application in confronting self-defeating beliefs following acquired physical disabilities in personal adjustment (Livneh & Sherwood, 1991) and family (Sweetland, 1990) adjustment. Application in adjustment to disability is done advisedly however. REBT is not heavily invested in a supportive relationship between client and counselor, and it treats extreme response to experience as "catastrophizing," with no way of alternatively dealing with extreme emotions because the loss was indeed catastrophic (Garske & Bishop, 2004). Calabro (1990) sees REBT applied later in the adjustment process, once the disability has been accepted as an activating event and actual irrational beliefs have begun to emerge (i.e., the "rational reencounter phase"), and differentially based on the physiological, security, affiliative, and self-worth priorities at play in the rehabilitation experience (Calabro, 1997).

Meta-analysis of REBT has established some claim to effectiveness (Engles, Garnefsky, & Diekstra, 1993) in the fundamentals across a variety of disorders across populations (David, Szentagotai, Eva, & Macavai, 2005). REBT is widely used in psychiatric support. REBT demonstrates a lasting therapeutic effect in treating major depressive disorder and is considered a first line therapy for nonpsychotic clients (David, Szentagotai, Lupu, & Cosman, 2008). It has been used as a technique in a group model of support for persons with psychiatric disabilities (Gilbert, Cicolini, & Mander, 2005). REBT arthritis counseling focuses on secondary beliefs that mediate coping and help-seeking behaviors (Sciacchitano, Linder, & McCracken, 2009). Reframing and retraining are employed to help people accept changing realities of vision loss. REBT includes socialization in the blind community as part of the process of building new, more constructive beliefs (Zaborowski, 1997). Chronic fatigue syndrome REBT has shown promise in group (Balter & Unger, 1997) contexts and work on secondary beliefs (Noonan, Lindner, & Walker, 2010). REBT's theorized relationship between irrational beliefs and maladaptive anger have been advanced in practice (Dryden, 1990) and supported in research (Martin & Dahlen, 2004). REBT enhanced outcomes in anger management programming for children with increasing control of anger, better social skills development, and a reduction in depressive symptoms (Flanagan, Allen, & Henry, 2010). REBT has been used in care facility in rehabilitation following stroke (Alvarez, 1997) and successfully adapted to help reduce stress among mothers of children with Down's syndrome (Greaves, 1997), along with CT, some of the most well-researched counseling strategies (Cormier & Nurius, 2003).

POSITIVE PSYCHOLOGY

Positive psychology is an emerging landscape for rehabilitation counseling interventions, and a promising one. Positive psychology is the pursuit of what is possible, from a client-centered perspective of strengths (Seligman & Csikszentmihalyi, 2000).

Positive psychology is in the DNA of rehabilitation counseling, but it required the scaffolding Seligman provided in the late 1990s:

> The field of positive psychology at the subjective level is about valued subjective experiences: well-being, contentment, and satisfaction (in the past); hope and optimism (for the future); and flow and happiness (in the present). At the individual level, it is about positive individual traits: the capacity for love and vocation, courage, interpersonal skill, aesthetic sensibility, perseverance, forgiveness, originality, future mindedness, spirituality, high talent, and wisdom. At the group level, it is about the civic virtues and the institutions that move individuals towards better citizenship: responsibility, nurturance, altruism, civility, moderation, tolerance, and work ethic (Seligman & Csikszentmihalyi, 2000, p. 5).

It is the inverse of traditional counseling psychology in its most central consideration. Rather than fix what is wrong, the core motivation of positive psychology is to nurture what is right (Peterson, 2000). It is not a radical displacement of traditional counseling psychology and its pathology focus, but a completion of the counseling view on the human condition.

Concepts

Positive psychology has much in common with humanistic theory, and in particular the Rogerian approach to client-centered counseling, with its assumption that all people tend to move toward optimal functioning (Joseph & Linley, 2006). Linley, Joseph, Maltby, Harrington, and Wood (2009) concede the similarity, providing these four assumptions to differentiate the approach between them:

- Positive psychology is concerned primarily with everyday problems of living, rather than extreme maladaptive behaviors.
- Clinical problems are normal problems, differing only in degree, and are part of the continuum of normal human function.
- Psychological problems are not analogous to biological problems or diseases in that they reflect problems in the person x environment interaction, not a problem wholly found within the individual.
- The primary role of positive psychology intervention is to promote human strengths and health as assets that buffer against psychological weakness or mental health issues.

One of the tenets of positive psychology is that psychologically healthy and well-adjusted people have a "positivity bias" (Peterson, 2000) that is reflected in the developing construct of optimism. We tend to assume that a totally rational approach to life is the pinnacle of the good life without a clear examination of the underlying psychology of health. A perfectly rational person who is optimally informed and engaged in life may rationally conclude that there is little to be happy about (consider Frankl, 1984). The positivity bias is the ingrained human tendency to think more positively about ourselves, about our world, and about the future than the evidence suggests.

What good is rationality in hard times if it does not make you happy? Positive psychology is about the pursuit of happiness and the definition of hope.

Early in the pursuit, happiness was described as a monolithic trait that was stable and relatively constant regardless of situational circumstance (i.e., "hedonic treadmill"). Positive psychology defines functional happiness as a developmental and complex construct (i.e. "subjective well-being") that is subject to both study and change (Diener, 2000). In positive psychology, we can learn to be happier, and being happier is therapeutic. Well-being in the face of life problems and crises requires what Lazarus (1983) called "positive denial" for healthy response and survival. Optimism is a cognitive reframing, a way of interpreting the world, and in particular the bad events that happen to us (Buchanan & Seligman, 1995; Seligman, 1991).

Positive psychotherapy (Seligman, Rashid, & Parks, 2006) focuses on positive emotions and strengths as a means to ameliorate symptoms of psychopathology. Early work suggests that it is as efficacious as traditional pharmacological interventions. Clinical approaches to growth following traumatic experiences are emerging with positive psychology themes (Linley et al., 2009) that provide a foundation for strategic theory and practice development.

Application

Positive psychology interventions include such things as positive writing (e.g., gratitude letters), practicing optimistic thinking, positive reminiscence, mindfulness, life coaching, rehearsal of positive statements, forgiveness, and socializing. Meta-analysis indicates that these techniques, considered in the aggregate, increase well-being and ameliorate depression as stand-alone treatment and exhibit a medium effect size (Sin & Lyubomirsky, 2009). Positive psychology has been applied to groups and the workplace as well. It has been used to build employee engagement on the job, which has demonstrated positive outcomes in reduced turnover and increased productivity (Harter, Schmidt, & Hayes, 2002). Life coaching is finding a theoretical base in positive psychology (Linley et al., 2009). Life coaching provides an accessible venue for positive therapies of interest to rehabilitation counselors.

Well-being therapy is a brief counseling strategy that emphasizes self-observation and journaling. This approach uses CBT techniques to interrupt thoughts that interfere with psychological well-being (Fava, 1999). Well-being therapy (Myers & Sweeney, 2008) demonstrates effectiveness with reducing symptoms of panic, anxiety, and agoraphobia (Fava, Rafanelli, Cazzarro, Conti, & Grandi, 1998; Fava et al., 2001, 2005).

Hope therapy (Snyder, 2002) involves a two-stage process of instilling and then increasing hope. Initial sessions focus on goal setting and storytelling (see Lambie & Milsom, 2010), with an eye on reframing the personal narrative from a positive perspective and establishing a baseline for the role of that hope plays in the client's life. Cognitive-behavioral and solution-oriented techniques are applied to achieving reasonable goals, building success and raising the expectations for success (hope) in the future.

The overlap between positive psychology and cognitive-behavioral techniques is apparent. Yet, the change in valence and subtle differences are demonstrably unique in their effect (see Fava et al., 2005; Rafanelli et al., 2000). Positive psychology, like reha-bilitation counseling, is inclusive. It can and probably should be adapted to all approaches without denying the need for traditional pathology-driven approaches (Chou, Lee, Catalano, Ditchman, & Wilson, 2009).

BRIEF THERAPIES

Brief therapies are different from the major schools of counseling thought in that they focus on a specific issue and intervene directly in the resolution of that issue in a very proactive and extremely time-limited fashion. There is little consideration of issue origins or connections to some larger personality problem (Gingerich & Eisen-gart, 2000). The brief approach has been interpreted through cognitive behavior (Byford et al., 2003), psychodynamic (Rogers, 1994), and Adlerian (Croake & Myers, 1989) therapies and would seem a very effective venue for using these theories in the time-limited context of rehabilitation counseling (see Back, Waldrop, Brady, & Hien, 2006). Three approaches that reflect the characteristic aspects of brief therapy are presented here to represent the large and growing specializations.

Solution-Focused Counseling

A brief therapy approach (de Shazer, 1985) with obvious connections to positive psychology emerged as a positive response to problem-solving models that focus on the persistence of problems. Solution-focused brief therapy is a "nonpathological, salutary, strengths- or competency-based approach to helping people..." (Lewis & Osborn, 2004, p. 38). In solution-focused counseling, clients have resources and strengths to resolve problems. Change is constant—the counselor's job is to identify and amplify the positive change. Small, positive, and constructive changes in complex and dysfunctional system can create a cascade of change for the better. Rapid change in a brief period of time is possible.

Solution-focused therapy focuses on what is possible and changeable rather than what is impossible and intractable (O'Hanlon & Weiner-Davis, 1989). Solutions are changes in perceptions or interactions that are client driven and cocreated (Berg & De Jong, 1996). Solutions are identified by focusing on nonproblematic examples or exceptions to the presenting problem. The client directs the process, by voicing pre-ferences (Walter & Peller, 2000). Techniques include asking the miracle question "If you woke up tomorrow and everything was put right, what would it look like, what would you do, etc." Scaling questions are used to objectify and quantify the underlying emotions (e.g., "on a scale of 1 to 10 . . ."). Looking for strengths and solutions, setting goals and homework are common techniques. The client and the counselor identify an issue that can be easily resolved, and set about applying the solutions. Negotiating a solvable problem creates a schema to solve similar problems in the future, and sets the stage for a positive reframing of position in life. Meta-analysis suggests a small but positive effect in general, with some representation of studies involving people with psychiatric disabilities and some outcome measures of anxiety and depression (Kim, 2010).

Reality Therapy/Choice Theory

Choice theory and reality therapy have evolved from Glasser's work (2000a; 2000b) as a brief form of psychotherapy. Choice theory contends that peoples choices and ability to choose are the most important characteristics affecting their mental health. Choice theory focuses on the internal needs that motivate people in their environments and the role of happiness as the indicator and outcome of their need fulfillment. There are five basic needs: survival, love and belonging, power, freedom, and fun. People choose everything they do, think, and feel. They even choose to be unhappy. Success and failure identities form around the fulfillment of these basic needs, or lack thereof. Reality therapy stresses personal responsibility and that which is under personal control. The behavior of others is beyond the client's control—how the client chooses to respond to the behavior of others is completely within the client's control. Involvement is the motivator behind all behavior and the engine of identity. Self-determination, once realized and properly trained, is the road to health and happiness (Glasser, 2005).

Reality therapy heavily depends on the therapeutic alliance focusing on the seven helping habits (support, encouragement, listening, acceptance, trust, respect for the client, and negotiating differences with the client) (Glasser, 2005). Counseling creates an environment for self-evaluation. What values are placed on current decisions? Does the client see himself or herself as a change agent or a victim of circumstance? The insight of reality therapy is that clients are more in control of their own happiness than they realize, and that with training they can evaluate their own behavior and make new decisions that bring them closer to happiness. Counseling strategy is basically to ask and explore: What do you want? What are you doing to get it? How effective is your strategy? What can you do differently? Based on this conversation, plans are formed, implemented, and evaluated. Clients select objectives by imagining the things they want most out of life and working toward them (i.e., "Quality World"; Glasser, 1998). Confrontation is often used as a means of improving the plan. "What can you do to improve the situation?" is used to disrupt victimization and refocus on an internal locus of control. Homework is involved in putting plans into action and evaluating the impact in sessions.

Reality/Choice therapy makes sense for rehabilitation counseling (Turpin & Ososkie, 2004) and applications have been suggested, such as a strategy for increasing physical activity for people with disabilities (Schoo, 2008), or teaching decision-making skills to clients with developmental disabilities (Lawrence, 2004). Actual research is rather scattered and thin, but positive for posttraumatic stress disorder (Prenzlau, 2006), increasing self-determination in persons with developmental disabilities (Lawrence, 2004), and a supplemental support in applied behavior analysis with autism spectrum disorder (Renna, 2004). There is little in the literature that is directly actionable for rehabilitation counselors, but some preliminary instrumentation has been proposed (Rapport, 2007).

Motivational Interviewing

Motivational interviewing (MI) is a philosophy of practice, not a theory (Lewis & Osborn, 2004). It was created as a technique for dealing with resistance in alcohol and substance abuse counseling. It evolved out of the States of Change Model

(Prochaska, DiClemente, & Norcross, 1992) that identifies a cycle of change processes that people go through in the process of recovery: (1) precontemplation, (2) contemplation, (3) preparation, (4) action, and (5) maintenance (prevent relapse, anchor gains). Movement through the model tends to be stepwise, but relapse is a common and expected outcome. MI is a particularly focused and effective tactic, rather than a strategy; it is a singular approach to a specific part of the process. Specifically, it is a "client-centered, directive method for enhancing intrinsic motivation to change by exploring and resolving ambivalence" (Miller & Rollnick, 2002, p. 25). MI emerges from the humanistic and positive psychologies that undergird rehabilitation counseling by way of Rogers (1957) and Seligman (1991). It starts with the counselor's lived philosophy. The counselor believes that all people have the ability to change, to grow, to throw off unproductive behaviors, and to be employed. The interviewer assumes that the only thing keeping the person from acting in his or her best interest is a lack of motivation.

In MI, the counselor seeks to honestly understand what the client likes and dislikes about substance abuse. If the client is ambivalent about substance abuse, or if the consequences of the behavior are at odds with the clients stated values, then these discovered discrepancies are investigated. As the client moves from precontemplation, to contemplation, to preparation, to plan, the counselor moves with the client and the issues of the session shift accordingly.

The key task within MI is "rolling with resistance." Consumer resistance can be as much a response to the counselor's approach as it is an internal struggle. Counselors actually become a barrier to the client's change process when they judge, admonish, and otherwise challenge the client's character and personal sovereignty. When the client is resistant to change, the counselor does not interject, but moves on, indeed, reassures the client that he or she are free to do as he or she pleases. The collaborative exploring of underlying motivation and the real value of the abusing behavior in the client's life continues. Supporting techniques include expressing empathy, avoiding argument, supporting self-efficacy, developing discrepancies, summarizing key steps taken, and affirming decisions made (Lloyd, Tse, Waghorn, & Hennessy, 2008). A specific technique that has demonstrated utility across settings is the "decisional balance sheet" exercise. In this exercise, decisions are mapped out in a 2×2 grid enumerating reasons for change and not changing (benefits versus cost). Of all of the techniques used in MI, the decisional balance sheet has demonstrated the most consistent relationship to positive outcomes (Apodaca & Longabaugh, 2008).

Evidence in application

Even though it is difficult to pin down the specific instrumental protocol(s) in this philosophical approach, it has amassed a sizeable body of evidence to support its efficacy in substance abuse treatment (see Carey, Carey, Maisto, & Henson; 2006; Carroll et al., 2006; Clark, 2002; Hettema, Steele, & Miller, 2005) and addictions such as gambling (see Carlbring, Jonsson, Josephson, & Forsberg, 2010; Petry, 2006). MI has been used successfully to change drinking behaviors among people with learning disabilities (Mendel & Hipkins, 2002). However, MI may not be equally effective in dual-diagnosed mental illness and substance abuse treatment across different addictions (Martino, Carroll, Nich, & Rounsaville, 2006).

Use has been expanding and differentiating in psychiatric recovery. MI has been used to improve engagement of women in mental health treatment (Grote, Zuckhoff, Swartz, Bledsoe, & Geibel, 2007). Barrowclough et al. (2001) found that MI and CBT in a family therapy intervention for a dually diagnosed client with schizophrenia and substance use disorders had significant improvement in general functioning compared with traditional care. MI and CBT in individual counseling settings with clients with anxiety disorders demonstrated better control over anxiety and improved homework productivity (Westra & Dozois, 2006).

Lloyd et al. (2008) proposed using MI for vocational rehabilitation of people with psychiatric disabilities. They draw a parallel between the concept of "motivational toxicity" (see McCown & Howatt, 2007), characterized by a dwindling ability to be motivated by anything but recovery, and the reluctance of many clients with psychiatric disabilities to engage in productive job-seeking strategies. MI can be used to explore client's perspective on the meaning and value of employment; rationale for including, or not including, employment as a recovery goal; origins of positive and negative motivations with regard to employment; short- and long-term employment goals; and expectations for employment's impact on recovery (Lloyd et al., 2008). A similar model has been developed to deal with employment ambivalence in support employment for clients with psychiatric disabilities (Larson, 2008).

CAREER COUNSELING: CHOICE AND DEVELOPMENT

Career counseling is a signature venue for rehabilitation counseling. It is the space in which most rehabilitation counseling occurs and concerns the most important outcomes of the professional mission. Parsons (1909) proposed that career development entailed gaining a full understanding of the person, a full understanding of the world of work, and a strategic matching of the two. Person × environment fit has become the foundation on which a variety of theories and models have emerged, each with its own perspective on the two primary themes of career choice and development. In the 1990s, a consortium of career theorists sought to unify the discipline through theory convergence (Savickas & Lent, 1994). While far from successful, the effort provided a more contiguous and connected sense to theory development. Szymanski, Enright, Hershenson, and Ettinger (2010) proposed an ecological model as a framework for creating a space where career theories could coexist, if not coalesce. In an increasingly complex and multicultural world, career counseling practice requires such a model to develop integrated and evidence-based practice.

Career choice and development is the core of all related theories. For the purposes of this chapter, we will describe three of the most popular and useful approaches to provide a sense of the spectrum of service possibilities.

Minnesota Theory of Work Adjustment

Person × environment fit models have largely been used in career theory and developed as an approach widely applied in the vocational rehabilitation of people with disabilities (Kosciulek, 1993; Szymanski & Hershenson, 1998). Foremost among these was the Minnesota Theory of Work Adjustment (MTWA; Dawis, England, & Lofquist, 1964). The MTWA was inclusive of people with disabilities in its study, development, and application. It is based on behaviorist concepts of stimulus, response, and reinforcement in the development of work personality, and characterized work adjustment in nine propositions.

1. An individual's work adjustment at any point in time is indicated by his concurrent levels of satisfactoriness and satisfaction.
2. Satisfactoriness is a function of the correspondence between an individual's abilities and the ability requirements of the work environment, provided that the individual's needs correspond with the reinforcer system of the work environment.
3. Satisfaction is a function of the correspondence between the reinforcer system of the work environment and the individual's needs, provided that the individual's abilities correspond with the ability requirement of the work environment.
4. Satisfaction moderates the functional relationship between satisfactoriness and the ability-requirement correspondence.
5. Satisfactoriness moderates the functional relationship between satisfaction and the need-reinforcer correspondence.
6. The probability that an individual will be forced out of the work environment is inversely related to his (or her) satisfactoriness.
7. The probability that an individual will voluntarily leave the work environment is inversely related to his (or her) satisfaction.
8. Tenure is a joint function of satisfactoriness and satisfaction.
9. Work personality—work environment correspondence increases as a function of tenure (Lofquist & Dawis, 1969, cited in Szymanski et al., 2010, pp. 50–53).

"Fit" is a fluid measure of the relationship between the two, the less the gap between the two, the better the outcome (Rounds & Tracey, 1990). The MTWA provides a strategy for conceptualizing the gap, developing an intervention plan, and evaluating progress along the way.

Holland's Theory

Holland's theory is a person—environment fit theory. Holland proposed six work characteristics that could be matched to corresponding interests of individuals. They are, in order around a hexagon, (R) realistic, (I) investigative, (A) artistic, (S) social, (E) enterprising, and (C) conventional. His theory proposes that people can be characterized based on these qualities, and that they would be attracted to and successful in jobs that mirrored these characteristics (Holland, 1997). The RIASEC hexagon is a common tool of career counseling and available for use by individuals without counseling intervention. As influential as the theory is, it has not always held up well under scrutiny (Tinsley, 2000). As a measure of personality it has demonstrated a "congruence problem" (Arnold, 2004), and in metaanalysis (job satisfaction and congruence), the effect size was small at best (Assouline & Meir, 1987; Spokane, Meir, & Catalano, 2000; Tranberg, Slane, & Ekeberg, 1993). The biggest challenge is the potential impact of disability in limiting expression of interests. Limitations of early experiences (career development issues) lead to a "flat" profile of no interests, which may or may not be clinically relevant. Still, Holland's theory has application and effect in generating career options and as a tool to help build a better understanding of self as worker (Holland, Fritzsche, & Powell, 1994), and utility as a planning tool (Szymanski et al., 2010).

Super's Life Span, Life Space Theory

Super's (1990) career development model conceptualizes both stages of life and expected roles. People move from stage to stage of life and the meaning and importance of the roles change. Life stages are growth (0–14), exploration (15–24), establishment (25–44), maintenance (45–64), and decline (65+). Of course, ages of transition are elastic, but changes do happen, and within each stage there are minicycles running through the same birth–growth–decline cycle. Super (1990) starts with the basic person × environment fit assumptions as with the MTWA and focuses on the change process over time. Self-concept can change with time and (work) experience but tends to be relatively stable. Change happens in cycles and minicycles. Career patterns are impacted by a confluence of personal and situational variables, including personal traits (aptitude, interests, achievement, personality [work and otherwise]), career maturity, and the opportunities that avail themselves. Career maturity is a central concept. It refers to both cognitive and affective dimensions of coping response. It is built through the stages, and things not learned become problematic. It is a difficult construct to nail down. Career development is the development and implementation of work self-concepts, the development of self-concept is dependent on the experience. The interaction between a person's self-concept and the realities the person faces is the point of counseling. The degree of appropriateness is important. Role-playing career situations is the primary mechanism in counseling, or psychosocial rehabilitation (PSR)-type support groups, or *in situ*. Work and life satisfaction depend on the full expression of the work–self concept. Beyond work satisfaction, one must stop to consider how central the work role is to the client. Other roles may be more prominent (Super, 1990).

Super's theory is very useful to rehabilitation counseling. The life stage perspective provides a means of evaluating the degree to which cycles are successfully completed, and career maturity is advanced. It illuminates the role of limited early experiences on future ability to make career plans and career decisions (i.e., career maturity; Szymanski et al., 2010). The theory allows the counselor to identify career maturity issues that become barriers to inclusion in career planning. It provides a fruitful perspective for understanding acquired disabilities. The acquisition of a disability and the disruption that it causes initiates a "minicycle" as the individual explores and develops a new career and consequent identity.

Applications

Vocational rehabilitation has been central to the theory and incorporated into it development and empirical support over the years (Brown, 1990; Lofquist & Dawis, 1991). The counseling approaches that evolve out of this model focus on Parsons' (1909) admonishment to know the client, know the world of work, and work toward a match. It relies on an astute vocational evaluation of the client's aptitudes, interests, abilities, and work personality, and the counselor's agency in facilitating client knowledge of the world of work and ability to make informed and autonomous decisions. The career counselor brings knowledge of work and specific employment to the planning phases, as well as resources and strategies for assistive technologies and potential accommodation. Individual career counseling has demonstrated the most effectiveness in generating client outcomes (Whiston, Sexton, & Lasoff, 1998; Oliver & Spokane, 1988). Career skill training has demonstrated efficacy as has career counseling tools for people with disabilities, in a model that reflected strong didactic and experiential components (Bolton & Akridge, 1995) and short-term workshops (Merz & Szymanski, 1997).

PSYCHOSOCIAL REHABILITATION

It is proper to conclude with PSR as it is, in a sense, a culmination of work and thought that puts counseling squarely in the center of the community. That is not to say that it is a new way of thinking or the latest. Indeed, as a profession rehabilitation counseling has early roots here (Wright, 1972). We will use the model of PSR that has developed around mental illness to describe the construct, but it had its origins in application to persons with physical disabilities and the work of Beatrice Wright (1983). Wright's original treatise is driven by a set of values that spring from the fundamental mission of full community inclusion and provides the foundation of PSR, and rehabilitation counseling's part in it.

1. *Every individual needs respect and encouragement; the presence of a disability, no matter how severe, does not alter these fundamental rights...*
2. *The severity of a handicap can be increased or diminished by environmental conditions...*
3. *Issues of coping and adjusting to a disability cannot be validly considered without examining reality problems in the social and physical environment...*
4. *The assets of the person must receive considerable attention in the rehabilitation effort...*
5. *The significance of a disability is affected by the person's feelings about the self and his or her situation...*
6. *The active participation of the client in the planning and execution of the rehabiliation program is to be sought as fully as possible...*
7. *The client is seen not as an isolated individual but as part of a larger group that includes other people, often family...*
8. *Because each person has unique characteristics and each situation its own properties, variability is required in rehabilitation plans...*
9. *Predictor variables, based on group outcomes in rehabilitation, should be applied with caution to the individual case...*
10. *All phases of rehabilitation have psychological aspects [emphasis added]...*
11. *Interdisciplinary and interagency collaboration and coordination of services are essential...*
12. *Self-help organizations are important allies in the rehabilitation effort...*
13. *In addition to the special problems of particular groups, rehabilitation clients commonly share certain problems by virtue of their disadvantaged and devalued position...*

14. *It is essential that society as a whole continuously and persistently strives to provide the basic means toward the fulfillment of the lives of all its inhabitants, including those with disabilities. . .*

15. *Involvement of the client with the general life of the community is a fundamental principle [emphasis added] guiding decisions concerning living arrangements and the use of resources. . .*

16. *People with disabilities, like all citizens, are entitled to participate in and contribute to the general life of the community [emphasis added]. . .*

17. *Provision must be made for the effective dissemination of information concerning legislation and community offerings of potential benefit to persons with disabilities. . .*

18. *Basic research can profitably be guided by the question of usefulness in ameliorating problems, a vital consideration in rehabilitation fields, including psychology. . .*

19. *Persons with disabilities should be called upon to serve as coplanners, coevaluators, and consultants to others, including professional persons. . .*

20. *Continuing review of the contributions of psychologists and others in rehabilitation within a framework of guiding principles that are themselves subject to review is an essential part of the self-correcting effort of science and the professions (Wright, 1983; pp. xi–xvii)*

These principles have guided us through the evolution of rehabilitation counseling and remain the core values of PSR today. In Wright's words, the need for rehabilitation counseling is invested through PSR, and its ultimate goal is full community inclusion.

Vocational rehabilitation is at the heart of PSR (Zahniser, 2005). PSR's fundamental goal is to obtain, maintain, and expand meaningful social roles for people with disabilities in communities of choice. The world of work is a choice community and employment is a pivotal social role. The model was developed largely from the perspective of psychiatric disabilities, but the message has possible application across rehabilitation counseling settings.

Recovery as Model

The spirit of PSR is clearly defined in the recovery model. Recovery is complex. Davidson, O'Connell, Tondora, Staeheli, and Evans (2005) describe a conceptual framework based on the four definitions of recovery. Recovery can mean a return to preimpairment status. This is most appropriate in describing recovery in acute, physical impairment. Recovery can refer to the process of recovering, incremental improvement over time. This is most applicable to the recovery experience related to trauma (coma, stroke, etc.). Recovery in substance abuse parlance is "something gained or restored," that is, sobriety. Recovery from severe mental disorder is reflected in the least common recovery definition "obtaining usable substance from unusable sources." Recovery is a socially constructed response to rehabilitation that can mean different things to different people, for different reasons. The recovery model most commonly associated with the term came from serving people with psychiatric disabilities. People affected by psychiatric disabilities wrestle with stigma, isolation, discrimination in housing, education, and employment. Learned helplessness is the key problem. Recovery comes through client empowerment. Empowerment takes place in the community through individualized and networked services. PSR's goal is recovery. Recovery is the model.

The core set of PSR recovery interventions (Frese, Stanley, Kress, & Vogel-Scibilia, 2005) for people with psychiatric disabilities include medication management, self-management, assertive community treatment, psychoeducational family, and supported employment. Anthony (2005) identified essential supporting services (Anthony, 2005) through which these interventions flow: treatment of symptoms, crisis intervention, case management rehabilitation (develop clients' skill and support), enrichment, rights protection and advocacy, basic support, self-help, and wellness/prevention.

Rehabilitation counseling is invested in every service to one degree or another. Just as vocational rehabilitation (VR) is the heart of PSR, recovery is in the heart of rehabilitation counseling.

Clients in the recovery model find relief and support in community:

- Reaching out for support—connecting with a nonjudgmental, noncritical person who is willing to avoid giving advice, who will listen while the person figures out for himself or herself what to do.
- Being in a supportive environment surrounded by people who are positive and affirming, but at the same time are direct and challenging—avoiding people who are critical, judgmental, or abusive.
- Peer counseling—sharing with another person who has experienced similar symptoms.
- Stress reduction and relaxation techniques—deep breathing, progressive relaxation, and visualization exercises. (Mead & Copeland, 2005, p. 75)

Clients have an active role to play in the process, and they play the central role in their own stories. Mental illness is not something that needs to be fixed, it is the client's lived experience; a normal, if challenging, aspect of the human condition. Clients (Mead & Copeland, 2005) believe in hope and actively pursue it in themselves and others. They take responsibility for personal wellness, not simply symptom reduction. Recovery is not curative; it is a lifelong process of becoming. Clients in recovery adhere to lifelong learning. Self-advocacy is often the context for counseling. Peer support is the birth of community as therapy.

Client tasks in recovery include generating hope; overcoming stigma; advocating for oneself and others; reclaiming identity—redefining oneself in one's own image; engaging in meaningful activities in self-directed venues; assuming control of one's affairs; linking into social support systems, managing symptoms (Davidson et al., 2005). Counselors have client-directed roles in this system. And clients have suggested guidelines for service delivery (Mead & Copeland, 2005):

- treat the person as an equal;
- never patronize, judge, or otherwise demean;
- focus on desires and empathy, not labels and diagnoses;
- break tasks down to small enough steps to be successful;
- limit the amount of advice giving;

- share simple, safe, effective, and inexpensive strategies and techniques that clients can use on their own;
- attend to and accept individual needs and preferences;
- personal choice is the bottom line, collaboration in the process;
- recognize strengths and progress;
- accept that a person's path is his or her own;
- listening is the first step toward recovery;
- look for barriers to wellness; and
- consider peer-to-peer support and service where productive.

Recovery is more philosophy than evidence, but the science is catching up (Frese et al., 2005). Recovery vision has become a growing moral anchor for service organizations; the integrated system approach to service delivery unites fragmented service for greater efficacy (Anthony, 2005).

Supported employment

The most established evidence-based VR practice is supported employment (Becker & Bond, 2004). Four core features are shared by all models: (a) competitive employment, (b) integrated setting, (c) serving workers with the most severe disabilities, and (d) ongoing service and support (Hanley-Maxwell, Maxwell, Fabian, & Owens, 2010). Client control as a step to empowerment includes goal setting, planning, and so on. Supported employment has been fitted to individual and group settings, with individualized supported employment being the classic and most efficacious. Supported employment is training focused, targeting client, employer, supervisor, and coworkers. Topics vary according to stakeholder needs and interests but focus on tenure topics, such as productivity, integration, problem solving, and so on.

Assessment is ecological, looking at the person, the job, and the support system in context. Job analysis evaluates essential functions of the job and potential supports. Training is an individualized, highly behavioral, process. Tasks are broken into teachable units and chained via systematic instruction into fully functional work behaviors. This approach has shown strong support for application with people with intellectual disabilities (Beyer, Brown, Akandi, & Rapley, 2010).

MODEL FOR INDIVIDUALS WITH PSYCHIATRIC DISABILITIES. Psychiatric illness presents many psychosocial issues that make employment problematic (Hanley-Maxwell et al., 2010). Symptoms create conflict. The stigma of mental illness creates other conflicts. Inadequate, inappropriate, or missing services (Wang, Demler, & Kessler, 2002) create conflicts. But they are not the same issues that confront people with developmental disabilities. They all have a character of their own, and supported employment has been interpreted rather successfully through this lens for this community. The evidence for supported employment for clients with psychiatric disabilities has been developed on seven principles: competitive work, fast job search and placement, integration of rehabilitation and mental health services, attention to consumer preference, consumer choice, no time limit on support, and benefits counseling (Bond, 2004).

Supported education

Supported education (SE) applies PSR principles to the goals of education, starting with normalization as a mindset and precondition for service. Normalization is the conscious rejection of unequal treatment at personal, interpersonal, group, and community levels. SE facilitates skill development, access to and mastery of support systems, including engagement in negotiating classroom accommodations and assistance for the purpose of maximizing success in class, course, or degree (Mowbray, Brown, Furlong-Norman, & Soydan, 2002). Empowerment is expressed through the strong self-determination of service planning and delivery, the generation of service options, development of client social networking capacity, support for group and individual advocacy, and the involvement of peer support (Soydan, 2004). SE programming generally includes initial orientation and assessment leading to a client-led plan beyond the identification of course work and certification goals to include support groups; training interventions with instructors, staff, and administrators; individual counseling; negotiating legally mandated accommodations; developing a SE consortium of agencies and key players; and organizing group efforts to combat stigma. While there is still a great deal of variation in competing models, SE has been identified as an exemplary service (Zahniser, 2005) and strongly supported in early research (Mowbray, Bybee, & Collins, 2001; Unger & Pardee, 2002).

Skills training

The ultimate goal for social skills training is enhanced community inclusion (Zahniser, 2005). Skills training can be on any topic that advances the cause, and tend to coalesce around issues of interpersonal (social) skills and skills for community living. Social skills training incorporates direct instruction, modeling, and rehearsal (Zahniser, 2005). Social skill training often includes cognitive behavioral interventions and MI components (Zahniser, 2005). Topics include work self-efficacy (Chou, Ditchman, Pruett, Chan, & Hunter, 2009), psychoeducation (re: disability and rehabilitation options), social skills, problem solving, coping (see Duchnik, Letsch, & Curtiss, 2009; Meichenbaum, 1985).

Peer support and consumer participation

The psychosocial model advocates for peer-to-peer support and the building of a supportive community (Zahniser, 2005). The presence of peers is an acknowledgment of their expertise and the power of shared experience. Peers, perhaps operating out of peer-run organizations, provide support groups, advocacy groups, and training groups—whatever is appropriate and called for. The importance of peer representation is as much political and sociological as it is psychological, and that is the point. Counseling cannot be isolated from any aspect of experience and maintain its legitimacy.

CONCLUSION

Rehabilitation counseling finds some value in every theory, differentially applied. Disability is a socially constructed phenomenon (Michailakis, 2003); no one theory captures the "truth" (Hansen, 2004) of it. We are eclectic, guided by theory; we are pragmatists (Hansen, 2006), guided by values. The common factors claim the bulk of therapeutic effect associated with counseling. Empathy, congruence, and unconditional positive regard are special cases of the ethos of community and communication. The working alliance and applied techniques are the tools of community inclusion at the atomistic level. Adlerian psychotherapy introduces a social identity, choices and lifestyle and neurosis as isolation, socialization, and family; the social development of personality and the potential for personality change. Humanist theory and practice provide philosophy at service and individual and levels. Person-centered counseling demonstrates the most pure interpretation of the common factors. It models the optimal counselor attitude toward the client, and an optimistic view of human drives to self-actualization. Logotherapy makes room for spirituality and the origins of social justice as a means to wellness. Behavioral, cognitive, and rational-emotive behavior therapies demonstrate the instrumental counseling applications. From differing positions along the A-B-C paradigm, they address the functional and possible in the here and now. Positive psychology has expanded the definition of counseling to include wellness (Meyers & Sweeney, 2008) and developed delivery methods that empower clients. Brief therapies open up the possibility that techniques across disciplines can be modified to work within a time-limited service such as rehabilitation. Solution-focused counseling, reality therapy/choice theory, and MI models focus on strength-based, client-centered, brief approaches with specialized potential for use in rehabilitation counseling. Career counseling explicates the central context for rehabilitation counseling and provides the framework for job placement and career development interventions. Person-environment fit models describe the process of choice and adjustment. Developmental models describe the dynamics of career growth and change. Ecological models of career theories demonstrate how disparate theories and practice can be integrated. PSR embeds rehabilitation counseling in a network of support, with maximal authority and responsibility in the hands of the client. The common factors of counseling and techniques are diffused through the network, becoming accessible egalitarian proactive community responses to wellness and inclusion.

A confluence of practice continues to flow through these constructs, and slowly, an evidence base is starting to form. Supported employment for people with psychiatric disabilities is the most established, but there is positive movement across the field. The utility of MI as a tool in substance abuse counseling, and the broad functional utility of cognitive-behavioral techniques are examples, but the spectrum of research and possibilities is much larger. Co-occuring psychiatric and substance abuse disorders remain a challenging issue. Psychosocial strategies will continue to evolve and may generate new techniques applicable to different populations.

This is the state of our identity as rehabilitation counselors. Our philosophy overreaches our evidence, but our practice is slowly coming into its own. The question of our identity is wrapped up in the answer to "what works and why" for rehabilitation counseling. Most specifically (Paul, 1967, p. 111), "*What* treatment, by *whom*, is most effective for *this* individual with *that* specific problem, and under *which* set of circumstances?" How rehabilitation counseling responds to Paul's question is the operational definition for the profession. For now, this is our answer, as incomplete as it is.

Rehabilitation counseling is driven forward by the fundamental mission of full community inclusion. The profession and its advocates will continue to explore what this mission means in our world, as our world expands.

REFERENCES

Aeschleman, S. R., & Imes, C. (1999). Stress innoculation training for impulsive behaviors in adults with traumatic brain injury. *Journal of Rational-Emotive & Cognitive-Behavior Therapy, 17*(1), 51–65.

Agras, W. S., Walsh, B. T., Fairburn, C. G., Wilson, G. T., & Kraemer, H. C. (2000). A multicenter comparison of cognitive-behavioral therapy and interpersonal psychotherapy for bulimia nervosa. *Archives of General Psychiatry, 57*, 459–466.

Alvarez, M. F. (1997). Using REBT and supportive psychotherapy with post-stroke patients. *Journal of Rational-Emotive & Cognitive-Behavior Therapy, 15*(3), 231–245.

Anthony, W. A. (2005). A recovery-oriented service system: Setting some system-level standards. In L. Davidson, C. Harding, & L. Spaniol (Eds.), *Recovery from severe mental illness: Research evidence and implications for practice* (Vol. 2, pp. 340–357). Boston, MA: Center for Psychiatric Rehabilitation.

Apodaca, T. R., & Longabaugh, R. (2008). Mechanisms of change in motivational interviewing: A review and preliminary evaluation of the evidence. *Addiction, 104*, 705–715.

Arnold, J. (2004). The congruence problem in John Holland's theory of vocational decisions. *Journal of Occupational and Organizational Psychology, 77*, 95–113.

Ashby, J. S., Rice, K. G., & Martin, J. L. (2006). Perfectionism, shame, and depressive symptoms. *Journal of Counseling & Development, 84*(2), 148–297.

Assouline, M., & Meir, E. I. (1987). Meta-analysis of the relationship between congruence and well-being measures. *Journal of Vocational Behavior, 31*, 319–332.

Back, S. E., Waldrop, A. E., Brady, K. T., & Hien, D. (2006). Evidence-based time-limited treatment of co-occurring substance-use disorders and civilian-related posttraumatic stress disorder. *Brief Treatment and Crisis Intervention, 6*, 283–294.

Balter, R., & Unger, P. (1997). REBT stress management with patients with chronic fatigue syndrome. *Journal of Rational-Emotive & Cognitive-Behavior Therapy, 15*(3), 223–230.

Barrowclough, C., Haddock, G., Tarrier, N., et al. (2001). Randomized controlled trial of motivational interviewing, cognitive behavior therapy, and family intervention for patients with comorbid schizophrenia and substance use disorders. *American Journal of Psychiatry, 158*(10), 1706–1713.

Basco, M. R., & Rush, A. J. (1996). *Cognitive behavioral therapy for bipolar disorder.* New York, NY: Guilford Press.

Beal, D., Kopec, A. M., & DiGiuseppe, R. (1996). Disputing clients' irrational beliefs. *Journal of Rational-Emotive & Cognitive-Behavior Therapy, 14*, 215–229.

Beck, A. T. (1999). *Prisoners of hate: The cognitive basis of anger, hostility, and violence.* New York, NY: Harper Collins.

Beck, A. T. (2008). The evolution of the cognitive model of depression and its neurobiological correlates. *American Journal of Psychiatry, 165*(8), 969–977.

Beck, A. T., & Emery, G. (1985). *Anxiety disorders and phobias: A cognitive perspective.* New York, NY: Basic Books.

Beck, A. T., & Weishaar, M. E. (2010). Cognitive therapy. In R. J. Corsini & D. Wedding (Eds.), *Current Psychotherapies* (9th ed.) (pp. 276–309). Belmont, CA: Brooks/Cole.

Becker, D. R., & Bond, G. R. (2004). *Supported employment implementation resource kit: User's guide.* Rockville, MD: Center for Mental Health Services, SAMHSA.

Berg, I. K., & De Jong, P. (1996). Solution-building conversation: Co-constructing a sense of competence with clients. *Families in Society, 77*, 376–391.

Beyer, S., Brown, T., Akandi, R., & Rapley, M. (2010). A comparison of quality of life outcomes for people with intellectual disabilities in supported employment, day services and employment enterprises. *Journal of Applied Research in Intellectual Disabilities, 23*, 290–295.

Bolton, B., & Akridge, R. L. (1995). A meta-anlaysis of skills training programs for rehabilitation clients. *Rehabilitation Counseling Bulletin, 38*, 262–273.

Bond, G. R. (2004). Supported employment: Evidence for an evidence-based practice. *Psychiatric Rehabilitation, 27*, 345–359.

Borkum, J. M. (2010). Maladaptive cognitions and chronic pain: Epidemiology, neurobiology, and treatment. *Journal of Rational-Emotive & Cognitive-Behavior Therapy, 28*(4), 4–24.

Bowers, W. A. (2001). Cognitive model of eating disorders. *Journal of Cognitive Psychotherapy: An International Quarterly, 15*, 331–340.

Bozarth, J. D., & Rubin, S. E. (1978). Empirical observations of rehabilitation counselor performance and outcome: Some implications. In B. Bolton & M. E. Jaques (Eds.), *Rehabilitation counseling: Theory and practice* (pp. 176–180). Baltimore, MD: University Park Press.

Brown, D. (1990). Trait and factor theory. In D. Brown & L. Brooks (Eds.), *Career choice and development: Applying contemporary theories to practice* (2nd ed.) (pp. 13–36). San Francisco, CA: Jossey-Bass.

Bruce, T., Spiegel, D., & Hegel, M. (1999). Cognitive-behavioral therapy helps prevent relapse and recurrence of panic disorder following alprazolam discontinuation: A long-term follow-up of Peoria and Dartmouth studies. *Journal of Consulting and Clinical Psychology, 67*, 151–156.

Buchanan, G. M., & Seligman, M. E. (Eds.) (1995). *Explanatory style.* Hillsdale, NJ: Erlbaum.

Butler, A. C., Chapman, J. E., Forman, E. M., & Beck, A. T. (2006). The empirical status of cognitive-behavioral therapy: A review of meta-analyses. *Clinical Psychology Review, 26*, 17–31.

Byford, S., Knapp, M., Greenshields, J., Ukoumunne, O. C., Jones, V., Thompson, S., et al. (2003). Cost-effectiveness of brief cognitive behaviour therapy versus treatment as usual in recurrent deliberate self-harm: The POPMACT study. *Psychological Medicine, 33*(6), 977–986.

Calabro, L. E. (1990). Adjustment to disability: A cognitive-behavioral model for analysis and clinical management. *Journal of Rational-Emotive & Cognitive-Behavior Therapy, 8*(2), 79–102.

Calabro, L. E. (1997). "First things first": Maslow's hierarchy as a framework for REBT in promoting disability adjustment during rehabilitation. *Journal of Rational-Emotive & Cognitive-Behavior Therapy, 15*, 193–213.

Carey, K. B., Carey, M. P., Maisto, S. A., & Henson, J. M. (2006). Brief motivational interventions for heavy college drinkers: A randomized controlled trial. *Journal of Consulting and Clinical Psychology, 74*, 943–954.

Carlbring, P., Jonsson, J., Josephson, H., & Forsberg, L. (2010). Motivational interviewing versus cognitive behavioral group therapy in the treatment of problem and pathological gambling: A randomized controlled trial. *Cognitive Behaviour Therapy, 39*(2), 92–103.

Carroll, K. M., Ball, S. A., et al. (2006). Motivational interviewing to improve treatment engagement and outcome in individuals seeking treatment for substance abuse: A multi-site effectiveness study. *Drug and Alcohol Dependence, 81*(3), 301–312.

Carroll, K. M., & Onken, L. S. (2005). Behavioral therapies for drug abuse. *American Journal of Psychiatry, 162*, 1452–1460.

Chan, F., Cardoso, E. D., & Chronister, J. A. (2009). *Understanding psychosocial adjustment to chronic illness and disability: A handbook for evidence-based practitioners in rehabilitation.* New York, NY: Springer.

Chou, C., Ditchman, N., Pruett, S. R., Chan, F., & Hunter, C. (2009). Application of self-efficacy related theories in psychosocial interventions. In F. Chan, E. D. Cardoso, & J. A. Chronister (Eds.), *Understanding psychosocial adjustment to chronic illness and disability: A handbook for evidence-based practitioners in rehabilitation* (pp. 243–276). New York, NY: Springer.

Chou, C., Lee, E., Catalano, D. E., Ditchman, N., & Wilson, L. M. (2009). Positive psychology and psychosocial adjustment to chronic illness and disability. In F. Chan, E. D. Cardoso, & J. A. Chronister (Eds.), *Understanding psychosocial adjustment to chronic illness and disability: A handbook for evidence-based practitioners in rehabilitation* (pp. 207–241). New York, NY: Springer.

Clark, A. J. (2007). *Empathy in counseling and psychotherapy: Perspectives and practices.* Mahwah, NJ: Erlbaum.

Clark, A. J. (2010). Empathy: An integral model in the counseling process. *Journal of Counseling & Development, 88*, 348–356.

Clark, D. M. (1996). Panic disorder: From theory to therapy. In P. Salkovskis (Ed.), *Frontiers of cognitive therapy* (pp. 318–344). New York, NY: Guilford Press.

Clark, H. W. (2002). Bridging the gap between substance abuse practice and research: The national treatment plan initiative. *Journal of Drug Issues, 32*, 757–768.

Cormier, S., & Nurius, P. S. (2003). *Interviewing and change strategies for helpers: Fundamental skills and cognitive behavioral interventions* (5th ed.). Pacific Grove, CA: Brooks/Cole.

Corrigan, P. W., & Liberman, R. P. (1994). Overview of behavior therapy in psychiatric hospitals. In P. W. Corrigan & R. P. Liberman (Eds.), *Behavior therapy in psychiatric hospitals* (pp. 1–38). New York, NY: Springer.

Croake, J. W., & Kelly, F. D. (2002). Structured group couples therapy with schizophrenic and bipolar patients and their wives. *The Journal of Individual Psychology, 58*(1), 77–86.

Croake, J. W., & Myers, K. M. (1989). Brief family therapy with childhood medical problems. *The Journal of Adlerian Theory, Research, & Practice, 45*(1), 159–168.

Cuipers, P. (1997). Bibliotherapy in unipolar depression: A meta-analysis. *Journal of Behavioral Therapy and Experimental Psychiatry, 28*, 139–147.

Daniels, T., & Ivey, A. E. (Eds.) (2007). *Microcounseling: Making skills training work in a multicultural world.* Springfield, IL: Charles C. Thomas.

David, D., Szentagotai, A., Eva, K., & Macavei, B. (2005). A synopsis of rational-emotive behavior therapy (REBT); fundamental and applied research. *Journal of Rational-Emotive & Cognitive-Behavior Therapy, 23*(3), 175–221.

David, D., Szentagotai, A., Lupu, V., & Cosman, D. (2008). Rational emotive behavior therapy, cognitive therapy, and medication in the treatment of major depressive disorder: A randomized clinical trial, posttreatment outcomes, and six-month follow-up. *Journal of Clinical Psychology, 64*(6), 728–746.

Davidson, L., O'Connell, M. J., Tondora, J., Staeheli, M., & Evans, A. C. (2005). Recovery in serious mental illness: Paradigm shift or shibboleth?L. Davidson, C. Harding, & L. Spaniol (Eds.), *Recovery from severe mental illness: Research evidence and implications for practice* (Vol. 1, pp. 5–26). Boston, MA: Center for Psychiatric Rehabilitation.

Dawis, R. V., England, G. W., & Lofquist, L. H. (1964). *A theory of work adjustment. Minnesota studies in vocational rehabilitation, 15* (Bulletin 38). Minneapolis, MN: University of Minnesota Industrial Relations Center.

de Shazer, S. (1985). *Keys to solution in brief therapy.* New York, NY: Norton.

Deale, A., Chalder, T., Marks, I., & Wessely, S. (1997). Cognitive behavior therapy for chronic fatigue syndrome: A randomized controlled trial. *American Journal of Psychiatry, 154*, 408–414.

Diener, E. (2000). Subjective well-being: The science of happiness and a proposal for a national index. *American Psychologist, 55*(1), 34–43.

Dixon, M. R., Hayes, L. J., Binder, L. M., Manthey, S. M., Sigman, C., & Zdanowski, D. M. (1998). Using a self-control training procedure to increase appropriate behavior. *Journal of Applied Behavioral Analysis, 31*, 203–210.

Dryden, W. (1990). *Dealing with anger problems: Rational emotive therapeutic interventions.* Sarasota, FL: Practitioner's Resource Exchange, Inc.

Dryden, W., & David, D. (2008). Rational emotive behavioral therapy: Current status. *Journal of Cognitive Psychotherapy: An international Quarterly, 22*(3), 195–209.

Duchnik, J. J., Letsch, E. A., & Curtiss, G. (2009). Coping effectiveness training during acute rehabilitation of spinal cord injury/dysfunction: A randomized clinical trial. *Rehabilitation Psychology, 54*(2), 123–132.

Ellis, A. (1962). *Reason and emotion in psychotherapy.* Secaucus, NJ: Citadel.

Ellis, A. (1997). Using rational emotive behavior therapy techniques to cope with disability. *Professional Psychology: Research and Practice, 1*, 17–22.

Ellis, A. (2004). Post-September 11th perspectives on religion, spirituality, and philosophy in the personal and professional lives of selected REBT cognoscenti: A response to my colleagues. *Journal of Counseling & Development, 82*(3), 439–442.

Ellis, A. (2008). Rational emotive behavior therapy. In R. J. Corsini & D. Wedding (Eds.), *Current Psychotherapies* (9th ed., pp. 196–234). Belmont, CA: Brooks/Cole.

Eng, W., Roth, D. A., & Heimberg, R. G. (2001). Cognitive behavior therapy for social anxiety. *Journal of Cognitive Psychotherapy: An International Quarterly, 15*, 311–319.

Engles, G. I., Garnefsky, N., & Diekstra, F. W. (1993). Efficacy of rational-emotive therapy: A quantitative analysis. *Journal of Consulting and Clinical Psychology, 6,* 1083–1090.

Farley, R. C. (1987). Rational rehavior [sic] problem-solving as a career development intervention for persons with disabilities. *Journal of Rational-Emotive Therapy, 5*(1), 32–42.

Farrugia, D. L. (1986). An Adlerian perspective for understanding deafness. *Individual Psychology: The Journal of Adlerian Theory, Research, & Practice, 42*(2), 201–214.

Fava, G. A. (1999). Well-being therapy: Conceptual and technical issues. *Psychotherapy and Psychosomatics, 68,* 171–179.

Fava, G. A., Rafanelli, C., Cazzarro, M., Conti, S., & Grandi, S. (1998). Well-being therapy: A novel psychotherapeutic approach for residual symptoms of affective disorders. *Psychological Medicine, 28,* 475–480.

Fava, G. A., Rafanelli, C., Ottolini, F., Ruin, C., Cazzaro, M., & Grandi, S. (2001). Psychological well-being and residual symptoms in remitted patients with panic disorder and agoraphobia. *Journal of Affective Disorder, 65,* 185–190.

Fava, G. A., Ruini, C., Rafanelli, C., Finos, L., Salmaso, L., Mangelli, L. et al. (2005). Well-being therapy of generalized anxiety disorder. *Psychotherapy and Psychosomatics, 74,* 26–30.

Ferguson, R. J., Cassel, A. G., & Dawson, R. F. (2010). Cognitive effects of cancer chemotherapy in adult cancer survivors: Cognitive-behavioral management. *Journal of Rational-Emotive & Cognitive-Behavior Therapy, 28,* 25–41.

Flanagan, R., Allen, K., & Henry, D. J. (2010). The impact of anger management treatment and rational emotive behavior therapy in a public school setting on social skills, anger management, and depression. *Journal of Rational-Emotive & Cognitive-Behavior Therapy, 28,* 87–99.

Frankl, V. (1984). *Man's search for meaning.* New York, NY: Washington Square Press.

Frankl, V. (1986). *The doctor and the soul: From psychotherapy to logotherapy* (3rd ed.). New York, NY: Vintage Books.

Frankl, V. (1988). *The will to meaning: Foundations and applications of logotherapy.* New York, NY: Meridan.

Freeman, S. C. (1993). Client-centered therapy with diverse populations: The universal within the specific. *Journal of Multicultural Counseling and Development, 21,* 248–254.

Frese, F. J., III, Stanley, J., Kress, K., & Vogel-Scibilia, S. (2005). Integrating evidence-based practices and the recovery model. In L. Davidson, C. Harding, & L. Spaniol (Eds.), *Recovery from severe mental illness: Research evidence and implications for practice* (Vol. 2, pp. 375–404). Boston, MA: Center for Psychiatric Rehabilitation.

Garske, G. G., & Bishop, M. L. (2004). Rational-emotive behavior therapy. In F. Chan, N. L. Berven, & K. R. Thomas (Eds.), *Counseling theories and techniques for rehabilitation health professionals* (pp. 177–195). New York, NY: Springer.

Gere, J., & MacDonald, G. (2010). An update of the empirical case for the need to belong. *The Journal of Individual Psychology, 66*(1), 93–115.

Gilbert, M., Cicolini, T., & Mander, A. (2005). Cost-effective use of rational emotive behavior therapy in a public mental health service. *Journal of Rational-Emotive & Cognitive-Behavior Therapy, 23*(1), 71–77.

Giles, G. M., Ridley, J. E., Dill, A., & Frye, S. (1997). A consecutive series of adults with brain injury treated with a washing and dressing retraining program. *American Journal of Occupational Therapy, 51,* 256–266.

Gillespie, K., Duffy, M., Hackmann, A., & Clark, D. M. (2002). Community-base cognitive therapy in treatment of posttraumatic stress disorder following the Omagh bomb. *Behaviour Research and Therapy, 40,* 345–357.

Gingerich, W. J., & Eisengart, S. (2000). Solution-focused brief therapy: A review of the outcome research. *Family Process, 39,* 477–498.

Glasser, W. (1998). *Choice theory: A new psychology of personal freedom.* New York, NY: Harper Collins.

Glasser, W. (2000a). *Counseling with choice theory.* New York, NY: Harper Collins.

Glasser, W. (2000b). *Reality therapy in action.* New York, NY: Harper Collins.

Glasser, W. (2005). *Defining mental health as a public health problem.* Chatsworth, CA: William Glasser Inc.

Gloaguen, V., Cottraux, J., Cucherat, M., & Blackburn, I. (1998). A meta-analysis of the effect of cognitive therapy in depressed patients. *Journal of Affective Disorders, 49,* 59–72.

Gould, W. B. (1993). *Viktor E. Frankl: Life with meaning.* Pacific Grove, CA: Brooks/Cole.

Greaves, D. (1997). The effect of rational–emotive parent education on the stress of mothers of young children with Downs syndrome. *Journal of Rational-Emotive & Cognitive-Behavior Therapy, 15*(4), 249–267.

Greenberg, L., Elliot, R., & Lietaer, G. (1994). Research on experiential psychotherapies. In A. E. Bergin & S. L. Garfield (Eds.), *Handbook of psychotherapy and behavior change* (4th ed., pp. 509–539). New York, NY: Wiley.

Griffiths, D., Feldman, M. A., & Tough, S. (1997). Programming generalization of social skills in adults with developmental disabilities: Effects on generalization and social validity. *Behavioral Therapy, 28*, 253–269.

Grote, N. K., Zuckhoff, A., Swartz, H., Bledsoe, S. E., & Geibel, S. (2007). Engaging women who are depressed and economically disadvantaged in mental health treatment. *Social Work, 52*(4), 295–308.

Hanley-Maxwell, C., Maxwell, K., Fabian, E., & Owens, L. (2010). Supported employment. In E. M. Szymanski, & R. M. Parker, *Work and Disability: Contexts, issues, and strategies for enhancing employment outcomes for people with disabilities* (3rd ed., pp. 415–453). Austin, TX: Pro-Ed.

Hansen, J. T. (2004). Thoughts on knowing: Epistemic implications of counseling practice. *Journal of Counseling & Development, 82*, 131–138.

Hansen, J. T. (2006). Counseling theories within a postmodern epistemology: New Roles for theories in counseling practice. *Journal of Counseling and Development, 84*(3), 291–297.

Harter, J. K., Schmidt, F. L., & Hayes, T. L. (2002). Business-unit-level relationship between employee satisfaction, employee engagement, and business outcomes: A meta-analysis. *Journal of Applied Psychology, 87*, 268–279.

Heimberg, R. G., Liebowitz, M. R., Hope, D. A., Schneier, F. R., Holt, C. S., Welkowitz, L. A. et al. (1998). Cognitive behavioral group therapy vs. phenelzine therapy for social phobia: 12 week outcome. *Archives of General Psychiatry, 55*, 1133–1141.

Hettema, J., Steele, J., & Miller, W. R. (2005). Motivational interviewing. *Annual Review of Clinical Psychology, 1*, 91–111.

Hjertaas, T. (2009). Rediscovering the construct of basic anxiety. *The Journal of Individual Psychology, 65*(1), 47–56.

Hofmann, S. G., & Spiegel, D. A. (1999). Panic control treatment and its applications. *Journal of Psychotherapy Practice and Research, 8*, 3–11.

Holland, J. L. (1997). *Making vocational choices: A theory of vocational personalities and work environments.* Odessa, FL: Psychological Assessment Resources.

Holland, J. L., Fritzsche, B. A., & Powell, A. B. (1994). *The self directed search (SDS) technical manual.* Odessa, FL: Psychological Assessment Resources.

Hollon, S. D., Stewart, M. O., & Strunk, D. (2006). Enduring effects for cognitive behavior therapy in the treatment of depression and anxiety. *Annual Review of Psychology, 57*, 285–315.

Horvath, A. O., & Symonds, B. D. (1991) Relation between working alliance and outcome in psychotherapy: A meta-analysis. *Journal of Counseling Psychology, 38*, 139–149.

Hunt, G. M., & Azrin, N. H. (1973). A community-reinforcement approach to alcoholism. *Behaviour Research and Therapy, 11*, 91–104.

James, I. A., Reichelt, F. K., Carlsonn, P., & McAnaney, A. (2008). Cognitive behavior therapy and executive functioning in depression. *Journal of Cognitive Psychotherapy: An International Quarterly, 22*(3), 210–218.

James, R. K., & Gilliland, B. E. (2003). *Theories and strategies in counseling and psychotherapy* (5th ed.). Boston, MA: Allyn & Bacon.

Johnson, M. H., & Kazantzis, N. (2004). Cognitive behavior therapy for chronic pain: Strategies for the successful use of homework assignments. *Journal of Rational-Emotive & Cognitive-Behavior Therapy, 22*(3), 189–218.

Joseph, S., & Linley, P. A. (2006). *Positive therapy: A meta-theory for positive psychology practice.* London, UK: Taylor & Francis.

Kanfer, F. H., & Goldstein, A. P. (Eds.) (1991). *Helping people change: A textbook of methods* (4th ed.). New York, NY: Pergamon Press.

Kaufman, J. A. (2007). An Adlerian perspective on guided visual imagery for stress and coping. *The Journal of Individual Psychology, 63*(2), 193–204.

Kazantzis, N. (2000). Power to detect homework effects in psychotherapy outcome research. *Journal of Consulting and Clinical Psychology, 68,* 166–170.

Kazdin, A. E. (2000). *Behavior modification in applied settings* (6th ed.). Belmont, CA: Wadsworth.

Kim, J. S. (2010). Examining the effectiveness of solution-focused brief therapy: A meta-analysis. *Research on Social Work Practice, 18*(2), 107–116.

Koch, L. C., McReynolds, C., & Rumrill, P. D. (2004). Basic counseling skills. In F. Chan, N. L. Berven, & K. R. Thomas (Eds.), *Counseling theories and techniques for rehabilitation health professionals* (pp. 227–243). New York, NY: Springer.

Kosciulek, J. D. (1993). Advances in trait-and factor theory: A person x environment fit approach to rehabilitation counseling. *Journal of Applied Rehabilitation Counseling, 24*(2), 11–14.

Kuntze, J., van der Molen, H. T., & Born, M. P. (2009). Increase in counseling communication skills after basic and advanced microskills training. *British Journal of Educational Psychology, 79,* 175–188.

Laidlaw, K., Thompson, L., Dick-Siskin, L., & Gallagher-Thompson, D. (2003). *Cognitive therapy with older people.* Chichester, UK: John Wiley.

Lambert, M. J., & Bergin, M. A. (1994). The effectiveness of psychotherapy. In A. E. Bergin & S. L. Garfield (Eds.), *Handbook of psychotherapy and behavior change* (4th ed., pp. 143–189). New York, NY: Wiley.

Lambie, G. W., & Milsom, A. (2010). A narrative approach to supporting students diagnosed with learning disabilities. *Journal of Counseling & Development, 88,* 196–203.

Larson, J. E. (2008). User friendly motivational interviewing and evidence-based supported employment tools for practitioners. *Journal of Rehabilitation, 74*(4), 18–30.

Lawrence, D. H. (2004). The effects of reality therapy group counseling on the self-determination of persons with developmental disabilities. *International Journal of Reality Therapy, 23*(2), 9–15.

Lazarus, R. S. (1983). The costs and benefits of denial. In S. Breznitz (Ed.), *The denial of stress* (pp. 1–30). New York, NY: International Universities Press.

Lewis, T. F., & Osborn, C. J. (2004). Solution-focused counseling and motivational interviewing: A consideration of confluence. *Journal of Counseling & Development, 82,* 38–48.

Lewis, F. D., & Bitter, C. J. (1991). Applied behavior analysis and work adjustment training. In B. T. McMahon (Ed.), *Work worth doing: Advances in brain injury rehabilitation* (pp. 137–165). Orlando, FL: Paul M. Deutsch.

Linley, P. A., Joseph, S., Maltby, J., Harrington, S., & Wood, A. M. (2009). Positive psychology applications. In S. J. Lopez, & C. R. Snyder (Eds.), *Oxford handbook of positive psychology* (2nd ed., pp. 35–47). New York, NY: Oxford University Press.

Livneh, H., & Wright, P. E. (1995). Rational emotive therapy. In D. Capuzzi & D. R. Gross (Eds.), *Counseling and psychotherapy: Theories and interventions* (pp. 325–352). Englewood Cliffs, NJ: Prentice Hall.

Livneh, H., & Sherwood, A. (1991). Application of personality theories and counseling strategies to clients with physical disability. *Journal of Counseling and Development, 69,* 525–538.

Lloyd, C., Tse, S., Waghorn, G., & Hennessy, N. (2008). Motivational interviewing in vocational rehabilitation for people living with mental ill health. *International Journal of Therapy and Rehabilitation, 15*(12), 572–579.

Lofquist, L. H., & Dawis, R. V. (1969). *Adjustment to work: A psychological view of man's problems in a work-oriented society.* New York, NY: Apple-Century-Crofts.

Lofquist, L. H., & Dawis, R. V. (1991). *Essentials of person environment correspondence counseling.* Minneapolis, MN: University of Minnesota Press.

Lukas, E., & Hirsch, B. Z. (2002). Logotherapy. In F. W. Kaslow, R. F. Massey, & S. D. Massey (Eds.), *Comprehensive handbook of psychotherapy, Vol. 3, Interpersonal/humanistic, existential* (pp. 333–356). New York, NY: Wiley.

Madle, R. A., & Neisworth, J. T. (1990). Mental retardation. In A. S. Bellack & M. Hersen (Eds.), *International handbook of behavior modification and therapy* (2nd ed., pp. 731–762). New York, NY: Plenum.

Marr, J. N. (1982). Behavioral analysis of work problems. In B. Bolton (Ed.), *Vocational adjustment of disabled persons* (pp. 127–147). Baltimore, MD: University Park Press.

Martin, D. J., Garske, J. P., & Davis, M. K. (2000). Relation of the therapeutic alliance with outcome and other variables: A meta-analytic review. *Journal of Consulting and Clinical Psychology, 68*(3), 438–450.

Martin, R. C., & Dahlen, E. R. (2004). Irrational beliefs and the experience and expression of anger. *Journal of Rational-Emotive & Cognitive-Behavior Therapy, 22*(1), 3–20.

Martino, S., Carroll, K. M., Nich, C., & Rounsaville, B. J. (2006). A randomized controlled pilot study of motivational interviewing for patients with psychotic and drug use disorders. *Addiction, 101,* 1479–1492.

McCown, W. G., & Howatt, W. A. (2007). *Treating gambling problems.* Hoboken, NJ: John Wiley & Sons.

McCracken, L. M. (1997). "Attention" to pain in persons with chronic pain: A behavioral approach. *Behavior Therapy, 28,* 271–284.

Mead, S., & Copeland, M. E. (2005). What recovery means to us: Consumers' perspectives. In L. Davidson, C. Harding, & L. Spaniol (Eds.), *Recovery from severe mental illness: Research evidence and implications for practice* (Vol. 1, pp. 69–81). Boston, MA: Center for Psychiatric Rehabilitation.

Meichenbaum, D. (1985). *Stress inoculation training.* New York, NY: Pergamon Press.

Mendel, E., & Hipkins, J. (2002). Motivating learning disabled offenders with alcohol-related problems: A pilot study. *British Journal of Learning Disabilities, 30,* 153–158.

Mendelowitz, E., & Schneider, K. (2008). *Existential Psychotherapy.* In R. Corsini & D. Wedding (Eds.), *Current psychotherapies* (8th ed., pp. 295–326). Belmont, CA: Thompson/Brooks Cole.

Merz, M. A., & Szymanski, E. M. (1997). The effects of a vocational rehabilitation based career workshop on committment to career choice. *Rehabilitation Counseling Bulletin, 41,* 88–104.

Meyers, J. E., & Sweeney, T. J. (2008). Wellness counseling: The evidence base for practice. *Journal of Counseling & Development, 86,* 482–493.

Michailakis, D. (2003). The system theory concept of disability: One is not born a disabled person, one is observed to be one. *Disability & Society, 18*(2), 209–229.

Miller, W. R., & Rollnick, S. (2002). *Motivational interviewing: Preparing people to change addictive behavior.* New York, NY: Guilford Press.

Morley, S., Eccleston, C., & Williams, A. (1999). Systematic review and meta-analysis of randomized controlled trials of cognitive behavior therapy and behavior therapy for chronic pain in adults, excluding headache. *Pain, 80,* 1–14.

Mosak, H. H., & Maniacci, M. (2010). Adlerian psychotherapy. In R. J. Corsini & D. Wedding (Eds.), *Current Psychotherapies* (9th ed., pp. 67–112). Belmont, CA: Brooks/Cole.

Mowbray, C. T., Brown, K. S., Furlong-Norman, K., & Soydan, A. S. (Eds.) (2002). *Supported education and psychiatric rehabilitation: Models and methods.* Columbia, MD: International Association of Psychosocial Rehabilitation Services.

Mowbray, C. T., Bybee, D., & Collins, M. E. (2001). Follow-up client satisfaction in a supported employment program. *Psychiatric Rehabilitation Journal, 24*(3), 237–247.

Myers, J. E., & Sweeney, T. J. (2008). Wellness counseling: The evidence base for practice. *Journal of Counseling & Development, 86,* 482–493.

Nieuwenhuijsen, K., Verbeek, J., de Boer, A., Blonk, R., & van Dijk, F. (2010). Irrational beliefs in employees with an adjustment, a depressive, or an anxiety disorder: A prospective cohort study. *Journal of Rational-Emotive & Cognitive-Behavior Therapy, 28,* 57–72.

Noonan, M., Lindner, H., & Walker, K. (2010). Chronic fatigue syndrome severity and depression: The role of secondary beliefs. *Journal of Rational-Emotive & Cognitive-Behavior Therapy, 28,* 73–86.

O'Hanlon, W. H., & Weiner-Davis, M. (1989). *In search of solutions: A new direction in psychotherapy.* New York, NY: W. W. Norton & Company.

Oliver, L. W., & Spokane, A. R. (1988). Career–intervention outcome: What contributes to client gain? *Journal of Counseling Psychology, 35,* 447–462.

Ososkie, J. N., & Holzbauer, J. J. (2004). Logotherapy. In F. Chan, N. L. Berven, & K. R. Thomas (Eds.), *Counseling theories and techniques for rehabilitation health professionals* (pp. 118–134). New York, NY: Springer.

Parsons, F. (1909). *Choosing a vocation.* Boston, MA: Houghton Mifflin.

Paul, G. L. (1967). Strategy of outcome research in psychotherapy. *Journal of Consulting Psychology, 31*(2), 109–118.

Peterson, C. (2000). The future of optimism. *American Psychologist, 55*(1), 44–55.

Petry, N. M. (2006). *Pathological gambling: Etiology, comorbidity, and treatment.* Washington, DC: American Psychological Association.

Pike, K. M., Walsh, B. T., Vitousek, K., Wilson, G. T., & Bauer, J. (2003). Cognitive behavior therapy in the post hospitalization treatment of anorexia nervosa. *American Journal of Psychiatry, 160,* 2046–2049.

Prenzlau, S. (2006). Using reality therapy to reduce PTSD-related symptoms. *International Journal of Reality Therapy, 25*(2), 23–29.

Prochaska, J. O., DiClemente, J. C., & Norcross, J. C. (1992). In search of how people change: Applications to addictive behavior. *American Psychologist, 47,* 1102–1114.

Rafanelli, C., Park, S. K., Ruin, C., Ottolini, F., Cazzaro, M., & Fava, G. A. (2000). Rating well-being and distress. *Stress Medicine, 16*(1), 55–61.

Rapport, Z. (2007). Using Choice Theory to assess the needs of persons who have a disability and sexual/intimacy/romantic issues. *International Journal of Reality Therapy, 27*(1), 22–25.

Renna, R. (2004). Autism spectrum disorders: Learning to listen as we shape behaviors blending choice theory with applied behavior analysis. *International Journal of Reality Therapy, 23*(2), 17–22.

Robertson, L. A., Smith, H. L., Ray, S. L., & Jones, K. D. (2009). Counseling clients with chronic pain: A religiously oriented cognitive behavior framework. *Journal of Counseling & Development, 87,* 373–379.

Robinson, M. E., & Riley, J. L., III. (1999). The role of emotion in pain. In R. J. Gatchel & D. C. Turk (Eds.), *Psychosocial factors in pain* (pp. 74–88). New York, NY: Guilford.

Rogers, C. (1957). The necessary and sufficient conditions of therapeutic personality change. *Journal of Consulting Psychology, 21,* 93–103.

Rogers, R. (1994). Brief psychodynamic therapy – part 1. *Harvard Mental Health Letter, 10*(9), 1–3.

Rogers, F. (1996). Behavioral therapy of substance abuse treatment: Bringing science to bear on practice. In F. Rogers, D. S. Keller, & J. Morgenstern (Eds.), *Treating substance abuse: Theory and technique* (pp. 174–201). New York, NY: Guilford.

Rounds, J. B., & Tracey, T. J. (1990). From trait-and-factor to person-environment fit counseling: Theory and process. In W. B. Walsh, & S. H. Osipow (Eds.), *Career counseling: Contemporary topics in vocational psychology* (pp. 1–44). Hillsdale, NJ: Erlbaum.

Rubin, S. E., & Roessler, R. T. (2001). *Foundations of the vocational rehabilitation process* (5th ed.). Austin, TX: PRO-ED.

Rule, W. R. (2004). Adlerian therapy. In F. Chan, N. L. Berven, & K. R. Thomas (Eds.), *Counseling theories and techniques for rehabilitation health professionals* (pp. 53–74). New York, NY: Springer.

Savickas, M. L., & Lent, R. W. (Eds.). (1994). *Convergence in career development theories: Implications for science and practice.* Palo Alto, CA: Consulting Psychologists Press.

Schoo, A. (2008). Motivational Interviewing in the prevention and management of chronic disease: Improving physical activity and exercise in line with choice theory. *International Journal of Reality Therapy, 27*(2), 26–29.

Sciacchitano, L., Linder, H., & McCracken, J. (2009). Secondary beliefs: A mediator between illness representations and coping behavior in arthritis suffers. *Journal of Rational-Emotive & Cognitive-Behavior Therapy, 27*(1), 23–50.

See, J. (1986). A person-centered perspective. In T. F. Riggar, D. R. Maki, & A. W. Wolf (Eds.), *Applied rehabilitation counseling* (pp. 135–147). New York, NY: Springer.

See, J., & Kamnetz, B. (2004). Person-centered counseling in rehabilitation professions. In F. Chan, N. L. Berven, & K. R. Thomas (Eds.), *Counseling theories and techniques for rehabilitation health professionals,* (pp. 76–97). New York, NY: Springer.

Seligman, M. E. (1991). *Learned Optimism.* New York, NY: Knopf.

Seligman, M. E., & Csikszentmihalyi, M. (2000). Positive psychology: An introduction. *American Psychologist, 55,* 5–14.

Seligman, M. E., Rashid, T., & Parks, A. C. (2006). Positive psychotherapy. *American Psychologist, 61,* 774–788.

Shifron, R. (2010). Adler's need to belong as the key for mental health. *Journal of Individual Psychology, 66*(1), 10–29.

Sigmon, S. B. (1986). The orthopedically disabled child: Psychological implications with an individual basis. *Individual Psychology: The Journal of Adlerian Theory, Research, & Practice, 42*(2), 274–279.

Sin, N. L., & Lyubomirsky, S. (2009). Enhancing well-being and alleviating depressive symptoms with positive interventions: A practice-friendly meta-analysis. *Journal of Clinical Psychology: In Session, 65*(5), 467–487.

Snyder, C. R. (2002). Hope theory: Rainbows in the mind. *Psychological Inquiry, 13*, 249–275.

Soydan, A. S. (2004). Supported education: A portrait of a psychiatric intervention. *American Journal of Psychiatric Rehabilitation, 7*(3), 227–248.

Spokane, A. R., Meir, E. I., & Catalano, M. (2000). Person-environment congruence and Holland's theory: A review and reconsideration. *Journal of Vocational Behavior, 57*, 137–187.

Stoll, J. L. (2004). Behavior therapy. In F. Chan, N. L. Berven, & K. R. Thomas (Eds.), *Counseling theories and techniques for rehabilitation health professionals* (pp. 136–158). New York, NY: Springer.

Stout, C. E., & Hayes, R. A. (Eds.). (2005). *The evidence-based practice: Methods, models, and tools for mental health professionals.* Hoboken, NJ: Wiley & Sons.

Strong, T., & Zeman, D. (2010). Dialogic considerations of confrontation as a counseling activity: An examination of Allen Ivey's use of confronting as a microskill. *Journal of Counseling & Development, 88*, 332–339.

Super, D. E. (1990). A life-span, life-space approach to career development. In D. Brown & L. Brooks (Eds.), *Career choice and development: Applying contemporary theories to practice* (2nd ed., pp. 197–261). San Francisco, CA: Jossey-Bass.

Sweetland, J. D. (1990). Cognitive-behavior therapy and physical disability. *Journal of Rational-Emotive & Cognitive-Behavior Therapy, 8*(2), 71–78.

Sysko, R., & Hildebrandt, T. (2009). Cognitive-behavioural therapy for individuals with bulimia nervosa and a co-occurring substance use disorder. *European Eating Disorders Review, 17*, 89–100.

Szymanski, E. M., Enright, M. S., Hershenson, D. B., & Ettinger, J. M. (2010). Career development theories, constructs, and research: Implications for people with disabilities. In E. M. Szymanski & R. M. Parker (Eds.), *Work and disability: Contexts, issues, and strategies for enhancing employment outcomes for people with disabilities* (3rd ed., pp. 87–131). Austin, TX: Pro-Ed.

Szymanski, E. M., & Hershenson, D. B. (1998). Career development of people with disabilities: An ecological model. In R. M. Parker & E. M. Szymanski (Eds.), *Rehabilitation counseling: Basics and beyond* (3rd ed., pp. 327–378). Austin, TX: Pro-Ed.

Thomas, K. R., Thoreson, R., Parker, R., & Butler, A. (1998). Theoretical foundations of the counseling function. In R. M. Parker & E. M. Szymanski (Eds.), *Rehabilitation counseling: Basics and beyond* (3rd ed., pp. 225–268). Austin, TX: Pro-Ed.

Tinsley, H. E. (2000). The congruence myth: An analysis of the efficacy of the person-environment fit model. *Journal of Vocational Behavior, 56*, 147–179.

Todman, L. C., & Mansager, E. (2009). Social justice: Addressing social exclusion by means of social interst and social responsibility. *The Journal of Individual Psychology, 65*(4), 311–318.

Tranberg, M., Slane, S., & Ekeberg, E. (1993). The relation between interest congruence and satisfaction: A meta-analysis. *Journal of Vocational Behavior, 42*, 253–264.

Turpin, J., & Ososkie, J. N. (2004). Reality therapy. In F. Chan, N. L. Berven, & K. R. Thomas (Eds.), *Counseling theories and techniques for rehabilitation health professionals* (pp. 196–209). New York, NY: Springer.

Unger, K. V., & Pardee, R. (2002). Outcome measures across program sites for postsecondary supported education programs. *Psychiatric Rehabilitation Journal, 25*(3), 299–303.

Waller, B., Carlson, J., & Englar-Carlson, M. (2006). Treatment and relapse prevention of depression using mindfulness-based cognitive therapy and Adlerian concepts. *The Journal of Individual Psychology, 62*(4), 443–454.

Walter, J. L., & Peller, J. E. (2000). *Recreating brief therapy: Preferences and possibilities.* New York, NY: Norton.

Wampold, B. E. (2000). Outcomes of individual counseling and psychotherapy: Empirical evidence addressing two fundamental questions. In S. D. Brown & R. W. Lent (Eds.), *Handbook of counseling psychology* (3rd ed., pp. 711–739). New York, NY: Wiley.

Wampold, B. E. (2001). *The great psychotherapy debate: Models, methods, and findings.* Mahwah, NJ: Erlbaum.

Wang, P. S., Demler, O., & Kessler, R. C. (2002). Adequacy of treatment for serious mental illness in the United States. *American Journal of Public Health, 92*, 92–98.

Westra, H. A., & Dozois, D. J. (2006). Preparing clients for cognitive behavioral therapy: A randomized pilot study of motivational interviewing for anxiety. *Cognitive Therapy and Research, 30*, 481–98.

Whiston, S. C., Sexton, T. L., & Lasoff, D. L. (1988). Career-intervention outcome: A replication and extension of Oliver and Spokane (1988). *Journal of Counseling Psychology, 45*, 150–165.

Wilson, G. T. (2000). Behavior therapy. In R. J. Corsini & D. Wedding (Eds.), *Current psychotherapies* (6th ed.). Itasca, IL: Peacock.

Wright, B. A. (1972). A value-laden beliefs and principles for rehabilitation psychology. *Rehabilitation Psychology, 19*, 38–45.

Wright, B. A. (1983). *Physical disability—A psychosocial approach*. New York, NY: Harper Collins.

Zaborowski, B. (1997). Adjustment to vision loss and blindness: A process of reframing and retraining. *Journal of Rational-Emotive & Cognitive-Behavior Therapy, 15*(3), 215–222.

Zahniser, J. H. (2005). Psychosocial rehabilitation. In C. E. Stout & R. A. Hayes (Eds.), *The evidence-based practice: Methods, models, and tools for mental health professionals* (pp. 109–152). Hoboken, NJ: John Wiley & Sons.

INSIDER PERSPECTIVE
The Story of Kristine Stebler

My journey into darkness began one day when I was about 7 years old, growing up in Pittsburgh, Pennsylvania, in a family of seven children. My parents, six siblings and I lived in a five-room house. Two of my siblings at that time were totally blind; my brother Keith, who is now a musician and my twin sister Korene, who is now a mother of two. Another brother, Kenn was visually impaired. On that fateful day in the spring of 1964, I was playing with my three sisters and decided to lie down after putting on a plastic headband. It was shaped like a horseshoe, with tiny teeth on the inside. Rolling over in bed, the headband jerked, cutting my eye. Surgery was performed but to no avail. Although the surgeons did not remove the eye, only light perception remained. As the years went by, I learned to adjust using one eye, and psychologically as a child adapting seemed to come naturally. My parents, who had already been raising three visually impaired children, attempted to enroll me in the Western Pennsylvania School for Blind Children in Pittsburgh, PA, to be with my brother, Keith, and sister, Korene, who were thriving there. It was determined, however, that like Kenn, I had "too much sight" to qualify for admission to the school for blind children and so I attended public school.

In elementary school, I wore glasses and had to sit up front to see the blackboard, which today would be considered a reasonable accommodation under the Americans with Disabilities Act. But in the 1960s, teachers just did this because a parent asked, or because it was necessary. Occasionally, other children would call me "four eyes" because I wore glasses, but for the most part I was included socially with my peers. I don't know how my parents did it; not only raising seven children but also managing the constant medical appointments and special needs of four visually impaired children. There were many emotionally challenging times for all of us. Like the period of time when my right eye that had been previously injured was beginning to grow large and disfigured. At 14, my parents and I had to make the excruciating decision to have that eye removed. Although it served no useful purpose and as a teen it was quite disfiguring, most of our discussions centered around saving the eye in the event that a "cure" for blindness may someday become available. Opting for surgery to remove the eye, this was done during the prime of my high-school education. Physical recuperation proved much easier, however, than psychological. There I was, a teen having a body part removed and being fitted for a glass eye.

In terms of my ability to see, however, things remained relatively stable, until 1974, when at the age of 16, not only my vision changed again but also my life as well. I have always loved sports, and in high school if there was a sport offered I wanted to play. School officials were reluctant to allow me to participate in sports, however, because having sight in only one eye, they feared liability if I should have an accident. I was persistent to the point of being obnoxious, so my parents signed waivers that allowed me to participate as long as I wore protective eye gear. Then one afternoon my friends and I were hitting tennis balls in the gym after school, and for some strange reason I chose not to wear my eye gear. We started slamming some balls on a wall in front of us and without ever seeing it, a ball careened off a wall and smashed into my glasses in my other eye. I felt the thick lens press into my eye and the pain was indescribable. Darkness came next, I screamed and wiped my eye with my hand, eventually winding up in the principal's office with my friends, where my parents and the paramedics were summoned.

What followed immediately was my first view of and interaction with the world as a totally blind person. I was guided down the steps of the high school and told to get into a rescue vehicle, which I thought was an ambulance. Disoriented with no sight and probably in shock, I began to fumble. I adjusted quickly and on the way to the hospital I began to tremble. The reality of what had happened was beginning to set in and I remember thinking, what will I do now? The surgeons were pessimistic about the prognosis of my eye. They repaired a cut that stretched half way around the eyeball and stitches made it impossible for me to open my eye for several weeks.

The physical insult of this injury was incredulous; in a mere second I was blind, but along with the injury came depression and social isolation. My friends, who were mostly active and sports minded, didn't visit. Being totally blind, returning to my high school in the short term was not an option. Not much help or advice came from medical professionals or school officials. Fortunately, my determined mother made some telephone calls and I was soon enrolled in a rehabilitation program at Pittsburgh Vision Services. There I learned skills to live and travel independently. There were lessons on how to cook, clean, read braille, and to type and write with various adapted devices. Mobility lessons (walking with a cane, enlisting a sighted guide and aid taking the bus) were very useful but challenging. I needed courage during this time and fortunately my family was there to help me find it.

During my rehabilitation, however, there was a gradual remarkable twist of fate. As the injury healed I could open my eye and I could see light, then shadows, forms, colors, and finally it all came together. About 4 months after the horror some of my vision came back. I was able to finish my last year at my previous high school, but it was hard as I could not play sports, so I lost most of my friends. It was unbearably lonely and my role as an active teenager had changed.

In the years after the accident, I was followed by ophthalmologists at the University of Pittsburgh Medical Center. Dr. Biglan, a pediatric ophthalmologist was able to correctly diagnose our family's eye conditions as kerataglobus, a very rare eye condition in which the cornea is unusually thin. He concluded that even minor insults to the cornea could rupture it, and we now understood that if we wore protective lenses and avoided contact sports, we could prevent further injury or blindness.

In terms of my visual acuity for the next 20 years following the accident, I lived as a legally blind person. There evolved a slow and continual deterioration of my sight, however, when a cataract began to form over the previously injured eye making it increasingly more difficult to see. Over the years seeing became laborious like looking through a keyhole that was fogged over. This, in turn, created a number of barriers to overcome, both physical and attitudinal. Reading was impossible without adaptations, and driving was not an option. Day-to-day tasks like grocery shopping took lots of effort and were visually exhaustive. The most challenging task by far though was trying to maneuver a shopping cart with many aisle mishaps, including running over a woman's coat while she was kneeling, and mistaking running over a loaf of bread for a screaming baby nearby. Fortunately, management at my supermarket has never banned me for being a public nuisance.

In terms of attitudinal barriers relative to my disability, I've had my share. For example, during my undergraduate education, there was a professor who decided that since I was visually impaired, I was unfit to graduate as an elementary school teacher. Her school of thought was that I would somehow injure students in a classroom since I could not see them and that no school district would hire me because I would be an "insurance liability." The irony in this situation was that elementary education was my minor and special education was my major.

Attitudinal barriers have been by far the hardest to overcome and accept more so than the physical. I have heard so many theories about my "dilemma" from so many people, including total strangers who take it upon themselves to give me unwanted advice, stereotype my situation, provide help I don't want or need, and tell me what's best for me. Despite this, and precisely because of these ignorant attitudes, I decided early on that if I excelled above and beyond, received a good education, and got as much work experience as I could, that some of these barriers would dissolve. In addition, I worked hard to develop openness about my visual impairment as well as a keen sense of humor. Oddly, the attitudes and misconceptions of other people have influenced the way I interact with people in life. As a result, I am very open about my visual impairment and willing to speak to anyone in an effort to educate them on how those of us with visual impairments live. I thank God everyday for whatever vision I have had, but in terms of barriers, navigating through the physical and attitudinal sighted world has sometimes been frustrating, lonely, physically dangerous, and psychologically challenging.

The story of my vision loss doesn't end here, however. In August 1998, my eyesight deteriorated to less than 20/200 and I was struggling visually to handle the everyday tasks in my life on the job as a licensed social worker and in my personal life. The cataract was continuing to grow larger, thereby robbing me of what limited vision I had. Desperate, I went to see Dr. Paul Freeman, a low vision specialist at Allegheny

General Hospital in Pittsburgh, PA. After examining my eye, he prescribed assistive devices that would help me to see (a monocular to read bus signs, store signs, street signs, and a closed-circuit television that would enlarge the print of any page, and reading glasses). These devices gave me improved, but still limited independence. I was also referred to Dr. Theirry Verstraeten who advised me that the odds for successful cataract removal surgery were 90% improved vision, 5% no change, and 5% total loss of vision. The thought of losing any remaining vision was scary. For a year I did multiple checks, and all the while the cataract was continuing to grow and my vision was deteriorating more rapidly. I was tripped and fell down more often despite using my walking cane. Life was becoming more and more challenging again, yet I was clinging to what precious little sight I had. It was an asset I did not want to part with.

In the fall in 1999, Dr. Verstreten advised that the cataract was turning yellow and could break apart and cause blindness. There was no choice at this point but to have the surgery. Falling back on the advice I had been giving my social work clients for 20 years, I turned to my family, friends, and faith and sought out as much information as possible. I also developed a "plan B" and began to request information on guide dog schools and other services in case I lost my eye sight to the surgery. The day before the surgery, I found myself fretting about whether I had made the right decision. I went for a walk to clear my head and crashed into a stranger without ever having seen him. It was at that moment that I realized it was time to let go and put this into God's hands.

The surgery went smoothly and I was to go home in bandages and return the next morning to remove them. When the patch was removed I sat there searching for courage to open my eye, then opened my eye in pleasant shock at how much I could see. I looked around the exam room and looked into my mother's beautiful face. As we left the hospital, I was laughing, crying, trembling, praying, and looking at absolutely everything. I was a sightseer looking at everything for the first time. Snow, cars, buildings, birds, the sky, people, you name it. I discovered quickly that I could see at night and in the middle of the winter, I went outside after dark in front of my apartment to take in the view. But I initially suffered from sensory overload and was still using my sense of hearing, smell, and touch that I used for almost 25 years to help me function. I could not shut off these senses that seemed like they were now in overdrive. The world was visually very loud and there were times when I actually found myself suffering from motion sickness. People were coming to visit me to celebrate my recovery, and I knew who they were by their voice, but visually I was newly introduced to them. It was fun to actually *see* people I had befriended while I had almost no sight and get reacquainted with what my family and old friends looked like. My vision at this point was 20/70, improved from 20/200 or less. I was discovering and rediscovering new things everyday.

For days, months, and even years after this surgery, I was able to see new things and my vision improved to 20/60. I cherished seeing raindrops and snow falling, puddles, birds in flight, and people sleeping in church. Have you ever noticed how bright an orange is? Losing my sight and the gift of getting it back had a physical, psychological, and spiritual impact on my life. Initially, I struggled psychologically when I got my sight back because my visually impaired siblings did not and in all probability never would. I will never know why each of us could not have a little slice of that pie. After the surgery I spoke with my siblings, who were all very happy for me, which allowed me to resolve this issue. In addition, physically and psychologically speaking I was no longer a disabled person and did not have to use my cane since the surgery. Spiritually, I thanked God everyday for this incredible gift. It perplexed me, however, as to the reason I was given my sight back; not once, but twice, and often prayed that I was able to use it in the manner in which God intended.

Life goes on with many twists and turns. Any human being would probably agree with this. As fate would have it, however, I once again began to lose vision rather rapidly in the Spring of 2003, and one morning fell down from steps fracturing my foot as I readied for work. It seemed like I had a lapse of consciousness. My PCP Dr. Knupp had a CAT scan done and delivered the surreal news that I had a benign brain tumor called meningioma, and it had to be removed immediately. By this time, my vision had deteriorated significantly because of the tumor. At this point, fear consumed me. I have never been so afraid in my life. But once again, my family and friends stepped up to the plate and literally held my hand through- out this ordeal. The tumor caused a significant vision loss that would never return. Managing my disabilities psychologically and financially as well as coping with the stress of my everyday life is a full-time job. In 2008, I lost my eyesight. But somehow, by the grace of God, a great support system and a talented group of medical providers, I have managed to somehow survive several trips to hell and back.

Key Messages for Those Working With People With Disabilities

Individuals and families with disabilities are vulnerable. There exists for us the physical impact of our disability such that the nature of the condition could be of sudden onset, or one that causes a gradual deterioration of function. There are added responsibilities like additional medical appointments, surgeries, or medications that take additional time, thought, and effort. We may be required to make difficult decisions, have increased financial burdens, or experience side effects to medications or procedures. Many times there exist transportation and/or communication barriers. In families with disabilities, caretakers can burn out with added physical responsibilities, difficul- ties in finding sitters/caretakers for disabled children or adults, and sometimes siblings are asked to take on adult responsibilities. All this can cause stress, can be frustrating, and can be exhausting at times. Reaction to a disability or lack of function/indepen- dence can vary among the individual, family members, and/or friends. Anger, fear, denial, and guilt are normal in some situations and differ from one individual and/ or family to the next. Some individuals or families with a disability may avoid public reaction to a disability, thus creating social isolation.

An area that is sometimes overlooked in the medical arena is the spiritual impact of a disability with patients. Spirituality is a coping mechanism that sometimes provides lifestyle motivation, a social network, and/or defines one's beliefs about their illness. When there is disability or illness in a family, their belief system may be questioned. Some may abandon their faith or stop attending church; others may need it more or opt to change their beliefs.

What Can Rehabilitation Counselors Do?

Recognize that all disabilities are as different as the individuals who possess them. Don't stereotype anyone with a disability. Remember that each person you encounter has different abilities and disabilities, and just because you have read about a disorder or work with others with my same disability doesn't mean you know what I can and cannot do. Be sure to look at my strengths when you are assessing my problems.

Obtain as much information as you can by asking *me* as many questions as possible. On several occasions, physicians, specialists, and counselors had ignored me and attempted to talk with my mother or sister who had accompanied me to appointments. Talk directly to your clients and acknowledge their presence. Express interest but *do not* pity them or any person with a disability; learn the difference between empathy and sympathy and use them both appropriately. Develop a rapport with us so that we feel comfortable telling you what we need and be honest and sincere. Tell us when you don't understand something or when you disagree.

Always include *our* perspective of the problem in your treatment plan and be honest and tell us what you do and do not know about our condition. Here I am reminded of a time when I had very little sight and went to the emergency room with an injured ankle. I made it a point to tell all of the health professionals I saw that day in the ER that I was visually impaired. The x-rays came back and my ankle was fractured. A young doctor came in and reported that he was ordering the ankle be cast and that I should have crutches. Despite my several protests that I could not use crutches as a visually impaired person, he refused to listen to my perspective. The ankle was cast and he gave me crutches. Frustrated, I politely took the crutches, and when I got home they went into the closet and I used my cane. In this situation, a treatment plan was designed without my input being acknowledged. When health professionals don't listen to patients, we do what we think is best and we're labeled "non-compliant" by those medical professionals. Remember I am the expert about my disability, my body, and my life. You are the expert in the field to help me adapt to my situation and we must have mutual respect of each other's opinions. Always remember that all problems cannot be solved and do not promise me what you cannot deliver. If professionals can understand and learn to accept this, we'll both be better off.

Summary

I hope that from the time you meet and assess your first and your last client/patient that first and foremost you will remember that I am not a disabled person, but a person who happens to be disabled. Understand that living in a world that values strength and perfect body images, that as a person with a disability, I have to put forth 150% effort everyday of my life just to survive in this world. Success in medicine, nursing, rehabilitation counseling, and social work depends on the success of interpersonal relationships between providers and clients/patients. When developing yourself as an expert, it's not enough to just pass tests, read textbooks, or learn procedures. True professionals learn how to treat patients with kindness, respect, and dignity as if their patients are their own mothers, brothers, children, or partner.

DISCUSSION QUESTIONS

1. How does the professional choose the eclectic path and why? What is required of them in the pursuit of mastery?
2. Why are the cognitive-behavioral approaches so pervasive? Can you imagine what counseling would be like without cognitive interventions?
3. Are working alliances all the same, or are they situationally and theoretically determined?
4. What is the future of positive psychology in rehabilitation?

EXERCISE

A. A pragmatic eclectic approach to rehabilitation counseling obliges the dedicated professional to a life time of study and skill training. Develop an action plan for developing your own skill set, assuming instant access and unlimited funds. What literature would you explore? What was your rationale for choosing these topics? How would it change your current practice?

THIRTEEN

Counseling Families

Michael Jay Millington

OVERVIEW

Rehabilitation counselors deal with families every time they meet with a client, whether they attend to them or not (Hall, 2003; Minuchin, 1980). Humans are social creatures born into a family, shaped and defined by our family experiences, nurtured and supported by our family networks, and obligated by our family roles. The family is the first-order community, an interdependent system of relationships, inseparable from the person of the client. Families have as much influence on the rehabilitation process as the client chooses to allow, sometimes more. The disability experience resonates from the individual and through the family as one. Disability mediates and moderates the relationships between family members and between the family and other social support systems, including rehabilitation counseling.

The family's importance to rehabilitation counseling is common wisdom. State agencies and community rehabilitation program administrators overwhelmingly support the idea that properly trained counselors should work with client families (Power, Hershenson, & Fabian, 1991). Educators in graduate programs concur on the need for family counseling content in the curriculum (Riemer-Reiss & Morrissette, 2002). Researchers support the inclusion of family in rehabilitation counseling plans and practice (see Alston & McCowan, 1994; Cottone, Handelsman, & Walters, 1986; Frain et al., 2007; Freedman & Fesko, 1996; Versluys, 1980). And yet, for all those who champion family inclusion in service (Kosciulek, 2004), little progress has been made in the development of research model implementation (Accordino, 1999; Bryan, 2009; Freedman & Fesko, 1996), professional training (May & Hunt, 1994), or policy (Kneipp & Bender, 1981). In the absence of a best practice, or much in the way of its pursuit, the family remains relegated to the periphery of rehabilitation. Families are a counseling afterthought and an addendum to service, despite calls to the contrary.

There are reasons for the slow progress toward family inclusion (Accordino, 1999; Cottone et al., 1986; May & Hunt, 1994; Power et al., 1991). Policy and circumstance create outsized caseloads, restrictive regulations, and ponderous documentation demands that diminish available resources for counselor training and skill implementation. Counselors are neither sufficiently trained in family counseling, nor do they have ready access to proper training through current preservice or in-service programs (Herbert, 1989; Sutton, 1985). Family counseling and support neither ranks high in the role and function studies that stand in for ideal service, nor high in the knowledge domains to be mastered through training. Essentially, family inclusion in service delivery has not developed because the rehabilitation counseling system does not reward it, the practitioners are not competent to provide it, and there are no established models that can make the case for a best practice. Finding the proper working relationships between family and client, between family and counselor, and between family and service delivery system is a difficult work in progress for the rehabilitation counseling profession.

An important early step in family inclusion will be to integrate current generic family counseling models into rehabilitation counseling practice. Traditionally, the purpose of family counseling is to disrupt and replace dysfunctional relationships, with the goal being a healthier and more stable family. For rehabilitation counseling, a healthier and more stable family is instrumental to the primary goals of full community inclusion for the client. And so the question for rehabilitation counselors is more specific: How do we optimize the natural supports families can offer in service of the rehabilitation plan? For the purposes of this chapter, we will first describe the family in relation to the experience of disability. We will then provide an overview of family counseling approaches that bring different perspectives to this particular family challenge. We will conclude with a discussion on the themes that unite these approaches under the rubric of rehabilitation counseling and implications for current practice.

FAMILY AND DISABILITY

What makes a family? In the past, psychologists in search of the "normal" held up the common nuclear family as the norm, that is, statistical model, and interpreted its common characteristics as normative, that is, preferred or superior to other characteristics (Walsh, 2003). This nuclear-centric worldview was a conceit of the ethnic majority of the United States in the past century ... more accurate then, statistically speaking, than now, but just as biased in effect. Narrow definitions of family are increasingly inappropriate for an increasingly diverse clientele (Kneipp & Bender, 1981). From today's postmodern, multicultural perspective, there is no normative family structure. The traditional nuclear family (mother, father, siblings) is one structure, but it is not the only means to quality family life (see Alston & Turner, 1994; Joosten-Weyn et al., 2008). Families described as extended, unmarried, same sex, and single parent satisfactorily fulfill the functions of family as well. With demographics trending away from the nuclear and toward diversity in family models (Sheridan & Burt, 2009), the search for "normal" structures has reached its unproductive end. The emphasis of enquiry has shifted from what a family is, to what a family does, not what makes a family normal or abnormal, but what makes a family productive or unproductive in its tasks (Walsh, 2003).

Family From a Counseling Context

The primary function of the family unit is to develop and maintain the psycho-social-biological health of its members. Family is a complex living system of relationships (Hanna & Brown, 1999) beyond biological relatives to include anyone who lives with, has a substantial interest in, or influence over, the client. Family is operationally defined through stakeholder roles (father, mother, sibling, etc.) and their transactions. Roles articulate familial expectations and are negotiated between members. A unique relationship arises out of the experiences of every dyad in the system (Cottone et al., 1986). The amalgam of these family relationships is, in a sense, the internal identity of the group. Family roles are also differentiated based on the need for external transactions with the network of families and organizations in the community. The character of the family is expressed in the history and consequences of these internal and external transactions.

Just as individuals within the family evolve through life stages and face different learning experiences and challenges along the way, so does the family cycle through a process of evolution (Becvar & Becvar, 1999). The individual grows within the context of the growing family, transitioning to new roles along the way. Cultural identity is passed down the generations through ritual, tradition, history (oral or otherwise), values, occupational choices, common conflicts, and approved resolution strategies (McGoldrick & Giordano, 1996). As roles change, the family changes. Individuals progress and expand experience through a parade of roles from child, to sibling, to spouse, to parent, to grandparent, to ancestor. Family system shapes the person and the person shapes the family system (Minuchin, 1980; Testa, Malec, Moessner, & Brown, 2006; Versluys, 1980).

The healthy family comprises individually healthy members, secure in themselves, with fully intact personalities and strong, yet flexible, personal boundaries (Lewis, Beavers, Gossett, & Phillips, 1976). Each family member is conscious of, and fully engaged in, his or her role. Members in healthy families enjoy reciprocal mutuality (Kaslow, 1982), that is, each individual provides value to the others through his or her works and is recognized for the contribution. Healthy family members see each other and themselves in congruent and supportive ways with emotional openness, warmth, and good humor (Lewis et al., 1976). They have shared goals and the expectation of success.

Family members create and sustain appropriate relationships within the family structure, based on relative role position (e.g., mother/daughter relationship, wife/husband relationship). Effective relationships are sustained through emotionally open, clear, direct, and congruent communication and a collaborative approach to problem solving. Healthy relationships are capable of trafficking in diverse views in pursuit of common ground (Sander et al., 2002). There is a stable, legitimate, and predictable power structure among the family roles. Rules are known and applied consistently. Healthy families are guided by shared traditions, rituals, and other expressions of shared values, such as those that make up sound parenting practices or marital management strategies (Becvar, 1985). Nurturance is consistently available to all family members as needed. Members are not isolated by the family, but move freely within other social groups.

All these qualities, in their absence, are as indicative of poor health as their presence suggests wellness and strengths. Families express a spectrum of functionality across tasks and time. Families negotiate their fortunes in the world, facing internal conflicts between family members and external conflicts with the world at large. Families differ widely on how well they cope with these challenges and their efforts in coping define them. As Beavers (1982) suggests, healthy families seek intimacy; midrange families seek control; and dysfunctional families flounder incoherently.

McMaster model

Health is evidenced in how families cope with change. The McMaster model looks at the function of family in the execution of family tasks and the dimensions of family function leading to healthy or unhealthy outcomes. It is based on empirical findings and provides a useful framework for understanding family values. According to the McMaster model (Epstein et al., 2003), the primary family functions are acted out in three task domains. The basic task domain involves all of the instrumental subroutines that sustain the family system (e.g., procuring and managing food, shelter, money, transportation). The developmental task domain includes growth and transition activities (graduation, marriage, procreation, death). The hazardous task domain deals with crisis and the unexpected (disability, job loss, bankruptcy, divorce, death). Family members' interactions are qualitatively described on six different dimensions that are directly relevant to internal health and external efficacy in dealing with the task area issues (Epstein et al., 2003): (a) problem solving, (b) communication, (c) role function, (d) affective responsiveness and involvement, and (e) behavior control.

Problem-solving effectiveness

Instrumental and emotional problems are experienced by every family. Family health is facilitated by effective problem-solving skills. This implies the presence and utilization of a stable decision-making process that moves stepwise through a rational progression. The problem must be first comprehended and described, and then communication must be established between the family stakeholders, options generated, and a plan developed, implemented, and evaluated. The effectiveness of family problem-solving strategy is a function of the number of steps attempted and the quality of response at each step (Epstein et al., 2003).

Communication

There are two general fields for communicating within the family. Instrumental communication transmits the logistical and concrete (what I do). Affective communication transmits the idiosyncratic and emotional (how I feel). The means and strategies in each field may differ, but the quality of communication is the same for both and they focus on two orthogonal qualities: (a) clarity of message and (b) directness to the intended recipient. Communication can be qualified in four different styles along these axes.

- Clear/direct: (a) Message meaning is conveyed with minimal loss or distortion of meaning; (b) message came directly from the source
- Clear/indirect: (a) Message meaning is conveyed with minimal loss or distortion of meaning; (b) message came through an intermediary
- Masked/direct: (a) Message meaning is distorted, diluted, hidden, or lost in translation; (b) came directly from the source without an intermediary
- Masked/indirect: (a) Message meaning is distorted, diluted, hidden, or lost in translation; (b) message came through an intermediary

Different situations and different cultures call for different emphases in these quadrants. The message is clearest in the clear/direct quadrant, and most obfuscated in the masked/indirect quadrant. Problems arise when there is a breakdown between contextual expectations and communication characteristics.

Role function

Families are a specialized system with differentiated roles. Each role has interactional functions, things shared with other members of the family. Basic roles include provision of (a) resources (breadwinner), (b) nurturance and support, (c) sex and intimacy, (d) personal development and advancement (e.g., career support), and (e) family management. Family management includes authority expressed through decision-making, boundary maintenance (family and world), distribution of resources, caregiving, role allocation (how tasks are meted out, clear instructions, and appropriate for the developmental stage and age), and role accountability (responsibility to the family and the authority within the family, self-monitoring, and concrete corrective consequences for violation of role).

Affective responsiveness and involvement

Responsiveness is the ability to react with appropriate emotionality. Affective responsiveness is communicated through the volume, intensity, duration, style, content, and appropriateness of the emotional response to family cues. Involvement is the degree to which individuals engage emotionally, intellectually, and physically with other members. Engagement runs a continuum from (a) complete isolation; to (b) emotionally detached, strictly intellectual interface; to (c) narcissistic engagement; to (d) empathetic engagement, a full emotional exchange; to (e) overinvolvement, overprotecting, and smothering; and finally to (f) symbiotic loss of identity. Obviously, optimal engagement is a balance between these dysfunctional poles.

Behavior control

Roles have rules that make behavior within the family predictable and safe. Families have protocols for appropriate behavior in crisis situations that are physically dangerous or threatening, in the expression of personal needs and drives, and in interpersonal social situations. Here again, implementation style runs along a continuum of functionality. At one extreme, behavioral control is complete with excessive, rigid, inflexible rules and no negotiating for alternate behaviors. A healthier level of behavioral control follows a thoughtful path with predictable and enforced rules that are open to negotiation and change in the present. A laissez-faire style decentralizes control, allowing members to freely follow their own standards. At the other dysfunctional extreme, behavioral control becomes a chaotic mix of unpredictable, unreasoned, and continuously shifting application of strategies (Epstein, Ryan, Bishop, Miller, & Keitner, 2003).

The Experience of Disability

Disability resonates through the family system (McKellin, 1995) and challenges its structures and processes (Ell, 1996). The experience of disability (in its bounded but infinite permutations of onset, etiology, functional limitations, course and prognosis, demands of treatment and care, and stigma) becomes both the object and mediator of family behavior.

Roles are disrupted (Yeates, Henwood, Gracey, & Evans, 2007). Sometimes it becomes impossible for family members to maintain their customary role as authority, provider, or spouse (Coles, Pakenham, & Leech, 2007; Deatrick, Brennan, & Cameron, 1998). The authority hierarchy is compromised, and strategies of control that worked in the past may no longer apply. Disruption in roles changes affective engagement among family members (Feigin, 1994), often isolating one family member from another. Family members take on new roles, particularly as primary caregivers and advocates on behalf of their child, spouse, or sibling with a disability. With new roles come new obligations and greater demands placed on personal and family resources. Family members must learn to cope with symptoms, respond to the demands of adjustment, and engage a service system that is not consistently responsive (Spaniol, Zipple, & Lockwood, 2006). Lack of information about and training in these new roles is stressful and can lead to conflicted, inadequate, misguided, and disempowering family decisions (Ell, 1996).

The change in roles is a long-term challenge to function and resilience. Chronic conditions requiring ongoing care increase stress and decrease caregiver quality of life (Greenwood, MacKenzie, Cloud, & Wilson, 2008) in the present and worry for the future (Degeneffe & Olney, 2008). The long-term effect of added stress feeds back into the system. Chronic stress reduces physical health, constricts community activity (Gallagher & Mechanic, 1996), erodes the caregiver's social network (Schmidt & Welsh, 2010), and isolates the client within the family (Magliano et al., 2005 [mental illness]; Kozloff, 1987 [traumatic brain injury]). Reduction in these qualities is a reduction in resilience. Lower resilience increases the susceptibility of the family to stress, potentially creating a spiral of diminishing health. Sibling care can be incessant, interminable, and increasingly demanding (Degeneffe, 2001; Degeneffe & Burcham, 2008). The lack of caregiver optimism and diminishing sense of self-efficacy can feed into the depressogenic context of caregiving (Degeneffe & Lynch, 2006).

The experience of disability changes the relationship of the family to its community. Established relationships change and diminish. New relationships are formed. The family moves in new disability-related circles. Stigma enters the home (see Moses, 2010) and becomes part of the emotional climate. Family attention shifts from daily routine to crisis management to stabilization. New skills are required to negotiate the service system. Disability becomes part of the family identity (see McKellin, 1995).

The introduction of disability into a family system ill equipped to handle the cumulative stress leads to inefficient care (Degeneffe & Lee, 2010), poor outcomes (Degeneffe & Lynch, 2006), and potential abuse (Forbat, 2002). And yet, the familial response to disability has been a largely uncontrolled variable in applied rehabilitation counseling. Rosenthal, Kosciulek, Lee, Frain, and Ditchman (2009) have responded to the general lack of models at the interface of family counseling and disability with a proposed integration of the "resiliency model of family stress, adjustment, and adaptation" (Kosciulek, McCubbin, & McCubbin, 1993); and the "risk and resistance model" (Wallander, Varni, Babani, Banis, & Wilcox, 1989), providing us with a point of reference for our consideration of family counseling applications to rehabilitation counseling.

The resiliency model of family stress, adjustment, and adaptation

The Kosciulek et al. model (1993) was itself an integration of earlier theories concerned with adjustment and adaptation. Early family response to nascent disability is an immediate and unfolding problem, even crisis. The experience of disability disturbs the equilibrium, stresses existing family vulnerabilities, and threatens to the throw the system into chaos. Families have varying degrees of vulnerability to stress that become instrumental in maintaining family function as the demand for resources and attention mounts.

Following the introduction of disability into the family system, the first response is to resurrect and stabilize predisability family structures and processes, that is, restore equilibrium with minimal change (bonadjustment). Families engage their resources and coping strategies, sometimes successfully, sometimes not. Sometimes family defenses are insufficient to deal with the problem. Sometimes, dysfunctional family processes exacerbate existing problems and create new ones. The experience of disability can overwhelm the family system. Mounting stress leads to a deterioration of established patterns, a loss of centeredness and self-control, and a threat to self-efficacy (see Bandura, 1997) in the extreme, to the point of hopelessness (maladjustment). Families struggle along this continuum until a new system starts to approximate equilibrium once again.

The introduction of disability into a family unbalances the system, but not forever. The system structure reorganizes in the adaptation phase. It reorients to a new way of being in, and interacting with, the world. Adaptation is a long-term process of learning how to be a family in the presence of a disability. Adaptation is developmental in its approach to equilibrium. Bonadaptation is characterized by reduced stress, improved physical and mental health/wellness, continued commitment to care, recovery, and development; optimal role function; the functional ease with which the family navigates the transitional stages (and challenges) of its "life"; and family cohesion, a sense of self-efficacy, and the proactive contemplation of future challenges. Maladaptation is characterized by a chronic imbalance between members of the family, resulting in repetitive and irresolvable conflicts, and family incompetence in self-advocacy and negotiating in the larger community (Kosciulek et al., 1993).

Family resilience is a multifaceted approach to adjustment and adaptation (McCubbin, Thompson, & McCubbin, 1996; Singer & Powers, 1993) at the interface of family problem-solving and coping skills; social supports and resources; personal appraisal (optimism); and function (Frain, Bishop, Tschopp, Ferrin, & Frain, 2009). Resilient families maintain control, identity, and integrity of boundaries. Communication in resilient families is open and lively with free expression of appropriate emotion. Family members share an optimistic view of the future and actively pursue an agenda that will fulfill their vision. Resilience embraces cognitive reframing as a means of perceptually transforming threats into challenges, stressors into learning events, and rigid worldviews into flexible ones (Antonovsky, 1987). Resilient families readily adapt roles and transfer tasks. Challenges are sought out and resolved with coordinated problem-solving, goal setting, troubleshooting, and crisis management strategies. Resilient families actively engage their support networks in collaborative relationships with service and resource professionals, trading with mutual respect, and positively assertive self-advocacy (Singer & Powers, 1993). Families that can effectively leverage their social networks move with more confidence and self-efficacy and less stress in confronting the disability-related challenges imposed on them (Sarason, Levine, & Pierce, 1990).

Risk and resistance model

The risk and resistance model focuses on the factors that contribute to family adjustment and adaptation to the experience of disability (Wallander et al., 1989). Vulnerability is articulated through factors that increase stress on the system. They include conditional factors surrounding the disability (diagnosis, prognosis, etiology, visibility of the condition, stigma, etc.), factors arising out of the loss of functional independence, and psychological stressors (dysfunctional affect, cognition, and behavior). Vulnerabilities can permeate the family system. They can be event driven, arising out of singular stress-inducing situations; or they can be ongoing chronic stressors that challenge system endurance over the long term.

Families respond to this differentiated challenge by diminishing its negative effect and transmuting the experience into a positive where possible. The family's identified coping strategies are the first line of resistance. Individual and intrapersonal coping skills are essential components. Socioecological factors enhance resistance through community-based resources. The social support network provides emotional, economic, and logistic help as well as access to expert networks of information, service, and public resources (Rosenthal et al., 2009). Considered together, these models provide the targeted processes and structures for psychosocial family counseling.

FAMILY COUNSELING ROOTS

Rosenthal et al.'s (2009) offering moves the discourse on the experience of disability within the family in a decidedly systemic direction and provides a workable context for exploring family counseling perspectives on adjustment and adaptation to disability. What follows is not meant to be a comprehensive explication of family counseling theory, but a representative cross section of its primary features. None of the family counseling theories we will discuss were created specifically for the issues of disability as they are understood by rehabilitation counselors, but they all speak to disability in some form or another. Every theory is a facet, incomplete but necessary for understanding the family dynamic in rehabilitation counseling.

Family counseling, like family, is given form by the voices and interactions of its component parts. It does not have a theory as such, just a systems approach and an amalgam of practice/knowledge sets interpreted from the panoply of psychotherapeutic interventions. Family counseling is framed as a pragmatic eclecticism that integrates across theories in service of the client (Lebow, 1997). Need drives the applicable theory in specific applications of practice. The question is what do the various theoretical viewpoints have to offer in the way of utility to the cause of rehabilitation counseling?

Psychodynamic Origins and Adlerian Family Therapy

The most relevant expression of the psychodynamic worldview in family therapy is arguably through object relations (Goldenberg, Goldenberg, & Pelavin, 2008). Object relations address the development and growth of the internal psychic landscape; how personality is formed through a developmental process by which the infant constructs an external reality and the ego's relationship to it. At birth, there is no "other" for the child; the newborn is awash in sensation and in a sense without boundaries. First objects to arise out of the chaos serve basic infant needs for warmth, contact, and sustenance. These are the early experiences with the mother. The infant constructs and completes the mother as an object, separates from the mother as a unique identity, and seeks rapprochement with the mother in a new relationship (Becvar & Becvar, 2009). This primal relationship is the first instance (Scharff & Scharff, 2006) of a deep human need to make contact with others. It points to the biological origins of our social nature and the centrality family in its development. Attachment is the development of healthy bonds of affection grown through shared experience . . . the first attachment (mother) is the template for future emotional relationships and efforts to build relationships (Ainsworth, 1989). People bring their past experiences to their present-day relationships, and introject the pain of remembered childhood loss and disappointment into the mix. Expectations for the relationship between family members are formed early and can crystallize into an ill-fitting pattern as family roles evolve. To break from being the "baby of the family" requires a change in all parties.

Psychodynamic approaches are individual by nature. Object relations theory provided the first best leap of psychodynamic practice from intrapsychic to interpsychic domains, from the individual-in-therapy to the relationship between individuals. The psychodynamic argument for relevance in family therapy is that the intra- and interpsychic domains are in constant exchange and mutual influence (Becvar & Becvar, 2009). The social nature of our identities grows as relationships expand and mature. Spouse function and behavior are shaped by their experiences vis-à-vis the family of origin. The unconscious works out issues of past family experience in the context of the current family experience. According to Walsh, "... family processes and psychopathology are conceptualized in terms of the interlocking of parental individual dynamics, multigenerational loyalties, conflicts, and losses, and transferences or unconscious role assignments" (Walsh, 2003, p. 37). Object relations represent a family approach by extension rather than design. Its value in this discussion is more philosophical than practical.

Adlerian family therapy was the first actual family therapy to come out of the psychodynamic tradition (Bitter, 2009). For Adler, family therapy was a natural evolution from the individual approach. Adler perceived clients as social beings whose identities are formed in the family and expressed through lifestyle and choices (Mosak & Maniacci, 2010). Family atmosphere (a concept comparable to organizational climate) is the emotional tenor of the complex of family relationships. Atmosphere gathers around the way members treat each other. Parents are the core and the model of decorum. The emotional atmosphere charges the connotative meaning in communication. Communication can be charged with hostility or caring, warmth or coldness, any manner of emotional content. These emotions color the meaning of information and the context in which it is delivered. The emotional charge of a message communicates family values (e.g., education, work, money, morality, politics, etc.) and become part of the scaffolding for individual growth. Family member transactions and member interpretation of the meaning of those transactions are the experiences on which self- and family identity is based (Bitter, Roberts, & Sonstegard, 2002).

Adler noted that birth order was an important organizing principle in child development in that the child's position within the family constellation preordains predictable roles and inevitable family interactions (Bitter, 2009). There are five basic birth order positions (i.e., the only, the oldest, the second-of-two, the middle, and the last child), each with its unique perspective, obligations, and benefits. The experience of growing in these roles and lessons learned shape personality in predictable ways. Adlerians investigate birth order as a function of family structure, transactions, and growth.

Adlerian Family Therapy is parenting oriented. It is often employed to deal with child misbehavior. Childhood misbehavior has goals ... mistaken goals, but goals nonetheless. The fundamental childhood goals are attention getting, struggle for power, revenge, assumed disability, getting, self-elevation, and avoidance (Bitter, 1991). When counseling children, Adlerians explore the child's motivations for the misbehavior. Usually the child lacks introspection and has no answer to the question "Why?" These common misdirected motivations are suggested to the child and become the topic of further investigation. The mistaken aspect of the goal is the child's assumptions behind the motivation. For example, a child desiring parental attention is pursuing an appropriate goal. The child's demand that parental attention be immediate and positive in a family system with eight siblings is mistaken in the pursuit of that goal. Adlerians suggest that there are adult mistaken beliefs that align with the parent–child interactions. The parent may desire to be seen as a "good parent" in the community, and vicariously fulfill this desire through the good works and public achievements of the child. The parent may misconstrue control over the maturing child, trumping the child's need for increasing independence and trust. The parent may be intent on exacting revenge for imagined slights in which the child is either the agent or object of revenge. Parents may feign parenting incompetence in the family system to avoid their responsibilities. Adlerians disclose these mistaken goals, elucidate underlying motivation, and bolster parents in their role as family leadership.

Parents are supported through reorientation and reeducation. Psychoeducational resources are used to teach the leadership role through the explication of the needs of the family system. Positive reframing is also employed to prompt parents to appreciate their family behavior as normal, their problems as resolvable, and the future as hopeful (Bitter, 2009). Genograms are often used to map out family constellations (Bowen, 1976) and provide a graphic framework for exploring shared meaning (Rigazio-DiGilio, Ivey, Grady, & Kunkler-Peck, 2005).

Experiential and Existential

Experiential and existential approaches are united in the Humanist tradition and steeped in the existential search for meaning and transcendence (Lantz, 1993). They are different approaches to free will in the pursuit of the authentic. They are grouped here to provide contrasting perspectives on how we find our place in the world.

The goal of experiential therapy is to encourage the open flow of appropriate emotion and to create growth experiences where very positive emotions are the appropriate response. Experiential counseling emphasis is on surfacing individual subjective needs and wants that will facilitate self-discovery and individuation. The premise of the experiential approach posits that if everyone in the family is well individuated and actualized unto themselves, optimal function will be the natural outcome of their interactions.

Existential family therapy holds the "will to meaning" as the universal motivational dynamic behind all individual and family behavior. Families seek meaningfulness for the family's sake. Meaning can only be taken from experience. The real-life problems that face us on a daily basis are the most authentic and powerful contexts for learning. Pain and struggle are not to be avoided *per se*; they are part of the human experience. We grow through our struggles and need to honor them. Families have the capacity to transcend environmental challenges and barriers, physical impairment and pain, and past experience (Lantz, 1993). And in transcending, the true nature of the family is revealed.

Both experiential and existential approaches are more philosophy than theory. Both center squarely on finding the humanity in the human. Whitaker (see Whitaker & Bumberry, 1988), the leading proponent of experiential family therapy, adopts a very strong commitment to the here-and-now as the moment of creation for identity, the place for the expression of individuation through enacted values, and the moment of therapeutic change. He takes this to an extreme antitheoretical stance, eschewing all theory as a barrier to his clinical work. Existential therapy's approach is more in the psychodynamic tradition in its operationalization of repression and resistance; its search is not for deep-seated memories, but for fundamental truths. Existential family therapy is engaged in the internal struggle for balance in the individuation/intimacy dialectic. The human condition has two seemingly opposite drives: to be expressed as an individual, separate and unique from the rest of the world ("I am"), and to be part of something larger than her/himself ("We are"). Meaning making is the work of family in therapy and the synthesis of these drives.

The experiential approach creates problems in a safe environment and then facilitates family problem solving through the experience. Engaging family members in expansive emotions such as creativity, playfulness, and humor lightens the mood, creates possibility of change, and provides hope for the future. The problems of the family are depathologized (Goldenberg, Goldenberg, & Pelavin, 2008), that is, reframed as part and parcel of the course of normal family experience. Sharing personal experience opens communication. Paradox and double binds are used as fodder for conversation. Silence has meaning in counseling. It is used for dramatic effect to impart subtext, raise emotion, or simply to bear witness without comment.

In existential therapy, the goal is to have the family address and process life events in search of hidden (repressed) meaning. Awareness dynamics exercises are used to surface repressed meaning by bringing attention to the patterns and meanings behind behavior, honoring and validating that found meaning and giving it credence by remembering it, and actualizing new meaning by employing it, leading to changing family interaction patterns that disrupt their ability to make use of the deeper meaning behind the behavior (Lantz, 1993).

Multigenerational Systems

Bowen (1966, 1976) was very influential in bringing family therapy into the mainstream. Bowen, in stark contrast to Whitaker, embraced theory and disciplined application in working with families and schizophrenia (Bitter, 2009). The resultant multigenerational systems approach has become the foundation of family counseling and the lens through which other theories are interpreted. Multigenerational systems theory posits that family members are systemically interdependent and linked (if not enmeshed) in their cognition, affect, and behavior within the family. Problems stem from issues of boundaries and identity. Personal dysfunction stems from the lack of differentiation between the individual and family members, leaving them vulnerable to emotional upheaval. The emotional unity of family members that promotes a sense of "oneness" can become "fusion" or an unhealthy lack of differentiation. Total fusion is to be undifferentiated from the family, that is, no identity outside of that context and little identity within it. Parents who themselves are poorly differentiated within the family system often transmit this dysfunction through their family interactions (Bitter & Corey, 2005). The fused family relationship engenders conflict as allegiances are formed and children are recruited as pawns in emotional civil war (i.e., triangulation). Fused individual become divorced from their authentic rational selves and cut off from their real emotions. They live in what Bowen (1976) called a pseudoself, built on emotional coercion and distorted reasoning. Fused families become locked in never-ending cycles of dysfunction. For instance, a fused family response to childhood disability: ". . . the child [with a disability] resonates the mother's instability and lack of confidence in herself as mother, which the mother interprets as a problem in the child. The mother therefore increases her attention to and overprotectiveness of the child, who thus becomes more impaired. The father's role, as the third leg of the triangle, is to seek to calm the mother and play a supportive role in dealing with the child" (Becvar & Becvar, 2009, p. 146). This position becomes stable, but not optimal for recovery, rehabilitation, or service effectiveness in general (Singleton, 1982).

Bowen emphasized the tendency of emotional systems to reproduce themselves from generation to generation (Goldenberg & Goldenberg, 2000). Sibling birth order prescribes a narrow and rigid role in a fused family (Bowen, 1976). Fused parents raise fused children who tend to seek out and marry fused partners and thus dysfunction can be compounded over time. Family problems have multigenerational roots.

Differentiation creates healthy boundaries between family members in their thoughts, emotions, and behaviors. Differentiation also refers to psychological boundaries within the individual, specifically reducing the conflation of thinking and behaviors. Differentiated family members are capable of maintaining autonomy while pursuing intimacy (Becvar & Becvar, 2009). As always, balance is the key to personal health and the health of the family.

Counselor focus is on the process of the family system, rather than the emotional content of the relationship. Therapy surfaces, analyzes, and confronts fusion issues buried in previous generations that create problems in the present family dynamic. Clients are tasked with renewing relationships in the present, armed with knowledge of differentiation, triangulation, and so on . . . to find insight into their own position within the family system. Client control over and responsibility for change is maximized. Inappropriate helpfulness is discouraged as it promotes helplessness (Bowen, 1976).

Genograms are graphic representations of family systems constructed of symbols that describe the position of family members in hierarchy, birth order, and the nature of the relationship between family members over the span of three generations (Bowen, 1976). They are a tool of assessment and counseling as clients direct the collection and interpretation of information and the construction of the genogram itself. Information integrated into the evaluation can include any characteristic of interest, such as ethnicity, culture, socioeconomic status, religion, geography, proximity to family members, frequency and type of family contacts, and the emotional content of interactions (Guerin & Pendagast, 1976). Genograms can be used to (a) assess family in culturally appropriate terms, (b) engage family (attention and action), (c) reframe and depathologize family problems, and (d) assess counselor/family fit (Estrada & Haney, 1998). Genograms are often collected over time to reveal the evolution of the nuclear family and provide a moving measure of fusion among members.

Counseling focuses on questions that reveal the mechanics of underlying dysfunctional family processes. The purpose is to analyze fusion and its consequences. Homework often entails experimenting with fused relationships to raise client awareness about the dynamics of the dysfunctional interactions (e.g., triangulation) and to test differentiation interventions. Family members practice "I-positions," statements of opinion or belief owned by the client and devoid of the affect, to disengage the pseudo-self and encourage a more rationale and authentic family identity. Coaching strategies are used in families that are relatively well differentiated and motivated to improve. The counselor's role is to provide training, encouragement, and feedback as families learn to identify and intervene of their own accord.

Structural

The structural approach, the most influential model of family therapy, focuses on the family as an integrated system of patterns, processes, and transactions (Becvar & Becvar, 2009). Family structure comprises the rules (written, formal, or otherwise) that set the stage for communication. Rules make themselves apparent in the interaction of the family members, who instinctively know and follow them. Family subsystems are the component interactive units within the family. There is the spousal subsystem, the parental subsystem, the sibling subsystem, the system of extended family members, and so on into the community. Each subsystem has its own structure (rules) for interacting within and between subsystems (sibling-to-sibling contrasted with sibling-to-parent). The spousal subsystem is created through marriage or its emotional equivalent through a process of accommodation and negotiation between two competing and collaborating family structures. The parental subsystem revolves around stability and change in the issues of child rearing. The sibling subsystem is a virtual social skills laboratory to test and explore boundaries, collaboration, problem solving, and so forth (Becvar & Becvar, 2009).

Emotional boundaries maintain identity and regulate the flow of information between family members and thereby mediate the quality, intensity, and frequency of family transactions. The identity, function, and patterns within a subsystem are impacted by identity, function, and patterns between subsystems, and vice versa. Emotional boundaries vary along a spectrum integration. At one extreme, rigid emotional boundaries signal a disengagement from family communication, a lack of interface, a resistance to change, and ultimately psychological isolation within the family. Isolation leads to conflict as transitions occur and require change. Isolation reduces family resilience as it diminishes social resources (Becvar & Becvar, 2009). At the other extreme, emotional boundaries between family members disappear and their respective identities become enmeshed. Enmeshed relationships force support where support is not needed. There is a violation of roles with too much accommodation and overinvolvement in the decisions of the other—resulting in the loss of independent identity, autonomy, and experimentation. Enmeshed families become growth impaired by lack of appropriate structure. Health strikes a balance somewhere between these extremes (Bitter, 2009). It is within this framework that the client navigates the expected (marriage, birth, graduation, death, etc.) and the unexpected (accident, homelessness, divorce, disability, etc.) but ever-present challenges to family stability. There is much room for variation and expression; normal response to crisis, however extreme, is not pathological (Becvar & Becvar, 2009).

Structural intervention does not require insight. The structural approach is a very here-and-now action-oriented approach to learning. Exploring the past is minimized as practically irrelevant. The goals of structural therapy are to facilitate the development of an effective parental hierarchy, a united parental front in child rearing, well-differentiated family members with clear boundaries and communication of appropriate frequency, duration, and content (Becvar & Becvar, 2009). In structural therapy, symptoms are "conflict diffusers" that allow more fundamental conflicts to remain submerged (Goldenberg et al., 2008). That is to say, family energies and attention are constantly appropriated in resolving surface problems rather than resolving the core problems that generate them.

The therapist enters and assumes a leadership role in the family to evaluate and change family function, not to solve family problems (Bitter, 2009). Family mapping (Minuchin, 1980) employs a graphic vocabulary of boundaries, structures, and subsystems in the evaluation of client family structure, derivative of the family system genograms discussed earlier. The augmented family leadership (parents and therapist) maps and analyzes family structure from an emic perspective, relying on spontaneously occurring family behavior patterns and staged family demonstrations of problem-solving methods (enactments). The therapist observes these behaviors *in situ* without direction or encouragement. Family mapping provides the venue within which therapist and parents forge a working alliance.

On the basis of these collaborative findings, family leadership formulates a plan to transform family structures. The therapist listens to parents in their leadership role, reframes, and transforms family interpretations into a structural (cognitive) framework, and focuses interventions on the here-and-now. Relationships can be manipulated from within the family, applying a variety of techniques to disrupt habituated dysfunctional exchanges, restructure boundaries, and unbalance stalemated arguments. Intervention in this model challenges rigid, counterproductive family transactions to get them to become more fluid and allow for family reorganization (Goldenberg et al., 2008). Specific interventions include (a) actively realigning boundaries; (b) facilitating independent problem-solving in dyads; (c) modifying the frequency of contact between members; (d) providing psychoeducational resources in applied structural theory; (e) cognitive reframing; and (f) use of paradox to challenge existing structures (Becvar & Becvar, 2009).

Cognitive-Behavioral

Behaviorism is a positivistic, empirical approach to counseling that deals exclusively with behaviors that can be observed and measured, and validates only those that can be repeated. Behaviors change in response to change in the pattern of reinforcers that sustain them. Classical conditioning demonstrates how neutral stimuli can be made to cue new behaviors (classic Pavlovian [CS/US > CR] response) and is generally used as the framework for "unlearning" unwanted conditioned responses in counseling situations. Operant conditioning demonstrates how new behaviors can actually be shaped through the manipulation of reinforcers and their schedules. In behavioral approaches maladaptive behaviors are analyzed. Behavioral plans are made to maintain, change, or extinguish behavior by manipulating or removing reinforcement altogether (Becvar & Becvar, 2009).

Social Learning theory (Bandura, 1977) provides the conceptual bridge that links learning with community, ushers behavioral approaches into family therapy, and introduces personal mediating variables between stimulus, response, and consequence. Where behaviorism presumes that environment causes behavior, Bandura recognized "reciprocal determinism" (Bandura, 1977) a continuous and reciprocal transactional process between the cognitions and behaviors of the individual and the family. In this expanded perspective, learning is embedded in the social milieu. Our identities, our worldview, and everything we know about ourselves are based on the models we are given by the social networks that contain and sustain us (Vygotsky, 1978). Social learning is observational, but not all observed behavior is learned. In order to pass from sensation to learning, the individual must (a) attend to the event, (b) interpret and retain it in some symbolic way (schema), (c) be able to reproduce the behavior in some fashion, and (d) possess the motivation to learn. There are three kinds of social models from which to learn: live modeling of behavior, descriptions of the modeled behavior (how to); or descriptive narrative in which the behavior is employed (case study). Similarly, learning rehearsals can be "symbolic" or acted out *in situ*. Motivation is the key in social learning theory. Social learning theory emphasizes intrinsic motivations beyond the extrinsic emphasis of behaviorism. People are motivated from within by idiosyncratic values and cognitions that shape their world. It is here that social learning theory completes the cognitive-behavioral bridge to the cognitive theories.

Cognitive therapy and rational-emotive therapy have contributed to the cognitive-behavioral family model. As a group, they posit that faulty cognitions about the self and the world, and faulty cognitive processes create problematic behaviors. Cognitive therapy uses an information processing approach to explain how distortions in information selection and interpretation lead to dysfunctional schemas and beliefs (Beck & Weishaar, 2010). In rational-emotive behavior therapy, the emphasis is on the systems-like development of second-order irrational beliefs and metaconsequences. In synthesis, the objectives of the cognitive-behavioral family counseling are to modify cognitions, teach new communication and problem solving behaviors, reduce cognitive vulnerabilities, and engage in the community.

In cognitive-behavioral family therapy, counselors work with families in three primary areas. Identifying and gathering data on maladaptive behavior engages the family in analysis of the character of the conflict, the players, and the pattern of events (antecedence, behaviors, and consequences). The approach is rational and scientific. Hypotheses are developed and tested. Target behaviors are quantified (frequency, intensity, etc.) to gauge the current state of family problems and as a benchmark for measuring progress. The second context for intervention is the interfamily communication process. Counselors are interested in the content of the messages, its intended connotative and denotative meaning; how the messages are communicated (medium, style, etc.); and the interpretation and response of the family members to the message received. Finally, counselors work with clients and family to understand and hopefully improve family problem-solving skill and style (Dattilio, Epstein, & Baucom, 1998).

Each member of the family brings predispositions to their relationships, that is, established cognitive schema that color interpretation and direct how the individual communicates and solves problems. A primary source of problems comes from the predispositions themselves. Dattilio (2005) identifies eight cognitive distortions common in family interactions.

- *arbitrary inference*, drawing conclusions from events without corroborating evidence;
- *selective abstraction*, actively distorting available information by interpreting it out of context, conflating erroneous details to create the appearance of a rational perspective, and ignoring or twisting evidence that would refute the conclusions reached;
- *magnification and minimization*, expanding and shrinking, respectively, attention to and value of information to fit the predisposition;
- *personalization*, interpreting events as personal affronts without corroborating evidence;
- *black and white thinking*, evaluating in the absence of any middle ground (hate or love, always or never, villain or victim);
- *labeling and mislabeling*, giving a label to someone based on limited observation that becomes a distorted and extremely limited stand-in for identity; and
- *mind reading*, attributing thoughts and reasoning to another based on speculation and using the premise to support the predisposition.

Counseling seeks out these cognitive distortions as the source of ongoing conflict. The task is to disrupt and replace them with more effective cognitive processes (Walsh, 2003). Dysfunctional communication and ineffective problem-solving skills are learned behavior that can be unlearned and replaced. Cognitive-behavioral family counseling is ahistorical; the problem is confronted in the present. Counselors are practitioner scientists who are only interested in what can be directly observed, in finding the determinants of current behavior, and in the analysis of the behavior and its component parts. Analysis reveals what is valued in the situation, what the reinforcers are, and what effect they have on the target behavior. What is valued is arbitrary; knowing its function in the system is enough.

Early steps in behavioral family counseling identify and support the natural leadership in the family, that is, the parental dyad (Dattilio & Epstein, 2005). Counselors work collaboratively with the parents throughout the process, strengthening their position and helping them get the tools necessary to provide the ongoing family learning environment. Behavioral analysis interviews evaluate family member responses to the problematic behavior, collecting baseline data in the process. The problem behavior is broken down into manageable subcomponents. Subcomponent objectives are developed based on changing a current and specific pattern of behavior. Collaborative planning follows, with parents receiving and providing psychoeducational support where feasible and counselor-facilitated behavioral interventions where necessary.

Counseling in the cognitive realm challenges automatic thoughts, cognitive distortions, and faulty schemas at the core of the family conflict and replaces them with functional schemas and processes that are based on reason rather than negative emotion. Self-report questionnaires are used to surface and draw attention to schema issues (Becvar & Becvar, 2009) that become the target of intervention. Counselors engage in cognitive-behavioral interviews that favor the Socratic method of investigation that reveals distorted assumptions and the automatic thoughts and responses that propagated the problem (Dattilio et al., 1998). The client and family are trained in the cognitive-behavioral model. The counselor is often in the role of educator, providing psychoeducational training in communication, problem-solving, and social learning theory. Across the cognitive-behavioral spectrum, interventions (e.g., skill training, self-monitoring and regulation, systematic desensitization, behavioral contracts) facilitate the learning of new coping skills. Homework is ever present and can be used to implement and record behavioral interventions.

Positive Psychology

Maslow coined the term "positive psychology" in 1954 (Lopez & Gallagher, 2009) in his observation that the science and practice of psychology was diminished by its preoccupation with dysfunction. Positive psychology would percolate for 40 years in the work of many, including Beatrice Wright, whose coping framework for rehabilitation (1983) is described elsewhere in this text. Positive psychology coalesced into a popular movement (Seligman & Csikszentmihalyi, 2000) in the late 1990s as Seligman organized a community of researchers and practitioners to the cause (Diener, 2009). Its momentum has increased over the ensuing decade and its influence has spread beyond the clinic and counseling session to businesses, schools, and human service agencies. Its interpretation into family counseling was an inevitable extension of its values (see Shapiro, 2004).

Positive psychology represents a rounding out of the whole of psychology and stands as an antithesis to the pathocentric tradition.

> ... Positive psychology at the subjective level is about valued experiences: well-being, contentment, and satisfaction (in the past); hope and optimism (for the future); and flow and happiness (in the present). At the individual level, it is about positive individual traits: the capacity for love and vocation, courage, interpersonal skill, aesthetic sensibility, perseverance, forgiveness, originality, future mindedness, spirituality, high talent, and wisdom. At the group level, it is about civic virtues and the institutions that move individuals toward better citizenship: responsibility, nurturance, altruism, civility, moderation, tolerance, and work ethic (Seligman & Csikszentmihalyi, 2000, p. 5).

Positive psychology is a philosophical position as much as a service (Maddux, Snyder, & Lopez, 2004). Positive psychology argues that there are human pursuits that make us stronger, values that are therapeutic, and aspirational goals that lead to greater family resilience. It is an extension of the humanist approach with its existential roots. It addresses common problems that can be reframed and treated as an opportunity to learn and grow. These interventions in minor challenges serve as models for dealing with more extreme and maladaptive behaviors. Ordinary problems are microcosms of clinical problems, and so developing solutions on the pedestrian scale prepares one for more traumatic encounters. The counselor's role is to help the family identify, develop, and employ their assets to best advantage, whether for enrichment or protection.

Assets are the building blocks of positive psychology (Chow, Lee, Catalano, Ditchman, & Wilson, 2009). Families are at the center of the client's social support network and offer the most immediate assets. Empirical research has identified 40 different assets for healthy child growth. Family strengths figure prominently in the mix. Family support, positive family communication, caring climate, involvement in child care and education, safety, family boundaries, adult role models, and time at home are stable assets that support the growth of the child to adolescence, though they change in expression with age. Specific parent behaviors are conducive to positive growth and good health. Warmth, sensitivity, responsiveness, and emotional availability facilitate the successful negotiation of challenging parental tasks and encourage empowerment and individual self-esteem (Sheridan & Burt, 2009).

Positive psychology is predicated on an ecological framework. Each family member is part of an irreducible system of nested micro- (personal), meso- (social), and exo- (societal) subsystems that govern transactions within and between subsystems. The pursuit of wellness and health spans across these three interactive systems with education and skill building, supporting family leadership in accessing optimal services, and empowering families to access all relevant and available interventions (see Marshall, 2008). Family-centered positive psychology recognizes the family's centrality in the promotion of strengths and positive growth in the face of challenge (Singer & Powers, 1993). The family-centered approach seeks to empower families through the promotion of self-determination at all stages of the process. The counselor is a supporting player primarily helping the family members to acquire communication, problem-solving, and other social skills that become part of the coping repertoire. The process builds on existing strengths (Dempsey & Dunst, 2004) by coordinating them in social support networks for optimum effect (Sheridan & Burt, 2009). Wellness and coping are the keys to increased resilience within the family that is expressed through sociability, self-esteem, autonomy, intelligence, creativity, special interests, hobbies, internal locus of control within the family, defined subsystems (parents, siblings etc.), structured rules, and trusting relationship with the parents (Hansson & Cederblad, 2004). Services are delivered *with* the families, neither "to them" nor "for them." The role of the counselor in this system is to develop skills and networks to support efforts at helping the client nurture and build on strengths (Seligman & Csikszentmihalyi, 2000). Positive therapeutic approaches (Linley, Joseph, Maltby, Harrington, & Wood, 2009) focus on well-being (Ruini & Fava, 2004), mindfulness (Brown & Ryan, 2003), and quality of life (Frisch, 2006), all very cognitive in their introspection and consideration of ecological circumstances.

Solution focused

Related to the strengths-based approach to conceptualizing the client/counselor experience, solution-focused approaches focus on the positive reframing of life events, finding and using what works, the encouragement of self-efficacy, perseverance, and the pursuit and celebration of progress (Nichols & Schwartz, 2006). Shifting focus from dysfunction to solutions opens up new possibilities and what can be celebrated along the way. It is a social constructionist approach to using language to change reality. The shift is to dialog about what is going well, what is possible, and how clients can move toward a better sense of self, accomplishment, and general well-being. The past and the present are minimized in favor of a revisioning of the future. By talking exclusively about solutions and success, the client begins to reframe in terms of solutions and success (Berg & de Shazer, 1993).

Solution-focused approach to family therapy is solidly anchored in cognitive reframing (Banks, 2005). Counselor engages the client in optimistic dialog about the future, about what might be possible, and to discover or rediscover strengths and strategies they did not consider. Seeking out stories, counselors invite a client narrative that reflects positive status, power, problem solving, happiness—whatever holds meaning for the client and family (Estrada & Beyebach, 2007). The collaboration works in the future tense by changing solutions into goals and goals into plans. Initial goals are small, meaningful, and doable with a high probability of success. Dialog revolves around imagining a more desirable present tense. The miracle questions introduce the concept of solution finding: "If your problem immediately went away, how would you know it was gone and resolved? What would be different? What would happen then?" The exception questions seek to find competencies that could be expanded: "Was there a time when you didn't have this problem? How was the world then? What did you do then?" Scaling questions quantify experience (emotion, mood, pain, etc.) for description and later comparison: "On a scale 0–10 with 0 being never and 10 being many times per day every day . . . How often do you actually find yourself in this negative state?" Questions of difference help focus on positive change and self-efficacy: "Can you identify positive self change as a result of your efforts? What is changing, how much? How fast?" Interaction is charged with compliments, never false or manufactured, but always observant of even the least of improvement and the competence that was required to make it happen. Hope is the model for cognitive reframing. Goals (direction) and agency (perceived ability to achieve) are part of self-efficacy and the two aspects of the construct of Hope (Snyder et al., 1991). Thus, hope is a positive cognitive appraisal strategy that responds to uncertainty (Mishel, 1999), reduces stress (McCubbin et al., 1996), and positively influences client experiences with recovery (Frain, Berven, Chan, & Tschopp, 2008; Scheier, Carver, & Bridges, 2001).

Family in a Psychosocial Approach

The psychosocial approach to rehabilitation counseling, with its focus on adjustment and adaptation to disability, provides the defining foundation for the field and context within which all counseling takes place. It originated in contemplation of the individual response to physical disability through three interrelated models. The somatopsychological model concerns itself with how the physical experience of disability changes the individual psyche. Positive adaptation comes with the containment of the impact of physical disability to the strictly functional and the revaluation, a reorganization of personal values, and a new perspective on self-worth based on assets rather than comparison to others (Wright, 1983). The work of adaptation moves through psychosocial stages as the experience of acquired disability is played out in the life of the individual. The experience of disability sets an unavoidable process of change in motion from impact of the initial event and the chaotic disruption of the established life, to the immediate mobilization of defenses to preserve the status quo, to the realization that irrevocable change has already occurred and must be addressed, to aggression and other outward projections of affective response to new realities, and finally (and hopefully) to the psychic reintegration of the person and the reintegration of the person in the environment (Livneh, 1986). The change processes of the stage model take place in the community (Livneh & Antonak, 1997) as ongoing and recursive transactions between persons (aspects of the disability, personality, sociodemographic variables, etc.) and their environment (cultural, economic, geographic variables, etc.).

Psychosocial rehabilitation has evolved out of this paradigm in response to the unique experiences and challenges of people with psychiatric disabilities and in the process introduced the family as an irreducible component of the social ecology. In the resultant model, adaptation is recovery, and rehabilitation is empowerment. The goal of psychosocial rehabilitation is to facilitate client choice, acquisition, maintenance, and growth in valued and meaningful community roles and thereby ... engender hope and optimism for the future (Zahniser, 2005). Employment is foremost among these valued roles and an impressive array of evidence-based practices has been developed for this purpose. Given that evidence-based practice in our profession is sorely lacking in every other respect, it gives one pause to consider the potential value of psychosocial rehabilitation in other venues.

The family is an important consideration in psychosocial rehabilitation, with counseling approaches being only a part of the overall family support strategy. Indeed, counseling is not the focus of therapeutic intervention here. This is psychosocial rehabilitation in a social–political frame. Psychiatric labels are the most stigmatizing of all disability labels. The history of people with psychiatric disabilities, and their families, has been one of abuse, isolation, and community exclusion. Psychosocial rehabilitation has been as much an organized consumer response to medical model disenfranchisement as a strategy for dealing with mental health. Empowerment and advocacy are therapeutic. Community building, including the family as first community, is an intervention.

Empowerment and advocacy

In the face of insufficient, ineffective, and/or inaccessible services, families must advocate on their own behalf, or succumb to the system. Advocacy is a bulwark against hopelessness (Spaniol & Zipple, 1984) and an actionable core value in counseling (Bryan, 2009; Gehart & Lucas, 2007). Pursuit of social justice is the context of counseling here. Advocating in solidarity with the family is the ultimate "working alliance." Teaching and supporting advocacy skills facilitate client growth and development (Smith, Reynolds, & Rovnak, 2009). Counselors set the stage for empowerment by intentional divesting whatever power differential exists in the relationship to the client family. This is accomplished in concert with an investment in the expertise of the family as caregivers, along with the respect and influence this entails (Holcomb-McCoy & Bryan, 2010). Family consultants possess valuable insight and are in a position to teach the rehabilitation counselor about working within on their family system (Spaniol et al., 2006). Empowerment is developed by reinforcing and nurturing family member sense of self-efficacy, building confidence and skill in self-advocacy, facilitating the rejection of stigma and the raising self-esteem, and developing skills in self-management and community transactions (Frain, Bishop, & Tschopp, 2009). Each of these tasks builds on one another through training and application in the community.

Psychoeducation

The term psychoeducation has been used elsewhere in this chapter to refer to educational interventions that empower families. Rationales for educational intervention may vary, based on the theory of the moment, but the outcomes are the same. The theoretical argument in psychoeducation is based on a stress model. Coping with recovery subjects the family to stressors (e.g., exasperation, discouragement with service, and worries about the future). Stressors are expressed as high emotion and conflict, which, in turn, increase the likelihood of relapse, social isolation, stigma, increased cost, and other debilitating effects. Stressors and their effects can be ameliorated by an active response from the social support network (Jewell, McFarlane, Dixon, & Miklowitz, 2005). Modifications in the environment (through advocacy and education directed at families and other support entities) leads to stress reduction, resulting in reduced negative consequences (Dausch & Saliman, 2009).

Families struggle to do the best that they can with the symptomology and secondary consequences of mental illness. They are engaged in trying to sustain or improve the situation, and are experts in their own experience. They are approached as valued frontline collaborators. Families are taught by professionals and peers (Walsh, 2003), and once educated, teach each other, becoming part of the social support network. Family psychoeducation in the traditional model is run by professionals and focuses on beneficial outcomes for the client. Multiple family models are peer run and focus on outcomes for the family. Topics vary broadly but tend to focus on the knowledge about the disability, its treatment, coping strategies, and accessing resources. Psychoeducational methodology includes role-playing, behavioral rehearsal, active listening, positive feedback, and constructive criticisms aimed at facilitating self-directed change (Jewell et al., 2005).

Psychoeducation is a coordinated component of the treatment plan and integrated into counseling focused on social well-being, medication management, planning/delivery partnerships, assessing family support strengths and limitations, exploring family expectations, resolving family conflicts, addressing loss and grieving, development and practice of explicit crisis plans, improving communication among family members, structured problem-solving techniques, facilitating family social support networks, and ensuring continuity of service (Jewell et al., 2005). The role of the counselor is diffused in this model, inseparable from the educator, case manager, and advocate. This is an incipient community-counseling model that seeks to decrease the negative impact of inevitable relapse, and increase family resilience to chronic stress (Dausch & Saliman, 2009; Miklowitz, George, Richards, Simoneau, & Suddath, 2003).

Multifamily focus

At last, we have interventions that do not require counselors at all. Multifamily psychoeducation is a tool within the social support network of likeminded families who have organized around the shared experience of disability, developed structures, and interventions of their own, including standardized training modules. These groups provide outreach to isolated families, bringing them into support groups where they can share experiences in a safe environment, review and evaluate their progress, and practice skills (McFarlane, 2002; Walsh, 2003). In this model, the problems that beset families are normalized. Often the first therapeutic event is to find out that you are not alone and that your experiences, however trying, are very common. Problems are a part of the natural human experience and the appropriate response is mastery of adaptation skills. Beyond the delivery of ongoing training/skill development and emotional support, multiple family groups include members in the development of social networks to expand access to resources and opportunities (Anderson, 1983), raise awareness of disability advocacy in the general public, and seek to engage professional service providers in responsiveness training for greater sensitivity to issues of recovery and empowerment (Spaniol et al., 2006). The original and most evolved multifamily model is the National Alliance on Mental Illness. They are a national organization that sponsors local, community-centered support groups to provide programmatic education (i.e., the Family-to-Family and Journey of Hope Program) and support. Multifamily groups are not necessarily as refined as this; they can spring up spontaneously as informal attempts of local families to find help in difficult times. Self help organizations demonstrate that resilience is a community event (Levine & Perkins, 1987; Singer & Powers, 1993).

DISCUSSION: WORKING WITH FAMILIES

There is a bit of a conundrum surrounding the issue of working with families in rehabilitation counseling. On one hand, the profound influence that families have on rehabilitation process and outcomes are well established (Power & Hershenson, 2003). Rehabilitation counseling must address this variable in service as a matter of scientist–practitioner integrity. It follows that counseling would be a primary means of intervention and that it could be used to (a) maximize family support in the client's rehabilitation goals, and (b) minimize counterproductive family actions due to fear, ignorance, dysfunction, or agenda. On the other hand, rehabilitation counseling is not family counseling. Families are not rehabilitation counseling clients. They are of value to the rehabilitation counselor only inasmuch as they are instrumental to the effective delivery of client-centered delivery of service and the achievement of client-centered goals. The rehabilitation counselors who wander unprepared into family dysfunction do so at great risk to their clients and their careers.

The cursory overview of family counseling approaches presented in this chapter is not an endorsement for practice. No direct translation is possible. However, the principles that undergird family counseling at large have inspired emerging practice in rehabilitation counseling and knowledge about them will make for more informed and strategic referral. Power and Dell Orto (2004) have proposed a model for working with families that sets the current tone for incorporating families into counseling, which we will use here as a point of departure for the concluding discussion.

Before the family enters, it is up to the client to establish the parameters of family involvement. Regardless of merit, it is the client's choice. It is for the counselor to create the opportunity for family inclusion, to provide the client with all of the information required to make an informed decision, and to facilitate the decision once reached.

The counselor joins the family in the sense of eschewing the expert role of power (Swain & Walker, 2003), becoming part of the group and its efforts on behalf of the client (Herbert, 1989). The earliest objective is to establish a working relationship with the family akin to the working alliance of counseling with its pursuit of collaboration, development of positive emotional bonds, consensus on goals and processes, and building motivation to succeed. In that vein, it is important to open clear and reciprocal channels of communication, bring strong problem-solving skills to the group, and project hopeful optimism about the future. The experience of disability is often traumatic and interpreted as a family tragedy. The family experience needs to be reinstated in the context of normal human behavior and circumstance. Starting with orientation and reinforced throughout, the tragedy is gently reframed as a (albeit severe) challenge that creates choices: There may be struggle but the family can still find happiness, fulfillment, and meaning. In the initial meeting, the counselor provides an orientation for the family, including appropriate educational materials. The counselor engages in relaxed conversation and ascertains family expectations for service and outcomes while observing the behavior of the group. The counselor seeks to identify the family decision makers and to get a sense of how the group communicates among its members.

The process of assessment involves three steps: (a) identify family needs for service and barriers to adjustment and adaptation; (b) building an understanding of the family situation through collaborative synthesis, and (c) engaging family in group planning and shared buy-in to its implementation. The focus is on identifying family assets and employing to best advantage. Power and Dell Orto (2004) noted that the topics of assessment depend on the family needs at the moment. The experience of disability and rehabilitation is fluid and evolving. The issues confronting families in acute care are different than outpatient, and questions shift accordingly. The issues relevant to rehabilitation counseling commonly arise around family communication, intimacy, changing roles in the family, caregiver challenges, and boundary issues that provide structure for assessment (Rolland, 1994).

Interventions with the family are limited to that which facilitates the plan. Interventions are collaborative partnerships, not therapeutic. Psychoeducation figures prominently as an intervention of choice. Knowledge about the disability, available resources, coping strategies, and any other information required or requested by the family can serve to build resilience. Rehabilitation counselors may introduce the family to multiple family advocacy and self-help groups. The counselor may meet with the family to track the progress made on the collaborative plan. Family members are treated as experts. The counselor is present to ensure family success, and encourage self-efficacy. Problem solving and communication can be modeled. Conflicts can be addressed. Should the rehabilitation counselor identify family systems dysfunction as problematic to the plan, appropriate referrals can be made to the appropriate family counseling service.

This is the extent of family integration into rehabilitation counseling at the moment. The degree to which family counseling models have informed our practice is modest and piecemeal. There are natural limits to how far we shall go, but there are a great many avenues for further exploration. Positive psychology with its strengths-based approach and the strong advocacy themes of the recovery model is a natural fit with the empowerment ethos of rehabilitation counseling. The tools of cognitive-behavioral therapy are universally applicable. Genograms could provide new ways of thinking about specific family issues, such as job search and employment support. Family systems theory forces us to face the ecological and unbreakable link between the rehabilitation client's goals and the people from where they came.

REFERENCES

Accordino, M. P. (1999). Implications of disability for the family: Implementing behavioral family therapy in rehabilitation education. *Rehabilitation Education, 13*, 287–293.

Ainsworth, M. D. S. (1989). Attachment beyond infancy. *American Psychologist, 44*(4), 709–716.

Alston, R. J., & McCowan, C. J. (1994). Family function as a correlate of disability adjustment for African Americans. *Rehabilitation Counseling Bulletin, 37*, 277–289.

Alston, R. J., & Turner, W. L. (1994). A family strengths model of adjustment to disability for African American clients. *Journal of Counseling and Development, 72*, 378–383.

Anderson, C. M. (1983). A psychoeducational program for families of patients with schizophrenia. In W. R. McFarlane (Ed.), *Family therapy in schizophrenia* (pp. 99–116). New York, NY: Guilford Press.

Antonovsky, A. (1987). *Unraveling the mystery of health: How people manage stress and stay well*. San Francisco, CA: Jossey-Bass.

Bandura, A. (1977). *Social learning theory*. Englewood Cliffs, NJ: Prentice Hall.

Bandura, A. (1997). *Self-efficacy: The exercise of control*. New York, NY: W. H. Freeman.

Banks, R. (2005). Solution-focused group therapy. *Journal of Family Psychotherapy, 16*(1), 16–21.

Beavers, W. R. (1982). Healthy, midrange, and severely dysfunctional families. In F. Walsh (Ed.), *Normal Family Processes* (pp. 45–66). New York, NY: Guilford Press.

Beck, A. T., & Weishaar, M. E. (2010). Cognitive therapy. In R. J. Corsini & D. Wedding (Eds.), *Current Psychotherapies* (9th ed., pp. 276–309). Belmont, CA: Brooks/Cole.

Becvar, D. S. (1985). Creating rituals for a new age: Dealing positively with divorce, remarriage, and other developmental challenges. In R. Williams, H. Lingren, G. Rowe, S. VanZandt, P. Lee, & N. Stinnett (Eds.), *Family strengths* (Vol. 6, pp. 57–65). Lincoln, NE: University of Nebraska-Lincoln Press.

Becvar, D. S., & Becvar, R. J. (1999). *Systems theory and family therapy: A primer*. Washington, DC: University Press of America.

Becvar, D. S., & Becvar, R. J. (2009). *Family therapy: A systemic integration* (7th ed.). New York, NY: Pearson Education.

Bitter, J. R. (1991). Conscious motivations: An enhancement to Dreikurs' goals of children's misbehavior. *Individual Psychology, 47*(2), 210–221.

Bitter, J. R. (2009). *Theory and practice of family therapy and counseling*. Belmont, CA: Brooks/Cole.

Bitter, J. R., & Corey, G. (2005). Family systems therapy. In G. Corey (Ed.), *Theory and practice of counseling and psychotherapy* (pp. 420–459). Belmont, CA: Brooks/Cole-Thomson.

Bitter, J. R., Roberts, A., & Sonstegard, M. A. (2002). Adlerian family therapy. In J. Carlson & D. Kjos (Eds.), *Theories and strategies of family therapy* (pp. 41–79). Boston, MA: Allyn and Bacon.

Bowen, M. (1966). The use of family theory in clinical practice. *Comprehensive Psychiatry, 7*, 345–374.

Bowen, M. (1976). Theory in the practice of psychotherapy. In P. J. Guerin, Jr. (Ed.), *Family therapy: Theory and practice* (pp. 42–90). New York, NY: Gardner Press.

Brown, K. W., & Ryan, R. M. (2003). The benefits of being present: Mindfulness and its role in psychological well-being. *Journal of Personality and Social Psychology, 84*, 822–848.

Bryan, J. (2009). Engaging clients, families, and communities as partners in mental health. *Journal of Counseling & Development, 87*, 507–511.

Chow, C. C., Lee, E. J., Catalano, D. E., Ditchman, N., & Wilson, L. M. (2009). Positive psychology and psychosocial adjustment to chronic illness and disability. In F. Chan, E. Cardoso, & J. Chronister (Eds.), *Understanding psychosocial adjustment to chronic illness and disability: A handbook for evidence-based practitioners in rehabilitation* (pp. 207–241). New York, NY: Springer Publishing.

Coles, A. R., Pakenham, K. I., & Leech, C. (2007). Evaluation of an intensive psychosocial intervention for children of parents with multiple sclerosis. *Rehabilitation Psychology, 52*, 133–142.

Cottone, R. R., Handelsman, M. M., & Walters, N. (1986). Understanding the influence of family systems on the rehabilitation process. *Journal of Applied Rehabilitation Counseling, 17*, 37–40.

Dattilio, F. M. (2005). Restructuring family schemas: A cognitive-behavioral perspective. *Journal of Martial and Family Therapy, 31*(10), 15–30.

Dattilio, F. M., Epstein, N. B., & Baucom, D. H. (1998). An introduction to cognitive-behavioral therapy with couples and families. In F. M. Dattilio (Ed.), *Case studies in couple and family therapy* (pp. 1–36). New York, NY: Guilford.

Dattilio, F. M., & Epstein, N. B. (2005). The role of cognitive-behavioral interventions in couple and family therapy. *Journal of Marital and Family Therapy, 32*(1), 7–13.

Dausch, B. M., & Saliman, S. (2009). Use of family focused therapy in rehabilitation for veterans with traumatic brain injury. *Rehabilitation Psychology, 54*(3), 279–287.

Deatrick, J. A., Brennan, D., & Cameron, M. E. (1998). Mothers with multiple sclerosis and their children: Effects of fatigue and exacerbations on material support. *Nursing Research, 47*, 205–210.

Degeneffe, C. E. (2001). Family caregiving and traumatic brain injury. *Health and Social Work, 26*(4), 257–268.

Degeneffe, C. E., & Burcham, C. M. (2008). Adult sibling caregiving for persons with traumatic brain injury: Predictors of affective and instrumental support. *Journal of Rehabilitation, 74*(3), 10–20.

Degeneffe, C. E., & Lee, G. K. (2010). Quality of life after traumatic brain injury: Perspectives of adult siblings. *Journal of Rehabilitation, 76*(4), 27–36.

Degeneffe, C. E., & Lynch, R. T. (2006). Correlates of depression in adult siblings of persons with TBI. *Rehabilitation Counseling Bulletin, 49*, 130–142.

Degeneffe, C. E., & Olney, M. F. (2008). Future concerns of adult siblings of persons with traumatic brain injury. *Rehabilitation Counseling Bulletin, 51*(4), 240–250.

Dempsey, I., & Dunst, C. J. (2004). Help-giving styles as a function of parent empowerment in families with a young child with a disability. *Journal of Intellectual and Developmental Disability, 29*(1), 50–61.

Diener, E. (2009). Positive psychology: Past, present, and future. In S. J. Lopez & C. R. Snyder (Eds.), *Oxford handbook of positive psychology* (2nd ed., pp. 7–11). New York, NY: Oxford University Press.

Ell, K. (1996). Social networks, social support and coping with serious illness: The family connection. *Social Science and Medicine, 42*, 173–183.

Epstein, N. B., Ryan, C. E., Bishop, D. S., Miller, I. W., & Keitner, G. I. (2003). The McMaster model: A view of healthy family functioning. In F. Walsh (Ed.), *Normal family processes: Growing diversity and complexity* (pp. 581–607). New York, NY: Guilford Press.

Estrada, B., & Beyebach, M. (2007). Solution-focused therapy with depressed deaf persons. *Journal of Family Psychotherapy, 18*(3), 45–63.

Estrada, A. U., & Haney, P. (1998). Genograms in a multicultural perspective. *Journal of Family Psychotherapy, 9*(2), 55–62.

Feigin, R. (1994). Spousal adjustment to a postmarital disability in one partner. *Family Systems Medicine, 12*, 235–247.

Forbat, L. (2002). 'Tinged with bitterness': Re-presenting stress in family care. *Disability & Society, 17*(7), 759–768.

Frain, M. P., Berven, N. L., Lee, G. K., Berven, N. L., Tansey, T., Tschopp, M. K., et al. (2007). Use of the resiliency model of family stress, adjustment and adaptation by rehabilitation counselors. *Journal of Rehabilitation, 73*, 18–25.

Frain, M. P., Berven, N. L., Chan, F., & Tschopp, M. K. (2008). Family resiliency, uncertainty, optimism, and the quality of life of individuals with HIV/AIDS. *Rehabilitation Counseling Bulletin, 52*, 16–27.

Frain, M. P., Berven, N., Tschopp, M., Lee, G., Tansey, T., & Chronister, J. (2007). Use of the resiliency model of family stress, adjustment and adaptation by rehabilitation counselors. *Journal of Rehabilitation, 73*(3), 18–25.

Frain, M. P., Bishop, M., & Tschopp, M. K. (2009). Empowerment variables as predictors of outcomes in rehabilitation. *Journal of Rehabilitation, 75*(1), 27–35.

Frain, M. P., Bishop, M., Tschopp, M. K., Ferrin, M. J., & Frain, J. (2009). Understanding the effects of cognitive appraisal, quality of life, and perceived family resiliency. *Rehabilitation Counseling Bulletin, 52*(4), 237–250.

Freedman, R. I., & Fesko, S. L. (1996). The meaning of work in the lives of people with significant disabilities: Consumer and family perspectives. *Journal of Rehabilitation, 62*(3), 49–55.

Frisch, M. (2006). *Quality of life therapy: Applying a life satisfaction approach to positive psychology and cognitive therapy.* Hoboken, NJ: John Wiley & Sons.

Gallagher, S. K., & Mechanic, D. (1996). Living with the mentally ill: Effects on the health and functioning of other household members. *Social Science Medicine, 42*, 1691–1701.

Gehart, D. R., & Lucas, B. M. (2007). Client advocacy in marriage and family therapy: A qualitative case study. *Journal of Family Psychotherapy, 18*(1), 39–56.

Goldenberg, I., & Goldenberg, H. (2000). *Family therapy: An overview* (4th ed.). Monterey, CA: Brooks/Cole.

Goldenberg, I., Goldenberg, H., & Pelavin, E. G. (2008). Family Therapy. In R. J. Corsini & D. Wedding (Eds.), *Current psychotherapies* (9th ed., pp. 417–453). Belmont, CA: Brooks/Cole.

Greenwood, N., MacKenzie, A., Cloud, G. C., & Wilson, N. (2008). Informal carers of stroke survivors—factors influencing carers: A systematic review of quantitative studies. *Disability and Rehabilitation, 30*, 1329–1349.

Guerin, P. J., & Pendagast, E. G. (1976). Evaluation of family system and genogram. In P. J. Guerin (Ed.), *Family therapy: Theory and practice* (pp. 450–464). New York, NY: Gardner Press.

Hall, A. S. (2003). Expanding academic and career self-efficacy: A family system framework. *Journal of Counseling & Development, 81*, 33–39.

Hansson, K., & Cederblad, M. (2004). Sense of coherence as a meta-theory for salutogenic family therapy. *Journal of Family Psychotherapy, 15*, 39–54.

Hanna, S. M., & Brown, J. H. (1999). *The practice of family therapy: Key elements across models.* Belmont, CA: Brooks/Cole-Thomson.

Herbert, J. T. (1989). Assessing the need for family therapy: A primer for rehabilitation counselors. *Journal of Rehabilitation, 55*(1), 45–51.

Holcomb-McCoy, C., & Bryan, J. (2010). Advocacy and empowerment in parent consultation: Implications for theory and practice. *Journal of Counseling & Development, 88*(3), 259–268.

Jewell, T. C., McFarlane, W. R., Dixon, L., & Miklowitz, D. J. (2005). Evidence-based family services for adults with severe mental illness. In C. E. Stout & R. A. Hayes (Eds.), *The evidence-based practice: Methods, models, and tools for mental health professionals* (pp. 56–84). Hoboken, NJ: John Wiley & Sons.

Joosten-Weyn Banningh, L., Kessels, R., Olde Rikkert, M., Geleijns-Lanting, C. E., & Kraaimaat, F. W. (2008). A cognitive behavioural group therapy for patients diagnosed with mild cognitive impairment and their significant others: Feasibility and preliminary results. *Clinical Rehabilitation*, *22*, 731–740.

Kaslow, F. (1982). Profile of the healthy family. *The Relationship*, *8*(1), 9–25.

Kneipp, S., & Bender, F. (1981). Services to family members by state vocational rehabilitation agencies. *Journal of Applied Rehabilitation Counseling*, *12*, 130–134.

Kosciulek, J. F. (2004). Family counseling. In F. Chan, N. Berven, & K. Thomas (Eds.), *Counseling theories and techniques for rehabilitation health professionals* (pp. 264–281). New York, NY: Springer.

Kosciulek, J. F., McCubbin, M. A., & McCubbin, H. I. (1993). A theoretical framework for family adaptation to head injury. *Journal of Rehabilitation*, *59*(3), 40–45.

Kozloff, R. (1987). Networks of social support and the outcome from severe head injury. *Journal of Head Trauma Rehabilitation*, *2*, 14–23.

Lantz, J. (1993). *Existential family therapy: Using the concepts of Victor Frankl*. Northvale, NJ: Jason Aronson.

Lebow, J. (1997). The integrative revolution in couple and family therapy. *Family Process*, *36*, 1–17.

Levine, M., & Perkins, D. V. (1987). *Principles of community psychology*. Oxford, UK: Oxford University Press.

Lewis, J. M., Beavers, W. R., Gossett, J. T., & Phillips, V. A. (1976). *No single thread*. New York, NY: Bruner/Mazel.

Linley, P. A., Joseph, S., Maltby, J., Harrington, S., & Wood, A. M. (2009). Positive psychology applications. In S. J. Lopez & C. R. Snyder (Eds.), *Oxford handbook of positive psychology* (2nd ed., pp. 35–47). New York, NY: Oxford University Press.

Livneh, H. (1986). A unified approach to existing models of adaptation to disability: Part 1: A model of adaptation. *Journal of Applied Rehabilitation Counseling*, *17*(1), 5–16.

Livneh, K., & Antonak, R. F. (1997). *Psychosocial adaptation to chronic illness and disability*. Gaithersburg, MD: Aspen Publishing.

Lopez, S. J., & Gallagher, M. W. (2009). A case for positive psychology. In S. J. Lopez & C. R. Snyder (Eds.), *Oxford handbook of positive psychology* (2nd ed., pp. 3–6). New York, NY: Oxford University Press.

Maddux, J. E., Snyder, C. R., & Lopez, S. J. (2004). Towards a positive clinical psychology: Deconstructing the illness ideology and constructing an ideology of human strengths and potential. In P. A. Linley & S. Joseph (Eds.), *Positive psychology in practice* (pp. 320–334). Hoboken, NJ: Wiley.

Magliano, L., Fiorillo, A., De Rosa, C., Malangone, C., Maj, M. & the National Mental Health Project Working Group (2005). Family burden in long-term diseases: A comparative study in schizophrenia vs. physical disorders. *Social Science & Medicine*, *61*, 313–322.

Marshall, C. A. (2008). Family and culture: Using autoethnography to inform rehabilitation practice with cancer survivors. *Journal of Applied Rehabilitation Counseling*, *39*(1), 9–19.

May, K. M., & Hunt, B. (1994). Family counseling training in rehabilitation education programs. *Rehabilitation Education*, *8*, 348–359.

McCubbin, H. I., Thompson, A. I., & McCubbin, M. A. (1996). *Family assessment: Resiliency, coping and adaptation*. Madison, WI: University of Wisconsin Press.

McFarlane, W. R. (2002). *Multifamily groups in the treatment of severe psychiatric disorders*. New York, NY: Guilford Press.

McGoldrick, M., & Giordano, J. (1996). Ethnicity and family therapy: An overview. In M. McGoldrick, J. K. Pearce, & J. Giordano (Eds.), *Ethnicity and family therapy* (2nd ed., pp. 1–27). New York, NY: Guilford Press.

McKellin, W. H. (1995). Hearing impaired families: The social ecology of hearing loss. *Social Science Medicine*, *40*, 1469–1480.

Miklowitz, D. J., George, E. L., Richards, J. A., Simoneau, T. L., & Suddath, R. L. (2003). A randomized study of family-focused psychoeducation and pharmacotherapy in the outpatient management of bipolar disorder. *Archives of General Psychiatry*, *60*, 904–912.

Minuchin, S. (1980). *Families and family therapy*. Cambridge, MA: Harvard University Press.

Mishel, M. H. (1999). Uncertainty in chronic illness. *Annual Review of Nursing Research*, *17*, 269–294.

Mosak, H. H., & Maniacci, M. P. (1998). *Tactics in counseling and psychotherapy.* Itasca, IL: F. E. Peacock.

Mosak, H. H., & Maniacci, M. P. (2010). Adlerian psychotherapy. In R. J. Corsini & D. Wedding (Eds.), *Current psychotherapies* (9th ed., pp. 67–112). Belmont, CA: Thomson Brooks/Cole.

Moses, T. (2010). Being treated differently: Stigma experiences with family, peers, and school staff among adolescents with mental health disorders. *Social Science & Medicine, 70,* 985–993.

Nichols, M. P., & Schwartz, R. C. (2006). *Family therapy: Concepts and methods* (7th ed.). Boston, MA: Allyn and Bacon.

Power, P. W., & Dell Orto, A. E. (2004). *Families living with chronic illness and disability: Interventions, challenges, and opportunities.* New York, NY: Springer.

Power, P. W., & Hershenson, D. B. (2003). Work adjustment and readjustment of persons with mid-career onset traumatic brain injury. *Brain Injury, 17,* 1021–1034.

Power, P. W., Hershenson, D. B., & Fabian, E. S. (1991). Meeting the documented needs of clients' families: An opportunity for rehabilitation counselors. *Journal of Rehabilitation, 57*(3), 11–16.

Riemer-Reiss, M., & Morrissette, P. J. (2002). Family counseling in vocational rehabilitation education. *Rehabilitation Education, 16,* 277–281.

Rigazio-DiGilio, S. A., Ivey, A. E., Grady, L. T., & Kunkler-Peck, K. P. (2005). *Community genograms: Using individual, family, and cultural narratives with clients.* New York, NY: Teachers College Press.

Rolland, J. S. (1994). *Families, illness, and disability.* New York, NY: Springer.

Rosenthal, D. A., Kosciulek, J., Lee, G. K., Frain, M., & Ditchman, N. (2009). Family adaptation to chronic illness and disability. In F. Chan, E. D. Cordoso, & J. A. Chronister (Eds.), *Understanding psychosocial adjustment to chronic illness and disability: A handbook for evidence-based practitioners in rehabilitation* (pp. 185–203). New York, NY: Springer.

Ruini, C., & Fava, G. A. (2004). Clinical applications of wellbeing therapy. In P. A. Linley & S. Joseph (Eds.), *Positive psychology in practice* (pp. 371–387). Hoboken, NJ: Wiley.

Sander, A. M., Caroselli, J. S., High, W. M., Jr., Becker, C., Neese, L., & Scheibel, R. (2002). Relationship of family functioning to progress in a post-acute rehabilitation programme following traumatic brain injury. *Brain Injury, 16,* 649–657.

Sarason, B. R., Levine, I. G., & Pierce, G. R. (1990). *Social support: An interactional view.* New York, NY: John Wiley & Sons.

Scharff, J. S., & Scharff, D. E. (2006). *The primer of object relations* (2nd ed.). New York, NY: Jason Aronson.

Scheier, M. F., Carver, C. S., & Bridges, M. W. (2001). Optimism, pessimism, and psychological well-being. In F. C. Chang (Ed.), *Optimism and pessimism: Implications for theory, research, and practice* (pp. 189–216). Washington, DC: American Psychological Association.

Schmidt, C. K., & Welsh, A. C. (2010). College adjustment and subjective well-being when coping with a family member's illness. *Journal of Counseling & Development, 88,* 397–406.

Seligman, M. E. P., & Csikszentmihalyi, M. (2000). Positive psychology: An introduction. *American Psychologist, 55,* 5–14.

Shapiro, A. (2004). The theme of the family in contemporary society and positive family psychology. *Journal of Family Psychotherapy, 15*(1), 19–38.

Sheridan, S. M., & Burt, J. D. (2009). Family-centered positive psychology. In S. J. Lopez & C. R. Snyder (Eds.), *Oxford handbook of positive psychology* (2nd ed., pp. 551–559). New York, NY: Oxford University Press.

Singer, G. H., & Powers, L. E. (1993). Contributing to resilience in families: An overview. In G. H. Singer & L. E. Powers (Eds.), *Families, disability, and empowerment: Active coping skills and strategies for family interventions* (pp. 1–25). Baltimore, MD: Paul H. Brookes.

Singleton, G. (1982). Bowen family systems therapy. In A. M. Horne & M. M. Ohlsen (Eds.), *Family counseling & therapy* (pp. 75–111). Itasca, IL: F. E. Peacock.

Smith, S. D., Reynolds, C. A., & Rovnak, A. (2009). A critical analysis of the social advocacy movement in counseling. *Journal of Counseling & Development, 87,* 483–491.

Snyder, R., Harris, C., Anderson, J. R., Holleran, S. A., Irving, L. M., Sigmon, S. T., et al. (1991). The will and the ways: Development and validation of an individual differences measure of hope. *Journal of Personality and Social Psychology, 60*(4), 570–585.

Spaniol, L., & Zipple, A. M. (1984). How professionals can share power with families: A practical approach to working with families of the mentally ill. *Psychosocial Rehabilitation Journal, 8*, 77–84.

Spaniol, L., Zipple, A., & Lockwood, D. (2006). The role of the family in psychiatric rehabilitation. In L. Davidson, C. Harding, & L. Spaniol (Eds.), *Recovery from severe mental illnesses: Research evidence and implications for practice* (Vol. 2, pp. 311–322). Boston, MA: Center for Psychiatric Rehabilitation.

Sutton, J. (1985). The need for family involvement in client rehabilitation. *Journal of Applied Rehabilitation Counseling, 16*, 42–45.

Swain, J., & Walker, C. (2003). Parent-professional power relations: Parent and professional perspectives. *Disability & Society, 18*(5), 547–560.

Testa, J. A., Malec, J. F., Moessner, A. M., & Brown, A. W. (2006). Predicting family functioning after TBI: Impact of neurobehavioral factors. *The Journal of Head Trauma Rehabilitation, 21*(3), 236–247.

Versluys, H. P. (1980). Physical rehabilitation and family dynamics. *Rehabilitation Literature, 41*, 58–65.

Vygotsky, L. S. (1978). *Mind and society: The development of higher mental processes.* Cambridge, MA: Harvard University Press.

Wallander, J. L., Varni, J. W., Babani, L., Banis, T. H., & Wilcox, K. T. (1989). Children with chronic physical disorders: Maternal reports of their psychological adjustment. *Journal of Pediatric Psychology, 13*, 197–212.

Walsh, F. (2003). Clinical views of family normality, health, and dysfunction: From deficit to strengths perspective. In F. Walsh (Ed.), *Normal family processes: Growing diversity and complexity* (3rd ed., pp. 27–57). New York, NY: Guilford Press.

Whitaker, C. A., & Bumberry, W. M. (1988). *Dancing with the family: A symbolic-experiential approach.* New York, NY: Brunner/Mazel.

Wright, B. (1983). *Physical disability: A psychological approach.* New York, NY: Harper Collins.

Yeates, G., Henwood, K., Gracey, F., & Evans, J. (2007). Awareness of disability after acquired brain injury and the family context. *Neuropsychological Rehabilitation, 17*, 151–173.

Zahniser, J. H. (2005). Psychosocial rehabilitation. In C. E. Stout & R. A. Hayes (Eds.), *The evidence-based practice; Methods, models, and tools for mental health professionals.* Hoboken, NJ: John Wiley & Sons.

INSIDER PERSPECTIVE
The Story of Kathleen Prime

When I was just 7 years old, I asked a question; an innocent, yet all-important, question that has shaped the course of my life ever since. I believe that the answer I received, with all its subsequent implications, has been responsible for my transformation from a timid and impressionable little blind girl into a determined and, I hope, compassionate woman. One day, I was sitting in my grandparents' basement listening to my grandfather read me a story. Suddenly, out of nowhere, a question popped into my head, and as a sensitive, curious 7-year-old, I felt compelled to ask it. I turned to my grandfather, and with words that must have stirred up many conflicting thoughts and feelings, I asked, "Does God love me, too? I'm different." My grandfather answered simply, yet profoundly, "Of course! God loves you very much." It would be many years before I would reflect back on those words and fully grasp their significance.

I was born 3 months before my parents expected me, and consequently was placed in an incubator where I was given too much oxygen. The result was total blindness, except for a bit of light perception in one eye. Since I myself have no experience as a parent, I can only imagine the pain and sadness my family must have felt on learning that their only daughter would have to face life without sight. However, my family's strength of character allowed them the insight they needed to realize that if given the opportunity and the necessary resources, I could live a life that would be as full and as meaningful as the life of any nondisabled person. They struggled to alleviate the fears and concerns of uninformed school officials who saw no place for a blind child in the public school system. Once that battle had been won, it was time for me to begin facing life in the "real world," with its innumerable joys and sorrows, challenges and triumphs, disappointments, hopes, and dreams.

As a young child growing up in East Patchogue, New York, I had many friends; more than I could count on both hands! I am sure this is because little children see with their minds and hearts, rather than with their eyes. To them, love and acceptance know no boundaries; all are included in their circle, whether Black, White, deaf, blind, physically challenged, or otherwise "different." As time went by, and I completed high school, college, and graduate school, I found that my circle of friends grew much smaller, and yet much closer. Like everyone else, I learned that friends come and go and that the essential thing is to have a few very dear friends who truly care. Thanks to them, as well as to the unfailing love and support of my family, I, now almost 27 years old, have come to view my visual limitation as a gift.

When asked what disability they would choose if such a choice were theirs to make, most people would only opt for blindness as the last possible resort. People simply cannot conceive of a life without sight. Well, if you want to know the truth, many of my visually impaired friends and I agree that being blind is the least difficult disability to live with. Even Helen Keller herself believed that while blindness separates people from things, deafness cuts them off from people. I also could not imagine my life without the freedom of mobility. Although I will be the first to admit that blindness has its share of challenges (some humorous and others not so easily brushed aside), it also has its special advantages! I can read in the dark, can type without looking at the keys, have an excuse for literally bumping into a nice guy, and am free from the daily pressures of having to drive on crowded, dangerous highways! By now I have learned that a sense of humor can take me a long way in overcoming any challenging situation that may arise. On a more serious note though, I believe that being without physical sight has given me a deeper kind of perception: the ability to know people as they really are, without the usual distraction of outward appearances.

Like any other life situation, blindness definitely has its ups and downs. In my view, three especially difficult issues are the problem of transportation, the dependence on others that is so often necessary, and the limitations on social interaction. Transportation systems are not always adequate, and we who are blind must often turn to others for help with tasks about which other people, whether disabled or not, don't have to think twice. As for socialization, one of the most painful challenges for me is to walk into a roomful of people, not knowing who is there and not being able to easily locate the people with whom I wish to speak. My knowledge of braille, computer technology, and white cane techniques has made communication and travel much more enjoyable. I have been fortunate enough to visit several countries and have always had friends from many parts of the world. I am blessed with a caring family and a wonderful balance of friends with and without disabilities—people who understand and accept me as I am, without expecting me to be any more or any less than I am capable of being. I also draw much strength from my participation in the American Council of the Blind, as well as in the Catholic parish to which I belong.

However, the basic challenges still remain: How do I overcome barriers to employment? How can I become a more independent traveler? And most of all, what would be the most fulfilling lifestyle for me? There are times when my longing to love and be loved by that special someone (whoever he may turn out to be) is very intense. This, I have found, is a struggle that I share with many disabled women in our often uncompromising society, which still secretly believes that women with disabilities cannot be good wives and mothers. However, there are other days when my appreciation of the unique freedoms of the single life is just as strong as my desire to be loved in that special way. It seems to me that this conflict of emotions is unique to my situation as a blind woman, yet at the same time, an experience that is common to everyone.

Overall, I have found that society's response to me as a blind person is one of tentative curiosity and sympathy, rather than wholehearted support. In general, people are uncertain how to approach someone with a disability and, therefore, are afraid or hesitant to do so. They are either amazed by our accomplishments or feel sorry for us because of the challenges we face. Neither of these approaches is healthy or desirable. The majority of people with disabilities do not consider themselves to be heroes; we are simply living our daily lives as others do, with some minor adaptations that conform to our individual need. On the other hand, the last thing we want is for people to pity us. This paternalistic attitude only serves to undermine the dignity for which we are continually striving in our everyday lives.

So this brings me to my final point; namely, that having a disability sets one apart from others in many ways, and yet when one looks beneath the surface, one cannot help concluding that almost all human experiences have the power to transcend physical limitations. I, as a blind person, have talents, gifts, and shortcomings that are uniquely mine, and yet I am, at heart, no different from my deaf friend or my nondisabled relative. This particular insight into my own situation has led me to conclude that my mission in this world is to do my best to help people with disabilities in their ongoing struggle to overcome communication barriers and societal misconceptions. I prefer to do this not by militant protests, but instead by setting an unobtrusive example of service to those in need.

Had I not been assured at an early age that I was loved unconditionally, I would never have come to the seemingly paradoxical realization that those who appear weakest in the eyes of the world possess within themselves a wonderful sense of empowerment. My life, with all its positive and negative experiences, has taught me that the most severe limitations I face are the ones that I place on myself. No wonder my grandmother, even today, counsels me with quiet confidence, "Never say you can't . . ."

Thus, there are two very important pieces of advice that I would offer prospective rehabilitation counselors. The first is that you should always view the person with a disability as a fully capable human being who just happens to have a certain limitation. In this way, he or she is no different from anyone else, as we all have our share of limitations to overcome. The person always comes first, and the disability is just one characteristic that he or she happens to have. By no means does the disability define everything about the person; it is merely one aspect of who that individual is. And secondly, I believe that the best way to approach your work with the disabled is to be as realistic as possible. Recognize that there are certain undeniable limitations, but also understand that most people with disabilities choose to see something positive about their life situation. Try to emphasize those positive perspectives, thereby assisting your clients in their journey toward greater independence and a deeper love of life itself. If you give your best effort, it is impossible to fail. Because for all we know, it may be enough to touch and transform the life of even one person . . .

DISCUSSION QUESTIONS

1. What are the deep ethical conflicts at the root of family work in rehabilitation? How do we proceed in an ethical manner?
2. Individuals with disabilities cope within families coping with disabilities. How do the client and caretaker perspectives inform each other? How do rehabilitation counselors use this to the client's best advantage?
3. Is advocacy therapeutic? Please expand on the thought.

EXERCISE

A. Create a genogram of your own family. What family problems do you need to address before you address the family problems of others? Under what conditions would you feel comfortable in using such a tool with your clients, and for what purpose?

FOURTEEN

Ethical Responsibilities in Working With Persons With Disabilities and Our Duty to Educate

Noreen M. Glover-Graf

OVERVIEW

Ethics is a term used to describe the principles involved in living a moral life that include righteousness, virtues, rules of conduct, and responsibilities as they apply to actions, thoughts, and relating to others (Beauchamp & Childress, 2001). The determination of the specific actions appropriate to various human service professions are written as codes of ethics that are based on ethical theories dating back to Socrates, Euripides, and Aristotle. The two ethical theories most commonly referred to in human services professions are consequential ethics and deontological ethics. Consequentialists believe that the determination of the correctness of actions is based on the outcome. Thus, civil disobedience might be justified if it led to laws that prohibited discrimination. For example, in 1977 persons with disabilities conducted a nationwide sit-in at government buildings in major cities; and in 1978, persons with disabilities sat on the streets refusing to allow buses to move for two days in Denver. These actions directly impacted the development and enforcement of accessibility. On the other hand, deontological ethics are concerned with the correctness of the actions leading to the consequences. In 2009, protestors blockaded the governor's office in California to protest cuts in services to people with disabilities ("Caregivers, disabled block Governor's office," 2009). Disobeying laws and restricting others' movements would be considered unethical, despite positive consequences under this ethical theory.

Recently, a feminist-based ethical theory that focuses on responsibility and social interconnectedness and collaboration, the *ethics of care*, has begun to emerge in the medical, social, and human services literature. This theory focuses less on moral judgments and more on caring, loving, sensitivity, and empathy (Davis, 1997; Edwards, 2009; Gatens-Robinson & Tarvydas, 1992; Tong, 1997; Ward & Gahagan, 2010). In an article that reviews the ethics of care, Gatens-Robinson and Tarvydas conclude that ". . . women's perspectives may significantly improve the quality of ethical practice in rehabilitation" (Robinson & Tarvydas, 1992, p. 26).

Ethical principles have to do with one's professional obligations and differ from morals that have to do with one's human obligations. Morals are personal beliefs based on universal understandings of goodness and goodwill toward others. A person's personal interpretation, adoption of, and incorporation of these beliefs make up his or her moral values, sometimes referred to as personal ethics. Ethical principles are somewhat consistent among human service and medical professions because they are in place to protect the client and to guide the professional. Rehabilitation counselor ethics include autonomy, which is a right held by clients to make their own decisions related to life choices. The remaining five principles are counselor obligations to the client and include beneficence, which instructs counselors to do good; nonmaleficence, which restricts counselors from causing harm to clients; justice, which involves being fair and equal distribution based on client need; fidelity, which involves being loyal, honest with clients, and keeping promises; and veracity, which insists that counselors be honest and truthful.

Ideally, ethics and morals should never come into conflict because ethics are based on goodness for the client and incorporate acting in the best interest of the client, fair and just treatment, being faithful to the client and keeping promises, respecting the client's right to be the director of his or her own life, and not imposing or coercing clients into making choices that are contrary to their desires. Unfortunately, these ethical principles can come into conflict, causing ethical dilemmas. Toriello and Benshoff (2003) defined ethical dilemmas as the existence of choices between two courses of action where significant consequences will result from choosing either course, and where each choice can be supported by an ethical principle. Choosing either course will compromise an ethical principle.

For example, the counselor may believe that what the client wants will cause the client to be harmed in some way or to fail, and may attempt to coerce the client into acting in his or her own best interest by withholding information or presenting information deceptively. In this case, doing good and allowing the client to be autonomous appear to be in conflict. The counselor may feel the need to oppose one principle to achieve the greater good. This is not an uncommon situation for counselors. In an examination of ethical dilemmas associated with client choice, Patterson, Patrick, and Parker (2000) found that balancing autonomy with justice and beneficence were frequent ethical dilemmas for vocational rehabilitation counselors, noting that counselor's assessment of the client's intelligence, work experience, aptitudes, and limitations might be inconsistent with client's vocational choices. Honoring the client's choice (autonomy) would be in direct conflict with client vocational success (beneficence) and use of taxpayer dollars (justice).

While many counselors will carefully examine their options and ethical responsibilities, they may fail to examine the extent to which their personal morals are involved in their decisions. They may also fail to examine the role of their personal values in their decision making. For example, the counselor might ask herself, "If I believe the client's choice will lead to failure, can I tolerate this failure? Can any good come from allowing the client to fail? Is my personal investment in this client causing me to personalize the potential failure? Does my personal need to control and succeed interfere with the client's need for autonomy?"

Another component of ethical decision making has to do with procedures, policies, regulations, and laws. For the most part professional accrediting bodies have made this an easy choice when ethics come into conflict with the law by giving priority to the law. Counselors are obligated to follow the law. However, when ethical conflicts arise from problems with policies and procedures, the line can become blurred for counselors. Codes of ethics are established to guide counselors and other professionals in behaviors and decision making. The Code of Professional Ethics for Rehabilitation Counselors provides general guidance for rehabilitation counselors but, like any code of ethics, is written to provide generalized instruction that can apply to a variety of situations. Unfortunately, the codes are limited in scope and unable to cover specific situations definitively enough, often leaving counselors confused and feeling forced into making difficult decisions without sufficient guidance. Counselors often fail to utilize a critical component of ethical decision making: that of consultation, which can involve consults with colleagues, supervisions, professional boards, regulators, and experts. Consultation is necessary in many situations to demonstrate that the counselor has sought appropriate education and advice to make competent and effective treatment choices (Shaw & Lane, 2008). Even so, at least among the approximately 16,000 certified rehabilitation counselors, relatively few ethical complaints have been made to the certifying body. Of the 141 complaints made between 1994 and 2010, the Commission on Rehabilitation Counselor Certification (CRCC) has formally reprimanded eight RCs, placed four on probation, suspended five certifications, and revoked 18 certifications due to ethical violations (Commission on Rehabilitation Counselor Certification, 2011).

The topic of ethics is vast and impossible to cover comprehensively in any single work. The intent of this chapter is to present some of the relevant and controversial topics in this arena. It is not intended to be a primer in ethics, although a good foundation in ethics theory and principles is essential for beginning counselors and can be found in the work of Howie, Gatens-Robinson, and Rubin (1993) and Wilson, Rubin, and Millard (1991). Rather, this chapter will focus on common ethical dilemmas, factors that influence counselor ethics, counselor competence and ethics, and current and debated ethical issues.

COMMON ETHICAL DILEMMAS

Ethical issues in rehabilitation counseling include numerous areas, for example, issues of confidentiality and privileged communication breaches, such as revealing private information to persons outside of the agency, including employers, medical professionals, third-party payees, and family members, without client consent. Counselors may also commit breaches in group counseling settings, or to the treatment team in debriefings and staffing by sharing more that what is necessary. Violations of informed consent occur when there is a failure to meet the obligation to give a detailed explanation of what information and with whom it will be shared, and to gain client permission to do so. This includes explaining the rights of third-party payees to receive summary information of services.

Counselors who administer any kind of counseling or services without established competence also commit an ethical violation. Counselors must be certain that the client has the capacity to understand fully what treatment and services will be administered and voluntarily, without coercion, agree to participate in services. They must be mentally competent to give consent or have a legal guardian act on their behalf. Relationship violations are unethical because they create a dual relationship that involves unequal power, setting the stage for coercion. The principles of justice, fidelity, and beneficence are compromised, risking psychological harm to the client.

The code of ethics allows for personal relationships with clients only after 5 years following the termination of services. Counselors must maintain awareness of the power dynamics created in the counseling relationship and attend to their own issues of paternalism and codependence that may lead to unduly influencing the client to act in a manner prescribed by the counselor without sufficient client input or deliberation.

Counselors may fail to disclose when a client is of harm to themselves or others in violation of their duty to warn. In this case, the responsibility to the intended victim becomes greater than the responsibility to client confidentiality. It is the responsibility of the counselor to make every effort to inform the intended victim directly and take crisis intervention measures by contacting appropriate agencies to intervene in a life-threatening situation.

In a 13-year review of 113 complaints filed with the CRCC, Saunders, Barros-Bailey, Rudman, Dew, and Garcia (2007) determined that complaints could be categorized as (1) competence and conduct, including dishonest communication, sexual intimacy, and abandonment; (2) business practices, including documentation and billing; and (3) professional practices, including lack of or inappropriate referrals for employment and counseling and nonprofessional relationships. Of the complaints filed, 37 violations were confirmed. Eight (21.1%) counselors received letters of instruction, eight were issued reprimands, three were placed on probation, four were suspended, and 15 counselor certifications were revoked.

FACTORS THAT INFLUENCE COUNSELOR ETHICS

The preamble to the code of ethics lists a number of counselor expectations regarding RCs professional functioning that include respecting human rights and human dignity, acting with integrity in professional relationships, seeking to alleviate distress and suffering, enhancing professional knowledge and effectiveness, appreciating diversity of experience and culture, and advocating for fair and adequate services (CRCC Code of Ethics, Preamble, 2009).

In addition to these professional behaviors, Corey, Corey, and Callanan (2007) listed a number of factors that, if not attended to, could be detrimental to the counse-lor-client relationship, including self-awareness regarding the influence of counselor personality traits and personal needs; counselor values; transference and countertrans-ference issues; and stress, burnout, and counselor impairment.

Personality Factors

Clearly, not everyone is suited to be a counselor. Not to say that only one type of person will make a good counselor because what and who works for clients will depend on their needs and preferences. Undeniably, clients will work better with, and be more open to, counselors who they feel connected to in some way. A part of this will be determined by counselor approach and skills, but another piece will have to do with counselor personality traits. Some studies have shown that counselor personality traits and relationship building have a greater impact on clients than do counselor knowledge and applied use of specific theories, techniques, and skills (Stein & Lambert, 1995; Stevens, Dinoff, & Donnenworth, 1998).

In a study to determine which personality traits were considered to be the most important for counselors, Pope & Kline (1999) solicited 10 counselor experts to rank order 22 personality traits and determined that the top 10 traits were acceptance, emotional stability, open-mindedness, empathy, genuineness, flexibility, interest in people, confidence, sensitivity, and fairness. Interestingly, the least important traits were resour-cefulness, sympathy, and sociability. Pope concluded that the essential traits should be present in students entering counselor education programs since they were not easily taught to students. Many of these traits reflect the client-centered necessary conditions established by Rogers as empathy, positive regard, genuineness, and congruence.

Specific to rehabilitation counselors, McCarthy and Leierer (2001) examined the traits that clients find the least and most important in their rehabilitation counselors. The top three traits were (a) having a consumer-first attitude and client advocacy (28.5%), (b) being nurturing and enhancing the counselor relationship (20%), and (c) being knowledgeable about disabilities and rehabilitation (14%). Interestingly, the bottom three traits, endorsed by only a small minority of consumers were (a) having a personal disability experience (4%), (b) educational background/credentials (2.5%), and (c) professional experience and maturity (1.5%). The relegation of the latter traits to the bottom of this list is particularly important because these components are frequently stress-producing for counselors in training and beginning counselors; they worry that clients will believe they are too young and inexperienced or that they cannot relate to disability because many RCs are not persons with disabilities. Rather, attitude, advocacy, relationship building, and knowledge are what clients desire, and these things can be taught and practiced immediately upon working with clients.

In addition to the influence of personality traits and skills, Corey et al. (2007) dis-cussed the influence of the personal needs of counselors, some of which appear altruistic in nature but may be motivated by issues of power, control, and a need for recognition. Counselors may meet a need for control by telling people what to do instead of working through issues with the client. They may take on too much of the responsibility for making changes in clients. The personal need for power may be met by a need to have all the right answers for clients, desiring to remove all pain and discomfort from clients. Counselors may have a strong need to be recognized and appreciated for their accomplishments, to experience the feeling of being valued.

Counselor Values

Counselor neutrality is more a myth than a reality. The idea that counselors can transcend their values would not only be a superhuman feat but also likely render the counselor dysfunctional and indecisive. Rather, counseling relationships are influenced by counselor values, even to the point of clients taking on or moving closer to the counselor's values, known as convergence, during sessions, and that counselor values have great influence on diagnosis, goals, treatment, and outcomes (Beutler & Bergan, 1991; Kelly & Strupp, 1992; Tjeltveit, 1986, 1999).

In reviewing and assimilating literature related to counselor values, Consoli, Kim, and Meyer (2008), classified counselor values into four categories that include personal, interpersonal, social, and environmental spheres:

- The personal sphere includes values of independence, autonomy, personal responsibility, and interdependence. Counselors place value on coping abilities, flexibility, self-expression, and self-esteem. They demonstrate self-control but are able to accept conflict and ambiguity.
- The interpersonal sphere includes the relational values of friendship, intimacy, working in cooperation, benevolence, diversity of opinion, and mutual consent. Counselors value supportive relationships and devalue relationships built on hierarchical arrangements and coercive or controlling interactions.
- The social sphere includes a de-emphasis on social power and influence, authority, and dominance over others. Counselors tend to devalue social conformity.
- The environmental sphere includes values of harmony and unity in relationships between nature and people. Counselors devalue control over nature.

In a national survey of counselor values ($n = 479$), Kelly examined universal values, mental health values, individualism/collectivism values, and religious/spiritual values. Within these domains, counselors were found to moderately value or highly value benevolence, self-direction, achievement, compassionate responsiveness, responsible self-expression, forgiveness, autonomy, personal development, sexual acceptance, disciplined personal living, collaboration, and spirituality. In the religious/spiritual value domain, nearly 90% of counselors indicated some spiritual or religious orientation. Spiritual values were more widely affirmed than religious values, although approximately 70% expressed some religious affiliation or orientation.

Transference and Countertransference

Transference and countertransference have long been a topic of discussion in the field of counseling because these relationships are built on feelings for other people that are projected onto the client or counselor. Transference refers to a client's feelings for another significant person that are projected onto the client. For example, a client may interact with the counselor as if the counselor were a parent and might become overly compliant or, contrarily, might become overly resistive. Clients can also develop romantic feelings for the counselor that are based on transference. Counselors must remain attentive to transference issues as it might be far easier to work with clients who are compliant regardless of their motivations, or prematurely terminate a resistive client if transference is not identified and worked through in the counseling setting.

Watkins (1983) identified five transference patterns in counseling that include the client relating to a counselor as:

1. An ideal person without flaws. While this can lead the counselor to experience feelings of pride and competence, the counselor recognition of the honeymoon period eventually leads to counselor frustration and a need to confront the client and tolerate the initial disappointment and possible anger.
2. A seer who has all of the correct answers due to a kind of mystical physiological knowledge. This type of transference may feed the ego of the counselor providing them with feelings of power and extraordinary expertise. Ultimately when the unrealistic image fails, the counselor may feel incompetent. The clients benefit from this transference in that they are able to let others make decisions for them and responsibility for failure falls on someone else. Clients must be moved toward risking making decisions and potential failures.
3. A nurturer who needs to emotionally sooth the client. Clients exhibit inept and helpless behaviors, excessive crying and expressed fears, and may make requests for holding, touching, and hugging. Counselors may respond with soothing gestures and behaviors and experience deep sympathy for the client. If counselors do not become aware of the transference, they will enter into a nonproductive and collusive counseling relationship. Confrontation of their dependency needs based on clients' beliefs that they are unable to make decisions and care for themselves will be necessary.
4. A frustrator who is viewed with suspicion and distrust. While the clients desire counseling assistance, they fear disappointment and distance themselves quickly from the process by missing appointments and being noncompliant. The counselor will feel anxious and uneasy and begin to distance from the client and may begin to feel hostility for the client. The counselor will need to work with the basic issues of trust and mistrust and perhaps delve into past experiences that contributed to current feelings and behaviors.
5. A nonentity who is void of feelings, needs, and hopes. Counseling sessions lack direction as client continually switches topics. Initially the counselor feels overwhelmed but may later come to feel manipulated, discounted, and resentful. Because these clients tend toward control and manipulation, the counselor must be firm and persistent in directing the session and confront clients on their intolerance of silence and lack of reflection. They may need to work with past unresolved issues to assist the client in moving to a more satisfactory life.

As indicated above, counselors are likely to have some reaction to the client's transfer response. On a good day, a counselor might immediately recognize the client's reactions as transference and then go on to make intentional choices aimed at confronting and disarming the transference. In reality, counselors may take some time to recognize transference, and they may revert to reacting from a personal standpoint, becoming, as Corey et al. (2007) point out, overly protective or benign, creating relationships that are more about advice giving and seeking client approval. They may come to develop a number of strong emotional feelings for the client, including romantic or sexual feelings, a desire for friendship with the client, or seeing themselves in the client, or they may reject the client. With the exception of the last, counseling relationships in which countertransference is present are at risk for (aside from being inauthentic and nonproductive) client exploitation and boundary violations.

The Exploitation Index Questionnaire was developed by Epstein and Simon (1990). It is a list of 32 counselor behaviors and feelings that might indicate client exploitations and includes items related to touching clients, accepting gifts, participating in social activities, entering into business deals, sharing counselor personal problems, romantic daydreaming, and a number of feeling indicators. In a study to examine potential exploitive behaviors using the Exploitation Index, Epstein, Simon, and Kay (1992) surveyed 532 psychiatrists and found that 43% indicated they related to at least one item that could be counterproductive to their treatment. The average number of potentially exploitive behaviors among these participants was 3.6 (range 1–17). Twenty-nine percent indicated they would make appropriate changes in future treatment practices.

Half or more of the respondents prescribed medications or acted in a professional capacity for family members, accepted gifts from clients, sought personal gratification from client achievement, disclosed exciting aspects of the client lives to others, made exceptions for clients out of fear or pity, and were gratified by feelings of power over their clients. The authors concluded:

> *Exploitation* can arise in any relationship. Unfortunately, the psychotherapy setting increases the potential for such *exploitation*. Close and repeated examination of the temptations and errors that occur in any therapeutic endeavor is likely to protect the therapist and facilitate a more beneficial treatment relationship. (Epstein et al., 1992, para 36)

Specific to sexual boundaries, Epstein and Simon (1990) concluded that about a third had romantic daydreams about their clients and/or were gratified by the client's seductive behaviors, about 5% felt that romance with the client would be beneficial, and about a quarter of participants made favorable comparisons of clients to their spouses. Results indicated that female psychiatrists were less likely to engage in sexual exploitation than males.

It is unlikely that many therapists, male or female, enter the counseling relationship with the intent of sexual exploitation; however, boundaries appear to erode gradually and without much notice. Counselors may be particularly vulnerable to these erosions when they experience personal problems and may become susceptible to patient idealization (Simon, 1995). Simon (1989) suggests that therapists become skilled at transference recognition, seek counseling for countertransference issues, consult with colleagues, educate clients on transference, and refer as appropriate.

Corey et al. (2007) describe covert forms of misconduct that can include sexual hugging and sexual gazes, seductive behaviors, and inappropriate attention to client appearance and dress. Overt behaviors may eventually emerge and include sexual comments, remarks, and jokes; "therapy" centered around learning to love; bonding and trust exercises; sexual touch; and exploring the client's sexual identity. These overt behaviors may then give way to romantic involvement and sex with the client.

In a survey study, to examine the prevalence of sexual intimacy between psychologists and clients, harm to clients, and client characteristics, Pope and Vetter (1991) determined that about half of the surveyed 647 psychologists reported having sexual intimacies with at least one client for a total of 950 individual clients. Most of the instances occurred prior to termination of the counseling relationship, and most resulted in harm to the client. In a review of client characteristics, 32% had histories of childhood sexual abuse, 20% were not charged for their therapy or were given a reduced fee, 14% had attempted suicide, 11% required hospitalization related in part to the sexual intimacy with the therapist, 10% had been victims of a rape, 5% were minor children, and 1% committed suicide. These authors conclude, "That half of the respondents in this study reported seeing at least one patient who was sexually intimate with a prior therapist is a stark reminder that we have unfinished business in this area that urgently requires our attention. We have many questions to explore and much work to do" (Pope & Vetter, p. 437). If, however, up to half of psychotherapists are willing to discard their codes of ethics, it may be time for new precedents to emerge, beginning with establishing a priority of matching counselors with sexually nonpreferential gender clients, lest our profession become tantamount to Catholic priests who have taken advantage of vulnerable children in their care, committing despicable and indefensible acts.

Stress, Burnout, and Lack of Personal Mental Health

Counselors, like all other humans, are likely to have times when life situations cause considerable stress and may impair the mental health of the counselor. As well, Corey et al. (2007) believe that the profession itself can put a counselor at risk for increased stress in addition to whatever life events may be occurring for them. When counselors have set high goals and expect perfection, they are likely to feel intense pressure to solve the clients' problems. If clients fail to make progress, the counselors may feel that they are not helping the clients and erroneously take on the full responsibility for this failure. Whether or not impacted by personal or professional situations that lead the counselor to become overwhelmed, impaired counselors will demonstrate a number of nonproductive behaviors and attitudes, including having a fragile self-esteem, a lack of intimacy in one's private life, and professional isolation. Counselors may demonstrate a need to be reassured and to rescue clients. Problems with substance abuse may also contribute to counselor ineffectiveness.

Counselor burnout has been described by Maslach and Jackson (1981) as a syndrome of emotional exhaustion, a lack of personal achievement, and depersonalization. Using cluster analysis and the Counselor Burnout Inventory (Lee et al., 2007) to measure components of burnout (subscales of Exhaustion, Incompetence,

Negative Work Environment, Devaluing Client, and Deterioration in Personal Life), Lee, Cho, Kissinger, and Ogle (2010) identified three counselor types in relation to burnout: well-adjusted, persevering, and disconnected counselor types. These types differed in self-esteem, job satisfaction, and locus of control. *Well-adjusted* counselors had the second-highest income and the highest job satisfaction. The *disconnected* counselors were moderately exhausted, indicated a negative work environment, and had deterioration in their personal lives. They scored high on Incompetence, Depersonalization, and Devaluing Clients. This group reported the lowest income, poorest self-esteem, and lowest job satisfaction. Finally, like the disconnected type, the *preserving* type had high Exhaustion, Deterioration in personal life, and a Negative work environment. However, scores on Incompetence and Devaluing Client were low to moderate. Counselors in this group were attentive to client needs and flexible even though exhausted in their professional and personal lives. These counselors had the highest income and self-esteem and the most experience, but were unsatisfied with their current position. These findings may indicate that some variables, such as experience and sufficient remuneration, may be sufficient to mediate the effects of burnout and suggest that experienced counselors may have developed coping skills that could benefit less experienced counselors from succumbing to burnout in a manner that affects interactions with clients.

ETHICS AND COUNSELOR COMPETENCE

Counselor competence includes being able to work with a variety of clients from various cultural backgrounds. Counselors must be willing to actively pursue enlarging the scope of their competence and comfort in dealing with clients who are different from them based on ethnicity and race, gender, age, sexual preference, and religious and spiritual beliefs, among others. Referring clients due to a lack of competence is demanded by ethical codes, but real scrutiny of these referrals may reveal that other factors play a role in counselors' refusals to engage with a particular client.

Counselor Referral of Clients

Referral of a client should be a carefully thought-out decision. The client will receive appropriate messages from the counselor, such as "I believe you need to see someone with more experience or expertise in this area, and am going to refer you to another counselor." The client's interpretation of that message may vary considerably. Clients may believe that their problems are beyond the scope of "normal" and may believe that the problems are really unfixable. Or they may interpret the message as meaning that they are not likeable or worth working with any longer. Corey et al. (2007) list a number of reasons for which a counselor might be ethically bound to refer clients, including when religious, moral, and political values are in conflict with those of the counselor and central to the client's problems; when the counselor is not competent in a necessary area or is in need of additional education or training; when a counselor is extremely uncomfortable with a client's values or beliefs that the counselor is imposing his or her values on the client; when unable to remain objective.

Relatively little research has been done in this area recently; however, Weinrach (1984) suggested that a lack of adequate time and expertise or a lack of rapport with the client were reasons for appropriate referral and additionally noted that the referral process should be both mutual and interactive. Clients should agree with and participate in the decision to refer. At the very least they should understand the reasons for the change. When counselors do refer, they should do so by preparing the client and following up to make certain the referrals were appropriate and effective. Referral should not occur as a result of counselor frustrations with a slow or seemingly failing process, or client attempts to sabotage the process through disruptive or manipulative behaviors. Rather, these are times to reevaluate the counseling process and the focus of sessions, perhaps directly addressing the behavior motivation.

Shiles (2009) examined referrals based on discrimination and bias against clients. For example, a counselor might refer a lesbian client because homosexuality is against the counselor's religious beliefs. Through her literature review, Shiles (2009) demonstrates that counselors may be using ethical standards to justify referral of clients (lack of competence) when they cannot tolerate the clients' attributes, but this is in conflict with standards that prohibit discrimination based on client characteristics. She states: "It is my belief that, currently, discriminatory referral practices within the field of psychology may be rationalized as ways of avoiding harming the client and working outside of one's competence while going unchallenged by the psychology community" (Shiles, 2009, p. 144). Stronger still, and thought provoking at the very least, Shiles challenges therapists to intensive self-examination of motivations for referrals:

> It is my contention that statements such as "It takes honesty and courage to recognize how your values affect the way you counsel, and it takes wisdom to determine when you are not able to effectively work with a client due to a clash of values" (Corey et al., 2007b, p. 106) overwhelmingly depict the referring psychologist as honest, courageous, and full of wisdom rather than possibly racist, prejudiced, or homophobic. These types of statements potentially reward the professional for making the referral, continue the pattern of cognitive dissonance, and allow the discriminatory referrals to go unnoticed and unchallenged in the field. (Shiles, 2009, p. 147)

Ethics and Cultural Competence

Diversity in counseling includes differences related to gender, age, race, culture, socioeconomic status, disability status, and sexual orientation. The idea that you have to understand "where a person is coming from" to counsel them is likely not resisted among counselors. But the follow-through with the work it takes to understand a variety of cultures is less enthusiastically embraced. For many counselors and the counseling profession, seeking to understand other viewpoints and cultural norms is either resisted or approached with hesitation. Sue (1996) categorized levels of "cultural encapsulation" or the ability to view the world only from one's own experiences and beliefs, noting four types of resistance to embracing cultural inclusion as follows:

(1) counselors who believe that they need to make no changes in standards or behaviors because rehabilitation counseling can be universally applied to all persons, regardless of their race, gender, culture, sexual orientation, or ethnicity; (2) counselors who believe that it is unrealistic to become culturally competent given the number and variety of cultures and cultural practices; (3) counselors who believe that cultural competence is important but wish to wait until written standards of practice are available for all culturally diverse groups; and (4) those who believe that cultural diversity is reverse discrimination, and standards discriminate against the majority population.

Middleton et al. (2000) argue: "Professional multicultural rehabilitation competencies and standards *are necessary* if persons with disabilities from diverse ethnic backgrounds are to be well served by rehabilitation counselors" (Middleton et al., 2000, p. 225). They state that majority counselors must dismiss their "cultural superiority" bias, assess their personal values and recognize the impact of those values on culturally diverse persons, take into account differences that account for underutilization of services, and assess counselor expectations and stereotyping related to client assimilation. In addition, minority counselors must remain aware that being a member of a minority culture does not qualify one as being culturally competent. These authors' recommend more than a required course on multicultural issues, but also challenge programs to incorporate the sociopolitical implications of living as a minority member and working toward moving beyond superficial understandings of differences toward cultural empathy through involvement with various cultural groups.

While the Code of Ethics demands respect for diversity and inclusive practices, the language is very broad. Middleton et al. (2000) call for (1) expanded awareness and greater sensitivity moving toward seeing other cultures as equally legitimate and valuable, (2) awareness of personal values, biases, and prejudices and how these affect clients, (3) awareness of overidentification or paternalistic behaviors and attitudes, (4) recognition of limitations that may require the counselor to refer a client to persons from their own race or culture, and (5) gaining comfort with cultural diversity and recognition of differences as positive.

Corey et al. (2007) also addressed the diversity needs related to counseling clients with minority sexual orientation, requiring counselors to be open to issues related to sexual orientation, and cognizant of their own assumptions, fears, stereotypes, and myths related to sexual orientation differences. Assumptions related to gay persons generally include some of the following:

- Gay people have particular mannerisms or physical characteristics.
- Most gay people can be cured by engaging in heterosexual sex.
- Most child molesters are gay.
- Being gay is a conscious decision.
- Gay adults attempt to convert younger persons to their lifestyle.
- Homosexuality can be cured by psychotherapy.
- In gay relationships, one partner usually takes a feminine role and the other takes the masculine role.
- Homosexuality is caused by a damaged gene.
- Homosexuality is unnatural and is not present in other species.

Essential and exemplary therapy requires the counselor to make no attempts to change sexual orientation without the client's expressed desire for change, advocating for clients through education of others and recognizing how prejudice and discrimination adversely affect clients.

Religion and Spirituality in Counseling

Avoiding the topic of religion and spirituality has long been justified by counselors as not wanting to impose personal preferences and opinions on clients; however, the avoidance of the topic also sends messages about the openness of the counselor and the counselor's belief about the importance, or rather unimportance of spirituality and religion, in counseling (Boyd-Franklin & Lockwood, 1999). If religion or spirituality plays an important role in the client's problem or condition, the omission of assessment of client needs and beliefs regarding this aspect of his or her life is potentially negligent.

The recent interest in addressing spiritual/religious values with clients in counseling is due, at least in part, to empirical findings. For example, Gallup (1996) found that 84% of U.S. Americans believe in God and a third or more had experienced miracles or mystical events that altered the course of their lives, and 90% of recovering alcoholics reported having spiritual experiences. Wallis (1996) reported nearly 80% of U.S. Americans believe that prayer can improve the course of illness. And, even though Oyama and Koenig (1998) found that 83% of patients wanted their physicians to discuss spiritual/religious issues with them, 91% of their sample stated that their physicians never inquired about their spiritual/religious beliefs. The desire to speak about spiritual issues with medical professionals was expressed by patients with life-threatening situations (77%), serious medical conditions (74%), and loss of a loved one (70%). Similarly, King and Bushwick (1994) determined that 94% of the patients believed that their spiritual health was as important as their physical health, but only 10%–20% of physicians had ever discussed spirituality with their patients; and Myers and Truluck (1998) found that 79% of the clients they surveyed indicated that spiritual and religious experiences and values were important to explore in counseling. Clearly, there is a disconnection between client beliefs and what the medical community and counselors are willing to consider as medically relevant and therapeutic.

In Levin's book *God, Faith, and Health: Exploring the Spirituality-Healing Connection* (2001), Levin uses over 200 epidemiological studies to address the effects of prayer/meditation, attending church, participating in church activities, and prayer healers in terms of mortality, illness and disability, mental health, and wellness practices. Benefits of religious affiliation are noted as:

1. Religious Americans have a mortality of approximately 7 years longer than non-believers of a higher power or being.
2. Religious affiliation benefits health by promoting healthy behavior, such as reduced smoking, drinking, drugs, suicide, or risky behavior (e.g., safe sex).
3. Participation in worship (e.g., prayer, meditation) benefits health through the physiological effects of positive emotions.

4. Faith benefits physical and mental health related to thoughts of hope, optimism, and positive expectation.
5. When persons who are prayed for by prayer groups (known as absent prayer) are compared with persons not prayed for, there is an indication of a health improvement due to perceived divine intervention.

Clearly, including spirituality in counseling may benefit some clients, and may even be essential for others since the exclusion of this topic may be a detriment to clients dealing with existential crises in relation to spirituality (Helminiak, 2001; Zinnbauer & Pargament, 2000). However, Steen, Engels, and Thweatt (2006) noted a number of ethical considerations related to the inclusion of spirituality, such as issues of client welfare, respecting diversity, personal needs and values, and professional competence, noting that the heart of these ethical issues center on clients' readiness and wiliness to be open to discussions that revolve around values and beliefs that may not match their own. These authors note that spirituality has long been an accepted area of personal growth and development, and exclusion of this area may neglect the counselor's obligation to "respect client dignity and promote client welfare and growth by being open to discussions of client spirituality" (Steen et al., 2006, p. 109). When spirituality and religion are framed within the context of diversity, it becomes the counselor's duty to have an understanding of spiritual/religious beliefs as a way of treating clients without discrimination and attending to multicultural differences. They note that the *Diagnostic and Statistical Manual of Mental Disorders* (American Psychiatric Association, 2000) include spiritual and religious issues in V codes, giving indication that an assessment of this area may be essential for some clients.

Professional and cultural competence therefore requires openness to clients' desires to discuss the meaning of religion and spirituality in their lives; developing competence in religious and spiritual beliefs within cultural contexts; inclusion of coursework in human services programs, directed at understanding various religious practices in relation to counseling; developing effective means of working with clients; and using clients religious and spiritual beliefs as positive assets and coping mechanisms. A counselor whose beliefs are rigid and inflexible and who cannot tolerate other's divergent beliefs is failing to recognize the importance of cultural competency.

CURRENT AND DEBATED ETHICAL ISSUES

Some ethical dilemmas seem inherent in the counseling process and are as likely to be encountered in the present day as they were in earlier generations. Others occur due to societal advancements and trends, new technologies, or catastrophic events or diseases that lead to increases in prejudice and discrimination. This section will cover current and debated ethical issues related to AIDS/HIV and duty to warn self-injuring clients, biotechnology advances, wrongful birth and wrongful life actions, decisions related to choosing disability, ethics and private sector rehabilitation, online and internet counseling, end-of-life counseling, and assisted suicide.

AIDS/HIV and Duty to Warn

Ethical dilemmas by definition are not easily resolved because they involve a weighing of various principles to determine the greater good. Contagious diseases such as AIDS and other STDs create dilemma with a great degree of difficulty. Currently, HIV is incurable and ultimately has a fatal outcome, and results in discrimination. However, with persons living longer lives with HIV, the contraction of the disease is no longer considered a death sentence because life expectancy in the United States has increased from about 11 years in 1996 to over 20 years in 2004 (Harrision, Song, & Zhang, 2008). This brings into question the duty-to-warn principle in contrast with a breaching confidentiality. The law remains unclear and gives little guidance to counselors facing a client who is unwilling to notify sex partners. Clearly, their lives are not in immediate danger even if they contract this disease.

In a study of 83 psychologists who were given hypothetical vignettes and asked whether they would breach the confidentiality of a client who was HIV-positive, had a partner, and was engaged in unsafe sex practices, 68% reported they would breach confidentiality. Factors related to their decisions included clients' perceived level of danger to their partners, clients' level of denial and unwillingness to enter into a safe-sex contract, and the counselors' belief in a moral obligation to the partners. The authors of this study make several suggestions to counselors faced with this dilemma, including taking a client sexual history; assessing dangerousness of client sexual practices; examining counselor objectivity, feelings, and judgments; and examination of relevant state laws, victim identification, and the importance of proper documentation. Finally, they state: "We would like to impress upon clinicians that the use of their professional training might be better utilized by helping the client cope with the complicated grief of living with HIV than to police behavior. Therapist actions that potentially sabotage the therapeutic relationship virtually eliminate the opportunity to influence behavior change in the future. Individuals living with HIV are at high risk for empathetic failure by our society. They require the very restoration of empathy that we are asking of them as clients to exercise with sexual partners during their most troublesome time" (DiMarco & Zoline, 2004, p. 84).

Knowledge of state law cannot be understated, particularly on the topic of duty to warn. For example, in the state of Texas, the courts have refused to impose duty to warn third parties in numerous cases, despite killings that resulted after making threats to therapists. In fact, the state of Texas will not protect therapists from civil liability that results from good-faith disclosures. The Texas health and safety code does, however, permit the disclosure of HIV to exposed persons. Similarly, the APA does not give a clear guidance for therapists because, while they do not endorse imposing a legal obligation on therapists to disclose HIV infection risk to third parties, they have not provided a clear policy. Therapists must continue to weigh the ethical obligations of respect for peoples' rights and dignity, concern for others welfare, and social responsibility to determine the actions they will take. "Unfortunately, the clinician hoping to find a clear edict for the professional standard of care in working with HIV clients who could spread the virus will be sorely disappointed. Thus, the issue remains a conundrum for those professionals treating such clients" (Huprich, Fuller, & Schneider, 2003, p. 278).

Self-Injuring Clients and Ethics

Nonsuicidal self-injury (NSSI) is of growing concern in the counseling professions in part because of a perception of an increase in this behavior trend, particularly among adolescents and young adults. Because self-injury can provoke negative reactions in counselors, a number of counselor behaviors may emerge that can cause neglect or harm to the client, including sadness, frustration, anger, helplessness, and disgust (Favazza, 1989). These clients perform socially unacceptable repetitive damage to their bodies that inflict superficial or moderate damage without the intent of suicide (Suyemoto & Kountz, 2000). Compared with the general population, where approximately 4% self-injure, in clinical populations (excluding persons with MR and DD), about 21% have been found to self-injure (Briere & Gil, 1998).

In a discussion on counselor ethical dilemmas, White, McCormick, and Kelly (2003) reviewed a client's right to act autonomously, such as the right to burn, cut, or otherwise injure themselves; they caution against transference, the counselor's need to have the client behave in a manner that suits the counselor's desires. Counselors may experience a strong desire to stop the client from self-harm. In doing so, counselors may unwittingly cause harm to the client, failing at the most fundamental ethical principle, nonmalfeasance. Rather, counselors need to be competent in this area since a substantial number of clients may exhibit self-injury and have an obligation to understand the functions and etiology of these behaviors.

Complications such as infections or serious injuries that threaten the life of the client must be otherwise considered as harmful to the client and may require a medical referral. However, referrals of clients to other counselors, because the counselor has little experience or is offended or intimidated by the client's behaviors, will be difficult because few counselors have taken the time necessary to become trained. Rather, it is essential that counselors become trained or risk providing inadequate treatment or avoiding treatment, both of which may harm the client.

Recent research suggests that NSSI is prevalent in 12% to 17% of college populations (Whitlock, Eckenrode, & Silverman, 2006). In a recent national study of 290 directors of college counseling centers, most reported recent increases in NSSI, and over half found that these clients were harder to treat than other clients. Only about a third of the participants felt that they were competent in this area, and about 75% felt that they needed to know more about the topic (Whitlock, Eells, Cummings, & Purington, 2009).

Biotechnology

The Human Genome Project, aimed at creating a complete, detailed map of the human DNA, has particular ethical ramification for persons with disabilities, specifically for persons with intellectual disabilities and birth defects. For the most part, eugenics has been successfully cloaked, hidden from public scrutiny, perhaps in part due to societal endorsement of the elimination of disability, as long as that elimination is prebirth. In an article to examine the ethics of abortions of fetuses with Down's syndrome, Glover and Glover (1996) pointed to the inconsistency in policy and practice. They note that while persons with disabilities are mandated to be treated equally under the law, in some states, abortions of fetuses with disabilities can be performed after viability (beyond 24 weeks). The same action to a fetus without a disability is a punishable crime and could be considered murder.

Advocates for disability rights express concerns about the implications of prenatal testing that they view as a return to the medical model philosophy of removing the "problem" instead of working on improving social discrimination against persons with disabilities. Rather, prevention of the birth of children with undesirable characteristics reinforces discrimination and prejudicial attitudes, and parents become unwilling to accept a departure from their dream for idealistic characteristics in their child, moving society further away from the idea that the problem is not with the person, but with the societal inability to effectively accommodate for differences. Choices to terminate a pregnancy based on disability exclude the idea that this otherwise wanted child would not have the potential for a significant quality of life and have benefits to offer the family and society (Parens & Asch, 2000).

The completion of the Human Genome Project further pushes the envelop, "... decisions about prenatal screening and selective abortion and, more recently, preimplantation genetic diagnosis and subsequent embryo selection occur every day without access to sufficient and accurate information about the life potential of people with disabilities" (Munger, Gill, Ormond, & Kirschner, 2007, pp. 123–124). Thus, selective abortion has the potential to become the back-up plan in the creation of the perfect child. On some levels, undeniably, the elimination of disabilities and chronic illness does sound good for society. But, it does not consider that disability has anything to do with the creation of greatness, of pushed potential, of compassion or love, of creative genius, or of what makes us human. Rather, it tells us that there is nothing to be gained from having to listen harder to people whose speech is impaired to hear what they have to teach us, to walk slower to keep pace with persons who are mobility impaired so we can see what they have to show us. Society does have the potential to move forward, back to a new kind of survival of the fittest, people who are super able-bodied, intelligent, and beautiful, who live long and healthy lives. The question is what do we lose and what do we become?

Wrongful Birth, Wrongful Life

Wrongful birth is a legal term that occurs when a negligent medical act results in the birth of an unplanned child who may or may not have a disability. Negligence can include a failure to warn parents of the risks of pregnancy following sterilization procedures, a failure to diagnose a pregnancy, a failure to inform parents about a condition that could or would result in disability for the child and would have led the parents to terminate the pregnancy, or failure to take reasonable care in performing abortions or sterilizations, or a failure to properly advise patients on the use on contraception. Lawsuits related to wrongful birth request the pregnancy and upbringing costs related to the birth of the unplanned child. Similarly, Wrongful Life is the result of medical negligence; had it not occurred, the child would not exist. For example, if there is a failure to diagnose rubella and the fetus is not terminated, and is born with a disability as a result of the failure, the term wrongful life could be applied. In this type of legal action, the child with a disability would sue for damages, including pain and suffering and financial costs associated with disability (Stretton, 2005).

In wrongful death and life cases, advocates for people with disabilities legally argue that the existence of a child with a disability is a burden, and that, had parents known of the disability, they would have aborted the fetus. While financial damages that result from medical negligence, leading to disability and adding to the cost of supporting a child, can be recovered in most states, emotional damage cannot. Wrongful life actions, which ask for emotional damages due to being alive with a disability, are generally unsuccessful. But, the idea of suing physicians for, in some way, allowing the birth of a person with a disability has much to say about the "progress" our society has made toward acceptance of persons with disabilities (Munger et al., 2007), as if to say that life with a disability is so undesirable that no life would be preferable.

Choosing Disability

Murphy (2009) examined the ethics of reproductive technologies as a means to have a deaf child. Usually, the ethical question of parents using biological interventions to create children who will have distinct advantages over others, such as superior intelligence, athletic abilities, and resistance to disease, is one of the rights to alter human nature and to respect differences versus the parents' decision to give their children as many advantages in life as possible. As well, there is an ethical question related to justice since only the wealthy have the financial means to enhance their children's traits through biological intervention. However, in the deaf community, the desire for deaf children is strong and the question of taking extraordinary measures as a means of increasing the possibility of deafness in their child is an entirely different debate. For many deaf couples, deafness is central to their way of life and to their identity. Parents may consider deafness an enhancement of the child's life, but Murphy (2009) argues that obstructing hearing capacity limits future capacities related to vocational choices, social interactions, social discrimination, and the ability to hear voices and music. Murphy argues that hearing people would not choose to deafen themselves and elective deafness is not in the child's best interests, but only in the parents' and the deaf community's best interests as a means of preserving the deaf culture.

Other reasons might also exist for parents wanting a deaf child, or parents wanting to create children with other disabilities. Some might wish to have children like themselves, or if one child with a disability is born into the nondisabled couple, they might wish to have a companion child with the same disability. These again, are in the parent's perceived best interest. Despite his stance, Murphy (2009) does not believe that laws should be put in place to stop people from making reproductive choices, even if they serve to create a child with a disability, arguing that a law protecting a child from having a disability could be used as justification for forcing a woman carrying a fetus with a disability to terminate the pregnancy in the name of protecting children from disabilities.

Ethics and Private Sector Rehabilitation

Private sector rehabilitation serves specific needs of clients while generating profit for rehabilitation specialists in the areas of medical case management that provides services for persons with catastrophic illness and injury. These services include *forensic testimony* that involves experts anticipating the extent of the injury and long-term consequences to help determine legal awards for damages incurred; *life-care planning* that includes detailed planning in terms of current needs and future needs and estimating the costs of living with a particular disability, including services, equipment, home modifications, and living arrangements, and so on; and *disability management* in which practitioners work with insurance companies and government agencies to control costs and facilitate recovery and return to work for injured persons. Individuals who work on a for-profit basis may encounter a number of unique ethical dilemmas that may not occur for those working for nonprofit agencies. For example, a private sector rehabilitation specialist who receives payment directly from an insurance company may be perceived as being unduly influenced by the desired outcome of the insurance company (Weed & Berens, 2011). Professional organizations provide codes of ethics for counselors in private practice to assist in such conflicts of interest. For rehabilitation counselors in private practice, the International Association for Rehabilitation Professionals (IARP) provides a Forensic Code of Ethics (International Association of Rehabilitation Professionals, 2007).

In a survey to assess the content and frequency of ethical dilemmas among rehabilitation counselors who work in private practice, Vaughn, Taylor, and Wright (1998) determined that six of the 33 dilemmas presented to a sample of rehabilitation counselors occurred for at least 75% of the participants, at least once per year. The most occurring dilemma (86.7%) was a conflict between a client's vocational objective and what the counselor believed to be a more realistic objective. Second, nearly 85% of counselors encountered difficulties in adhering to referral source guidelines versus providing optimal services to the client. Third, counselors struggled with informing insurance companies about the vocational capacities of clients, knowing that this information would likely mean an end to funding for services. Fourth, counselors sought to resolve a conflict between specific training services requested by the clients and those recommended in the evaluation reports. Fifth, counselors encountered differences between the clients' desired services and services they believed would increase the clients' vocational potentials. Finally, counselors had difficulty with encouraging clients to act on their own behalf in seeking medical treatment and obtaining medical treatment for the client.

These dilemmas are specific to private sector rehabilitation because the conflicts in principles are determined within the confines of the funding agency, where adhering to case management guidelines may be in conflict with the optimal services to the client. Additionally, counselors are obligated to work with clients for the shortest amount of time possible to achieve closure due to cost containment practices of managed care organizations.

In an article to examine ethics within the managed care environment, Kontosh (2000) identified three sources of potential conflict between the Code of Ethics for Rehabilitation Counselors and the private practice system that contracts the services or RCs or hires RCs as employees. These include counselors' inability to impose the ethical standards of their professional organization, a lack of independence on the part of the RC, and no recourse for violations of ethical principles.

Online and Internet Counseling

Online counseling has advantages for clients, such as anonymity and the convenience of private communications from home at client-designated times. Clients who otherwise would be greatly inconvenienced or unable to attend counseling, such as those who are mobility impaired, who are without transportation, or who live at great distances, can easily participate in online counseling, if they have access to a computer. However, counselors are trained to attend to vocal tone and body language and positioning to understand the intent and meaning of client messages, and without these sources of additional information, the counselor may have serious hurdles to overcome. For example, a counselor cannot know if a client is holding pills or a weapon when they are interacting over a computer. They also cannot tell if the client is writing with a joking, sarcastic, or a deadly serious intent. For these reasons, Bloom (1998) suggests that online counseling is not appropriate for counseling clients for sexual abuse, violence or violent relationships, serious psychiatric problems, and eating disorders.

Shaw and Shaw (2006) examined the ethical issues pertinent to online counseling and addressed the following important areas: trustworthiness and accountability, duty to warn and to protect, adolescent issues, and confidentiality concerns. They recommend that trust and accountability should initially involve sharing credentials with clients, including institutions attended and academic degrees, licenses and certifications, (including providing the certification or license number to the client), professional associations, and a means of making emergency contact with the counselor. Accountability also includes the establishment of a plan to attend to clients with speed and regularity and letting clients know what to expect in terms of responses.

While little precedence has been set regarding counseling online, counselors have been charged with client abandonment for being unavailable and unreachable between appointments, failing to respond to emergency treatment requests, failure of having an alternate counselor available when the counselor is absent for an extended period of time, and unilateral termination of counseling. Corey, Corey, and Callanan (2011) suggest that online counseling be combined with face-to-face sessions used alternately or in combination. In addition, they suggest that online counseling may be more appropriate for some types of problems than others. For example, they suggest that "deeply personal concerns or interpersonal issues" (Corey et al., 2011, p. 186) may be best served by face-to-face counseling.

The duty to warn others of a client's malicious intent to cause them physical harm demands that counselors know the identity, address, and contact information of the client. While some clients may prefer to remain anonymous, counselors who become aware of an intent to harm and do not have client-identifying information may need to contact their Internet provider to try to access this information or risk being held liable for a failure to inform in a timely manner. As well, without identifying information it will be difficult to impossible to respond effectively if a suicide assessment is required. Anonymity is also problematic for counselors because the intake process requires a signed consent form that informs the client of instances where client confidentiality will be breached (Shaw & Shaw, 2006).

Online counseling of adolescents also presents ethical concerns, particularly for those teens under the age of 18. A substantial number of adolescents have been shown to be more comfortable discussing sensitive topics using electronic communication than face-to-face discussions (Lenhart, 2001). Despite attempts to screen out underage clients through internet requirements and warnings, it is still essential that counselors require clients to provide them with their ages and dates of birth at intake. Unfortunately, teens may choose to lie and continue in a counseling relationship that is not suited to them. Counseling a teenager while assuming adulthood does not allow for adequate age-appropriate protection or advice based on life-stage development. Studies have determined that adolescents who use the internet tend toward greater depression and social isolation (Kraut et al., 1998; Sanders, Field, Diego, & Kaplan, 2000) that may increase the likelihood of depression, anxiety, and suicide ideation (Shaw & Shaw, 2006). Online counseling for these teens would be inappropriate.

Zack (2008) warns that simply renaming counseling services (i.e., e-health) will not protect the counselor from litigation if those services include counseling. Second, counselors must be aware that issues of jurisdiction may come into question if their clients live in states other than their own. Since most states require that therapists be state licensed, in the case of a lawsuit, it may be determined that the counselor was practicing illegally if a client lives in another state. While the laws that regulate counselor behaviors are the same for face-to-face counseling, it may be substantially more difficult to provide an appropriate standard of care should the client enter into crisis. Violations of counseling duties most often occur in the areas of competence, consent, and confidentiality. Since all counselors are required to provide competent care, Zack (2008) advises all mental health counselors to receive training in online counseling as a means of establishing additional competence. In terms of consent, disclosure is essential; in relation to online counseling, counselors need to disclose "additional risks" due to the online medium, inadvertent disclosers of confidential information, risk of losing communication before the session ends due to electronic problems, and possibility of misunderstandings. Counselors should disclose that online counseling is a newer, innovative therapy and disclose information about choices to engage in standard practice, face-to-face counseling.

Finally, confidentiality issues for online counseling require particularly close attention. All health providers, including counselors are subject to the Health Insurance Portability and Accountability Act (HIPAA) regulations that prohibit disclosure of client information without consent and subject the counselor to large fines and up to a year in prison for breaches. Internet communication offers a number of confidentiality concerns, because although counselors are obligated to safeguard clients against unintended disclosures of information shared in confidence, key logging software that tracks keystrokes is also available for hacking into electronic communications. Additionally, systems administrators are able to view e-mails and Web sites that have been visited, and many government agencies and private companies monitor employee use of the Internet. In addition, electronic communications can be intercepted when e-mails are not encrypted by a secure site. Counselors using the Internet for counseling need to use secure sites or encryption software (Shaw & Shaw, 2006) and inform clients of the potential for e-mail interception and advise them not to use shared computers or computers provided by employers.

While the above online issues are the most immediate and relevant for online counselors, there are a number of additional issues, such as client record keeping, which subjects every word typed by the counselor to potential legal scrutiny. Additional legal issues related to referral fees, third-party payments, intellectual property, and advertising are further discussed in relation to online counseling by Zack (2008).

In addition to online counseling ethical guidelines offered by numerous codes of ethics for various professions, the ACA also offers guidelines on the maintenance of counselor World Wide Web sites that include regular checking of links operation, backup communication outlets if the site is not working, links to licensure and certification boards, methods of identifying clients, written consent from legal guardians of minors or incompetent adults, accessibility options for persons with disabilities, and translation options for clients with different primary languages to help clients understand the reliability and validity of information available on the Internet (ACA, 2005).

End-of-Life Counseling and Assisted Suicide

A recent addition to the CRCC Code of Ethics has been the inclusion of end-of-life care, creating an ethical mandate that rehabilitation counselors prepare to assist clients with end-of-life issues and concerns. Wadsworth, Harley, Smith, and Kampfe (2008) suggest that therapeutic, advocacy, and assessment skills learned in training and education programs will transfer to end-of-life issues, but are insufficient in terms of creating competency for end-of-life counseling. They suggest a need to develop self-care support networks that may include family, friends, colleagues, support groups, and spiritual leaders; gaining awareness of the death experience from multicultural perspectives; developing the ability to communicate about death and dying issues in a culturally appropriate manner; and developing appropriate expectations through recognizing effective outcomes, for example, including nonmeasurable components such as counseling that leads to values clarifications and hopeful feelings.

In a study of missed opportunities to discuss end-of-life issues among physicians during family conferences, the most commonly identified missed opportunities included listening and responding to the family concerns, acknowledging and addressing emotions, exploring of patient preferences for palliative care, explaining surrogate decision making, and assurance of nonabandonment. The most frequently missed opportunities were related to listening and responding (Curtis et al., 2005), clearly a strength of well-trained counselors.

Aside from dealing with emotional issues, counselors will need to have familiarity with topics such as hospice care that is provided for terminally ill persons near the end of life; palliative care that aims to reduce symptoms of illness, especially pain; living wills/advanced directives that dictate the client's wishes regarding medical treatment limitations; and durable power of attorney designating a person to act on the client's behalf should the client become unable to make medical decisions (Pace, 2000).

Assisted Suicide

The name Jack Kevorkian has become synonymous with assisted suicide for having assisted in the deaths of approximately 130 persons. In an examination of the medical conditions of 69 of the persons Kevorkian assisted in dying, only 25% were found to be terminally ill. The remainder of persons were disabled, chronically ill, in pain, and depressed (Roscoe, Malphers, Dagovic, & Cohen, 2000). In 1997, the Detroit Free Press ran a series of articles that detailed the results of an investigation into the lives of 47 of Kevorkian's assisted suicide patients. They concluded that the majority were not terminally ill but had physical health problems that included multiple sclerosis, chronic pain, rheumatoid arthritis, stroke, mental illness, substance dependence, Alzheimer's, and quadriplegia. In addition, investigators concluded that there was a failure to recognize financial and family problems, including spousal abuse (Cheyfitz, 1997). In a video describing the suicide machine that he invented, Kevorkian states, "If a person feels in this own mind that he is *crippled* and suffering in some way where life no longer for him or her is worthwhile, then it's up to me to help no matter what I think personally" (docktordeath, 2010).

In an article that discussed the disability community's opposition to legalization of assisted suicide, Golden and Zoanni (2010) pointed to the disability-related effects stating that assisted suicide is based on bias and fear of disability. While many people believe that assisted suicide is a preferred alternate to a painful death, it is legal in all states for persons dying in discomfort to be sedated. In Oregon, where assisted suicide is legal, persons requesting assisted suicide do so for reasons other than pain, primarily, fear of loss of body function and loss of dignity. It is not a fear of pain, but a fear of disability, indignity, and not wanting to burden others. But this reaction assumes that persons who need assistance lack dignity and that death is preferred over reliance on others for assistance. It is a fear reaction, but it also feeds the prejudice and discrimination against persons with disabilities, the belief that it is better off to be dead than live with disability or chronic illness.

Another ethical dilemma centers on managed health care and assisted suicide. Oregon lists lethal injections as "comfort care." It has cut many medical services for people with disabilities but retained the relatively inexpensive lethal injection as a treatment. Services (chemotherapy, radiation, surgery) and more expensive medications may be denied if the patient has less than a 5% chance of living another 5 years. Other ethical problems involve the possibility of coercion from relatives who would benefit from the death of a person before their inheritance is drained, and persons opting for suicide due to a lack of social supports, adequate living arrangements, and health insurance. Also disturbing is that patients can receive lethal drugs only 15 days after the diagnosis of a terminal condition. Disability experts would argue that this is insufficient time for patients to adjust and make rational decisions. Interestingly, of the 627 personal prescribed lethal medication between 1998 and

2008, 401 died using the medications, 162 died within a year of the illness, and 101 were still alive a year later. These figures demonstrate that 16% of persons predicted to die within 6 months, which qualified them to receive the drug, were misdiagnosed in terms of how long they had to live, and lead to this question: "How many of the 401 might have chosen otherwise if they believed they had longer to live?" The important issue here, though, is the question, how can disability come to be viewed as more dignified and less burdensome? (Golden & Zoanni, 2010).

In an article that reviews the impact of depression among persons with chronic illness and disability and the role it plays in assisted suicide, Gill (2004a) concluded:

> Acquiring a disability seems so catastrophic to Americans that much of the public and many health professionals believe that disability should be separated out and handled differently from other human conditions in matters of life and death. Proponents of assisted suicide for people with incurable illnesses and disabilities generally exempt this class of individuals from the routine protections extended to citizens in despair. To support the exemption, they submit the idea that the hopelessness impelling some persons with disabilities toward death is a more rational brand of hopelessness than that experienced by non-disabled persons seeking death. Most would never suggest that suicide intervention should be suspended for "healthy" people, regardless of the severity or irreversibility of their loss. In effect, they seem to be saying that it is right to feel hopeless if you have a severe disability .... The message that people with chronic illnesses and disabilities are burdens conveys a sense of stigma that may more powerfully erode a person's will to live than does any physical condition. (Gill, 2004a, pp. 186–187)

CONCLUSION

Counselor ethics are based on moral values and provide guidelines for assisting in choosing actions that result in the greatest good and least harm to the client and society at large. Principles intended to guide counselors in their decision-making process include those of *nonmalfeasance, beneficence, autonomy, justice, fidelity, and veracity*. It is important to recognize that a number of other variables have the potential to influence counselor ethical decision making, such as personality factors, personal values, transference, stress, and counselor well-being. Counselors face a number of additional challenges related to ethics and maintaining competence that involve understanding a variety of cultures and life preferences. Additionally, they must sustain awareness of current and emerging ethical issues that are based on trends and societal advances to remain informed, educated, and competent.

REFERENCES

American Counseling Association. (2005). *ACA Code of ethics and standards of practice*. Alexandria, VA: Author.

American Psychiatric Association. (2000). *Diagnostic and statistical manual of mental disorders* (4th ed., text rev.). Washington, DC: Author.

Beauchamp, T., & Childress, B. T. (2001) *Principles of biomedical ethics* (5th ed.) New York: Oxford University Press, Oxford.

Beutler, L. E., & Bergan, J. (1991). Value change in counseling and psychotherapy: A search for scientific credibility. *Journal of Counseling Psychology, 38*, 16–24.

Bloom, J. W. (1998). The ethical practice of Web Counseling. *British Journal of Guidance and Counselling, 26*, 53–59.

Boyd-Franklin, N., & Lockwood, T. (1999). Spirituality and religion: Implications for psychotherapy with African American clients and families. In F. Walsh (Ed.), *Spiritual resources in family therapy* (pp. 90–103). New York, NY: Guilford Press.

Briere, J., & Gil, E. (1998). Self-mutilation in clinical and general population samples: Prevalence, correlates, and functions. *American Journal of Orthopsychiatry, 68*, 609–620.

Caregivers, disabled block Governor's office (2009, July 7). *Disability Rights California.* Retrieved from http://www.disabilityrightsca.org/news/KCRA_3-2009-07-07.htm

Cheyfitz, K. (1997, March 3). Suicide machine, Part 1: Kevorkian rushes to fulfill his clients' desire to die. *Detroit Free Press.* Retrieved from http://www.freep.com/article/20070527/NEWS05/70525061/Suicide-Machine-Part-1-Kevorkian-rushes-to-fulfill-his-clients–desire-to-die#ixzz16mo0JkJg

Consoli, A. J., Kim, B. S. K., & Meyer, D. M. (2008). Counselors' values profile: Implications for counseling ethnic minority clients. *Counseling & Values, 52*, 181–197.

Corey, G., Corey, M. S., & Callanan, P. (2007). *Issues and ethics in the helping professions.* Pacific Grove, CA: Brooks/Cole Publishing.

Corey, G., Corey, M. S., & Callanan, P. (2007b). Values and the helping relationship. In *Issues and ethics in the helping professions* (2nd ed., pp. 72–106). Belmont, CA: Thomson Brooks/Cole.

Commission on Rehabilitation Counselor Certification. (2009). *Code of professional ethics for rehabilitation counselors.* Schaumburg, IL: Author.

Commission on Rehabilitation Counselor Certification. (2011). *Actions taken against CRCs/CCRCs.* Retrieved from http://www.crccertification.com/pages/actions_taken/41.php

Curtis, J. R., Engelberg, R. A., Wenrich, M. D., Shannon, S. E., Treece, P. D., & Rubenfeld, G. D. (2005). Missed opportunities during family conferences about end-of-life care in the intensive care unit. *American Journal of Respiratory and Critical Care Medicine, 171*, 844–849.

Davis, A. H. (1997). The ethics of caring: A collaborative approach to resolving ethical dilemmas. *Journal of Applied Rehabilitation Counseling, 28*, 36–41.

DiMarco, M., & Zoline, S. S. (2004). Duty to warn in the context of HIV/AIDS-related psychotherapy: Decision making among psychologists. *Counseling & Clinical Psychology Journal, 1*, 68–85.

docktordeath (poster). (2010, October 14). *Assisted Suicide-Jack Kevorkian [video].* Retrieved from http://video.search.yahoo.com/search/video;_ylt=A0S00MxwsDdNeQ8AGtH7w8QF;_ylu=X3oDMTBncGdyMzQ0BHNlYwNzZWFyY2gEdnRpZAM-?p=assisted+suicide+jack+kevorkian&ei=utf-8&n=21&tnr=21&y=Search

Edwards, S. D. (2009). Three versions of an ethics of care. *Nursing Philosophy, 10*, 231–240.

Epstein, R. S., & Simon, R. I. (1990). The Exploitation Index: An early warning indicator of boundary violations in psychotherapy. *Bulletin of Menninger Clinic, 54*(2), 450–463.

Epstein, R. S., Simon, R. I., & Kay, G. G. (1992). Assessing boundary violations in psychotherapy: Survey results with the Exploitation Index. *Bulletin of the Menninger Clinic, 56*(2), 150–166. Retrieved from EBSCOhost

Favazza, A. R. (1989). Normal and deviant self-mutilation. *Transcultural Psychiatric Research Review, 26*, 113–127.

Gatens-Robinson, E., & Tarvydas, V. M. (1992). Ethics of care, women's perspectives and the status of the mainstream rehabilitation ethical analysis. *Journal of Applied Rehabilitation Counseling, 23*, 26–33.

Gallup, G. H. (1996). *Religion in America: Will the vitality of the church be the surprise of the 21st century?* Princeton, NJ: Princeton Religion Research Center.

Gill, C. J. (2004a). Depression in the context of disability and the "Right to Die". *Medicine and Bioethics, 25*, 171–198.

Glover, N. M., & Glover, S. J. (1996). Ethical and legal issues regarding selective abortion of fetuses with Down syndrome. *Mental Retardation, 34*, 207–214.

Golden, M., & Zoanni, T. (2010). Killing us softly: The dangers of legalizing assisted suicide. *Disability and Health Journal, 3,* 16–30.

Harrision, K. M., Song, R., & Zhang, X. (2008, August). *Life expectancy after HIV diagnosis based on United States national HIV surveillance data.* Paper presented 17th AIDS International Conference, Mexico City. Abstract retrieved from http://www.aids2008.org/Pag/Abstracts.aspx?AID=1778

Helminiak, D. (2001). Treating spiritual issues in secular psychotherapy. *Counseling and Values, 45,* 163–189.

Howie, J., Gatens-Robinson, E., & Rubin, S. E. (1993). Applying ethical principles in rehabilitation counseling. In M. Nagler (Ed.), *Perspectives on disability* (pp. 533–547). Palo Alto, CA: Health Markets Research.

Huprich, S. K., Fuller, K. M., & Schneider, R. B. (2003). Divergent ethical perspectives on the Duty-to-Warn principle with HIV patients. *Ethics & Behavior, 13,* 263–278.

International Association of Rehabilitation Professionals. (2007). *IARP code of ethics, standards of practice, and competencies.* Glenview, IL: Author.

Kelly, E. W., Jr. (1995). Counselor Values: A National Survey. *Journal of Counseling & Development, 73,* 648–653.

Kelly, T. A., & Strupp, H. H. (1992). Patient and therapist values in psychotherapy: Perceived changes, assimilation, similarity, and outcome. *Journal of Consulting and Clinical Psychology, 60,* 34–41.

King, D. E., & Bushwick, B. (1994). Beliefs and attitudes of hospital inpatients about faith healing and prayer. *Journal of Family Practice, 34,* 349–352.

Kontosh, L. G. (2000). Ethical rehabilitation counseling in a managed-care environment. *The Journal of Rehabilitation, 66,* 9–24.

Kraut, R., Patterson, M., Lundmark, V., Kiesler, S., Mukopadhyay, T., & Scherlis, W. (1998). Internet paradox: A social technology that reduces social involvement and psychological well-being? *American Psychologist, 53,* 1017–1031.

Lee, S. M., Baker, C. R., Cho, S. H., Heckathorn, D. E., Holland, M. W., Newgent, R. A. et al. (2007). Development and initial psychometrics of the Counselor Burnout Inventory. *Measurement and Evaluation in Counseling and Development, 40,* 142–154.

Lee, S. M., Cho, S. H., Kissinger, D., & Ogle, N. T. (2010). A typology of burnout in professional counselors. *Journal of Counseling & Development, 88,* 131–138.

Lenhart, A. (2001, June 21). Teenage life online: The rise of the instant-message generation and the Internet's impact on friendships and family relationships. *Pew Internet & American Life Project.* Retrieved from http://www.pewinternet.org/Press-Releases/2001/The-Rise-of-the-InstantMessage-Generation.aspx

Levin, J. (2001). *God, faith, and health: Exploring the spirituality healing connection.* Hoboken, NJ: Wiley & Sons.

McCarthy, H., & Leierer, S. J. (2001). Consumer concepts of ideal characteristics and minimum qualification for rehabilitation counselors. *Rehabilitation Counseling Bulletin, 45,* 12–23.

Maslach, C., & Jackson, S. E. (1981). The measurement of experienced burnout. *Journal of Occupational Behavior, 2,* 99–113.

Middleton, R. A., Rollins, C. W., Sanderson, P. L., Leung, P., Harley, D. A., & Ebener, D. (2000). Endorsement of professional multicultural rehabilitation competencies and standards: A call to action. *Rehabilitation Counseling Bulletin, 43,* 219–240.

Munger, K. M., Gill, C. J., Ormond, K. E., & Kirschner, K. L. (2007). The next exclusion bebate: Assessing technology, ethics, and intellectual disability after the Human Genome Project. *Mental Retardation and Developmental Disabilities, 13,* 121–128.

Murphy, T. F. (2009). Choosing disabilities and enhancements in children: A choice too far? *Reproductive Biomedicine Online, 18*(1), 43–49.

Myers, J. E., & Truluck, M. (1998). Health beliefs, religious values, and the counseling process: A comparison of counselors and other mental health professionals. *Counseling and Values, 42,* 106–123.

Oyama, O., & Koenig, H. G. (1998). Religious beliefs and practices in family medicine. *Archives of Family Medicine, 7,* 431–435.

Pace, B. (2000). Decisions about end-of-life care. *The Journal of the American Medical Association*, *284*(19), 2550.

Parens, E., & Asch, A. (2000). *Prenatal testing and disability rights*. Washington, DC, USA: Georgetown University Press.

Patterson, J. B., Patrick, A., & Parker, R. M. (2000). Choice: Ethical and legal rehabilitation challenges. *Rehabilitation Counseling Bulletin*, *43*, 203–208.

Pope, K. S., & Vetter, V. A. (1991). Prior therapist-patient sexual involvement among patients seen by psychologist. *Psychotherapy: Theory, Research, Practice, Training*, *28*, 429–438.

Pope, V. T., & Kline, W. B. (1999). The personal characteristics of effective *counselors*: What 10 experts think. *Psychological Reports*, *84*, 1339–1344.

Princeton Religion Research Center. (1996). *Religion in America: Will the vitality of the church be the surprise of the 21st century?* Princeton, NJ: The Gallup Organization.

Roscoe, L. A., Malphers, J. E., Dagovic, L. J., & Cohen, D. (2000). Dr. Jack Kevorkian and cases of euthanasia in Oakland County, Michigan, 1990–1998. *New England Journal of Medicine*, *343*, 1735–1736.

Sanders, C. E., Field, T. M., Diego, M., & Kaplan, M. (2000). The relationship of Internet use to depression and social isolation among adolescents. *Adolescence*, *35*, 237–242.

Saunders, J. L., Barros-Bailey, M., Rudman, R., Dew, D. W., & Garcia, J. (2007). Ethical complaints and violations in rehabilitation counseling: An analysis of commission on rehabilitation counselor certification data. *Rehabilitation Counseling Bulletin*, *51*, 7–13.

Shaw, H. E., & Shaw, S. F. (2006). Critical ethical issues in online counseling: Assessing current practices with an ethical intent checklist. *Journal of Counseling & Development*, *84*, 41–53.

Shaw, L. R., & Lane, F. (2008). Ethical consultation: Content analysis of the advisory opinion archive of the Commission on Rehabilitation Counselor Certification. *Rehabilitation Counseling Bulletin*, *51*, 170–176.

Shiles, M. (2009). Discriminatory referrals: Uncovering a potential ethical dilemma facing practitioner. *Ethics & Behavior*, *19*(2), 142–155.

Simon, R. I. (1989). Sexual exploitation of patients: How it begins before it happens. *Psychiatric Annals*, *19*(2), 104–112.

Simon, R. I. (1995). The natural history of therapist sexual misconduct: Identification and prevention. *Psychiatric Annals*, *25*(2), 90–94.

Steen, R. L., Engels, D., & Thweatt, W. T. (2006). Ethical aspects of spirituality in counseling. *Counseling and Values*, *50*, 108–118.

Stein, D. M., & Lambert, M. J. (1995). Graduate training in psychotherapy: Are therapy outcomes enhanced? *Journal of Consulting and Clinical Psychology*, *63*, 182–196.

Stevens, H. B., Dinoff, B. L., & Donnenworth, E. E. (1998). Psychotherapy training and theoretical orientation in clinical psychology programs: A national survey. *Journal of Clinical Psychology*, *54*, 91–96.

Stretton, D. (2005). The birth torts: Damages for wrongful birth and wrongful life. *Deakin Law Review*, *10*, 319–364.

Sue, D. W. (1996). Multicultural counseling: Models, methods & actions. *The Counseling Psychologist*, *24*, 279–284.

Suyemoto, K., & Kountz, X. (2000). Self-mutilation. *The Prevention Researcher*, *7*(4), 1–4.

Tjeltveit, A. C. (1986). The ethics of value conversion in psychotherapy: Appropriate and inappropriate therapist influence on client values. *Clinical Psychology Review*, *6*, 515–537.

Tjeltveit, A. C. (1999). *Ethics and values in psychotherapy*. New York, NY: Routledge.

Tong, R. (1997) *Feminist approaches to bioethics: Theoretical reflections and practical applications*. Boulder, CO: Westview Press.

Toriello, P. J., & Benshoff, J. J. (2003). Substance abuse counselors and ethical dilemmas: The influence of recovery and education level. *Journal of Addictions and Offender Counseling*, *23*, 83–98.

Vaughn, B. T., Taylor, D. W., & Wright, W. R. (1998). Ethical dilemmas encountered by private sector rehabilitation practitioners. *Journal of Rehabilitation*, *64*, 47–52.

Wadsworth, J., Harley, D., Smith, S. M., & Kampfe, C. (2008). Infusing end-of-life issues into the rehabilitation counselor education curriculum. *Rehabilitation Education*, *22*, 113–124.

Wallis, C. (1996). Faith and healing. *Time, 147,* 58–63.

Ward, L., & Gahagan, B. (2010). Crossing the divide between theory and practice: Research and an ethic of care. *Ethics & Social Welfare, 4,* 210–216.

Watkins, C. E., Jr. (1983). Transference phenomena in the counseling situation. *Personnel & Guidance Journal, 62,* 206–210.

Weinrach, S. G. (1984). Determinants of vocational choice: Holland's theory. In D. Brown, & L. Brooks & Associates (Eds.), *Career choice and development* (pp. 61–93). San Francisco: Jossey-Bass.

Weed, R. O., & Berens, D. E. (2011). Private sector rehabilitation. In J. H. Stone & M. Blouin (Eds.), *International encyclopedia of rehabilitation.* Retrieved May 17, 2011, from http://cirrie.buffalo.edu/encyclopedia/article.php?id=11&language=en

White, V. E., McCormick, L. J., & Kelly, B. L. (2003). Counseling clients who self-injure: Ethical considerations. *Counseling and Values, 47,* 220–229.

Whitlock, J., Eells, G., Cummings, N., & Purington, A. (2009). Nonsuicidal self-injury in college populations: Mental health provider assessment of prevalence and need. *Journal of College Student Psychotherapy, 23,* 172–183.

Whitlock, J. L., Eckenrode, J. E., & Silverman, D. (2006). Self-injurious behavior in a college population. *Pediatrics, 117*(6), 1939–1948.

Wilson, C. A., Rubin, S. E., & Millard, R. P. (1991). Preparing rehabilitation counselors to deal with ethical dilemmas. *Journal of Applied Rehabilitation Counseling, 22,* 30–33.

Zack, J. S. (2008). How sturdy is that digital couch? Legal considerations for mental health professionals who deliver clinical services via the Internet. *Journal of Technology in Human Services, 26,* 333–359.

Zinnbauer, B., & Pargament, K. (2000). Working with the sacred: Four approaches to religious and spiritual issues in counseling. *Journal of Counseling & Development, 78,* 162–171.

INSIDER PERSPECTIVE

The Story of Patricia (Allen) Konczynski

My name is Patricia (Allen) Konczynski, and I am 53 years of age. I was born, raised, and educated in San Francisco, and moved to Staten Island, New York, on my marriage 31 and a half years ago. I graduated from San Francisco State University in 1969, with a BSW (Bachelor's of Social Work) cum laude. I recently graduated from Long Island University with an MPA (Masters of Public Administration). I have three children: one 28 years old, and 25-year-old twins. I am currently employed at A Very Special Place, a nonprofit agency on Staten Island, which serves the needs of developmentally disabled individuals. I am currently the Director of Quality Assurance, a position that I was recently promoted to 6 weeks ago. I now work in administration and am an internal auditor for the agency. Prior to this position, I was the Program Director for the vocational training program for 9 years. In this position, I created and implemented two vocational programs, and developed "real" jobs for individuals with learning/developmental disabilities in the community.

Before working at A Very Special Place, I worked out of the College of Staten Island Special Student Services Department as a transition coordinator to assist a high-school senior with disabilities with the transition to college. I worked there for 14 months, and then became a Job Coach with Job Path, a Vocational Rehabilitation agency in Manhattan for 2.5 years. I also work at H&R Block part-time during the tax season. My expertise is assisting deaf clients with their taxes. While my children were in elementary school, I worked at Block as a tax preparer and instructor on a full-time seasonal basis.

I was born hearing impaired. My mother's placenta separated prior to delivery, and caused auditory nerve damage. I was born with 55% hearing in my right ear and 45% in my left ear. I lost more hearing later on as an adult when I contracted chickenpox and became quite ill from the virus. The loss was not obvious at first, but a year later it was confirmed that I had lost 25% more hearing and have since been considered "profoundly" deaf. I have never heard a bird sing, raindrops falling, or a cat meow. I love music and love to dance as I sense the vibrations; however, I cannot understand the lyrics to songs. I have tried hearing aids, but they only amplify the sound and do not increase my comprehension of language or sounds.

I hear on the phone with a phone amplifier at the highest volume, and will often perceive names and numbers incorrectly. I am alerted that the phone is ringing by a light that goes off. Staff and coworkers at work have been supportive and will assist me if I have difficulty with a phone call. In addition, before the miraculous invention of closed caption, my perception of television show plots was very different. I prefer to watch rented movies in closed caption at home rather than to attend a movie in a theater. I never like to spend megabucks to go to a Broadway play that I cannot understand. Recently, however, I did attend the closed caption performance of "Phantom of the Opera" and it was one of the most "awesome" experiences of my life.

My mother denied my hearing loss all my life. She never went past the initial grieving process that a parent of a child with a disability normally goes through. She was stuck on the initial stage all her life. Due to this denial, my speech pattern was affected and I never received speech therapy until kindergarten. My mother justified my speech pattern by saying it was "just baby talk." My mother's denial and confusion was somewhat understandable, as I became an expert lipreader at an early age and that was my survival technique in dealing with the world. Even when I became an adult, my mother would say to people, "You see, there is nothing wrong with my daughter. She is a college graduate and married with children. So what is wrong with her?"

How am I perceived by society? If you see me in the street, I look quite "normal," average, and nondisabled ... until I start to speak. Depending on who the listener is, some individuals say that my speech is marvelous for someone who can't hear herself talk. Others will react by saying: "I simply don't understand you!" (and believe it or not, this is the comment I received over the phone from an American Red Cross representative the other day). I have trouble obtaining jobs in spite of the ADA because of "communication problems." This is difficult for me to prove because I have been told that a candidate with more experience has been selected for a particular position.

Even in the medical profession I have difficulty with medical personnel's reactions. I recently went for a mammography and couldn't understand the technician. I asked her to look at me while speaking and she started to mouth her words. This was not my first occurrence with a medical professional. This is the Number #1 reason why I dislike telling a stranger about my deafness, because the immediate response is the mouthing of words and talking very loudly. If you just talk naturally,

I will understand you. (After all, family members will ask me what coaches say on the sidelines during televised games.) Also, volume does not affect how I comprehend language.

There are times when individuals do not truly "believe" that I have a severe hearing loss since I am able to cope with it. For example, a new coworker in my new office needed someone to be a witness for a conference call. No one was available except for me. He asked me if I could assist him and I informed him that conference calls are just incomprehensible noise to me. He said, "But I see you talking on the phone. You can hear." I informed him that I could hear with the assistance of an amplifier, but that a conference call cannot be carried on next to my ear. The purpose of a conference call is to have a discussion among parties with an audience.

When my children were younger and I would go strolling with them, I would be asked by strangers why my speech was difficult. Strangers have reacted to me by saying things such as "So, how come your children talk normally? (They did have an involved father and a large extended family in their lives.) "How could your husband think of marrying you?" (Said to me by an angry parent of a child with a disability.)

My childhood was difficult because of my speech impediment. Children are very honest to the point of being cruel. I was nicknamed "Eskimo yo-yo" because in the 1950s, Alaska was not a state and Eskimo were considered foreigners. I was always lonely during elementary school. I was the last picked on teams and had no real friends. I was someone's friend for a day, when their best friend was temporarily angry with him/her and ignoring him/her. In junior high, I was friends with a clique of "rejects" (two obese individuals and a stutterer). We gave each other much needed support.

When I was in high school, however, I made friends with a very caring and supportive group of individuals with whom I am still friends with today. This group gave me the confidence to successfully run for student government offices, to develop leadership skills, and to increase my self-confidence. I am forever grateful to this unique group of individuals.

How do I deal with my disability today? By just being myself. If people cannot accept me for who I am, then I will not waste my time associating with them. If a comment is made, such as "I simply can't understand you." I then tell the person, "I am hearing impaired, which has caused my speech impediment. Please, just be patient and listen to me closely." In today's fast paced world, people do not want to stop and wait, or listen. People who know me well do not even think about my speech impediment. I have to often tell family members, "Please look at me," as they are walking around casually talking.

There are times when things are out of my control, and I am affected by my hearing loss. When I was working at Job Path in 1981 and I was leaving the office one day, I got stuck in an elevator alone for 1.5 hours. I was unable to access the elevator phone, and I was unable to get anyone's attention. Finally, the fact that only one of the two elevators was working came to someone's attention. Notes were passed under the door to me. Fortunately I am not claustrophobic, and so I sat on the floor and did paperwork. But after the incident I became depressed for a few days because it made my disability all the more real and it was a time I could not use any creative coping skills to get myself out of the situation.

The greatest assets of my life are my husband and children. My husband has always made me feel that I could do anything I put my mind to and would not tolerate feeble excuses on my part. My children, because of my disability, are sensitive to other individuals with disabilities. My oldest daughter currently teaches preschool autistic children. My younger daughter is a high-school English teacher and sometimes teaches classes of students with learning disabilities. One of the greatest influences of my life was my high-school history teacher, Saul Barnett. I was all set to go to nursing school because I wanted to be in a helping profession. Saul Barnett told me that I could go further than nursing school and I should go to college. He said, "You know you have the ability to be anything you want to be." He was one teacher who saw the potential in me and made me look into myself. Most of all, he accepted me as a nondisabled student.

The greatest barrier in my life was my mother's denial of my hearing. If I had gotten speech therapy at the age of two, then my speech impediment would not have been as obvious. It is a barrier that I cannot undo and must deal with it creatively whenever a situation occurs.

The key message I would like to give to prospective counselors is **treat anyone with a disability just as you would like to be treated yourself. Treat them as a unique human being, with feelings and emotions.** You never know when someday, in your personal life, you will have a family member with a disability. I have been told by people that their lives are perfect and "disability-free"; however, at a later point in time a grandchild with a disability is born and their whole perspective changes.

In dealing specifically with persons who are hearing impaired, speak naturally and directly to them. Do not stand by a light or window as that light affects lipreading. For men, be aware that facial hair may somehow impede lipreading. Please do not mouth words as it is an insult. Take the time to listen and don't be in a hurry.

In terms of working with individuals with disabilities, you may find that you may be more comfortable working with one disability over another. I prefer working with developmentally disabled individuals who have a good command of speech and conversation so that I can understand them. I have difficulty working with individuals who have speech difficulties because I cannot understand them due to my own disability.

It is often said that we are put on this Earth for a purpose. My purpose has been to improve the quality of lives of developmentally disabled individuals through jobs and monitoring quality of agency services.

DISCUSSION QUESTIONS

1. Have students make a list of their top personal values and then discuss the impact of personal values on counseling and decision making.
2. Discuss anyone's experience with disliking someone because they were reminded of someone else they knew. Relate these experiences to client transference.

3. Ask students to identify persons they would be most likely to refer to another counselor, and discuss the professional and personal reasons for these referrals. Identify appropriate and inappropriate referral differences.

4. Discuss the case of a person who is HIV-positive, has a partner, and is practicing unsafe sex in the context of duty to warn and students' personal ideas about moral obligations.

5. Solicit student stories about experiences with online communication that led to misunderstandings. Relate these stories to potential problems with online counseling.

EXERCISES

A. For a class activity, have students attend activities that are outside of their culture, such as religious services or social events.

B. Have students make a personal biases and prejudices list based on their cultural norms and discuss how these might affect their future counseling.

C. Have students form teams to debate the ethics of pregnancy termination based on disability status.

FIFTEEN

Basic Do's and Don'ts in Counseling Persons With Disabilities

Michael Jay Millington

OVERVIEW

A class of future rehabilitation counselors listened intently to the guest speaker, a gentleman from England, who was describing his experiences in supervising a supported employment program. When the time came for questions, an earnest student asked, "What do you call them?" The speaker was confused. The student clarified, "Your clients, what do you call them?" Still not quite understanding the question, he answered, "It depends, Nigel, Sarah, Robert . . .?" The student was looking for an answer to a far larger question than she knew. Underneath it all she was asking, "How do we treat people with disabilities?" And the answer was, appropriately, "Like human beings." The rest of this chapter is nothing more than commentary on that basic truth.

Counseling is predicated on a working alliance built on empathy, congruence, and unconditional positive regard. We couch these as counseling skills and appropriate them for the profession, but they are actually quite common. These are the skills of being human and treating others humanely. More than techniques, they are an expression of our values as counselors.

In this chapter, we are tasked with reviewing the do's and don'ts of interacting with people with disabilities, not as clients but as human beings. A collection of suggested behaviors, a disability etiquette, has emerged from the collective experience of people with disabilities and is widely available in brochures and on the Internet. While disability etiquette is an important read for anyone in the field, it is not, by itself, sufficient for the rehabilitation counselor. The profession's obligation to the people we serve runs deeper than manners. We are a value-driven profession. We share allegiance to the fundamental mission of full community inclusion for people with disabilities. We act with our clients and on their behalf to help individuals achieve standing in their communities and to advance a more inclusive world for all people with disabilities. Disability etiquette is only the superficial expression of professional values that have much deeper roots and higher aspirations. We are compelled by the value-laden principles of our profession to do much more.

VALUE-LADEN PRINCIPLES AND PROFESSIONAL ETHOS

When Beatrice Wright put 20 value-laden principles in the preface of her seminal work (1983), it was to infuse values into the evolving professional discourse. Values undergird and sustain a profession; without their guidance, science and practice are prone to corruption by passing fads and personal agendas. The 20 principles have stood for decades without significant revision, and still represent the core and guiding light of rehabilitation psychology and counseling. As such, they provide the professional ethos that shapes the relationship between counselor and client. We repurpose the 20 value-laden principles verbatim for a contemplation of their implications for the counselor/client relationship. Taking each one in turn, we consider the obligations it places on the professional. Taken in the aggregate, these obligations form the deep rationale behind disability etiquette.

1. *Every individual needs respect and encouragement; the presence of a disability, no matter how severe, does not alter these fundamental rights.*

    The value of human life is not determined by its length or productivity. It is valued in the act of living. In a living system, equilibrium is dynamic—satiation is a fleeting pursuit. We move in the world seeking sustenance, challenged by threat and need. Nowhere is life more in evidence, more fully expressed, than when life responds to challenge. Challenge is the essence of disability and so we honor our clients for all they have to teach us about what it means to be alive. Respect is grounded in this fundamental truth. Treating people with the deep respect required of this value goes beyond being polite. First and most difficult for the professional is to give up the pretense of positional power. Your job is to serve, and it is your honor to do so. You must assiduously work on your own issues of self-centered thinking and cognitive distortions before you can effectively counsel others. You must recognize that the person before you is the expert in the subject at hand (his or her life), and you are the student. Show respect by honoring the teacher. Show respect by being prepared, timely, and responsive. Show respect by anticipating needs and accommodations.

    Encouragement is the act of bringing hope, courage, and confidence to the lives of others. Hope is the dare to dream of the possible . . . to imagine that there are better times ahead and to be sustained through present trials by it. Courage is the ability to face fearful challenges and persist despite trepidation. Confidence is challenge met with self-assurance and the expectation of success. Encourage first by being a model of these things in your own life. Start and stay positive in all communication. Focus on solutions, options, and opportunities.

2. *The severity of a handicap can be increased or diminished by environmental conditions.*

    Environmental barriers are the artifacts of societal disregard for its own citizens. They can be architectural, attitudinal, educational, economic, and affective. They are often deeply engrained in the culture and practically invisible to those not excluded. But they are everywhere, and at every turn they communicate, even propagate, exclusion. First, accept that you do not know the depth and extent of these barriers unless you have experienced them for yourself. Know that your clients may not even be aware of what is oppressive, if all they have ever known is oppression. Be with your clients as they navigate the various service systems and bear witness to their challenges. Failing that, listen to their stories and empathize ... walk a mile in their shoes. Seek out the barriers that impede client progress in the home, in the community, and especially in the service you provide, and advocate for change. Change in your own service is the most difficult to address. We generally start with the assumption that our present model is somehow sacrosanct when it is only the current approach to a far-from-perfect service delivery system. The intransigence of high unemployment rates for people with disabilities signals that we may well be part of the problem. We should be admonished by our own lack of progress to reject the status quo as good enough.

3. *Issues of coping and adjusting to a disability cannot be validly considered without examining reality problems in the social and physical environment.*

Rehabilitation counseling is community based and empowerment oriented. Coping and adjustment issues in rehabilitation counseling arise out of the complex dynamics of affective, cognitive, and behavioral responses and interactions of multiple individuals in the client's social network (individual, family, and community) within the context of culture, history, and physical environment. Focus on practical solutions to concrete problems in the here-and-now. Teach coping skills in the real world. Encourage community building around client support.

4. *The assets of the person must receive considerable attention in the rehabilitation effort.*

Assets are the organizing principle of a positive, empowering approach to rehabilitation counseling. Everyone has assets; sometimes they need help seeing it. Rehabilitation counselors look for practical knowledge, skill, ability, attitude, personality, and wisdom that can translate into resources. Help clients see the value in what they have and the strategic path to what they want. The counselor communicates from the affirmative, imagines possibilities, sees opportunities, and plans for success.

5. *The significance of a disability is affected by the person's feelings about the self and his or her situation.*

Emotions color disability experiences in infinite shades. There is a developmental arc of emotional responses to acquired disabilities, from inception to resolution, and an infinite number of paths across it. Emotions can become issues in themselves as individuals and families cope with resentment, anger, guilt, shame, anxiety, and worries about the future. It can take time to heal. Where the emotional burden is chronic, healing is constant, and perseverance is strength. Listen to their stories and bear witness to suffering where it occurs. Be patient, consistent, and encouraging.

6. *The active participation of the client in the planning and execution of the rehabilitation program is to be sought as fully as possible.*

Full community inclusion starts in service delivery. To the degree possible, given the unique circumstances of the particular, the professional role is to facilitate the planning process, not to direct it. No one knows more about the client than the client. The client needs information, training, technical assistance, and support from the counselor. As partners in rehabilitation, clients inherit both authority and responsibility for the path chosen and the ends reached. Nowhere is communication more important. Make sure that you are fully understood by the client and that the client is fully understood by you. Make sure that clients are fully informed and take care to equip them with the decision-making and problem-solving skills they will require for success. In a word, empower with every decision and action.

7. *The client is seen not as an isolated individual, but as part of a larger group that includes other people, often the family.*

The client's family is the first community; it is where the individual learns his or her identity. It is the source of social support, the first line of caregiving, and the gateway to the larger community. Coping and adjustment, whether optimal or problematic, is nested in the family dynamic. Family involvement is encouraged, but the choice remains with the client. To the degree and in the spirit of family involvement desired by the client, the family members can have roles in the plan, tasks to perform, and a share in the outcomes.

8. *Because each person has unique characteristics and each situation its own properties, variability is required in rehabilitation plans.*

Science and experience suggest that certain patterns of behaviors and conditions are associated with patterns of problems/challenges and their conco-mitant solutions. This is the basis of rehabilitation counseling science and practice. In application, we must guard against the devolution of practice when experience becomes habit, generalizations slip into stereotype, and informal algorithms replace critical thinking. Work toward more cognitively complex decision-making, a more complete and thoughtful case conceptualiz-ation with plenty of hypothesis testing. Approach each client as a unique person with unique characteristics and circumstances, a person who will require a network of services capable of an articulated, appropriate, and potentially unique response.

9. *Predictor variables, based on group outcomes in rehabilitation, should be applied with caution to the individual case.*

The most common purpose of a predictor variable is to estimate the prob-ability of future success in some identified endeavor. Considered in isolation from other information, predictor variables do not make allowances for accom-modations, learning, adapting, and alternate strategies. Improper interpretation of suspect data inevitably leads to fewer choices and a bleaker employment outlook. Vocational evaluations, popular in rehabilitation counseling, should focus on description and generating options instead. Counselors focus on evalu-ation *in situ* for example, situational assessments, job try-outs and shadowing, be-havioral observations, and interviews. The most useful information is the most immediate to the experience. The best predictor of future performance is current performance. The best judge of whether or not a person can do something is to give them the opportunity to try.

10. *All phases of rehabilitation have psychological aspects.*

Coping, adjustment, and adaptation are the psychological themes that thread through the rehabilitation experience. Over time and across contexts, the client and family deal with evolving (and sometimes devolving) emotional and cognitive responses to the events of their lives. Educational context sets the stage for one set of psychological stressors. Vocational context sets the stage for another, and so on for all venues. Approach every client initiative to advance practical goals with a counselor's thoughtfulness, discipline, and empathy. Applied counseling in the community can find therapeutic value in the tasks and homework of the plan.

11. *Interdisciplinary and interagency collaboration and coordination of services are essential.*

Just as the client has a support network, the services that surround the client should be networked as well. Part of empowerment is creating access to and control over all the extant services that will advance the plan. The counselor brings these people together and works with them to coordinate their efforts across services. Form your own community of practice and work on its effectiveness.

12. *Self-help organizations are important allies in the rehabilitation effort.*

Communities grow out of shared concern and the mutual benefit enjoyed by members. People with disabilities, who organize in support of themselves, to share their combined wisdom and reach out to others make a profound statement about the nature of rehabilitation and its outcomes. When we encounter such initiatives we fulfill our philosophy by building strong partnerships with them.

13. *In addition to the special problems of particular groups, rehabilitation clients commonly share certain problems by virtue of their disadvantaged and devalued position.*

Special problems are disability specific, such as the communication issues of the deaf. Other problems stem from the generic disenfranchisement common to minority groups. Rehabilitation counselors need to attend to both. Strategies for the former are based in counseling and case management. Strategies for the latter are based in community advocacy as well.

14. *It is essential that society as a whole continuously and persistently strives to provide the basic means toward the fulfillment of the lives of all its inhabitants, including those with disabilities.*

Our profession is overtly evangelical in championing the cause of full community inclusion in all aspects of life in all quarters of governance. In order to maximize the efficacy of service for the client in our presence, we advocate for more and better service in housing, education, transportation, recreation, and health. Advocate through public service on councils and boards. Advocate as a citizen on behalf of policy. Advocate through professional organizations. Join with other advocate groups building toward a movement. In this way we strengthen our own professional support network.

15. *Involvement of the client with the general life of the community is a fundamental principle guiding decisions concerning living arrangements and the use of resources.*

Independent living in the community begins with the home. Intensity and scope of support needed to sustain a person's home in the community need to be flexible and constantly adjusting to the need of the client. Living needs to be integrated, as much as possible, in the community and not be isolated on the edge or constrained by the walls of institution. The more intensive the intervention, the greater attention needs to be paid to sustaining a balance of service and optimal integration. Client desire for self-determination trumps the convenience and profits of nursing homes and other residential service providers.

16. *People with disabilities, like all citizens, are entitled to participate in and contribute to the general life of the community.*

      The ultimate purpose of rehabilitation counseling service is to advance full community inclusion in society, one individual client at a time. Facilitate client opportunities for expanding social life and influence beyond employment. Model inclusion and universal access in all aspects of professional and private life. Support inclusive organizations and accessible businesses.

17. *Provision must be made for the effective dissemination of information concerning legislation and community offerings of potential benefit to persons with disabilities.*

      Knowledge is power. Access to knowledge is empowerment. Help clients access knowledge about disability, best practices, available services, ancillary resources, support groups, advocacy, and their rights under the law. Encourage proactive recruitment to bring clients and knowledge together, and raise awareness in public. Seek and utilize existing information dissemination resources, through national clearinghouses, training centers, and local agencies.

18. *Basic research can profitably be guided by the question of usefulness in ameliorating problems, a vital consideration in rehabilitation fields, including psychology.*

      The value of research is measured by its usefulness. Usefulness should direct the formulation of research, its implementation, interpretation, and the application of its findings. Client-centered counseling requires client-centered research.

19. *Persons with disabilities should be called upon to serve as co-planners, co-evaluators, and consultants to others, including professional persons.*

      The clarion call of empowerment in rehabilitation counseling is, "Never about me, without me." At every level, in every aspect of service, the people served should be represented. They should be called upon for leadership, consulted in policy, included in every partnership and community of practice, represented on every board and committee. Treat clients as colleagues in the common pursuit of creating a more inclusive world.

20. *Continuing review of the contributions of psychologists and others in rehabilitation within a framework of guiding principles that are themselves subject to review is an essential part of the self-correcting effort of science and the professions.*

      Wright concluded the list of value-laden principles by linking them to a process of continuous improvement in a scientist practitioner model that leaves practice, research, and values open and responsive to new knowledge. Thus, the final implication for rehabilitation counseling is that the counselor is obligated by her values to constantly seek to improve practice in a value-driven profession . . . part of a larger community of professionals that share different aspects of the same goal, the same fundamental mission of full community inclusion through research, education, management, advocacy, and service.

DISABILITY ETIQUETTE

Full community inclusion shapes our mission. The value-laden principles shape our practice. Living our professional values in the day-to-day provides the challenge by which we can continuously hone our own skills in the mundane and specific. What follows is an accumulation of common tips on etiquette, taken from brochures designed to raise public awareness (Easter Seals, 2011; United Cerebral Palsy Association, 2010) and compliance (Federal Communications Commission, 2008). They have been compiled and organized here to provide an overview of accepted decorum as it might be applied to the counselor's relationship with the client.

Relax

If you are a student of community inclusion, every encounter with clients is an opportunity to learn and explore. If you do not know what to do in a particular situation, simply put yourself in the place of the referent and consider how you'd like to be treated—and do that. Other than the rules surrounding the use of disability labels, people with disabilities are generally not hypersensitive to the colloquial turn of phrase. Deaf people want to "hear the news." People with visual impairments will look forward to "seeing you again." You honor people by being yourself. It is more important to have the right intent than to say the right thing . . . as long as you learn from your mistakes.

Think "Common Courtesy"

Again, treat people with disabilities as you would be treated, show them the respect everyone deserves in a polite society. Validate the person's social presence through eye contact and physical cues. Offer the appropriate greeting regardless of your assumptions concerning the person's ability to respond. Make efforts to include them in group conversations; create a space in that conversation for the person to participate. As an advocate, seek out persons with disabilities in the social milieu that appear isolated and engage them. Introduce them to others.

In casual conversation do not broach subjects that impinge on the boundaries of privacy that we all enjoy. You would not question an acquaintance about his or her sex life, bowel movements, income, and medical problems, nor would you regale others with the details of your hygiene regime. If the topic is appropriate in content and delivery, it will likely be appropriate regardless of disability status. Everyone has something to share, topics of interests, and small talk. Do not assume that people with disabilities want to talk about disability; their interests range as far and wide as everyone else.

Treat adults with the respect they deserve. When formal titles are appropriate, use them for everyone. Do not single out persons with disabilities with diminutive nicknames. Address them directly in conversation, make eye contact and communicate attention and interest in their responses. Do not speak over them to an aide or defer to a caretaker/significant other when the issue at hand belongs to the person with a disability. Do not patronize or insult with demeaning praise. Do not make your acquaintance be a tragic hero, plucky mascot, or any other stereotype that distances the real person from the conversation. It is a fact that people with disabilities need assistance from time to time. So do we all. If you perceive that help is needed, offer your assistance ... but wait for your offer to be accepted and allow the person to instruct you in how to proceed. Do not grab, push, or otherwise interfere with the person's autonomy without expressed permission.

Be Patient, Plan Ahead

As a student of full community inclusion, one of the best teachers is public experience. When you have friends with disabilities, your routine adapts accordingly. Learn patience. It takes longer to navigate access to buildings with a wheel chair. It takes longer for a person with cerebral palsy to order off the menu. Let your friend set the pace. When planning events involving persons with disabilities, consider their needs ahead of time. If an insurmountable barrier exists, let them know about it prior to the event and make alternate plans.

Create an Accessible Environment

Identify barriers within your own organization and make plans to ameliorate them, or improve on the merely adequate. Improve physical access to work stations, restrooms, break areas, parking lot, and so on. Be aware that a person with chemical sensitivity may have a reaction to smoke, perfume, or other toxins in the environment. Acoustics and lighting can diminish participation of persons with hearing or visual disabilities if not addressed.

Taking a cue from pro-inclusion businesses, we can create accessible organizations by advocating development on a myriad of points. Engender a commitment to accessibility from executive management. Generate policies, procedures and practices that specifically mention accessibility. Recruit board members with disabilities and seek to hire workers with disabilities at all skill and management levels. Market your services or products to customers with disabilities. Train staff on disability awareness. Create alternate formats for training materials, such as large print, braille, and captioning. Employ workers with disabilities as mentors for new hires who do not have disabilities. Provide ongoing and current information on issues of disability and accessibility to staff. Build partnerships with community resources that serve people with disabilities. Create an internal work group that discusses disability issues and makes recommendation to management on the appropriate steps toward universal access. Work with coworkers to create a disability-friendly culture in your organization.

Vision issues

When meeting persons with a visual impairment, greet them by name immediately as they enter the room. Speak directly to them, not through a companion or guide. Use a natural conversational tone and speed. Identify yourself with whatever information is appropriate for the situation (often including your affiliation when attending meetings or conferences). If they are joining a conversation already in progress, identify and introduce the other participants. It is sometimes helpful to provide a directional cue associated with the person being introduced ("that's Kelly Green to your right . . ."). Cue the person with a visual disability when the group moves from one place to another. Make the end of the conversation apparent with closing statements and leave-taking.

Describing the surroundings is often helpful. Be precise, descriptive, and thorough in your descriptions of individuals, places, or things. When dining with a friend with visual disability, you could read the menu, or describe the items on the plate. When shopping, provide a commentary on displays, sales and other visual input that is of interest. Should you observe a blind person who is unwittingly moving toward a dangerous situation, remain calm and speak in a firm voice to alert them to the danger.

Offer to guide people who are blind or visually impaired by asking if they would like assistance. Allow them to accept or decline as it suits them. If they accept, allow the person to take your arm. Guide, do not lead, the person. Do not leave a person with a visually standing in "free space." If you must be separated momentarily, navigate to a place where the person is in contact with something substantial like a wall or table. Describe surroundings as you proceed, identifying hazards and facilitating navigation along the way. Be descriptive and specific ("approaching a flight of stairs in about twenty feet"). When traveling with a guide dog, remember that service animals are finely trained assistants employed in serving their masters. They are not pets in the common sense. Do not distract them from their work or interact with them without permission.

Hearing issues

When meeting people with hearing disabilities it may be necessary to wave or tap them lightly on the shoulder to get their attention. Look directly at the person and speak clearly, slowly, and expressively to facilitate lip reading. If lipreading is being used, make sure that your mouth and face are well lit and not obscured in shadow or by any object. Expressive body language also helps convey your meaning. If a sign language interpreter is present, speak directly to the person with the hearing impairment, not the interpreter. If the person is wearing a hearing aid, do not assume that it effectively delivers your speaking voice to the person. Do not yell—it does not help. Written notes can also be used to augment communication.

Mobility issues

Balance is a challenging issue for people who use canes or crutches. Ambulating across uneven terrain, opening doors, negotiating steps, moving in traffic can present difficult and precarious situations. Falling is a constant concern. Attempting to help may actually create accidents. Grabbing at people can throw them off balance. Opening doors unexpectedly can take away a temporary support. Do not intervene in their efforts without permission. Always ask before offering help. Keep floors clean, dry, and unobstructed. Consider the ease of transferring in and out of any chair that is offered. Often times, a chair with an elevated seat is preferable. Canes, walkers, crutches, any equipment used are an extension of the person's personal space. They should be kept within easy reach, and not touched, moved, or used unless permission is given.

When communicating with a person in a wheelchair, make sure the person is physically included in the space of conversation. Sit down to carry on the conversations at eye level when possible. In informal group socializing, adjust space between speakers so that the individual in the wheelchair does not have to arch her neck to engage the group. When giving directions to a person in a wheelchair, consider distance, weather conditions, and physical obstacles such as stairs, curbs, and steep hills.

A wheelchair is a mobility tool used by an expert who needs it for freedom of movement. It is not a piece of incidental furniture; it is part of the personal space of the wheelchair user. Treat that personal space with respect. Do not sit in it, put things on it, lean against it, push, pull, or otherwise engage it for any purpose unless instructed by its owner to do so. There are times when you may be asked to help collapse, stow, retrieve, and assemble portable wheelchairs for friends and acquaintances. It behooves the professional to become familiar with the mechanics of these chairs to make sure that assembly is complete and the chair is safe. There may be times when the wheelchair user needs some assistance in negotiating a curb, rough terrain, or other environmental barriers. Do not intervene without permission and some instruction on how to proceed.

Communication issues

There are a variety of disabilities that involve speech and language impairments, each with their own unique challenges. The presence of even the most severe communication barrier is not an indication of intellectual deficit. It does, however, require considerable effort from both parties to overcome. A variety of strategies are available, including sign language, writing, speaking, using a communication device, or a combination of methods. Find what works and is comfortable for the person.

When communicating verbally with a person who is difficult to understand, move to a quiet place and focus attention on his or her efforts. Keep your manner encouraging rather than correcting. Be patient when the person speaking and do not interrupt or attempt to finish his or her sentences. Do not pretend to understand if you are having difficulty. Repeat what you do understand, and attempt to clarify what you do not. Often, there is enough information to form some hypotheses that the person can verify or reject with simple nods or short answers. You can work together in this manner in successive approximations until the content and message is fully understood. Work on your communication skills with the individual. Communication gets easier with practice.

If the person communicates through an attendant, remember to address the speaker not the translator. If the person uses a communication device, make sure it is readily available to them and that you are familiar with its application. When phone conversations are necessary, a speech-to-speech relay service through a trained professional can facilitate communication.

Cognitive/affective issues

Do not assume that a person with a learning disability is not paying attention because he or she does not offer the traditional cues. Do not assume agreeableness and understanding when the person with mental retardation answers every question in the affirmative. Avoid nuanced and abstract communication style; speak concretely and verify understanding through open-ended questions and summary. Remain age appropriate in content and delivery. Do not patronize or diminish the person's autonomy.

Psychiatric disabilities are the most stigmatized. Respect, unconditional regard, and fidelity are important characteristics in relationship building. Become knowledgeable about the recovery process and the role of relapse. Become part of the support community and involved in local support groups.

CONCLUSION

In the end, disability etiquette is about ethics (see Miller & Millington, 2002). Not the capital 'E' ethics of dilemmas and ethical codes, but the pedestrian ethics of our character as reflected in the way we treat our clients. That we have a collection of do's and don'ts for day-to-day client interactions is proof of our ethos. That we need one is evidence of how far we have to go to live up to our aspirations. A cursory view of the contents of this collection of polite admonishments is enough to see that it is spotty, incomplete, and vague around the edges. A comprehensive tome of decorums would be encyclopedic; its value as a guide to daily life questionable. You can never capture every instance of proper protocol in the universe of possible contexts and popular trends. The only constants are our values. Beneath all values is a single golden axiom: "Treat others as you would wish to be treated." Follow this (it is more difficult that one can imagine) and you will find the human being in the client and in yourself.

REFERENCES

Easter Seals. (2011). *Disability Etiquette*. Retrieved from http://www.easterseals.com/site/PageServer?pagename=ntl_etiquette

Federal Communications Commission. (2008). *Section 504 programs & activities accessibility handbook* (2nd ed.). Washington, DC: Consumer and Government Affairs Bureau.

Miller, D. J., & Millington, M. J. (2002). What is required of us? Rethinking ethical conduct in the practice and profession of vocational rehabilitation. In J. D. Andrew & C. W. Faubion (Eds.), *Rehabilitation services: An introduction for the human services professional* (pp. 278–295). Osage Beach, MO: Aspen Professional Services.

United Cerebral Palsy Association. (2010). *The ten commandments of communicating with people with disabilities*. Retrieved from http://www.rehab.cahwnet.gov/workplace/comand10.htm

Wright, B. (1983). *Physical disability: A psychosocial approach*. New York, NY: Harper & Row.

INSIDER PERSPECTIVE

The Story of Michael Hineberg

Every disability is unique, just as every person is unrepeatable. My observations about life as a person with a disability apply to me alone. I take ownership of my hopes, dreams, fears, and failures. I will not attribute my life reactions to my disability. Yet, my disability-related challenges have taken me down a path I would have never traveled had it not had been for my constant companion called Disability.

I acquired a disability at the age of 16. I was the typical teenager, filled with the invincibility, idealism, and dreams of an adolescent. "I have the world by the tail," I boasted in my juvenile arrogance. I owned a brand new Kawasaki motorcycle, I had a girlfriend and was on my way to becoming a plumber. I was active in high-school gymnastics. I placed 7th in a city tournament on parallel bars and 13th in the State of Wisconsin on rings. I even sported a mustache. My father and I enjoyed weekend hunting trips in Wisconsin. I was thrilled by all that life had to offer.

On the evening of January 11th, 1976, my father, a neighbor, and I were returning from hunting rabbits. It was a blustery and biting winter day. A lady in the oncoming lane suffered a heart attack, crossed the centerline, and hit the car I was driving. The head-on crash killed my father, our neighbor, and the driver of the other car. As a result of the collision, I fractured my jaw, collarbone, hip, leg, and knee. More seriously, I suffered a traumatic brain injury. Once my condition stabilized, I was transported to Milwaukee County General Hospital. For days my survival was uncertain. If I did survive, my outcome was unknown.

I remained comatose for 4 weeks, then, gradually, I regained consciousness. I had no idea of what happened, or how much time had passed. Everyone was instructed not to talk about the accident until I brought it up. Eventually, I asked for my father, because I noticed he wasn't coming to visit me. I scribbled out his name on paper because a tracheotomy prevented me from talking. I was told that he was killed in the accident.

The news of his death ripped right through me. "What do you mean he's gone?" I cried in a daze. A minute ago, I could reach out and touch him. He can't be gone. I didn't get to say good bye. Suddenly, I was overwhelmed with guilt. How would I know it is not my fault since I didn't remember anything about the accident? Maybe we stopped for a beer, as we occasionally did. Maybe *I* crossed the centerline and caused these terrible deaths. I felt as if I had something to hide. I wept uncontrollably. Relatives brought copies of the accident report and tried to convince me that it wasn't my fault. Eventually, I was persuaded but it didn't ease the pain. I remained in the hospital for 3 months. I went to summer school, but stayed in high school an extra year.

As time went by, the denial about my brain-injury yielded to reality. My deficits became more apparent and the permanence of my disability became certain. I possessed the typical head-injury sequelae: distractibility, impaired organizational skills, retrieval deficit, and difficulty sequencing activities. My left arm and leg were partially paralyzed, and I have a visual field cut, which eliminates the left visual hemisphere in both eyes. I was determined to return to as much of my former lifestyle as possible. I tried many different jobs, as I attempted to reenter the work force. My deficits manifested themselves differently in each situation. Consequently, I needed to develop compensatory strategies for each new job, depending on what was required of me. For example, checklists, reminders, filing systems, reachers, and grabbers were all employed to assist me. It became clear that plumbing was not an appropriate career, and so I set my sights toward college in spite of my difficulty in reading.

I completed an Associate of Arts degree at Concordia College and decided to study physical therapy, because of all the therapy I received. I successfully completed 2 years of course work in physical therapy at the University of Wisconsin-Madison.

I was terminated from the program during my clinical internships, for disability-related reasons. I was six credits short of finishing my degree, when my physical and cognitive impairments prevented me from performing adequately in the clinic. I was not able to make the quick decisions and abstract problem solving needed in the clinic. I went back to school and finished an alternate degree: a Bachelor of Science in Allied Health.

Life was most difficult during the time period immediately following my injury. As an adolescent, I lacked the tools needed to cope with the loss of my father during a very formative time period. I was in the process of finding my own identity when I was suddenly thrust into having to redefine myself as a former teenage athlete to a survivor of traumatic brain injury. My circle of friends changed greatly the first year. Most relationships are built on mutual interests and activities. Since my friends and I had little in common after I acquired my disability, friends drifted away. Furthermore, my teenage friends were uncomfortable about all the changes I was going through, and they choose to avoid the discomfort.

As time progressed I matured, and my peers developed better interpersonal skills and relationships became more natural. Maturity brought self-acceptance and self-acceptance provided interpersonal comfort. Relationships became my way of feeling connected to a world that seemed to be continuously changing.

I consider myself extremely fortunate to have had such a high level of recovery, yet a "high-level" of recovery has its own unique challenges. For the most part, my disability is not "visible." Therefore, on first glance, most people do not know I have a disability. My leg brace is not visible, and my gait is pretty good. As a result, my impairments are not obvious. For example, I cannot use my left hand very well, and so unless a task requires both hands, my motor problems go undetected. Likewise, my cognitive problems are situation specific. Unless I am performing a task that requires a damaged skill, my distractibility, impaired organizational skills, retrieval deficit, difficulty-sequencing activities will also escape notice.

People eventually notice my disability, but I am very aware of my disability at *all times*. Therefore, I appreciate when someone inquires about my disability, as long as his or her inquiry is not motivated by morbid curiosity. Once my disability is out in the open, I am relieved because I don't have to pretend not to be disabled. I can tell someone when I do need help and when I am able to be independent. The timing of this self-disclosure is personal judgment based on trust and acceptance.

I became a Christian as a result of my accident and my relationship with Christ is my main support in a turbulent world, where I am constantly required to adapt. Many of my other coping techniques are the same used by most people, such as physical exercise, and healthy diversions, such as hobbies and volunteering. I have a strong drive to assist people with disabilities, which is exactly what I do at Independence*First*.

As an independent living center, Independence*First* promotes independence among people with disabilities. The philosophy is to empower people with disabilities to exercise control and choice over matters affecting his or her personal life. (This job is a far cry from my goal of becoming a plumber.) I also make a deliberate effort to focus on helping other people, and I concentrate on the positives in my life. I worked in a Brain-Injury Rehabilitation Clinic for 4 years. This position was a tremendous object lesson for me, as I worked with many survivors of brain injury, who did not have as fortunate a recovery as I did.

My attitude is my greatest trigger. If my attitude is right I can weather almost anything. I can focus on the things I have going for me. But when I have the wrong attitude, I am defeated by anything and everything. For example, when my outlook is wrong, I can be oversensitive toward anything remotely pertaining to my disability. In fact, I tend to attribute foibles that are well within the normal scope of human experience to my disability. We all know how a bad attitude plays havoc on self-acceptance too. My attitude can be my best friend or my greatest enemy.

Several other things really irritate me. I hate being treated like a child. I hate when people are impatient with me and do things for me—to suit their convenience. It is what I call the parental attitude, which says I can see you are having trouble, so let me do it for you *(it's faster)*. Likewise, I dislike when people pity me. Nothing is more demeaning than someone giving you his or her pity, as if pity will mend. Everyone appreciates empathy. Empathy empowers, but pity degrades.

I find true empathy supportive, but I hate the presumptuous, patronizing, "I know how you feel." Believe it or not, people still say this to me. It is much more supportive to hear, "Tell me how you feel, I want to understand."

My greatest asset is my attitude, for which I give God all the glory. I see everyday as borrowed time. I try to focus on all the things I have going for me instead of all the things gone wrong. My motto is: *You have to make the most of what you've got.*

I am also fortunate to have my communication skills and relationship skills intact. Family and friends provide a lot of help coping. Fortunately, I am the type of person who finds it helpful to talk through things. Even though most of my friends do not have disabilities and may never truly understand my struggles, a genuine ear is extremely supportive.

The Me-and-Them Mentality

Many people with disabilities develop what I call the me-and-them mentality. Individuals with disabilities have a tendency to view the world in terms of me-and -"Them" (Me, being the person with a disability, and them as those out there who do not have my disability). People with disabilities must be careful, because this attitude tends to turn people off. If you want to be accepted as an equal in the workplace, you must guard against this attitude.

Most people who have a disability do not want preferential treatment. Stereotypes exist that portray people with disabilities folks as expecting handouts. One of the ways people with disabilities can prevent this perception is to make sure you do not develop the "me-and-them" mentality. Focus on your abilities, and what you have in common with people, not on how you are different.

Self-acceptance is a journey, not a destination. It is not like traveling to a distant country, where eventually you arrive. It is a companion who is sometimes at your side and sometimes nowhere to be found, depending on the situation, on your mood, and on your support systems.

Physical and mental impairments can affect many aspects of the human experience. Employment, recreation, mobility, communication, and self-care may be different when an individual has a disability. But a disability goes much further than limited job options, or requiring the use of a wheelchair to get around. The greatest limitation created by a disability is the invisible one. It is the *social isolation* created by a world geared for the able-bodied person. Until there is a barrier-free world, people with disabilities will be isolated. Buildings without wheelchair ramps are not available to everyone. People are disconnected when they are warehoused away in congregate housing.

People with disabilities are removed from the mainstream when public transportation does not afford them the opportunity to go where others can go. People with disabilities will be isolated as long as there continue to be members of the society who perpetuate the me-and-them mentality. The greatest impairment of a disability is social isolation. Remember that the person with an acquired disability may have a pervasive sense of loss not experienced at the same depth as the person who has a congenital disability.

I consider myself extremely fortunate to have achieved such a high level of recovery, yet there are many unsuspected frustrations that accompany such a fortune. People unaware of my limitations expect me to be able to do everything the "average" person can do. If I had a sign on me that read "Disabled" I feel people could see I have a disability. Furthermore, my level of functioning causes me to feel that I have a foot in two different worlds: the world of those with disabilities and the world of people without disabilities. I have a very real disability, yet I am more able bodied than most people with disabilities are—therefore, I straddle two worlds. On the positive side, I possess a perspective from both sides of the fence. On the negative side, I often feel like I do not fit in either world.

Another common theme I see among people with disabilities centers on control. Everyone I know wants to maintain as much control as possible over his or her life. Disabilities often reduce a person's control. Disability often robs a person of control, whether it is dressing, communicating, eating, or mobility. Therefore, it is essential for a person with a disability to exercise as much control over choices in matters that impacts his or her life.

One of my biggest pitfalls is the comparison trap. There is a great tendency for people with acquired disabilities to compare themselves with their nondisabled peers or the way they were before their injury is great. Comparison that leads to self-improvement is healthy. Comparison to that leads to self-abasement is destructive.

Most people with acquired disabilities have a profound sense of how near everyone is to experiencing a disability. *Those who are not disabled are temporarily "abled."* Such an insight provides a unique life perspective. If every "able-bodied" person realized that they are only a heartbeat away from disability, they might not view people with disabilities as foreigners from a world. Disability is not as far away as people might like to think.

Sometimes, people may avoid individuals with disabilities because they are reminded of his or her own vulnerable humanity. Thankfully, ADA has brought more people with disabilities into public view. My hope is for people to become more comfortable around their fellow human beings, who happen to have disabilities, so that people with disabilities can feel fully assimilated into society as equal citizens. Barriers can be structural and attitudinal. As able-bodied people realize the temporal nature of their health, people with disabilities would not seem so different.

Advice

- A person is more than his or her disability, but that disability is an integral part of who they are. In order to understand a person with a disability you truly must understand their story. You must know their journey and know how they see the world, and how they perceive they are seen by the world.
- People with disabilities want a level playing field—not preference. Equality is desired not parentalism.
- Foster independence. No one with a disability wants to be treated as an inferior. Encourage independence by giving the person with a disability the right to fail. Do not be overprotective.

Conclusion

In summary, remember that people with disabilities want to be treated as equals. They do not want preferential treatment, and they do not want a parent. They are a mixture of hopes, dreams, fears, and aspirations—like everyone else. They are just inside of a slightly different package.

DISCUSSION QUESTIONS

1. This chapter implies that there are underlying values that all rehabilitation counselors must share, although it does not directly list them. What are the unifying values of the profession? What are your values? How do your values affect your relationship with rehabilitation counseling clients?
2. What values are apparent in the do's and don'ts of disability etiquette? Are they reflected in the 20 value-laden principles?
3. Disability etiquette is an accumulation of guidelines, obviously incomplete … a work in progress with no organized plan for completion. What might an unabridged collection of etiquette guidelines look like? What purpose could it serve?

EXERCISE

A. Disability etiquette is an extension of etiquette in general. Observe public behavior in any venue where there is a lot of activity. How do people treat each other? What kind of deference is given to the elderly, children, and others who obviously need a little help? Consider how this general level of social accommodation helps or hinders people with disabilities. Discuss.

SIXTEEN

What We Counsel, Teach, and Research Regarding the Needs of Persons With Disabilities: What Have We Been Missing?

Irmo Marini

OVERVIEW

With almost 100 years of state-federal programs aimed at working with the vocational goals of persons with disabilities, and over half a century of specialized attention addressing the vocational, psychosocial, and independent living needs of this population, have we gotten it right, or do we as a profession need to stop for a moment and reflect on important issues we have missed out on or paid little attention to (Chubon, 1994; Leahy, Rak, & Zanskas, 2009; Olkin, 1999; Rubin & Roessler, 2008; Wright, 1988)? Stubbins (1991) appealed to the profession of rehabilitation psychology to gain knowledge of related disciplines and how they view disability. Olkin (1999) called for a holistic counseling approach to working with persons with disabilities she describes as disability affirmative therapy. This approach encompasses empowering clients, recognizing that there are valid complaints of discrimination and social injustice that must be acknowledged, and learning to work and network with multiple, and often fragmented health care services.

In this chapter, we explore and synthesize a number of topics that have not generated much discussion or related research in working with persons with disabilities in the rehabilitation counseling and education field. Indeed, an extensive literature review on the topic of social justice found only one article by Alston, Harley, and Middleton (2006). Similarly, topics such as advocacy, empowerment, participatory action research (PAR), and positive psychology in relation to persons with disabilities are rare. Greenleaf and Williams (2009) call for a paradigm shift toward a more ecological, holistic counseling perspective and approach to working with generally oppressed and discriminated minority groups. People with disabilities, and specifically minority persons with disabilities, unquestionably have been, and continue to be, the most disenfranchised group in America. As such, this final chapter serves as a call to all related rehabilitation professionals who work with persons with disabilities to literally begin providing a "holistic approach" to educational training and counseling when we clearly have not.

Our definition of a holistic approach needs to extend beyond sitting behind a desk, developing rapport, providing services, and then holding our breath hoping that our clients with disabilities will succeed. Philosophically and statistically, there is no question that rehabilitation counselors, educators, and researchers have clearly made a positive difference in the lives of millions of persons with disabilities. To that end, we can clearly pat ourselves on the back and claim the glass is half full. But what about the glass that continues to be half empty? What about the statistics we have all memorized but become desensitized to, including the 70% unemployment rate among this population (Houtenville, 2000), underemployment (National Organization on Disability, 2004), higher high-school dropout rates (National Organization on Disability, 2004), higher poverty rates (McNeil, 2001), poorer and inadequate health care (Berk, Schur, & Cantor, 1995), social oppression and discrimination (Ratts, D'Andrea, & Arredondo, 2004), and continuing physical access barriers (Graf, Marini, & Blankenship, 2009), all in comparison with the general population. In order to fill the proverbial glass further, we need to now explore and hopefully put into practice the following principles.

SOCIAL JUSTICE

The American Counseling Association (ACA) has led the way only recently in considering social justice to be a valid counseling specialization. Specifically, in its 2005 revised code of ethics, ACA cites "when appropriate, counselors advocate at the individual, group, institutional, and societal levels to examine potential barriers and obstacles that inhibit access and/or growth and development of clients" (ACA, 2005, p. 5). The ACA has also approved the new Division for Counselors for Social Justice within ACA. On its 2010 homepage defining what social justice counseling entails, it cites:

> Social justice counseling represents a multifaceted approach to counseling in which practitioners strive to simultaneously promote human development and the common good through addressing challenges related to both individual and distributive justice. Social justice counseling includes empowerment of the individual as well as active confrontation of injustice and inequality in society as they impact clientele as well as those in their systemic contexts. In doing so, social justice counselors direct attention to the promotion of four critical principles that guide their work; equity, access, participation, and harmony. This work is done with a focus on the cultural, contextual, and individual needs of those served (http://counselorsforsocialjustice.com).

Greenleaf and Williams (2009) discuss the view that the counseling profession has been largely driven or entrenched by the medical model paradigm, one that focuses exclusively on the individual and treating his or her impairments. This represents a pathological orientation to diagnosis and treatment described earlier, and is perhaps no better evident than our reliance on the *Diagnostic and Statistical Manual of Mental Disorders* (American Psychiatric Association, 2000). However, to truly consider a holistic approach toward working with people with disabilities, we must consider the 75-year-old writings of Kurt Lewin (1936) concerning the person–environment interaction discussed in Chapter 5. Specifically, our behavior is a function of our individual traits and characteristics in response to our interactions with our environment ($B = f[P \times E]$). Numerous empirical studies have shown that regardless of how strong a character someone has, with a perceived discriminatory social environment, the individual's physical and mental health may be negatively affected (Dohrenwend, 2000; Gee, 2002; Li & Moore, 1998; Rumbaut, 1994; Williams & Williams-Morris, 2000).

In further exploring the mental and physical health implications for individuals who are, or perceive to be, oppressed and/or discriminated against, a number of interesting studies show the significance of the person–environment interaction and its implications. Aguinaldo (2008), for example, studied the concept of gay oppression as a determinant of gay men's health, citing the premise, "homophobia is killing us." In his literature review, Aguinaldo notes the mental and physical health problems of gay men living in a society that oppresses, discriminates, and is blatantly prejudice toward them. The resulting fear, physical and verbal abuse, felt hatred, and anger gay males often endure by others carries a heavy psychological toll, sometimes resulted in depression, anxiety, lacking self-worth, shame, self-destructive behaviors such as suicide, inferiority, and self-defeating behaviors (Dempsey, 1994).

Generalized stress and stress-related illnesses have also been linked to others who are oppressed and feel discriminated against (Dohrenwend, 2000; Turner & Avison, 2003). Dohrenwend (2000) assessed the rates of psychological and physical stress-induced problems in ethnic/racial groups regarding perceived prejudice and discrimination, and found that those who felt discriminated against expressed higher rates of depression and anxiety than the nondisadvantaged or majority group. Similarly, Turner and Avison (2003) found that African Americans reported higher occurrences of discriminatory experiences including violence, death, and daily discrimination resulting in chronic stressors, when compared with White study participants. Perlow, Danoff-Burg, Swenson, and Pulgiano (2004) noted how discrimination negatively impacts one's sense of control, and feelings of hopelessness can ultimately lead to a variety of mental health disorders.

If societal discrimination and oppression simply stopped there, the negative physical and mental health impact of oppressed individuals would be alarming in and of itself. Unfortunately, the peripheral implication of perceived prejudice toward an individual or group has further negative ramifications that can exacerbate health problems (Kessler et al., 2003; Krieger, 1999). Numerous studies show the resulting ripple effect of discrimination, including unemployment or underemployment, lower socioeconomic status, poorer health care, lower educational attainment, and poverty (Eaton & Muntaner 1999; Kessler et al., 2003; Krieger, 1999; Williams, Yu, Jackson, & Anderson, 1997).

The Social Justice Counselor

The paradigm shift in how we work with clients must extend beyond simply working with them and their families, to ultimately exploring what, if any, societal and environmental barriers may likely block their goals (Neville & Mobley, 2001). It has been suggested that social advocacy is the "fifth force" within the counseling profession, essentially an extension and complement to the multicultural movement (Ratts et al., 2004, p. 28). The ecological approach to counseling acknowledges the impact that an unfriendly environment can have on the well-being of clients (Wilson, 2003). Ivey and Ivey (1998) describe the Developmental Counseling and Therapy model, noting how external stressors can impact intrapsychic changes in clients. The authors cite the progression and reciprocal effect of these interactions, including: (a) environmental or biological insult may lead to; (b) stress and physical/emotional pain, which may lead to; (c) sadness/depression, which may lead to; (d) defense against the pain, possibly mental disorders.

In providing a holistic approach to helping clients with disabilities, counselors must be willing to not only acknowledge social injustice exists but willing to also go the extra mile to do something about it. As the Division for Counselors of Social Justice Web page indicates, "Social justice counseling includes empowerment of the individual as well as active confrontation of injustice and inequality in society as they impact clientele as well as those in their systemic contexts." In defining exactly what "active confrontation of injustice and a quality in society" means, counselors must be aware of what their job's contractual limitations are, if any, regarding Congressional letter writing, advocacy, peaceful protests, and other legal remedies to confront injustice and inequality. The ACA has been quite effective over the years in rallying its 43,000 plus constituents by providing them with legislative alerts, synopsis of relevant legislative bills being introduced for passage, who their Congressional leaders are, and sample letters for counselors to use as a template. The ACA Advocacy Competencies (Lewis, Arnold, House, & Toporek, 2003) concerning social justice advocacy in counseling recognizes the ecological model; oppression and discrimination are socially constructed and has damaging physical and mental health impact on individuals who are functioning within a toxic reciprocal person–environment atmosphere (Bronfenbrenner, 1977; Wilson, 2003).

Several recent school counselor education publications have addressed active steps in preparing counselors for social justice (Bemak & Chung, 2008; Steele, 2008). Bemak and Chung (2008), for example, describe ACA Advocacy Competencies in relation to promoting systems advocacy, student empowerment, identifying specific advocacy strategies to communicate to colleagues, and stressing the need to further disseminate information to other constituents. These competencies emphasize strength in numbers and group action in promoting equality in educational funding, adequate resources, and a safe learning environment. To passively sit back and counsel students in a dysfunctional or antiquated learning environment is inadequate. The authors cite potential counselor concerns as to why they may not want to become involved in remedying social injustice problems. Some obstacles include general apathy, labeled as a troublemaker, fear of retribution, a sense of powerlessness, and anxiety that can lead to guilt for not advocating. Bemak and Chung offer recommendations to assist counselors, for example, aligning social justice advocacy with organizational mission and goals, using data-driven strategies, having the courage to speak out, taking calculated risks, recruiting colleagues and others in the cause, developing political partners, becoming politically knowledgeable, and keeping faith (Bemak & Chung, 2008, pp. 379–380).

In considering social justice regarding persons with disabilities, counselors and case managers can influence a number of possible inequities in health care, education, and employment. Persons with disabilities and especially those of minority status are statistically the most disenfranchised population in the United States (National Organization on Disability, 2004). Counselors have to acknowledge environmental inequities as well as the implications that oppression and discrimination can have on clients who can succumb to and give up trying (Dempsey, 1994; Dohrenwend, 2000; Gee, 2002). Thesen (2005) discusses how he and other physicians often knowingly or unknowingly treat patients in a dehumanizing and oppressive manner. He indicates that this type of behavior is counterproductive to patient health and can leave them feeling powerless and without any control. Thesen calls for medical professionals to instead empower their patients by including them in the decision-making process, educating them, and acknowledging their concerns. Bham and Forchuk (2008) illustrated empirically Thesen's (2005) premise in their interview of 336 current and former psychiatric and/or physically disabled clients. Specifically, the authors found that patients with comorbid conditions of a psychiatric and physical disability perceived themselves to be more discriminated and oppressed by health care professionals. This, in turn, positively correlated with psychiatric problem severity, self-rated general health, and poorer life satisfaction and well-being. Counselors should be prepared to step in and advocate for clients when they witness the negative attitudes of health care professionals.

In other life domains concerning clients with disabilities, counselors and case managers should be prepared to tackle social injustice issues that impede client progress in the social and vocational realm. Despite the 20-year-old Americans with Disabilities Act (ADA), environmental barriers still exist that have been shown to result in some persons with disabilities feeling frustrated, angry, socially anxious, and depressed at times (Charmaz, 1995; DiTomasso & Spinner, 1997; Graf et al., 2009; Hopps, Pepin, Arseneau, Frechette, & Begin, 2001; Li & Moore, 1998; Marini, Bhakta, & Graf, 2009). Counselors can assist clients in constructing letters to business owners demanding removal of access barriers, filing complaints with the Office of Civil Rights, referring clients to Client Assistance Programs (CAPs), and finding an ADA lawyer if necessary (Blackwell, Marini, & Chacon, 2001; Blankenship, 2005; Marini et al., 2009). There appears to be little doubt from numerous empirical studies showing negative or perceived hostile environmental conditions can, and do, have a negative impact on client well-being. For counselors to concern themselves just with assisting clients to deal with living in an able-bodied world, it is a job that is left unfinished or incomplete.

ADVOCACY

Social justice and advocacy are sometimes used interchangeably and are often considered synonymous concepts. The primary difference, however, is that social justice is a broader concept recognizing unequal power, unearned privilege, and oppression (Alston et al., 2006). Advocacy is more behavioral and action oriented, and is an activity that often involves actions to correct some social injustice. As such, several authors discuss social justice advocacy in relation to some perceived social inequity. O'Day and Goldstein (2005) interviewed 16 disability advocacy and research leaders regarding the top contemporary advocacy issues concerning persons with disabilities. Disability advocacy organizations, such as the Consortium of Citizens with Disabilities (CCD), Not Dead Yet (NDY), Americans with Disabilities for Attendant Programs Today (ADAPT), American Association of People with Disabilities (AAPD), and others, are involved with grassroots advocacy, ongoing events, rallies, and information dissemination regarding important legislative issues toward enhancing full inclusion of persons with disabilities. O'Day and Goldstein found the top five contemporary issues included affordable and accessible health care, employment, access to assistive technology, long-term care, and civil rights enforcement concerning Titles II and III (public services and public accommodations) of the ADA. Similar concerns have been reported elsewhere (Graf et al., 2009; Marini et al., 2009).

Advocacy can take several forms in terms of action. The simplest form of advocacy involves letter writing to local and state constituents in attempts to bring attention to some social inequity, such as accessible housing. Arguably, more extreme forms can involve peaceful protests, such as occupying lawmaker's offices and sometimes subsequent citations for trespassing. The group ADAPT has been relentless and fairly successful over the past several decades in promoting disability rights, with its successful start in the early 1980s fighting for public accessible transportation in major cities, including city buses, subways, and Greyhound bus lines. The group would organize, and primarily the wheelchair users would block buses and chain themselves and otherwise occupy legislators' offices to be heard. In time, the majority of their efforts were successful in bringing major change across America, where persons with physical disabilities were unable to use public transportation. During the past decade or so, ADAPT has focused its fight on community-based care, whereby persons who require assistance with activities of daily living do not have to live in a nursing home. Their motto is "free our people," arguing that over two-thirds of federal and state monies are successfully lobbied into nursing homes instead of the money following the person who chooses to live at home. For counselors and case managers who work for the state or federal government, the central question becomes whether this type of advocacy to support such causes has any job repercussions. If conducted on our own time, there generally is no adverse impact; however, counselors are encouraged to be familiar with their agencies workplace policies. Too often when we advocate, we do so for our own interests and to protect our jobs or territory and disguise it as client beneficence.

Ericksen (1997) indicates that advocacy is conceptually a cross between public policy, public relations, and conflict resolution. Bradley and Lewis (2000) and Lee

(1998) define advocacy as becoming the voice of the clients and taking action to make environmental changes that may impede barriers to a client's career, academic, personal, or social goals. Semivan and White (2006) noted that the skills needed for effective advocacy include passion, fact-finding, knowledge, data-based research, and goal-oriented concrete objectives. They must also know the limits of their professional roles and be able to separate highly charged emotions from their actions. Stewart, Gibson-Semivan, and Schwartz (2009) cited practical advocacy strategies to include: (a) identifying the target population and the nature/facts of the injustice; (b) developing a rationale as to how advocacy will affect the advocate and target population chosen; (c) developing clearly and concisely how advocating will fit the therapist's role, and fits within the scope of practice or ethics for the counselor; (d) conducting research on the background and nature of the social injustice thoroughly, including speaking to individuals who have been affected by it; (e) developing a list of references and resources for dissemination; (f) outlining the broader and then individual measurable goals of the advocacy project and review them regularly for refining if necessary; and (g) after selecting goals, determining what the first steps are and whose responsibility it is to carry out each activity (Stewart et al., 2009, p. 58).

So how can rehabilitation educators, researchers, and counselors either directly or indirectly become better advocates for persons with disabilities? For educators, teaching students about relevant advocacy community services, such as CAPs, legal aid, guardianship, and services provided by Centers for Independent Living (CILs), becomes important in knowing about nonmedical services that can help in social injustice situations (Blankenship, 2005; Marini et al., 2009). In addition, educators can teach students about legislation pertaining to persons with disabilities, provide legislative alerts, and show students how to write to legislators on behalf of persons with disabilities. Two organizations that are extremely effective in providing information and education on these topics are the National Rehabilitation Association and the American Counseling Association. Educators can also have letter-writing campaigns for important legislation as part of a class grade, and/or attending or developing local information sessions about impending legislation. Currently, there is only a handful of Council on Rehabilitation Education (CORE) accredited programs that offer a course on advocacy. Overall, teaching students how to advocate effectively can then be passed on to teaching clients with disabilities once students graduate.

For rehabilitation education researchers, studying the impact of teaching and empowering persons with disabilities about how to advocate for themselves can minimize years of dependency on others who have traditionally made decisions for them (Brinckerhoff, 1994). Brinckerhoff noted how teaching adolescents affected by learning disability self-advocacy skills regarding effectively managing their college experience can be self-empowering and enhance self-esteem (Van Reusen & Bos, 1990). Research topics could include a control and experimental group design, provide the experimental group with tangible training skills to become more proficient at some self-advocacy task, then measuring the psychosocial impact of empowerment, locus of control, and self-efficacy. Anecdotally, it would seem self-evident that individuals who are taught skills to become more proficient in mastering or controlling parts of their environment would enhance client self-esteem and self-confidence.

Counselors working directly with persons with disabilities in a variety of settings and in a variety of ways can work with clients directly regarding advocacy and self-empowerment issues. Although many counselors have been empowering clients for years regarding job clubs, job search strategies, interview skills training, and so on, others may tend to "do for" rather than "do with" clients; that can be counterproductive. Brodwin, Star, and Cardoso (2007), for example, discuss the importance of including clients in selecting assistive technology or adaptive equipment, because otherwise without client input, many clients will not use or will discard the device. As noted with educators, counselors can refer clients to appropriate advocacy agencies, assist in writing letters of complaint or letters to congressional leaders, and teach assertiveness and advocacy skills in presenting their case.

PARTICIPATORY ACTION RESEARCH

This concept again involves rehabilitation educators, researchers, and counselors. PAR pertains to directly involving the individual(s) researchers are interested in finding more about, from study inception to conclusion. Mmatli (2009) and others have expressed a greater need for PAR-designed studies, particularly in the social sciences, and specifically with regard to persons with disabilities (Graf et al., 2009; Turnbull, Friesen, & Ramirez, 1998). In arguing the merits of PAR, Mmatli writes, ". . . if disability research were to acknowledge and recognize respondents' lived experiences, viewpoints, and aspirations, then the policies, programs, services, and new approaches resulting from the research would be client informed, and more likely to be meaningful to them" (Mmatli, 2009, p. 17). Mmatli argues the merits of qualitative research in gaining a deeper appreciation for the value-laden circumstances of peoples' lives, and the need for researchers to involve them to determine the direction of the research. Radermacher, Sonn, Keys, and Duckett (2010) interviewed 12 disabled and able-bodied persons regarding barriers in participation to an organizational planning activity, aptly titling their study *Disability and Participation: It's About Us but Still Without Us,* finding that the participants with disabilities felt excluded from the process.

Oliver (1992) noted that PAR also serves to empower persons with disabilities because they perceive their voices and opinions being counted. Quantitative research despite having merit has never had the capacity to fully capture the many confounding variables regarding participant experiences. In many studies, researchers end up with snapshots of how depressed some group is without knowing why, but make the disability salient to the emotion. As Olkin (1999) argues, some researchers focus on caregiver burden without noting the caregiver has been unsuccessful in obtaining funding for support that could otherwise remedy the burden perception. Oliver (1992) indicates that researchers need to break the artificial distinction between the researcher and those being researched, while Graf et al. (2009) add that researchers need to look outward at the environmental barriers that negatively affect the client and/or the family's well-being.

In a PAR study, Garcia-Iriarte, Kramer, Kramer, and Hammel (2008) involved 14 members with intellectual disabilities of People First in a group advocacy project to promote their chapter over a 15-month period. Focus groups and individual qualitative interviews were conducted. Results indicated that members expressed having a sense of control over providing input and influencing the outcome, ultimately improving their capacity to self-advocate. Overall, including persons with disabilities in PAR appears to accomplish several desirable goals, such as sense of control and empowerment if conducted effectively.

Revisiting Wright's Fundamental Negative Bias

Researchers should heed Wright's (1988) cautions in her classic paper, *Attitudes and the Fundamental Negative Bias: Conditions and Corrections* regarding how attitude research is conducted. She noted how some researchers begin with preconceived ideas, ignore nonsignificant findings that are clinically meaningful (e.g., persons with disabilities are more similar, in many ways, to people without disabilities), and somehow interpret positive findings into negative ones. Wright argued that disability researchers studying attitudes often make the disability the most salient feature and are motivated to publish statistically significant findings that show differences, but do not report nonsignificant similarities they perceive may not be publishable.

Insider Versus Outsider Perspective: Dembo, Leviton, and Wright (1956, 1975), and Wright (1983) also address an often ignored phenomenon by researchers; what they termed the "insider versus outsider" perspective, the "fortune phenomena," and the "mine–thine" problem. These fascinating concepts overlap and have been confirmed in subsequent studies centering on the almost totally divergent perspectives that persons with and without disabilities believe about disability circumstances. The insider versus outsider perspective focuses on how people with disabilities (insiders) view their lives in comparison with how those without disabilities (outsiders) perceive those with disabilities must think, feel, and behave. Overall, persons without disabilities often view the lives of persons with disabilities very negatively, and in some instances not worth living (Bogdan & Taylor, 1989; Grayson & Marini, 1996; Singer, 2000). Conversely, persons with disabilities who have had their disabilities for some time most often do not view their disabilities negatively (Whiteman & Lukoff, 1965; Wright & Howe, 1969; Wright & Muth, 1965). For them, it is a lifestyle they have long since adapted to and essentially moved on emotionally and mentally. However, for those without disabilities looking in, to them the disability is salient and new, and as a result can infer a number of erroneous assumptions regarding disabled individuals' lifestyles, quality of life, and life satisfaction.

The fortune phenomenon is a similarly overlapping concept in which outsiders view persons with disabilities as less fortunate, while those with disabilities do not view themselves in the same way (Wright & Howe, 1969). The authors had women from four groups (patients from psychiatric hospitals, welfare recipients, college students, and middle-class housewives) rate themselves on an 11-point scale of being very fortunate to very unfortunate. The hospital patients and welfare recipients rated themselves average or above average in being fortunate; however, the housewives and college students rated them as unfortunate. Similar findings were reported by Wright and Muth (1965), where persons with physical disabilities rated themselves at least average in being fortunate, but outsiders viewed them as being unfortunate.

The "mine–thine" (Wright, 1983) concept also reflects insider versus outsider perspectives. With this concept, persons with disabilities, when given choices regarding hypothetically choosing to have their own disabilities or opting for other disabilities, consistently choose their own. Wright describes why individuals consistently reclaim their own disabilities in such studies due to the fact that they are familiar and have adapted to their situation. Persons who are blind generally will choose to remain blind as opposed to becoming physically disabled, and vice versa. Perhaps even more remarkable, are the studies in which persons with disabilities are queried as to whether, if available, they would take a magic pill to become able bodied (Hahn & Belt, 2004). Earlier studies have found that indeed many persons with disabilities would not want to be cured due to having become accustomed to their lifestyle (Weinberg & Williams, 1978; Weinberg, 1988). Many persons who are deaf, for example, refuse to have cochlear implants for fear of losing their signing ability and connection with the deaf community (Jankowski, 1997; Niparko, 2000). In Hahn and Belt's (2004) study of 156 ADAPT activists, members were asked, "Even if I could take a magic pill, I would not want my disability to be cured," with responses ranging from strongly agree to strongly disagree. Results indicated that 47% expressed that they would not want to be cured, 8% were ambivalent, and 45% disagreed with the statement. The authors found that those who would refuse a cure, scored higher in having a strong disability identity, whereas those who would take the cure rejected the disability identity affirmation. In addition, those who were injured longer were less likely to want a magic cure.

CONCLUDING INSIGHTS

The field of rehabilitation counseling and education have in the past been unduly influenced by the medical model paradigm, however, perhaps not so much as psychology, social work, and related health professions. Although contemporary rehabilitation counseling and psychology have over the past decade begun to recognize that we have placed much of our past efforts on the pathological orientation of disability, focusing on what's wrong and how to fix it, many of us have advanced into a new era of viewing disability as a socially constructed phenomenon (Mackelprang & Salsgiver, 2009; Olkin, 1999; Smart, 2009; Vash & Crewe, 2004). In this contemporary approach, we are reminded of Frank Bowe's (1978) sentiment that it is often the negative attitudes of Americans that further handicaps people with disabilities. And as we have observed with the numerous study findings throughout this book, people with disabilities can be negatively affected by an otherwise unfriendly environment. At the same time, if many people with chronic illness and/or disabilities do not otherwise have any demonstrative psychological problems living with their disabilities, how then, and why can we continue to justify the same recycling of issues to tackle to validate our jobs?

When asked, many people with disabilities indicate that their negative emotions (e.g., anger, frustration, depression, anxiety, loneliness) are directly or indirectly facilitated by environmental barriers, negative attitudes, and lack of available funding for services. Rehabilitation professionals may choose to continue helping those with disabilities to adapt to an able-bodied world and basically get used it. Or, we can collectively go further and actively advocate socially and politically to correct social injustice, conduct more PAR-type studies to really explore the problems and how to correct them, and finally to focus more on a salutogenic approach of positive psychology and posttraumatic growth. It is our hope that you have realized where many of the real problems for persons with disabilities lie, and are prepared to move forward in providing a holistic approach to serving this population.

REFERENCES

Aguinaldo, J. P. (2008). The social construction of gay oppression as a determinant of gay men's health: "Homophobia is killing us". *Critical Public Health, 18*(1), 87–96.

Alston, R. J., Harley, D. A., & Middleton, R. (2006). The role of rehabilitation in achieving social justice for minorities with disabilities. *Journal of Vocational Rehabilitation, 24*, 129–136.

American Counseling Association. (2005). *ACA code of ethics.* Alexandria, VA: Author.

Bemak, F., & Chung, R. C. (2008). New professional roles and advocacy strategies for school counselors: A multicultural/social justice perspective to move beyond the nice counselor syndrome. *Journal of Counseling & Development, 86*, 372–382.

Berk, M. L., Schur, C. L., & Cantor, J. C. (1995). Ability to obtain health care: Recent estimates from the Robert Wood Johnson Foundation National Access to Care Survey. *Health Affairs, 14*, 139–146.

Bham, A., & Forchuk, C. (2008). Interlocking oppressions: The effect of a comorbid physical disability on perceived stigma and discrimination among mental health consumers in Canada. *Health and Social Care in the Community, 17*(1), 63–70.

Blackwell, T. M., Marini, I., & Chacon, M. (2001). The impact of the Americans with Disabilities Act on independent living. *Rehabilitation Education, 15*(4), 395–408.

Blankenship, C. J. (2005). Client assistance programs and protection and advocacy services. In W. Crimando & T. F. Riggar (Eds.), *Community resources: A guide for human service workers* (pp. 218–224). Long Grove, IL: Waveland Press.

Bogdan, R., & Taylor, S. (1989). Relationships with severely disabled people: The social construction of humanness. *Social Problems, 36*, 135–148.

Bowe, F. (1978). *Understanding America: Barriers to disabled people.* New York, NY: Harper & Row.

Bradley, L., & Lewis, J. (2000). Introduction. In J. Lewis & L. Bradley (Eds.), *Advocacy in counseling: Counselors, clients & community* (pp. 3–4). Greensboro, NC: ERIC Clearinghouse on Counseling and Student Services.

Brinckerhoff, L. C. (1994). Developing effective self-advocacy skills in college-bound students with learning disabilities. *Intervention in School & Clinic, 29*(4), 229.

Brodwin, M. G., Star, T., & Cardoso, E. (2007). Users of assistive technology. In A. E. Dell Orto & P. W. Power (Eds.), *The psychological and social impact of illness and disability* (pp. 505–519). New York, NY: Springer.

Bronfenbrenner, U. (1977). Toward an experimental ecology of human development. *American Psychologist, 32*, 513–531.

Charmaz, N. (1995). The body, identity, and self: Adapting to impairment. *The Sociological Quarterly, 36*, 657–680.

Chubon, R. A. (1994). *Social and psychological foundations of rehabilitation.* Springfield, IL: Charles C Thomas.

DiTomasso, E., & Spinner, B. (1997). Social and emotional loneliness: A re-examination of Weiss' typology of loneliness. *Personality and Individual Differences, 22*, 417–427.

Dembo, T., Leviton, G. L., & Wright, B. A. (1956). Adjustment to misfortune: A problem of social–psychological rehabilitation. *Rehabilitation Psychology, 2*, 1–100.

Dembo, T., Leviton, G. L., & Wright, B. A. (1975). Adjustment to misfortune: A problem of social–psychological rehabilitation. *Artificial Limbs, 3*, 4–62.

Dempsey, C. L. (1994). Health and social issues of gay, lesbian, and bisexual adolescents. *Families in Society: The Journal of Contemporary Human Services, 75*(3), 160–167.

Dohrenwend, B. P. (2000). The role of adversity and stress in psychopathology: Some evidence and its implications for theory and research. *Journal of Health and Social Behavior, 41*, 1–19.

Eaton, W. W., & Muntaner, C. (1999). Socioeconomic stratification and mental disorder. In A. V. Horwitz & T. L. Scheid (Eds.), *A handbook for the study of mental health: Social contexts, theories, and systems* (pp. 259–283). New York: Cambridge University Press.

Ericksen, K. (1997). *Making an impact: A handbook on counselor advocacy.* Washington, DC: Taylor & Francis/Accelerated Development.

Garcia-Iriarte, E., Kramer, J. C., Kramer, J. M., & Hammel, J. (2008). 'Who did what?': A participatory action research project to increase group capacity for advocacy. *Journal of Applied Research in Intellectual Disabilities, 22*(1), 10–22.

Gee, G. C. (2002). A multilevel analysis of the relationship between institutional racial discrimination and health status. *American Journal of Public Health, 5*, 109–117.

Graf, N. M., Marini, I., & Blankenship, C. (2009). 100 words about disability. *Journal of Rehabilitation, 75*(2), 25–34.

Grayson, E., & Marini, I. (1996). Simulated disability exercises and their impact on attitudes toward persons with disabilities. *International Journal of Rehabilitation Research, 19*, 123–131.

Greenleaf, A. T., & Williams, J. M. (2009). Supporting social justice advocacy: A paradigm shift towards an ecological perspective. *Journal for Social Action in Counseling and Psychology, 2*(1), 1–12.

Hahn, H. D., & Belt, T. L. (2004). Disability identity and attitudes toward cure in a sample of disabled activists. *Journal of Health and Social Behavior, 45*(4), 453–464.

Hopps, S., Pepin, M., Arseneau, I., Frechette, M., & Begin, G. (2001). Disability related variables associated with loneliness among people with disabilities. *Journal of Rehabilitation, 67*(3), 42–48.

Houtenville, A. (2000). *Economics of disability research report #2: Estimates of employment rates for persons with disabilities in the United Sates by state, 1980 through 1998.* Ithaca, NY: Cornell University, Research and Rehabilitation Training Center for Economic Research on Employment Policy for Persons with Disabilities.

Ivey, A. E., & Ivey, M. B. (1998). Reframing DSM-IV: Positive strategies from developmental counseling and therapy. *Journal of Counseling and Development, 76*, 334–350.

Jankowski, K. (1997). *Deaf empowerment: Emergence, struggle, and rhetoric.* Washington, DC: Gallaudet University Press.

Kessler, R. C., Berglund, P., Demler, O., Jin, R., Koretz, D., Merikangas, K. R. et al. (2003). The epidemiology of major depressive disorder: Results from the National Comorbidity Survey Replication. *Journal of the American Medical Association, 289*, 3095–3105.

Krieger, N. (1999). A review of concepts, measures, and methods for studying health consequences of discrimination. *Journal of Health Services, 29*, 295–352.

Leahy, M. J., Rak, E., & Zanskas, S. A. (2009). A brief history of counseling and specialty areas of practice. In I. Marini, & M. A. Stebnicki (Eds.), *The professional counselor's desk reference* (pp. 3–13). New York, NY: Springer.

Lee, C. C. (1998). Counselors as agents for social change. In C. C. Lee & G. R. Walz (Eds.), *Social action: A mandate for counselors* (pp. 3–16). Alexandria, VA: American Counseling Association.

Lewin, K. (1936). *Principles of topological psychology.* New York, NY: McGraw-Hill.

Lewis, J., Arnold, M. S., House, R., & Toporek, R. (2003). *ACA Advocacy Competencies.* Retrieved from http://www.counseling.org/Publications/

Li, L., & Moore, D. , 1998. Acceptance of disability and its correlates. *Journal of Social Psychology, 138*(1), 13–25.

Mackelprang, R., & Salsgiver, R. (2009). *Disability: A diversity model approach in human service practice.* Pacific Grove, CA: Brooks/Cole.

Marini, I., Bhakta, M. V., & Graf, N. (2009). A content analysis of common concerns of persons with physical disabilities. *Journal of Applied Rehabilitation Counseling, 40*(1), 44–49.

McNeil, J. (2001). *Americans with disabilities 1997. Current population reports* (pp. 70–73). Washington, DC: U.S. Census Bureau.

Mmatli, T. O. (2009). Translating disability-related research into evidence-based advocacy: The role of people with disabilities. *Disability and Rehabilitation, 31*(1), 14–22.

National Organization on Disability (2004, June 24). *Landmark survey finds pervasive disadvantages* [press release]. Washington, DC: NOD.

Neville, H. A., & Mobley, M. (2001). Social identities in contexts: An ecological model of multicultural counseling psychology processes. *The Counseling Psychologist, 29*, 471–486.

Niparko, J. K. (2000). Culture and cochlear implants. In J. K. Niparko, K. I. Kirk, N. K. Mellon, A. McConkey-Robbins, D. L. Tucci, & B. S. Wilson (Eds.), *Cohlear implants: Principles and practices* (pp. 371–379). Philadelphia, PA: Lippincott Williams & Wilkins.

O'Day, B., & Goldstein, M. (2005). Advocacy issues and strategies for the 21st century. *Journal of Disability Policy Studies, 15*(4), 240–250.

Oliver, M. (1992). Changing the social relations of research production. *Disability Handicap and Society, 7*, 101–114.

Olkin, R. (1999). *What psychotherapists should know about disability.* New York, NY: The Guilford Press.

Perlow, H. M., Danoff-Burg, S., Swenson, R. R., & Pulgiano, D. (2004). The impact of ecological risk and perceived discrimination on the psychological adjustment of African American and European youth. *Journal of Community Psychology, 32*, 375–389.

Radermacher, H., Sonn, C., Keys, C., & Duckett, O. (2010). Disability and participation: It's about us but without us! *Journal of Community & Applied Social Psychology, 20*(5), 333–346.

Ratts, M., D'Andrea, M., & Arredondo, P. (2004). *Social justice counseling: "Fifth force" in field.* Retrieved from http:/www.counseling.org/content/NavigationMenu/Publications/Counselingtodayonline/July2004/SocialJusticeCounsel.htm.

Rubin, S. E., & Roessler, R. T. (2008). *Foundations of the vocational rehabilitation process.* Austin, TX: Pro-Ed.

Rumbaut, R. (1994). The crucible within: Ethnic identity, self-esteem, and segmented assimilation among children of immigrants. *International Migration Review, 28*, 748–794.

Semivan, S. G., & White, M. A. (2006). *Advocacy: The key to a counselor's success.* Poster session presented at annual American Counseling Association Conference, Montreal, Canada.

Singer, P. (2000). *Writings on an ethical life.* New York, NY: Ecco/Harper Collins.

Smart, J. (2009). *Disability, society, and the individual.* Austin, TX: Pro-Ed.

Steele, J. M. (2008). Counselor preparation: Preparing counselors to advocate for social justice: A liberation model. *Counselor Education & Supervision, 48*, 74–85.

Stewart, T. A., Gibson-Semivan, S., & Schwartz, R. C. (2009). The art of advocacy: Strategies for psychotherapists. *Annuals of the American Psychotherapy Association, 12*(2), 54–59.

Stubbins, J. (1991). The interdisciplinary status of rehabilitation psychology. In R. P. Marinelli & A. E. Dell Orto (Eds.), *The psychological & social impact of disability* (pp. 9–17). New York, NY: Springer.

Thesen, J. (2005). From oppression towards empowerment in clinical practice-offering doctors a model for reflection. *Scandinavian Journal of Public Health, 33*(66), 47–52.

Turnbull, A. P., Friesen, B. J., & Ramirez, C. (1998). Participatory action research as a model for conducting family research. *Research and Practice for Persons with Disabilities, 23*, 178–188.

Turner, R. J., & Avison, W. R. (2003). Status variations in stress exposure: Implications for the interpretation of research on race, socioeconomic status, and gender. *Journal of Health and Social Behavior, 44*, 488–505.

Van Reusen, A., & Bos, C. (1990). I plan: Helping students communicate in-planning conferences. *Teaching Exceptional Children, 22*(4), 30–32.

Vash, C. L., & Crewe, N. M. (2004). *Psychology of disability* (pp. 288–299). New York, NY: Springer.

Weinberg, N. (1988). Another perspective: Attitudes of people with disabilities. In E. Yuker (Ed.), *Attitudes toward persons with disabilities* (pp. 141–153). New York, NY: Springer.

Weinberg, N., & Williams, J. (1978). How the physically disabled perceive their disabilities. *Journal of Rehabilitation, 44*(3), 31–33.

Whiteman, M., & Lukoff, I. F. (1965). Attitudes toward blindness and other physical handicaps. *Journal of Social Psychology, 66*, 135–145.

Wilson, F. R. (2003). *What is ecological psychotherapy?* [Electronic Version], pp. 1–3. Retrieved from http://ecologicalcounseling.org/wilsonart2,html

Williams, D. R., & Williams-Morris, R. (2000). Racism and mental health: The African American experience. *Ethnicity and Health, 5,* 243–268.

Williams, D. R., Yu, Y., Jackson, J. S., & Anderson, N. B. (1997). Racial differences in physical and mental health: Socioeconomic status, stress, and discrimination. *Journal of Health Psychology, 2,* 335–351.

Wright, B. A. (1983). *Physical disability: A psychosocial approach* (2nd ed.). New York, NY: Harper & Row.

Wright, B. A. (1988). Attitudes and the fundamental negative bias: Conditions and corrections. In H. E. Yuker (Ed.), *Attitudes toward persons with disabilities* (pp. 3–21). New York, NY: Springer.

Wright, B. A., & Howe, M. (1969). *The fortune phenomenon as manifested in stigmatized and non-stigmatized groups.* Unpublished manuscript, University of Kansas, Lawrence, KS.

Wright, B. A., & Muth, M. (1965). *The fortune phenomenon with rehabilitation clients.* Unpublished manuscript, University of Kansas, Lawrence, KS.

INSIDER PERSPECTIVE
The Story of Shannon Nettles

My name is Shannon Nettles. I am 25 years old, single, 5 ft. 2 in. 108 lbs., and have brown hair and brown eyes. I am a recently licensed attorney and currently live with my parents, 22-year-old brother, and a 20-year-old family friend. This living arrangement will continue until I find a job or go crazy, and hopefully, the former. Plus, did I mention that I am hearing and visually impaired?

I have no vision in my right eye, it is a prosthesis (aka "fake" eye because no one in my family can say prosthesis.) I have 20/200 in my left eye corrected with glasses and contacts worn at the same time. I have no idea what the vision is with no correction. I also wear two hearing aids, which corrects my hearing.

I was born legally blind in both eyes, but doctors did not discover this until I reached the age of two. At four, my doctors told my parents to find a special school for me, but they did not listen and I attended public school all the way through high school. In kindergarten, the school discovered I had a hearing loss and I received a hearing aid, which I refused to wear because it picked up too much background noise. I did not wear a hearing aid until college and I functioned very well. In college, I began having difficulty hearing my professors and thought I had lost more hearing. Actually, the size of the classrooms had become larger and this made it more difficult for me to hear, and so I began wearing two hearing aids. The technology had improved and the benefits of the hearing aids outweighed the small amount of background noise.

In seventh grade, my eye doctor discovered that I had lost all but shadow vision in my right eye due to a detached retina. My parents, doctors, and I decided that I should have surgery to attempt to reattach the retina, but the surgery did not succeed and it caused me glaucoma. I lost all the sight in my right eye. Three years later, as a sophomore in high school, I chose to have my right eye removed. I use the word "chose" lightly because by this time it had become a necessity. I could not hold my head up or watch television because my eye had become so photosensitive. Approximately, two-and-a-half months later, I received my first prosthesis.

I began college in the fall of 1994, and graduated from Sam Houston State University in 1997, with a bachelor's in political science and history. In the fall of 1997, I fulfilled my lifelong dream when I began law school at Texas Tech School of Law.

I graduated with a JD in May 2000, took the Bar Exam in July, and received my license to practice law in November.

Although my road has not always been smooth, society has generally perceived me favorably. However, society's perception of me depends on which aspect of my life one looks at—that is, school, social, or everyday life. Also, no matter which aspect one looks at, I cannot separate the manner in which I cope and deal with my disability and society's perception of me. The reason for this is because society's perception of me is a product of the way I present myself to society.

For example, in school I had little trouble with classmates or teachers. I believe that this is because I was successful in school. In high school I often broke the curve, was in the National Honor Society, and in the top 10% of my class. At this stage of my life, I had not developed the sense of humor I now use to get me through difficult times. In college and law school I used this sense of humor more than anything else to cope with difficult situations. I did not find the fact that I could not see well amusing, plus I had my eye removed at the age of 15. Fifteen is a difficult age for anyone and when you add a disability to the equation, it even becomes more so, and thus I used my extracurricular activities to project myself favorably. I participated in marching band, took piano, and championed AIDS education. These activities combined to earn respect, if not acceptance, of my peers.

In college, I began to develop my sense of humor and a social life. By choice, necessity, or fate, I don't know, but my social life in high school was limited. College proved another story, although not an easy one. I had an eclectic group of friends in college—all races, sizes and personalities. From them, I discovered a sense of humor and a kind of acceptance only my family and best friend had given me before—unconditional. We laughed and made fun of each other and everyone else. This taught me how to project myself in a way that made others accept me. By laughing at myself, I realized other people saw I was just like them and this made them more comfortable with me.

My friends and I did everything from hanging out in our dorm rooms to going to dance clubs. I met all kinds of people and became more comfortable with myself. As I became more comfortable with myself, others became more comfortable with me. This ability to make others comfortable around me permeated all aspects of my life and I was able to project myself favorably in school and every day life. This served me especially well in law school because I moved where no one knew me, and I had to cultivate new friendships and relationships.

Law school took every coping mechanism I had and the development of some I did not have. It also introduced me to parts of everyday I had not hitherto experienced, since I lived by myself for 2 years and shared a house for a year. I ran into people who did not or would not try to understand my disability, and I discovered these people in the most mundane and unusual places—airports, malls, school, and restaurants. The two problems that occurred most often were people who refused to believe I could not see because I got around so well and people who felt I received special treatment I did not deserve. However, I quickly learned how to project myself so that people viewed me as I viewed myself—a law student who had worked hard to get there and who was proud of that accomplishment. This usually resulted in respect and acceptance even if it did not enhance the education of others regarding my disability.

I believe that I have been luckier than many disabled people because I learned early and quickly to project my perceptions of myself onto others. I also learned not to care what people thought of me. I always tell people that you cannot control other people's reactions to you, you can only control you. I believe that this maxim is the reason I have succeeded and gone as far as I have.

Law school proved an excellent example of the generally favorable perception I have received. I was welcomed with open arms and listened to with respect regarding any needs I might have by both the faculty and students. I was expected to produce the same amount work and participate in class discussions, and everyone believed I would have few or no problems. Most professors called on me without regard to my disability, although I have a sneaking suspicion one or two were afraid to call on me because they did not want to be perceived as picking on me. I also had a professor who did not call on me until he knew I had a reader, which I found refreshing and kind.

In college, I truly started to come into my own. I was always referred to as the "designated driver" and frequently offered to drive wherever we went. Since I exercised at night, the entire University Police Department knew me by name. (They provided escorts to any student after dark.) All of them enjoyed harassing me because I actually made them work. I also learned how to laugh at my mistakes. I often waved or spoke to people who were actually speaking to a person behind me. Finally, I learned how to gracefully recover from an embarrassing fall since the campus was full of stairs and hills.

Law school proved an entirely different and much more difficult experience. I was devastated when I was put on academic probation after my first semester and I had to learn about that, too. I laughed at the irony of the academic advisor I was given—I made a D+ in his class and often got caught snoozing. I laughed when I had "adventures" because I took a wrong bus or got off at the wrong stop. My friends worried about me, but laughed when I related my weekend "adventures."

Law school also taught me to relearn and rethink the way I did certain things. By the end of my first semester, I knew I could not keep up with the reading on my own as I had in college. I lined up readers from my study group during finals, and although I knew that I had to use readers, it took me a year before I felt comfortable learning this way. I had always studied out loud, but counted on written notes to learn initially. When the time came to study for the Bar Exam, I felt so comfortable listening to tapes that I relied on them extensively.

Aside from readers, my family got me through law school, as well as college and the rest of my life. I like to say that I was absent the day God handed out eyes and ears, but was first in line the day He handed out parents. My parents expected me to do my best no matter what that was. They would have been proud of me if I had been a C student who barely got through college, but because I am more than that, they are continually amazed and more proud of me everyday. Imagine being told that your four-year-old child must go to a special school and have her end up graduating from law school 21 years later. Not only are my parents proud of me but also is my entire extended family—including my younger cousins who love to tell their friends that I am a lawyer. When I get down, my mom gives me two options: sit there and feel sorry for yourself or get up and live your life. I am proud to say that for the most part, I have chosen to live my life. My parents continue to provide their love and support as I look for a job, and as always, they have more confidence in me than I do.

My family has been my greatest tool in dealing with my disability. Right now, I am extremely frustrated because I cannot find a job. For the first time in my life I care about what people think of me. I am afraid they will think I am lazy and not looking hard enough, but my parents stand proud by me with every confidence that I will find a job and it will suit me perfectly.

Other than that, it is the little things that get me down. I like to have control over as much as possible because there are so many things I cannot control. For example, I cannot drive and so I like to plan things out so I can accomplish my errands or get to class. People who are late or a sudden change in plans will throw me off-balance and I panic. Not being able to go where I want when I want has been a real issue for me since I have moved home. We live in the country and that makes it more difficult to get into town because we have no public transportation. I have begun planning my days with things I enjoy at home because I can control that. I also try to get involved in things so I will have a network of friends to help me. This worked well in law school. I had someone I attended church with, someone to take me to class, someone to take me grocery shopping, and if all else failed, public transportation.

While transportation is the major issue that gets me down, people's ignorance is another. I also consider this to be a major barrier in my life. I try to use it as an opportunity to educate people, but they must be open to new ideas. People who refuse to open up to new ideas frustrate me more than anything else. Also, people who have many misconceptions about disabled people in general, will approach me with fear or belittle me. I try to remember that others will follow me when I deal with people obviously not used to being around disabled people.

Stairs and dimly lit areas are also barriers for me. I find myself frequently commenting on good stairs (the ends are a different color or texture) or bad stairs (they are all the same color). Areas of the sidewalk that have been overgrown also cause problems. These physical barriers can be dealt with easily by walking with someone or using my cane in an unfamiliar area.

As for assets, I believe empathy (not sympathy because I do not believe in it), perseverance, and honesty are my greatest assets. I cannot always understand where a person is coming from because I do not know their story, but I do understand not being understood. Thus, I can emphasize with people in difficult situations. And, having dealt with difficult situations, I have learned to persevere. My best friend gave me a framed quote about perseverance for Christmas. She has watched me go through many difficult situations and come out on top or, at least, still standing. Due to this perseverance, I have learned that honesty is truly the best policy. I make sure the people around me in school or work environments are aware of my disability. They do not always know how to act, but most people respect my honesty and view it as a sign that I am comfortable with myself. Therefore, in their dealings with me they use the same straightforward honesty by asking me if I need help and giving it when I request it.

And so, I say to future rehabilitation counselors—be honest with your clients. We are just like everyone else. Our disability does not define us; it is part of us, just as our hair and eye color. Also, remember two things that may help your clients. Everyone (not just those with disabilities) has two choices everyday: (1) feel sorry for yourself or live your life; and (2) no one is a mind reader . . . if you need help, ask for it.

DISCUSSION QUESTIONS

1. Discuss and open for debate whether counselors should become actively involved with client social injustice advocacy on their own time, or whether such activities are simply not a part of their job.

2. How strong is the argument that some, or much of, clients' circumstances is due to oppressive and discriminatory social barriers?

3. Is there really an insider versus outsider perspective or do people with disabilities just exaggerate and complain the glass is half empty, especially after all the legislation protecting them?

4. Is there really any value in conducting PAR studies, and if so, what are they?

EXERCISES

A. As part of class assignment, have them research which disability related bills are coming before Congress, and engage in a letter-writing campaign to support its passage.

B. Have students visit, interview staff, then write reaction papers re: services provided by local CAPs and CIL. How do these entities advocate for persons with disabilities and what are commonly recurring issues.

C. Locate and participate in a community action project designed to bring awareness and change to some oppressed group. Note what the issues are and monitor the group's procedures for organizing.

Index